Essentials of Pediatric Emergency Medicine

Essentials of Pediatric Emergency Medicine

Edited by Rahim Valani, MD

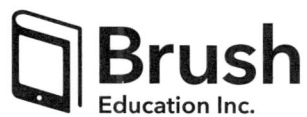

Brush
Education Inc.

Brush Education Inc.
www.brusheducation.ca
contact@brusheducation.ca

Editorial: Nicholle Carrière, Kay Rollans
Indexing: François Trahan

Cover design: Dean Pickup; Cover image: Dreamstime (Saiyood Srikamon)
Interior design: Carol Dragich, Dragich Design
Illustration: Chao Yu

Library and Archives Canada Cataloguing in Publication
    Essentials of pediatric emergency medicine / [edited by] Rahim Valani, MD.
Includes bibliographical references. Issued in print and electronic formats. ISBN 978-1-55059-
694-6 (hardcover).--ISBN 978-1-55059-695-3 (PDF).-- ISBN 978-1-55059-696-0 (Kindle).--
ISBN 978-1-55059-697-7 (EPUB)
    1. Pediatric emergencies--Handbooks, manuals, etc. 2. Emergency medicine-- Handbooks,
manuals, etc. I. Valani, Rahim, editor
RJ370.E88 2018   618.92'0025   C2018-902052-0   C2018-902053-9

We acknowledge the support of the Government of Canada | Canadä
Nous reconnaissons l'appui du gouvernement du Canada

To my parents and brothers for their support and inspiration over the years, and supporting my ideas; my teachers, mentors, and colleagues who have taught me the ropes of being a physician and an educator; and my friends for their understanding and support.

To the nurses and physicians for their unrelenting dedication towards the care of their patients in the Emergency Department.

In memory of my father – a source of inspiration in my life. His integrity, work ethic, and compassion have shaped me to be the individual I am.

Contents

Section 18: Trauma

Section 19: Toxicology

Section 20: Environmental Emergencies

Acknowledgements

I would like to express my appreciation to several people who have made this book possible. To all the contributing chapter authors across the country for their time in helping to put this book together in addition to their already demanding schedule. To my colleagues at McMaster Hamilton Health Sciences Centre and William Osler Health Centre, I am grateful for their patience as I continued to work on completing this book. To Lauri Seiditz and her amazing team of editors for their guidance and review process.

A special thanks to Dr. Anna Jarvis for the opportunity to be a part of the Pediatric Emergency Medicine community. Her mentorship and guidance is the inspiration for this book.

Introduction

Pediatric Emergency Medicine is a relatively new specialty with expanding competency requirements. Having an organized approach to managing patients that is consistent with best practices is essential. As clinicians, we are always looking to expand our knowledge and skills, and to use the best evidence to ensure excellent care for our patients. *Essentials of Pediatric Emergency Medicine* brings together the knowledge and expertise of clinicians from academic and community centres across Canada in a succinct format for easy reference.

This handbook is designed to provide the reader with a quick synopsis of the major topics in PEM. It is divided into 20 sections. The chapters in section 1 deal with undifferentiated acute presentations. This section also includes topics such as child life, non-accidental trauma and pain management which are important in the daily practice of emergency medicine. Despite the ongoing growth of knowledge and experience in these fields, there are currently few reference materials available on these topics and this guide will help to fill a significant void in pediatric emergency medicine resources. The remaining sections deal with specific pathologies and specific body systems. These chapters allow the reader to review the pathophysiology and management of specific diseases or medical conditions that are most common or life threatening.

One book, however, cannot cover everything, and for this reason several topics were also intentionally left out. Acute resuscitation is one of these subject areas. While resuscitation is the foundation of emergency medicine, there are excellent resources such as Pediatric Advanced Life Support (PALS) and Advanced Pediatric Life Support (APLS) which are most up to date and provide an excellent reference.

As with any reference source, there are always opportunities to improve. I invite feedback so that this handbook can continue to evolve and provide a guide both for those newly entering into practice, as well as seasoned practitioners who manage pediatric emergencies.

Note on Units

In the text, the symbol *mcg* is given instead of *µg* to avoid confusion with the symbol *mg*. In addition, all lab values in this text book are given in SI units, unless the conventional units are most commonly used. In order to assist the reader, a conversion table is provided at the end of the book.

Disclaimer

The publisher, authors, contributors, and editors bring substantial expertise to this reference and have made their best efforts to ensure that it is useful, accurate, safe, and reliable.

Nonetheless, practitioners must always rely on their own experience, knowledge and judgment when consulting any of the information contained in this reference or employing it in patient care. When using any of this information, they should remain conscious of their responsibility for their own safety and the safety of others, and for the best interests of those in their care.

To the fullest extent of the law, neither the publishers, the authors, the contributors, nor the editors assume any liability for injury or damage to persons or property from any use of information or ideas contained in this reference.

1.1

Pediatric Triage

Rodrick Lim

- Emergency departments (EDs) are inherently chaotic, unpredictable, and filled with risk. They involve multiple care providers, different areas of care, and differing availability of resources depending on the time of day, day of the week, and time of the year.
- Currently, EDs must cope with issues related to:
  » Overcrowding
  » Increasing patient volumes
  » Limited resources
  » Humanitarian and natural disasters
  » New infectious diseases
- EDs require a reliable triage system that allows for the timely and accurate assessment of patients to minimize risk.
  » The role of triaging is not to conduct a complete history and physical exam; rather, triaging is a means of identifying where patients would be best placed for their initial assessment.
- Triaging is particularly important for the most vulnerable populations, including children.
  » Pediatric deaths in hospital often occur within the first 24 hours of admission, and some of these deaths could be prevented if the severity of a patient's condition was identified upon their arrival at the health facility.

HISTORY OF TRIAGE

- Triage was thought to have originally been developed during Napoleonic times by Dominique Jean Larrey to quickly access multiple casualties.
  » *Triage* is a word derived from the French verb *trier*, meaning "to sort."
- During subsequent wars, frontline medics would divide the wounded into 3 categories:
  1. Those likely to live without immediate care
  2. Those requiring immediate care to survive

3. Those that would likely die of their wounds despite care being provided
- Commonly used triage systems worldwide for children include:
  » Manchester Triage System (MTS)
  » Emergency Severity Index (ESI)
  » Australasian Triage Scale (ATS)
  » Canadian Triage and Acuity Scale Paediatric Guidelines (PaedCTAS)

GOALS OF TRIAGE

- The goals of pediatric triage are:
  » To quickly identify patients with life-threatening conditions or who require timely medical care
  » To determine the most appropriate treatment area in which to receive care in an ED
  » To improve flow and reduce congestion in the ED
  » To provide a priority and a mechanism for ongoing patient assessment to prevent decompensation
  » To provide information to patients and families about what to expect and the approximate waiting time
  » To provide metrics and objective information defining the state of a department, and its anticipated safety and workload

CONSIDERATIONS SPECIFIC TO PEDIATRIC TRIAGE

- Pediatric triage must take into account age-dependent differences in physiology, anatomy, and development.
- The normal ranges of vital signs vary with age, so it is necessary to use age-specific standardized charts.
- Triage providers must be comfortable assessing children across the age spectrum and must be aware of pediatric-specific presentations and diseases that place

these patients at higher risk or may be unique to pediatric patients.

- Patient history and other important information may be unavailable or acquired second-hand through a primary caregiver, increasing the level of risk.
- Pain scoring is difficult to properly assess in children, so pain often goes untreated.
- Pediatric triage affords an opportunity to detect issues that make children vulnerable, such as nutrition, immunization status, and neglect or abuse.

TRIAGE SYSTEMS

- The Manchester Triage System (MTS):
  » Was developed in the United Kingdom
  » Uses flowcharts with different presenting complaints
  » Has specific complaint discriminators using the signs and symptoms of the patient, as well as general discriminators such as pain, bleeding, level of consciousness, and temperature
- The Emergency Severity Index (ESI):
  » Was developed in the United States
  » Uses specific pediatric flowcharts
- The Australasian Triage Scale (ATS):
  » Was developed in Australia
  » Is formally known as the National Triage Scale
  » Uses a combination of observation of general appearance, a focused history that identifies chief presenting complaint and risk, and psychological data
- The Canadian Paediatric Triage and Acuity Scale (PaedCTAS):
  » Was developed in Canada
  » Uses a combination of vital signs, presenting complaint, and primary and secondary modifiers

PAEDCTAS

- PaedCTAS is the most common triage system used in Canada.
- Initial triage is based on a critical look (i.e., pediatric assessment using the pediatric assessment triangle [PAT]; see "Triage Process," below).
- Triage modifiers are added for the following physiologic parameters:
  » First-order modifiers:
    › Level of consciousness with Glasgow coma scale (GCS) score (see *Table 18.1.1*, page 316) or appropriate alternative
    › Respiratory rate and effort
    › Circulatory status, including heart rate
  » Second-order modifiers:
    › Temperature, especially if patient < 3 months old or looks unwell
    › Mechanism of injury

  › Pain score
    · Use a scale that is age appropriate, such as the OUCHER, the Faces Pain Scale — Revised (FPS-R), or the visual analogue scale (VAS).
  › Glucose, particularly for known diabetic patients and those with altered mental status
- For PaedCTAS, the suggested times for initial physician assessment are:
  » CTAS 1 — immediate
  » CTAS 2 — within 15 minutes
  » CTAS 3 — within 30 minutes
  » CTAS 4 — within 1 hour
  » CTAS 5 — within 2 hours

TRIAGE PROCESS

- Triage systems are designed to be easy and quick to apply, and reproducible with good interpersonal reliability.
- Most systems assign a triage level of 1 to 5, with 1 being most severe and 5 being nonurgent.
  » Triage levels can be tied to expectations for time to physician assessment.
  » Triage levels correlate with the percentage of patients who subsequently require admission or suffer a critical event.
- Triage systems start with a quick check of the patient.
  » Many systems use an adaptation of the PAT to identify high-risk patients.
    › The PAT consists of 3 parameters:
      1. Airway and appearance
      2. Work of breathing
      3. Circulatory status
- Algorithms exist, depending on the triage system, that use a mix of physiologic parameters, presenting complaint, historic modifiers (e.g., mechanism), and/or additional physiologic or measured parameters (e.g., glucose).
- The use and interpretation of vital signs, including a properly obtained temperature (ideally a rectal temperature for children < 1 year of age, if there are no contraindications; see Chapter 2.4, "Pediatric Fever"), are essential to proper triage and are integrated into the assignment of triage categories.

PITFALLS OF TRIAGE

- The training and assessment of triage providers as part of ongoing quality assurance is important.
- Awareness of specific subpopulations is often lacking; for example, patients with conditions such as metabolic disorders or hemophilia who may have established care plans.

- Triage is for the initial assessment of patients and, regardless of initially-assessed category, requires timely and recurrent reassessments.
- Infants present a difficult group of patients who, despite best efforts, can still have poor correlation between initial triage score and final outcome.

REFERENCES

Elshove-Bolk J, Mencl F, van Rijswijck BT, Simons MP, van Vugt AB. Validation of the Emergency Severity Index (ESI) in self-referred patients in a European emergency department. *Emerg Med J.* 2007;24(3):170–174. https://doi.org/10.1136/emj.2006.039883. Medline:17351220

Gilboy N, Tanabe P, Travers D, Rosenau AM. Emergency severity index (ESI): a triage tool for emergency department care, version 4. Implementation handbook 2012 edition [PDF]. (AHRQ) Publication No. 12-0014. Rockville, MD: Agency for Health Care Research and Quality; 2011. Available from: https://www.ahrq.gov/sites/default/files/wysiwyg/professionals/systems/hospital/esi/esihandbk.pdf

Mackway-Jones K, Marsden J, Windle J; Manchester Triage Group. *Emergency triage.* 2nd ed. Oxford: Blackwell Publishing; 2006.

van Veen M, Moll HA. Reliability and validity of triage systems in paediatric emergency care. *Scand J Trauma Resusc Emerg Med.* 2009;17:38.

Warren DW, Jarvis A, LeBlanc L, Gravel J; CTAS National Working Group; Canadian Association of Emergency Physicians; National Emergency Nurses Affiliation; Association des Médecins d'Urgence du Québec; Canadian Paediatric Society; Society of Rural Physicians of Canada. Revisions to the Canadian Triage and Acuity Scale Paediatric Guidelines (PaedCTAS). *CJEM.* 2008;10(3):224–232. https://doi.org/10.1017/S1481803500010149. Medline:19019273

World Health Organization. Updated guideline: paediatric emergency triage, assessment and treatment, care of critically ill children. Geneva: World Health Organization; 2016 [cited 2016, Nov. 22]. Available from: http://apps.who.int/iris/bitstream/10665/204463/1/9789241510219_eng.pdf?ua=1

1.2

Pediatric Airway

Rahim Valani

- Assessment of the pediatric airway begins with an understanding of the differences between adult and pediatric airways.
- Children have:
  » A larger occiput, which influences head and neck positioning
  » Large adenoids and hypertrophied tonsils, which can result in upper airway obstruction
  » More cephalad larynx (C2/3) compared to adults (C4/5), making it better to use a straight blade for intubation
  » The narrowest part of their airway at the cricoid cartilage, predisposing the area to edema and scarring
  » Smaller-caliber lumens, which makes small amounts of mucus or blood more likely to cause obstruction, and also causes increased resistance to airflow
  » A floppy, omega-shaped epiglottis
  » Vocal cords at the lower end of C4 and with a more anterior attachment than in adults, which may cause endotracheal tubes (ETTs) to rest against the anterior commissure
  » Highly compliant larynx, trachea, and bronchi, which can result in easy distortion of the tissues
  » Poor neck tone
  » A large tongue relative to the oropharynx

Management

- Management of respiratory distress or airway problems can begin with noninvasive airway maneuvers, including:
  » Chin lift
    › The chin lift maneuver extends the head at the atlantooccipital joint, straightening the airway.
  » Jaw thrust
    › The jaw thrust maneuver moves the genioglossus anteriorly and opens the airway.
  » Lateral positioning
    › Lateral positioning helps to prevent aspiration if the patient vomits.
    › It is also useful when the pharynx and larynx are obstructed.

Initial Ventilation

- To prevent hypoxia, it is important to begin ventilating the patient as soon as possible, and while setting up for a definitive airway.
- Use a bag valve mask (BVM) for initial ventilation.
  » BVM is an easy skill to teach and develop.
  » It may be challenging to use with children < 4 years of age because of the smaller face, larger tongue, and easy compression of the soft tissues of the neck.

» Airflow may be further improved with:
› Chin lift
› Jaw thrust
- Consider oral or nasal airway as a further airway adjunct; ensure appropriate size.

Definitive Airway Management

- While BVM ventilation is underway, ensure that the following equipment is available for definitive airway management:
» Suction equipment
» Oxygen source and BVM
» Airway equipment, including blades and tubes of different sizes
› Miller straight blade is commonly used for pediatric patients (see *Table 1.2.1*).

Table 1.2.1. LARYNGOSCOPE BLADE SIZES

Miller blade size	Age
0	Preterm infants and neonates
1	Newborn to 2 years of age
2	2 to 10 years of age
3	> 10 years of age

» ETT (see "Endotracheal Tube," below, for sizing)
» Intubating aids:
› Stylet, forceps, and bougie
» Medications for sedation and paralysis as required
» Complete cardiorespiratory monitoring
» Advanced airway equipment

ENDOTRACHEAL TUBE

- Prepare tubes one size above and below the estimate from a formula or Breslow card.
- Either cuffed or uncuffed tubes can be used.
» A good rule of thumb is Cole's formula for uncuffed tubes:

› $\text{Internal diameter} = \dfrac{Age\ in\ years}{4} + 4$

» Sizing of a cuffed tube is based on a modification of Cole's formula:

› $\text{Internal diameter} = \dfrac{Age\ in\ years}{4} + 3.5$

- The advantages of using a cuffed tube include:
» No increased risk of airway complications
» Better precision for end-tidal CO_2 monitoring
» The possibility of using higher pressures to ventilate
» A theoretical decrease in aspiration risk
- Insertion depth of ETT (tube marker at the lips) may be calculated in two ways:

» $\text{Insertion depth} = \dfrac{Age\ in\ years}{2} + 12$

» Insertion depth = 3 × tube internal diameter

- A laryngeal mask airway (LMA) can be used as an alternative for airway management.
- LMA sizing is based on the weight of the patient (see *Table 1.2.2*).

Table 1.2.2. LARYNGEAL MASK AIRWAY SIZING

Patient weight in kg	LMA size
< 5	1
5 to 10	1.5
10 to 20	2
20 to 30	2.5
30 to 50	3

RAPID SEQUENCE INTUBATION

- Rapid sequence intubation (RSI) is a quick sequence of steps for emergent definitive airway management.
» Ensure the patient is appropriately monitored and has IV access.
» Have a plan ready for a failed attempt.
» Have advanced airway equipment ready or nearby.
» Preoxygenate the patient with 100% oxygen.
» Choose an appropriate induction agent (see *Table 1.2.3*).

Table 1.2.3. COMMON INDUCTION AGENTS FOR RAPID SEQUENCE INTUBATION

Agent	Dose (mg/kg)	Advantages	Disadvantages
Ketamine	1 to 2	• Maintains cardiovascular stability	• Hypersalivation • Emergence reactions
Propofol	2.5 to 4	• Reduces ICP without affecting CPP • Decreases nausea/vomiting	• Hypotension • No analgesic properties • Pain on injection • Propofol infusion syndrome • Egg based — use with care in patients with egg or soy allergies
Etomidate	0.2 to 0.3	• Maintains cardiovascular stability	• Adrenal suppression

ICP intracranial pressure. **CPP** cerebral perfusion pressure.

» Facilitate the intubation with a neuromuscular blockade agent:
› Depolarizing agent — succinylcholine 1.5 to 2 mg/kg
› Nondepolarizing agent — rocuronium 0.6 to 1.0 mg/kg
» Use BVM if needed.
- When intubating:
» Insert the ETT

» Always confirm tube placement with **more than one** of the following:
  › Listen to both lung fields
  › Monitor end-tidal CO_2
  › Mist in the tube
  › Ensure the absence of breath sounds over the epigastrium
  › Directly watch the tube pass the cords during intubation
- Postintubation care involves:
  » Obtaining a chest X-ray (CXR) to confirm tube placement
  » Determining the need for oro- or nasogastric tube
  » Evaluating the need for postintubation sedation and analgesia

DIFFICULT AIRWAY MANAGEMENT

- For a difficult airway, consider whether the patient should be taken to the operating room (OR) and intubated using anesthesia.
- Be especially careful with patients who have congenital syndromes that make airway management a challenge. These include:
  » Pierre-Robin syndrome — micrognathia, glossoptosis, and cleft palate
  » Treacher-Collins syndrome — hypoplasia of the maxilla and mandible
  » Hemifacial macrosomia
  » Klippel-Feil syndrome — cervical vertebral fusion
- Cervical spine abnormalities can also result in a difficult airway. These include:
  » Congenital — Down syndrome, Klippel-Feil syndrome, torticollis
  » Traumatic — fracture, subluxation
  » Inflammatory — rheumatoid arthritis
  » Metabolic — mucopolysaccharidosis
- Intubation options in difficult cases include:
  » Lighted stylet
  » Fiberoptic intubation (rigid or flexible)
  » Bullard laryngoscope
  » Retrograde intubation
  » Percutaneous needle cricothyrotomy
    › This is reserved for emergency situations.
    › It carries risk of subsequent laryngeal stenosis and permanent speech problems.
    › It helps with oxygenation but does nothing for ventilation.

COMPLICATIONS OF AIRWAY MANAGEMENT

HYPOTENSION

- Treat hypotension with fluid bolus.
- Consider vasopressors.

BRADYCARDIA

- Determine the underlying cause.
- Administer atropine 0.02 mg/kg (minimum dose 0.1 mg, maximum dose 0.5 mg).

LARYNGOSPASM

- Laryngospasm is a self-protective response — laryngeal muscles contract, causing complete airway obstruction during inspiration.
- Increased risk factors include:
  » Recent upper respiratory tract infection (URTI)
  » Second-hand smoke exposure
- Laryngospasm can be differentiated into partial and complete obstruction.
  » Partial obstruction
    › Stridor can still be heard, which indicates a small amount of air entry.
    › To manage partial obstruction:
      · Employ the jaw thrust maneuver
      · Use positive pressure ventilation (PPV)
      · Apply pressure over Larson's notch (laryngospasm notch)
      · Deepen the anesthesia
      · Consider a paralytic agent and intubate the patient
  » Complete obstruction
    › Hypoxemia develops rapidly.
    › Consider PPV while preparing for intubation with a sedative and paralytic agent.

BURN AND INHALATION INJURIES

- See also Chapter 18.8, "Pediatric Burns."
- Pulmonary insufficiency is a major cause of morbidity and mortality in burn patients.
- Early intubation is key.
- The smoke inhalation injury complex consists of 4 components:
  1. Hypoxia from low inspired FiO_2
     › Decreased oxygen tension results in hypoxic ischemia to end organs.
  2. Carbon monoxide / cyanide toxicity
     › Carbon monoxide shifts the oxygen dissociation curve to the left, which impairs oxygen offloading.

› Cyanide impairs adenosine triphosphate (ATP) production.
3. Upper airway obstruction from edema
   › This usually presents a few hours after injury.
   › Burns to the face can distort the face and neck, and oral edema causes soft tissue and tongue swelling.
4. Chemical burn to oral and respiratory mucosa
   › Water-soluble gases (e.g., ammonia, chlorine) react with water in the mucosa, resulting in chemical burns and impaired ciliary clearance.

- In addition to compromising the airway, burns to the chest impair chest wall compliance.

Physical Exam

- Clinical findings suggestive of smoke inhalation injury are:
  » History of a closed space explosion / burn environment
  » Facial burns
  » Wheezing or stridor
  » Carbonaceous sputum
  » Persistent cough
  » Singed nasal or facial hair
  » Hypoxia
  » Carbon monoxide confirmed by cooximeter

Management

- Initiate RSI for burn patients.
  » Succinylcholine can be used safely in the first 24 hours without triggering a hyperkalemic response.
  » Rocuronium is a preferred alternative.

REFERENCES

Bisonnette B. *Pediatric anesthesia*. Shelton, Connecticut: People's Medical Publishing House; 2011.

Coté CJ, Lerman JL, Todres ID. *A practice of anesthesia for infants and children*. Philadelphia: Saunders Elsevier; 2009.

Davis PJ, Cladis FP, Motoyama EK. *Smith's anesthesia for infants and children*. Philadelphia: Elsevier Mosby; 2011.

Demlong RH, LaLonde C. *Burn trauma*. New York: Thieme Medical Publishing; 1989.

Litman RS. *Pediatric anesthesia*. Philadelphia: Elsevier Mosby; 2004.

Longnecker DE, Brown DL, Newman MF, Zapol WM. *Anesthesiology*. 2nd ed. New York: McGraw Hill; 2012.

1.3

Child Life: Developmental Considerations in the Emergency Department

Tracy Lynn Akitt, Sheryl Christie, Elana Jackson, Karen Paling

- Attending to developmental considerations when treating children and adolescents is an imperative task for all healthcare providers working in the emergency setting.
- A visit to the emergency department (ED) is unexpected and distressing, particularly for children who may have little familiarity with the setting.
- Patient and family anxiety is decreased and better care is provided by:
  » Providing simple and concrete explanations of what to expect
  » Adapting communication to the temperament and coping style of the patient
  » Encouraging parent involvement
  » Being sensitive to the developmental needs of each patient

ROLE OF THE CHILD LIFE SPECIALIST

- Certified child life specialists (CCLSs) are professionals who provide psychosocial support to children and their families, most commonly in healthcare settings.
- They are specifically trained to work with children and families in stressful situations.
- As part of their scope of practice, CCSLs:
  » Assess patient development, coping, and responses to hospitalization
  » Provide patient and family education and emotional support
  » Prepare and support patients and families for procedures and treatments
  » Assist families to understand the ED process and facilitate patient flow

- Implementing child life programs in the ED has been shown to:
  » Relieve stress and anxiety for patients and families
  » Improve coping
  » Improve patient and parent satisfaction
  » Decrease medications required for sedation or analgesia
  » Improve staff efficiency
- The goal of child life programs is to decrease environmental stressors and support patients' coping needs.

ASSESSMENT CONSIDERATIONS

- Assessment of a pediatric patient can present numerous challenges due to the nature of the unexpected visit, the patient's response to strangers, being in a new environment, and pain.
- The goals of an assessment informed by a developmental approach are to:
  » Provide a positive experience
  » Enhance the accuracy of assessment
  » Maximize cooperation
  » Decrease the anxiety of the patient and parent(s)
- Before beginning any physical examination or procedure, look for clues as to the patient's and family's:
  » Emotional state
    › How closely does the patient stay to the parent(s)?
    › Who answers questions?
    › Do the patient and parent(s) appear calm and content, irritated, or distraught?
  » Level of activity
    › What were the patient and parent(s) doing prior to you entering the room?
    › Was the patient sleeping, engaged in an activity, or crying on a parent's lap?
  » Past medical experiences
    › Ask the parent(s) to describe the patient's typical response to healthcare procedures.
      · How does the patient cope at the dentist?
      · What calms the patient or has been helpful in the past?

BEGINNING THE ASSESSMENT

- Approach slowly and in a gentle manner, noting the patient's response.
- Speak softly and at the patient's eye level — you may need to sit or crouch down.
- If the patient appears withdrawn or anxious, address the parent(s) first then slowly engage the patient.
- Give the patient a task to gain their interest and direct their attention to a positive alternate focus (e.g., playing peekaboo or opening a package of gauze).
- Incorporate strategies to promote familiarization with the environment and with medical equipment, such as:

  » Demonstrating the equipment first on yourself or a parent
  » Allowing the patient to manipulate the equipment to enhance trust and build familiarity
  » Touching uninjured areas before touching areas that are painful
- Be mindful of language.
  » Avoid jargon — when necessary, explain acronyms and unfamiliar terms (e.g., bolus, flush IV, NPO).
  » Use developmentally sensitive language and avoid anxiety-provoking words and phrases (e.g., shot, "don't cry," "this will burn").
  » Avoid having the patient translate information for family members who do not speak English — engage the services of a professional translator whenever possible.

COMMUNICATION STRATEGIES

USING POSITIVE COMMUNICATION TECHNIQUES

- Allow the patient to express questions and concerns.
- Follow the patient's lead.
- Acknowledge and validate the patient's feelings.
- Be honest and model honest communication.
- Use descriptive praise to tell the patient what they are doing well (e.g., "You are doing a great job holding your arm still!" instead of simply, "Great job!").
- Use affirmative language — tell the patient what they can do rather than what they cannot do (e.g., "Take a deep breath while you hold your hand still," instead of, "Don't move").
- Provide a choice only when a choice is possible (e.g., "Do you want to hop onto the bed or should mom lift you?" instead of, "Are you ready to get onto the bed?").
- Use the third-person technique (e.g., "Some children tell me that …").
- Assess the patient's understanding and adapt language or explanations as needed.

SUGGESTIONS FOR BUILDING RAPPORT

- Identify the patient's interests.
  » Discuss favorite activities, sports, or TV shows to help shift attention away from the procedure or examination and build familiarity between the healthcare provider and the patient.
- Involve parents.
  » Give parents a task to focus on, such as engaging the patient in a rhyming game during a procedure.
  » Encourage the patient to sit on the parent's lap or

beside the parent if they wish in order to minimize separation anxiety and distress.

» Provide preparation for parents prior to any assessment or procedure.

› Include a description of what to expect, suggestions as to how the parent can support their child, and children's typical responses to the test or procedure.

- Show respect for privacy and independence.

» Respect the patient's growing need for autonomy.

» Look for opportunities to support the patient's healthcare mastery, such as encouraging them to ask questions and praising coping efforts for tests and procedures.

» Be mindful of closing curtains.

» Give adolescents time to ask questions, and offer adolescents the opportunity to speak with the healthcare provider without parents present.

» Involve adolescents in decision-making and encourage their participation when providing information about their illness or treatment.

PATIENT AND PARENT PREPARATION

- Preparation involves providing a simple, accurate, honest, and clear explanation before beginning an assessment or procedure.

- Preparation helps to:

» Decrease the patient's fear and anxiety

» Promote coping

» Establish a foundation for positive future healthcare experiences

» Build trust with a healthcare provider

- Preparation must be customized for each patient and family, with considerations for:

» Timing — When is it appropriate to deliver information?

› Some patients benefit from having preparation immediately before the procedure, so they have less time to develop anticipatory anxiety.

› Other patients benefit from having more time between preparation and the assessment or procedure to provide an opportunity for processing information and asking questions.

» Previous healthcare experiences or painful experiences

» The patient's developmental stage, temperament, and coping style (e.g., information seeker, avoider, sensitizer)

› Too much detail can create unnecessary anxiety.

› Assess the patient's developmental level and coping style to determine how much information will be helpful (i.e., Do they cope better with a lot of information or less?).

» Patient's and/or family's current emotional state

» Family's beliefs and/or cultural values

» What the patient and/or family have already been told

- Other practical considerations for preparation include:

» Determining the type of materials to use (e.g., authentic equipment, photos)

» Locating a quiet place to do the preparation

» Deciding who other than the patient should be present for the preparation (e.g., parents, siblings)

» Recognizing the time available for the preparation (what is feasible in the ED may be an important factor)

» Honoring the patient's need for repetition and reinforcement of the information communicated

- Information communicated during preparation should include:

» The reason for the test or procedure (why it needs to be done / what its purpose is)

» The steps involved (i.e., sequence of events)

» The length of the test or procedure

» Sensory information (sights, sounds, smells, and sensations)

» The development of a coping plan and choices

› Identify with the patient and family what coping strategies will be used (e.g., deep breathing, countdown, planned distraction, patient's choice to watch or look away).

› Define the patient and parent's role during the procedure or test.

› Discuss a position for comfort or implement the position required.

› Ensure the coping plan is relayed to everyone involved in the procedure.

DEVELOPMENTAL CONSIDERATIONS

INFANTS (0 TO 12 MONTHS)

- Involve parents as often as possible to provide comfort and decrease separation anxiety.

- Utilize comfort items (e.g., pacifier, blanket).

- Although the patient is too young to be prepared, preparation should be offered to parents to enhance their coping and increase their knowledge of ways to support their infant.

TODDLERS (1 TO 3 YEARS)

- Toddlers learn through exploration of their environment; it is therefore important to provide opportunities for familiarization with medical equipment and the setting.

- Ensure the procedure's efficiency.

» Set the room up for the procedure prior to having

the patient and family enter, or set up as much as possible outside the room prior to entering the room to begin the procedure.

- Although the patient has limited ability to be prepared, preparation should be offered to parents to enhance their coping and support of their child.

PRESCHOOLERS (3 TO 5 YEARS)

- Ensure the procedure's efficiency.
  » Set the room up for the procedure prior to having the patient and family enter, or set up as much as possible outside the room prior to entering the room to begin the procedure.
- Clarify any "magical thinking" around what caused the medical encounter (i.e., Was the medical issue preventable, unavoidable, contagious, etc.?).
- Be mindful that the concept of "inside the body" is too abstract for the patient to understand.

SCHOOL AGE (6 TO 11 YEARS)

- Clarify any "magical thinking" around what caused the medical encounter (i.e., Was the medical issue preventable, unavoidable, contagious, etc.?).

- Note that the patient **can** understand the concept of "inside the body."
- Keep in mind that this is a great age to teach active coping techniques.

TEENS (12 YEARS AND OLDER)

- Teens are often overlooked for preparation but benefit from understanding procedures and developing and practicing coping skills.
- Always ensure part of the assessment is done without parents to ensure honest answers (e.g., risk of pregnancy, STIs, drug use, etc.) and to provide opportunities for youth to practice self-advocacy.
- Allow the patient to have the option of having parents present for support.

COMMON EMERGENCY DEPARTMENT PROCEDURES

- Refer to *Table 1.3.1* for language, positioning, procedural, and developmental considerations, and suggestions for common medical procedures in the ED.

Table 1.3.1. COMMON EMERGENCY DEPARTMENT PROCEDURES: SUGGESTIONS FOR SUCCESSFUL COPING

Name of procedure	Language considerations	Positioning considerations	Procedural support and suggestions	Developmental considerations
Bloodwork / IV insertion	• The physician may say "straw" instead of "catheter" or "cannula."	• Facilitate a position for comfort close to parent when possible. • Allow patient to sit upright, as lying supine can feel threatening.	• Show medical equipment and steps (e.g., flexibility of "straw" and "how tiny it is") when preparing for an IV.	• Use the patient's nondominant hand or hand that the infant does not suck, when possible.
Casting / splinting	• The physician may say "holds bones, muscles and tendons safely in the correct position so they can heal."	• Consider the body part being casted or splinted and tailor coping strategies around the required position. • Facilitate a position for comfort with patient sitting or lying with a parent.	• Offer choices when possible (e.g., color of cast) and ensure adequate clothing (e.g., that clothing can be removed when patient returns home). • Provide headphones for cast removal and inform patient that it may sound like a vacuum.	• Reassure patient that cast/splint may feel warm as it is drying, and that it is not permanent. • Explain that the cast is removed using a special vibrating tool that cuts cast material, not skin (demonstrate if possible).
Laceration repair	• The physician may say "string" instead of sutures; "skin glue" instead of topical skin adhesive; "skin clips" instead of staples. • If patient requires lidocaine injection, describe sensation of lidocaine injection as "warm" instead of "stingy" and "burning."	• Consider body part being repaired and determine if it is ideal for patient to observe during procedure. • Offer a drape or visual block if patient does not want to observe. • Facilitate a position for comfort with patient sitting or lying with a parent.	• Consider removing any clothing that may get wet during irrigation. • Avoid getting water in patient's eyes, ears, and nose. • Wait until you are ready to begin the procedure before holding the body part with the laceration in the required position for repair. • Use pharmacological pain management, and test area to ensure medication is effective before starting laceration repair.	• With support from a CCLS, even toddlers can be supported through procedures without needing sedation. • Restraining a child can be emotionally traumatic, therefore it is important to only use restraint when safety is a concern and other options have been explored.

Table 1.3.1 continues on next page.

Name of procedure	Language considerations	Positioning considerations	Procedural support and suggestions	Developmental considerations
Nerve block	• Describe the sensation of the lidocaine injection as "warm" instead of "stingy" or "burning."	• Consider body part being treated and determine if it is ideal for patient to observe during procedure. • Offer a drape or visual block if patient does not want to observe. • Facilitate a position for comfort with patient sitting or lying with a parent.	• Apply ice to help with pain management at the injection site. • Employ an active coping strategy to cope with injection (e.g., deep breathing, squeezing a hand or stress ball, or coughing). • Remind the patient that the warm feeling will go away quickly (often can count with the patient to 10 or 15), and that often patients report feeling gentle "pushing," "pulling" or "pressure."	• Be aware that adolescents may appear to understand but may resist asking questions out of fear or embarrassment. • Be aware that adolescents may fear showing emotion and can have difficulty coping immediately after procedure (e.g., fainting).
Oral rehydration therapy (ORT)	• The physician may describe ORT as "drinking fluid slowly to help your body get better."	• Young children can be cradled in parent's arms if needed.	• Families of young children benefit from a demonstration of how to put fluid into the back corners of the mouth. • Offer choices for fluids if appropriate. • Syringes help families offer controlled volumes. • Some patients may require distraction or other coping strategies.	• Offer incentives if needed.
Sedation	• Avoid saying "put to sleep" or "knock you out." • The physician may say "give you medicine to make you sleepy so you don't feel anything."	• Position a parent close to the beside on the side opposite from the patient's IV to provide support while patient is being sedated.	• How a patient falls asleep is often how they wake up, therefore a quiet, calm conversation or watching a favorite movie is ideal. • Only begin the procedure when sedation is fully effective. • Ensure adequate analgesia.	• If the patient appears anxious, it is best not to mention what will happen during sedation portion of procedure, just talk to the consenting adult outside room.
Urine catheter	• The physician may say "tube" instead of "catheter."	• Position parent(s) at the head of the bed to provide relaxation and support.	• A urine catheter is often required to obtain a sterile urine sample from infants and toddlers. • Many patients benefit from distraction and relaxation techniques.	• Ensure adequate preparation for parent. • Ask parents what words they use for genitals with the patient.
Diagnostic imaging				
MRI	• Avoid saying "going into a tunnel." • The physician may say "the bed moves into the camera." • The physician may say "a large camera that makes sounds when taking the pictures."	• Discuss the importance of staying still and consider sedation, especially for younger children or procedures over 20 minutes. • Ask if a parent can be present at bedside to provide support. • Consider letting the patient listen to music. • Consider using deep breathing and relaxation techniques.	• Include a description of sounds in preparation. • Inquire what is available at your facility for headphones or distraction options in the MRI unit.	• Discuss with parents the use of a hand-held emergency call button, which is often a ball, and whether their child would understand how to use it appropriately (i.e., only squeezing the ball if they feel they need help, and only using their voice to answer questions when asked while in the MRI).

Table 1.3.1 continues on next page.

Name of procedure	Language considerations	Positioning considerations	Procedural support and suggestions	Developmental considerations
Diagnostic imaging				
CT scan	• Avoid saying "cat scan." • The physician may say "a large camera in the shape of a doughnut used to take pictures."	• The positioning required will vary depending on the body part being scanned. • Discuss the importance of staying still. • Infants may benefit from being swaddled. • Ask if a parent can be present at bedside (using lead precautions) to remind the patient to remain still.	• Utilize deep breathing and/or guided imagery. • Offer distraction when appropriate (i.e., a passive coping strategy to ensure the patient remains still) such as watching a movie, listening to music, or having a parent sing a song or tell/read a story. • Parents should avoid asking questions with a "yes" or "no" response. • Offer a warm blanket. • If the patient is receiving IV contrast, describe that they may feel warm or like they have urinated on themselves; provide age-appropriate reassurance.	• Consider nonsedation if the test does not take a long time and/or the patient is cooperative, calm, able to follow directions, and able to hold still. • School-age patients and adolescents are often able to remain still and cope well. • Infants, toddlers and preschoolers may require further support with staying still. Infants may benefit from being swaddled in a warm blanket. If possible, encourage parents to feed the infant and/or get the infant to sleep. Dim the lighting in the CT room.
Ultrasound	• The physician may say "a special camera that looks like a small wand or computer mouse to take pictures of a part of your body."	• Consider required positioning and tailor coping strategies around this position. • Facilitate a position for comfort with the patient sitting or lying down with a parent.	• Ensure appropriate clothing for all ages. • Offer coping strategies such as reading a story or looking at a book, singing songs, or watching a movie on a portable device. • Show the patient the camera wand and allow the patient to feel the gel prior to use. • Use warm gel when available.	• Privacy is of utmost importance to adolescents; discuss with adolescents during preparation that their privacy will be maintained.
X-ray	• The physician may say "take a picture of your bones and organs."	• Ask if a parent may wear lead and help with positioning or comfort.	• Ensure appropriate clothing for all ages. • Discuss the length of the procedure. • Explain that the machine is large, but it does not touch the body when it takes a picture. • For CXRs, have patient practice taking deep breaths and holding them.	• School-age children may begin to understand the concept of "inside the body" and often will benefit from seeing their X-ray and reviewing it with the ED physician.

CCLS certified child life specialist. **CXR** chest X-ray. **ORT** oral rehydration therapy.

• Coping is impacted by how prepared and supported a patient feels and how much pain they experience (see Chapter 1.4, "Pain Management").

• To maximize coping, it is ideal to divert a patient's view away from the procedure location when possible (e.g., if the laceration is on the left side, the distraction should be on the right side).

» Always honor a patient's coping preferences, as some patients cope better when they are allowed to observe the procedure.

REFERENCES

Bankhead K, Knefley C. Survival and success: emergency department interventions for the child life specialist. Paper presented at: Child Life Council 2011. Proceedings of the 29th Annual Conference on Professional Issues; 2011 May 26-29; Chicago, IL.

Duff AJ. Incorporating psychological approaches into routine paediatric venepuncture. Arch Dis Child. 2003;88(10):931–937. https://doi.org/10.1136/adc.88.10.931. Medline:14500318

Gaynard L, Wolfer J, Goldberger J, Thompson R, Redburn L, Laidley L. Psychosocial care of children in hospitals: a clinical practice manual from the ACCH child life research project. Arlington, VA: Child Life Council; 1998. 159 p.

Humphreys C, LeBlanc CK. Promoting resilience in paediatric health care: the role of the child life specialist. In: DeMichelis C, Ferrari M, eds. Child and adolescent resilience within medical contexts. New York: Springer; 2016. p. 153–173. https://doi.org/10.1007/978-3-319-32223-0_9

Koller D. Preparing children and adolescents for medical procedures [Internet]. Arlington, VA: Child Life Council; 2007 [cited 2018 Jan]. 24 p. Available from: https://www.childlife.org/docs/default-source/research-ebp/ebp-statements.pdf?sfvrsn=2

Krauss BS, Krauss BA, Green, SM. (2016). Managing procedural anxiety in children. N Engl J Med. 2016(374):e19.

McGrath PJ. Annotation: aspects of pain in children and adolescents. J Child Psychol Psychiatry. 1995;36(5):717–730. https://doi.org/10.1111/j.1469-7610.1995.tb01325.x. Medline:7559841

Oczkowski SJ, Mazzetti I, Cupido C, Fox-Robichaud AE, Canadian Critical Care Society. Family presence during resuscitation: a Canadian Critical Care Society position paper. Can Respir J. 2015;22(4):201–205. https://doi.org/10.1155/2015/532721. Medline:26083541

1.4

Pain Management

Naveen Poonai

- Pain often goes unrecognized and is suboptimally managed in the pediatric emergency department (ED) setting.
- The World Health Organization has mandated that adequate pain management should be a fundamental human right, and the American Academy of Pediatrics reaffirmed its position that adequate analgesia should be provided for children in healthcare settings.
- Evidence supports the use of nonopioid, opioid, and nonpharmacologic approaches to effectively manage acute pain in children.
- Multiple clinical practice guidelines support the use of validated tools for the assessment of pain by healthcare providers across all age groups.
- The emerging challenge facing clinicians and investigators is that of providing comprehensive pain management in the postcodeine era, particularly in environments where opioids are often scrutinized due to concern about the potential for dependence and other unintended effects.

- When assessing pain and options available for its management, consider the patient's:
  » Age and developmental level
  » Communication skills
  » Prior experiences and fears
  » Cognitive skills to comprehend the clinical procedures that need to be carried out
- See Chapter 1.3, "Child Life," for further information about developmental considerations in pediatric populations in the ED.

ASSESSMENT OF PAIN IN CHILDREN

- *Table 1.4.1* summarizes scales that have been extensively validated for observational assessment (by a healthcare provider) and self-assessment of pain in children.

Table 1.4.1. SCALES FOR PAIN ASSESSMENT IN CHILDREN

Age range* Authors (year)	Instrument	Metric	Context
0 to 18 years Merkel et al. (1997)	Face, legs, activity, cry, consolability (FLACC) scale	• 5 items scored 0 to 2 • Range 0 to 10	• Procedural pain • Brief painful events • Postoperative pain in hospital
4 months to 17 years McGrath et al. (1985)	Children's Hospital of Eastern Ontario pain scale (CHEOPS)	• 6 items scored 0 to 3 • Range 4 to 13	• Procedural pain • Brief painful events
0 to 7 years Fournier-Charrière (2012)	EVENDOL pain assessment scale	• 5 items scored 0 to 3 • Range 0 to 15	• Musculoskeletal, abdominal, headache, ear, and throat pain
0 to 17 years Ambuel et al. (1992)	COMFORT behavior scale	• 8 items scored 1 to 5 • Range 8 to 40	• On ventilator or in critical care unit
Self-report scales			
4 to 12 years Hicks et al. (2001)	Faces pain scale—revised (FPS-R)†	• Scored 0, 2, 4, 6, 8, and 10	• Procedural pain • Brief painful events
6 years and up McGrath et al. (1996)	Visual analog scale (VAS)	• Scored from 0 to 100 using a vertical tick mark on a 100 mm horizontal line	• Procedural pain • Brief painful events
7 years and up Castarlenas et al. (2017)	Numerical rating scale (NRS-11)	• Scored from 0 to 10	• Wide range of painful stimuli

* This represents the age range studied in research subsequent to initial scale development.

† The FPS-R is available in multiple languages from http://www.iasppain.org/fpsr/.

NONPHARMACOLOGIC APPROACHES TO ACUTE PAIN MANAGEMENT IN CHILDREN

- Many nonpharmacologic approaches can be used by caregivers, nurses, physicians, and certified child life specialists (CCLSs).
- The cornerstone is a child-friendly, nonthreatening relationship with the child and caregivers.
- Across all age groups, nonpharmacologic interventions should be considered an adjunct to:
  » Any painful or anxiety-provoking intervention
  » Procedural sedation to decrease preprocedural anxiety and sensitivity to pain

DISTRACTION

- Distraction is an option for children who have difficulty comprehending verbal explanations.
- The child needs to understand the clinical procedures and steps that are about to take place.
- Functional neuroimaging studies provide evidence of pain modulation through distraction.
- Evidence supports the effectiveness of distraction and hypnosis for needle-related pain in children and adolescents.
- Bubbles, toys, pinwheels, deep breathing, guided imagery, audiovisual techniques, and smartphone apps are active distraction techniques. These may be more effective than passive techniques such as watching television.

POSITIONING

- Upward (seated rather than reclining) positioning on the caregiver's lap in a gentle hug, either facing the caregiver or facing outward, is effective for procedural distress.

CAREGIVER HOLDING AND PRESENCE

- Skin-to-skin contact has shown benefits in preterm and term neonates.
- Holding may reduce anxiety for infants to patients in middle childhood for brief procedural pain (e.g., a heel lance).
- Provision of anticipatory guidance empowers caregivers and allows them to participate in the pain management process.

SUCROSE AND NONNUTRITIVE SUCKING

- Evidence supports the use of 24% to 30% sucrose for minor procedures in children < 1 year of age.

- Breastfeeding during painful procedures has been shown to decrease physiological indicators of pain in children < 1 year of age.

NONPHARMACOLOGIC DEVICES

- Physical devices that involve topical cooling or vibration (e.g., the Buzzy device) are effective for needle-related pain in children.

PHYSICAL RESTRAINT

- Physical restraint is sometimes called "physical immobilization."
- The technique can involve "active restraint" (involving another person) or "passive restraint" (using a device).
- Restraint can cause physical and/or psychological harm.
- Most guidelines agree restraint should be limited to an uncooperative child who requires an immediate, medically mandatory, and short procedure.

PHARMACOLOGIC APPROACHES TO ACUTE PAIN MANAGEMENT IN CHILDREN

- Pharmacologic agents should be used in conjunction with nonpharmacologic strategies to lessen the components of fear and anxiety that contribute to the experience of pain in children.

TOPICAL AGENTS FOR SKIN PUNCTURING PROCEDURES

- Eutectic mixture of local anesthetics (EMLA):
  » Is a combination of lidocaine 2.5% and prilocaine 2.5%
  » Is effective at numbing intact tissue 6 to 7 mm below skin if applied for 30 to 60 minutes
  » Has its maximal effect at 60 minutes with occlusive dressing
  » Has a duration of action of 1 to 2 hours
  » Carries a risk of methemoglobinemia with repeated doses, open wound, and < 3 months of age
  » May be used in cases of:
    › Venipuncture
    › Lumbar puncture
- Lidocaine, epinephrine, tetracaine (LET):
  » Is effective if applied for at least 20 minutes
  » Has a duration of action of 30 minutes
  » May be used in cases of open wound closure
  » Does not work well for intact skin
- Tetracaine hydrochloride 4% gel (Ametop):
  » Is a superior analgesia to EMLA for IV insertion in

children, but it is not associated with improved facilitation of IV insertion

» May cause local erythema, pruritus, and hypersensitivity reaction with repeated doses
» Becomes effective in 30 minutes (venipuncture) or 45 minutes (IV insertion) with occlusive dressing
» Has a duration of action of 4 to 6 hours
» Carries no risk of methemoglobinemia
» May be used for:
  › IV insertion
  › Venipuncture

- 4% liposomal encapsulated lidocaine (Maxilene):
  » Should be avoided in children < 1 month of age
  » Should not be applied to an area greater than the child's abdomen for children < 10 kg
  » Becomes effective in 30 minutes
  » Has a duration of action of 1 hour
  » Has the key advantages of not containing prilocaine (which has been implicated in cases of methemoglobinemia) and carrying less risk of vasoconstriction or local reactions
  » May be used for:
    › Venipuncture
    › IV insertion

NONOPIOID ANALGESIA

- Nonopioid analgesia is a great option for headaches, soft tissue injuries, otalgia, and pharyngitis.

Table 1.4.2. NONOPIOID ANALGESICS

Agent	Dose	Comments
Acetaminophen	• PO: 10 to 15 mg/kg (maximum 1000 mg) • PR: 15 to 20 mg/kg	• Maximum daily dose: 75 mg/kg (infants); 100 mg/kg (< 40 kg); 3 to 4 g (> 40 kg) • Only option for children < 3 months of age • Issues with liver toxicity in high doses
Ibuprofen	• PO: 10 mg/kg (maximum 800 mg) every 6 to 8 hours	• Maximum daily dose: 40 mg/kg (< 40 kg); 2400 mg (> 40 kg) • Limited efficacy and safety data on children 6 to 12 months • Cautionary use in children with renal disease • Theoretical risk of increased bleeding posttonsillectomy
Naproxen	• PO: 5 to 7 mg/kg (maximum 400 mg) every 12 hours	• Maximum dose 600 mg for children ≥ 12 years • Limited efficacy and safety data on children 6 to 12 months • Cautionary use in children with renal disease • Increased risk of bleeding posttonsillectomy
Ketorolac	• IV: 0.25 to 1.0 mg/kg (maximum 30 mg) every 6 to 8 hours	• Limited efficacy and safety data on children 6 to 12 months • Cautionary use in children with renal disease • Increased risk of bleeding posttonsillectomy

OPIOID ANALGESIA

- Use opioids for moderate to severe pain, especially in cases of:
  » Fracture
  » Dislocations
  » Sickle cell pain crisis
  » Abdominal pain / peritonitis
- Consider a lower dose for opioid-naïve patients and a dose adjustment for patients with hepatic or renal impairment.
- There is no ceiling effect, but be careful of side effects (e.g., respiratory depression and hypotension).

Table 1.4.3. OPIOID ANALGESICS

Agent	Dose	Comments
Morphine	• IV/SC: 0.05 to 0.2 mg/kg (maximum 2 to 10 mg) every 1 to 4 hours • Can be given as an infusion: 0.05 to 0.1 mg/kg per hour • PO: 0.2 to 0.5 mg/kg (maximum 15 to 20 mg) every 4 hours	• May cause respiratory depression and hypotension • Longer half-life in neonates
Hydromorphone	• IV: 0.01 to 0.015 mg/kg (maximum 0.2 to 1 mg) every 3 to 6 hours • PO: 0.03 to 0.08 mg/kg (maximum 1 to 4 mg) every 2 to 4 hours	• Select dose carefully as it is 5 to 8 times more potent than morphine • May cause respiratory depression and hypotension
Fentanyl	• IV: 0.5 to 2.0 mcg/kg (maximum 25 to 100 mcg) every 2 to 4 hours • IN: 1 to 2 mcg/kg (maximum 50 to 100 mcg)	• 100 times more potent than morphine • May cause chest wall rigidity (with rapid IV push) and respiratory depression • Minimal to no effect on blood pressure

OTHER AGENTS

Table 1.4.4. OTHER ANALGESIC AGENTS

Agent	Dose	Comments
Subdissociative dose ketamine	• IN: 1 mg/kg	• Found to provide adequate analgesia without sedation and minimal side effects
Sucrose 24% solution	• 2 mL given 2 minutes prior to procedure	• Great for infants and neonates < 6 months of age

LOCAL ANESTHETICS

- Provide local anesthesia to the region requiring the procedure (laceration repair, hematoma block, etc.).
- The characteristics of the agent chosen depend on:
  » pKa — the amount of the anesthetic that penetrates through the tissue

» The amount of protein binding
» The partition coefficient — how lipid soluble the compound is (greater potency with higher partition coefficient)
» The type of intermediate chain:
  › Amino ester (e.g., cocaine and tetracaine)
  › Amide ester (e.g., lidocaine and bupivacaine)
- Pain at the injection site can be decreased by:
  » Using topical anesthetic first (e.g., LET gel)
  » Using distraction techniques
  » Using a smaller-gauge needle
  » Infiltrating slowly
  » Warming the solution to body temperature
  » Buffering with sodium bicarbonate
- Some agents are premixed with epinephrine to increase the duration of action and help with hemostasis.

Table 1.4.5. LOCAL ANESTHETIC AGENTS

Drug	Lidocaine (Xylocaine)	Bupivacaine (Marcaine)
Class	Amide	Amide
Onset	10 minutes	30 minutes
Duration	1 to 2 hours	2 to 8 hours
Maximum dose (with epinephrine)	4 mg/kg (7 mg/kg)	2.5 mg/kg (3 mg/kg)
Adverse effects	• Fasciculations; seizures; CNS, respiratory, or cardiovascular depression* • Contraindicated if patient allergic to PABA	• Highest risk of systemic toxicity (see lidocaine)
Relative potency (to procaine)	Medium	High

CNS central nervous system. **PABA** paraaminobenzoic acid.

* Higher risk comes with intravascular injection.

Toxicity and Pathophysiology

CENTRAL NERVOUS SYSTEM (CNS) TOXICITY

- Symptoms can vary from lightheadedness, paresthesias, and agitation, to seizures and altered level of consciousness.
- Treat seizures with benzodiazepines.

CARDIAC TOXICITY

- Cardiac toxicity is due to sodium channel blockade resulting in hypo- or hypertension.
- Bradycardia or tachycardia (including ventricular tachycardia and ventricular fibrillation) may occur.
- Manage cardiac toxicity as per pediatric advanced life support (PALS) guidelines.
  » Amiodarone is the agent for ventricular arrhythmias (avoid lidocaine or procainamide).

» Intralipid therapy (20%) is recommended if the patient is unresponsive to standard therapy (consult poison center control).
  › Administer a 1.5 mL/kg bolus followed by infusion of 0.25 mL/kg for 10 minutes.

ALLERGIC REACTION

- True allergy to the local anesthetic is rare; however, allergic reactions may occur with:
  » Esters — usually from the metabolite PABA
  » Amides — from the preservative methylparaben

———

ACKNOWLEDGEMENT

The author of this chapter would like to acknowledge Carl von Baeyer for his input on the pain scales.

———

REFERENCES

Ambuel B, Hamlett KW, Marx CM, Blumer JL. Assessing distress in pediatric intensive care environments: the COMFORT scale. *J Pediatr Psychol.* 1992;17(1):95–109.

American Academy of Pediatrics Committee on Pediatric Emergency Medicine. The use of physical restraint interventions for children and adolescents in the acute care setting. *Pediatrics.* 1997;99(3):497–498. https://doi.org/10.1542/peds.99.3.497. Medline:9041311

Baxter A. Common office procedures and analgesia considerations. *Pediatr Clin North Am.* 2013;60(5):1163–1183. https://doi.org/10.1016/j.pcl.2013.06.012. Medline:24093902

Brennan F, Carr DB, Cousins M. Pain management: a fundamental human right. *Anesth Analg.* 2007;105(1):205–221. https://doi.org/10.1213/01.ane.0000268145.52345.55. Medline:17578977

Castarlenas EJM, von Baeyer CL, Miró J. Psychometric properties of the Numerical Rating Scale to assess self-reported pain intensity in children and adolescents: a systematic review. *Clin J Pain.* 2017;33(4):376–83.

Chiaretti A, Pierri F, Valentini P, Russo I, Gargiullo L, Riccardi R. Current practice and recent advances in pediatric pain management. *Eur Rev Med Pharmacol Sci.* 2013;17(Suppl 1):112–126. Medline:23436673

Cramton RE, Gruchala NE. Managing procedural pain in pediatric patients. *Curr Opin Pediatr.* 2012;24(4):530–538. https://doi.org/10.1097/MOP.0b013e328355b2c5. Medline:22732639

Fein JA, Zempsky WT, Cravero JP; Committee on Pediatric Emergency Medicine and Section on Anesthesiology and Pain Medicine, American Academy of Pediatrics. Relief of pain and anxiety in pediatric patients in emergency medical systems. *Pediatrics.* 2012;130(5):e1391–e1405. https://doi.org/10.1542/peds.2012-2536. Medline:23109683

Folkes K. Is restraint a form of abuse? *Paediatr Nurs.* 2005;17(6):41–44. Medline:16045005

Fournier-Charrière E, Tourniaire B, Carbajal R, Cimerman P, Lassauge F, Ricard C, Reiter F, Turquin P, Lombart B, Letierce A, Falissard B. EVENDOL, a new behavioral pain scale for children ages 0 to 7 years in the emergency department: design and validation. *Pain.* 2012;153(8):1573–82.

Hansen MS, Mathiesen O, Trautner S, Dahl JB. Intranasal fentanyl in the treatment of acute pain: a systematic review. *Acta Anaesthesiol Scand.* 2012;56(4):407–419. https://doi.org/10.1111/j.1399-6576.2011.02613.x. Medline:22260169

Hicks CL, von Baeyer CL, Spafford PA, van Korlaar I, Goodenough B. The faces pain scale–revised: toward a common metric in pediatric pain measurement. *Pain.* 2001;93(2):173•83.

Lander JA, Weltman BJ, So SS. EMLA and amethocaine for reduction of children's pain associated with needle insertion. *Cochrane Database Syst Rev.* 2006;19(3):CD004236. Medline:16856039

McGrath PA, Seifert CE, Speechley KN, Booth JC, Stitt L, Gibson MC. A new analogue scale for assessing children's pain: an initial validation study. *Pain*. 1996;64(3):435–43.

McGrath PJ, Johnson G, Goodman JT, Schillinger J, Dunn J, Chapman J. CHEOPS: a behavioral scale for rating postoperative pain in children. *Adv Pain Res Ther*. 1985;9:395–402.

Merkel SI, Voepel-Lewis T, Shayevitz JR, Malviya S. The FLACC: a behavioral scale for scoring postoperative pain in young children. *Pediatr Nurs*. 1997;23(3):293–7.

Moadad N, Kozman K, Shahine R, Ohanian S, Badr LK. Distraction using the BUZZY for children during an IV insertion. *J Pediatr Nurs*. 2016;31(1):64–72. https://doi.org/10.1016/j.pedn.2015.07.010. Medline:26410385

Murphy A, O'Sullivan R, Wakai A, et al. Intranasal fentanyl for the management of acute pain in children. *Cochrane Database Syst Rev*. 2014;(10):CD009942. Medline:25300594

Poonai N, Kilgar J, Mehrotra S. Analgesia for fracture pain in children: methodological issues surrounding clinical trials and effectiveness of therapy. *Pain Manag*. 2015;5(6):435–445. https://doi.org/10.2217/pmt.15.41. Medline:26399275

Pywell A, Xyrichis A. Does topical amethocaine cream increase first-time successful cannulation in children compared with a eutectic mixture of local anaesthetics (EMLA) cream? A systematic review and meta-analysis of randomised controlled trials. *Emerg Med J*. 2015;32(9):733–737. https://doi.org/10.1136/emermed-2014-204066. Medline:25351196

Ruest S, Anderson A. Management of acute pediatric pain in the emergency department. *Curr Opin Pediatr*. 2016;28(3):298–304. https://doi.org/10.1097/MOP.0000000000000347. Medline:26974975

Stevens B, Yamada J, Lee GY, Ohlsson A. Sucrose for analgesia in newborn infants undergoing painful procedures. *Cochrane Database Syst Rev*. 2013;1(1):CD001069. Medline:23440783

Uman LS, Birnie KA, Noel M, et al. Psychological interventions for needle-related procedural pain and distress in children and adolescents. *Cochrane Database Syst Rev*. 2013;(10):CD005179. Medline:24108531

von Baeyer CL, Spagrud LJ. Systematic review of observational (behavioral) measures of pain for children and adolescents aged 3 to 18 years. *Pain*. 2007;127(1-2):140–150. https://doi.org/10.1016/j.pain.2006.08.014. Medline:16996689

Yeaman F, Oakley E, Meek R, Graudins A. Sub-dissociative dose intranasal ketamine for limb injury pain in children in the emergency department: a pilot study. *Emerg Med Australas*. 2013;25(2):161–167. https://doi.org/10.1111/1742-6723.12059. Medline:23560967

1.5

Procedural Sedation

Suzan Schneeweiss

- Procedural sedation is a technique in which sedative or dissociative agents are administered to induce a state that allows a patient to tolerate unpleasant procedures.
  » Ideally, the sedative / dissociative agent is given with analgesic agents for pain control.
- The goals for patient safety in the emergency department (ED) setting include the following:
  » Ensure that protective airway reflexes are intact and that the patient can maintain a patent airway independently and continuously
  » Maintain cardiovascular stability
- The careful titration of medications to the desired clinical effect are important to avoid excessive sedation.
  » Individual patient responses vary; patients may progress to a deeper level of sedation than intended.
- Ensure that safeguards such as sedation guidelines are in place to minimize adverse events.

SELECTION OF DEPTH OF SEDATION

- Minimal, moderate, and deep levels of sedation are a continuum that leads to general anesthesia (see *Table 1.5.1*).

Table 1.5.1. LEVELS OF SEDATION

	Level of consciousness	Airway reflexes / patent airway	Response to verbal commands and/or physical stimulation
Minimal	Impaired	Present	Appropriate
Moderate	Depressed	Present	Appropriate
Deep	Depressed or unconscious	Partial or complete loss	Inappropriate or absent

- The intended depth of sedation will vary according to patient needs and procedure.
- Target a minimal to moderate sedation level to maintain airway reflexes and patency.
- Dissociative state is not easily classifiable with a level of sedation but is generally considered moderate sedation.
  » Dissociative state is a trance-like, cataleptic state induced by the dissociative agent ketamine.
  » Patients experience profound analgesic and amnestic effects.
  » Patients generally retain protective airway reflexes, spontaneous respirations, and cardiopulmonary stability.

INDICATIONS FOR PROCEDURAL SEDATION AND ANALGESIA

- The most common indications for procedural sedation of pediatric patients in the ED are:
  - » Fracture reduction
  - » Dislocations
  - » Laceration repair
  - » Abscess incision and drainage
  - » Foreign body removal
  - » Lumbar puncture
  - » Burn debridement
  - » Dental trauma

GUIDELINES FOR PROCEDURAL SEDATION

PREPROCEDURAL ASSESSMENT

History

- Follow AMPLE:
  - » **A**llergies
  - » **M**edications
  - » **P**ast medical history
  - » **L**ast meal
  - » **E**xisting circumstances (e.g., American Society of Anesthesiologists [ASA] physical status classification)

Physical Exam

- Conduct a physical examination that includes:
  - » Baseline vital signs
  - » Cardiovascular and respiratory exam
  - » Focused airway assessment with Mallampati classification
- Establish ASA status.
  - » Procedural sedation should ideally only be used with ASA I and II patients.
- Consider the age of the patient.
  - » Use caution in infants < 6 months of age due to increased risk of airway instability.
- Obtain informed consent.
- Communicate appropriate fasting guidelines.
  - » For elective procedures, patients should fast for 8 hours from solids, 6 hours from formula, 4 hours from breast milk, and 2 hours from clear fluids.
  - » For emergency procedures, apply institutional policies.
    - › Do not delay procedural sedation in adults or pediatric patients in the ED based on fasting time.
    - › Preprocedural fasting for any duration has not demonstrated a reduction in the risk of emesis or aspiration when administering procedural sedation or analgesia.

Indications for Anesthesia Consultation

- Anesthesia consultation is indicated if the patient:
  - » Is ASA III or IV
  - » Has a history of known airway problems (e.g., snoring, obstructive sleep apnea, large tonsils or adenoids, tracheomalacia) or current upper respiratory tract infection or wheezing
  - » Has cardiovascular (CV) disease (cyanosis, congestive heart failure)
  - » Has a severe neurologic disease, hypotonia, increased intracranial pressure, poorly controlled seizures, or central apnea
  - » Has severe renal or liver disease
  - » Has severe gastroesophageal reflux, previous esophageal injury, or esophageal surgery
  - » Is at increased risk of pulmonary aspiration
  - » Has a potential neck injury or limitations in movement of neck / opening of mouth or jaw
  - » Has a history of known sedation failure
  - » Has sickle cell disease (SCD)
  - » Is morbidly obese
  - » Has baseline vital signs indicating $SaO_2 < 95\%$ in room air
  - » Is < 3 months of age

PRESEDATION INTERVENTIONS

Equipment

- Ensure that appropriate monitoring and resuscitation equipment is available based on the patient's weight and size.
- Ensure that facilities are equipped for emergency resuscitative measures.

Table 1.5.2. MONITORING EQUIPMENT

S	**S**uction (Yankauer catheter)
O	**O**xygen mask (spontaneous breathing) or BVM with O_2 (supported breathing)
A	**A**irway (GlideScope/laryngoscope + sized blade, ETT with stylet in situ, tape, syringe for cuff tubes, rescue devices [e.g., nasal/oral airways, LMA])
P	**P**ositioning patient to support intubation (ear to sternal notch) Preoxygenate whenever possible
ME	**M**edications (prepared and labeled) **E**quipment (SaO_2 monitor, cardiac monitor, blood pressure cuff, end-tidal CO_2 device)

BVM bag valve mask. **ETT** endotracheal tube. **LMA** laryngeal mask airway.

Personnel

- A nurse or other qualified individual must be present to monitor the patient continuously. This qualified individual must:
  - » Monitor appropriate physiologic parameters and assist in any supportive or resuscitation measures

» Have, at a minimum, basic life support (BLS) certification
» Have a specific role assignment in the event of emergency
» Have knowledge of the emergency resuscitation cart (medications and airway equipment)

- A provider must be present to perform the procedure; ideally, this individual should be different from sedation practitioner.
- A sedation practitioner must be present who:
  » Is responsible for treatment of patient, administering drugs, monitoring, and managing complications related to the sedation
  » Must have advanced airway management skills
  » Must be able to rescue the patient from one level deeper than the intended level of sedation

PROCEDURAL SEDATION

- Obtain a baseline set of vital signs; repeat vital signs and monitoring as defined by level of sedation.
  » Minimal sedation (anxiolysis)
    › Not specified unless high risk
  » Moderate sedation
    › Continuous monitoring
    › Cardiac monitoring
    › Pulse oximetry
    › Capnography (recommended)
    › Sedation score (e.g., Bromage sedation score)
- Consensus guidelines recommend documenting the above parameters every 5 to 10 minutes once sedation is established.

POSTPROCEDURAL EVALUATION

- Use clearly defined discharge criteria. Consider use of scoring system to assess readiness for discharge (e.g., Modified Aldrete Scoring System).
- A patient ready for discharge should:
  » Be alert and oriented
  » Have stable vital signs and satisfactory airway patency
  » Tolerate fluids
  » Be able to talk, walk, and sit as developmentally appropriate
  » Be adequately hydrated
- Discharge patients with a responsible adult who has been informed about sedation complications.
- Provide written instructions for when to return to the ED.

Management

- Adverse events may arise during procedural sedation and must be managed.
- Sedation guidelines aid in reduction of adverse events but may not eliminate them.

- Children are more predisposed to respiratory complications, including airway obstruction.
- Practitioners must be aware of potential adverse events and be prepared to intervene.

Complications

- Common adverse events and their management include:
  » Vomiting
    › Provide ondansetron.
    › Have patient sniff isopropyl alcohol (place alcohol swab against nose for 2 or 3 breaths).
  » Oxygen desaturation
    › Provide supplemental oxygen.
    › Reposition airway.
- Rare adverse events and their management include:
  » Partial airway obstruction
    › Reposition airway.
    › Consider bag valve mask (BVM) ventilation.
  » Laryngospasm — stepwise approach
    › Suction excessive secretions and reposition airway.
    › Apply continuous positive airway pressure (CPAP) with 100% oxygen.
    › For partial laryngospasm:
      · Consider deepening sedation, knowing you will have to use BVM to support them
    › For complete laryngospasm:
      · Consider jaw thrust or pressure in laryngospasm notch to convert to partial laryngospasm; rapidly consider paralytic agent (succinylcholine) and atropine
  » Central apnea
  » Cardiovascular events (e.g., hypotension)
    › Consider underlying cause.
    › Treat hypotension with IV fluid bolus.
- Very rare adverse events include:
  » Pulmonary aspiration
  » Complete airway obstruction
  » Chest wall and glottic rigidity (from fentanyl)

Steps to Avoid Complications and Adverse Events

- Choose your patient carefully. Patients should:
  » Be healthy
  » Be ASA I and II
  » Have no intercurrent illness (e.g., upper respiratory tract infection)
- For all drugs, know the:
  » Appropriate medication titrations
  » Dose limits and potential adverse effects
- Monitor patient carefully and continue monitoring until patient returns to baseline.
- Be prepared to intervene with age appropriate resuscitation equipment, reversal agents, and personnel with

Table 1.5.3. SEDATIVE AND ANALGESIC AGENTS

Drug	Method of administration	Dose	Comments
Minimal sedation (anxiolysis)			
Midazolam	PO	• Weight < 20 kg: 0.5 to 0.75 mg/kg • Weight > 20 kg: 0.3 to 0.5 mg/kg (maximum 20 mg) • May cause paradoxical reactions (hyperactive)	• No analgesia • May not immobilize patient
	IN	• 0.2 to 0.5 mg/kg (maximum volume 0.5 mL per nostril in infants and 1.0 mL per nostril in older children)	• Consider for children > 6 months of age • Use lower doses for nonpainful procedures or if combined with analgesic agents
Nitrous oxide	Inhaled	• 30% to 50% nitrous oxide blended with oxygen — **or** — • Preset mixture with minimum of 50% O_2 (may be self-administered by demand-valve but requires a cooperative child)	• Avoid in pneumothorax, bowel obstruction, otitis media • Combine with other analgesic agent for painful procedures
Moderate sedation			
Midazolam	IV	• Initially 0.05 to 0.1 mg/kg up to 0.15 mg/kg (maximum 10 mg)	• Synergistic with opioid analgesic; may need to decrease dose • No analgesia
Ketamine	IV	• 0.5 to 1.5 mg/kg slowly over 1 to 2 minutes to reach dissociative state (maximum 100 mg)	• **Not reversible** • Analgesia, dissociation, amnesia, motion control
		• May repeat in 0.5 mg/kg increments every 5 to 10 minutes to maximum 2 mg/kg	• Not for use if cardiovascular disorder (increased BP), ICP, airway instability, active pulmonary infection or disease, procedures resulting in increased secretions, patient < 3 months of age, psychiatric disorder, increased intraocular pressure (e.g., glaucoma, globe rupture)
	IM	• 4 mg/kg	• Use **50 mg/mL concentration**
Deep sedation			
Propofol	IV	• 1 to 4 mg/kg, usually starting dose 1 mg/kg IV slow push; titrate dose to effect	• No analgesia; consider ketamine or fentanyl for analgesia
		• May repeat 0.5 mg/kg increments every 3 to 5 minutes • May cause CV depression and hypotension • Avoid if patient has an egg or soybean allergy	• May cause rapidly deepening sedation
Analgesic agents for use with sedative agents			
Ketamine	IV	• 0.5 mg/kg	• Combined with propofol ("ketofol" — propofol sedation with ketamine analgesia — start propofol 0.5 mg/kg and titrate to effect)
Fentanyl (Note: dosage in micrograms [mcg]. 1 mg = 1000 mcg)	IV	• 0.5 to 1.0 mcg/kg, administered slowly in incremental doses every 1 to 2 minutes to desired effect; maximum 3 mcg/kg; maximum initial dose 100 mcg	• Apnea, skeletal muscle rigidity (with rapid IV push), chest wall rigidity with higher doses • Midazolam and fentanyl have synergistic effects; reduce dosages of each if combined
	IN	• 1.5 mcg/kg (maximum 0.5 mL per nostril in infants, 1.0 mL per nostril in older children)	• Larger volumes are not reliably absorbed in the nose due to saturation of mucosal surfaces and drug loss in the oropharynx (ideal volume 0.2 to 0.3 mL)
Morphine	IV	• 0.05 to 0.1 mg/kg over 1 minute (maximum 15 mg) • Dose may be repeated once at 10 min	• Peak effect in 10 to 20 minutes • CNS and respiratory depression, nausea, vomiting, hypotension, bradycardia, pruritus, vasodilation, histamine release
Reversal agents (note: if used, must monitor for at least 3 hours)			
Naloxone	IV, IM	• 0.001 to 0.01 mg/kg; titrate dose for partial opioid reversal; may repeat as required	• For **narcotic** reversal, duration of action 45 minutes; may require repeated doses • Maximum 0.01 mg/kg per dose • Dose limit for full reversal 2 mg per dose
Flumazenil	IV	• 0.01 mg/kg over 15 seconds, repeat every 1 to 3 minutes to maximum 5 doses (maximum 1 mg)	• For **benzodiazepine** reversal, duration of action 30 to 60 minutes; may require repeated doses

BP blood pressure. **CNS** central nervous system. **CV** cardiovascular. **ICP** intracranial pressure.

advanced pediatric life support and airway management skills.

REFERENCES

American Society of Anesthesiologists. ASA physical status classification system. (Last updated: Oct 15, 2014). Available at: https://scholarlykitchen.sspnet.org/2017/08/11/game-thrones-copyeditors-edition/

Bhatt M, Johnson DW, Tajjaard M, et al; Association of preprocedural fasting with outcomes of emergency department sedation in children. *JAMA Pediatr.* 2018; online first publication. https://doi.org/10.1001/jamapediatrics.2018.0830.

Coté CJ, Wilson, S; American Academy of Pediatrics; American Academy of Pediatric Dentistry. Guidelines for monitoring and management of pediatric patients, before during and after sedation for diagnostic and therapeutic procedures: update 2016. *Pediatrics.* 2016;138(1):e20161212. https://doi.org/10.1542/peds.2016-1212. Medline:17142550

Fein JA, Zempsky WT, Cravero JP; Committee on Pediatric Emergency Medicine and Section on Anesthesiology and Pain Medicine. Relief of pain and anxiety in pediatric patients in emergency medical systems. *Pediatrics.* 2012;130(5):e1391–e1405. https://doi.org/10.1542/peds.2012-2536. Medline:23109683

Godwin SA, Burton JH, Gerardo CJ, et al; American College of Emergency Physicians. Clinical policy: procedural sedation and analgesia in the emergency department. *Ann Emerg*

Med. 2014;63(2):247–58.e18. https://doi.org/10.1016/j.annemergmed.2013.10.015. Medline:24438649

Green SM, Roback MG, Kennedy RM, Krauss B. Clinical practice guideline for emergency department ketamine dissociative sedation: 2011 update. *Ann Emerg Med.* 2011;57(5):449–461. https://doi.org/10.1016/j.annemergmed.2010.11.030. Medline:21256625

Kennedy RM. Sedation in the emergency department: a complex and multifactorial challenge. In: Mason KP, editor. *Pediatric sedation outside of the operating room.* New York: Springer-Verlag; 2015. p. 263–331.

Langhan ML, Mallory M, Hertzog J, Lowrie L, Cravero J; Pediatric Sedation Research Consortium. Physiologic monitoring practices during pediatric procedural sedation: a report from the Pediatric Sedation Research Consortium. *Arch Pediatr Adolesc Med.* 2012;166(11):990–998. https://doi.org/10.1001/archpediatrics.2012.1023. Medline:22965648

Mace SE, Brown LA, Francis L, et al; EMSC Panel (Writing Committee) on Critical Issues in the Sedation of Pediatric Patients in the Emergency. Clinical policy: critical issues in the sedation of pediatric patients in the emergency department. *Ann Emerg Med.* 2008;51(4):378–399.e57. https://doi.org/10.1016/j.annemergmed.2007.11.001. Medline:18359378

Wolfe TR, Braude DA. Intranasal medication delivery for children: a brief review and update. *Pediatrics.* 2010;126(3):532–537. https://doi.org/10.1542/peds.2010-0616. Medline:20696726

1.6

Technologically Dependent Children

Nicole Anderson, Jonathan Duff

- An increasing number of children with chronic disease are living with some form of technology that allows management of their care.
- Hospital readmission is frequent in this population due not only to their fragile medical state, but also the risk of technology malfunction.
- Tracheostomies, enteral feeding tubes, ventricular shunts, and central venous access are some of the common technologies seen in the emergency department (ED).

TRACHEOSTOMIES

- There are several steps that should be carried out with every tracheostomy patient in the ED.
  » Identify the type and size of the tracheostomy tube.
  » Suction the tracheostomy.
    › This should be done using a premarked suction catheter (half the diameter of the tracheostomy tube) to avoid epithelial damage.
    › This step should be carried out prior to attempting

bag-valve ventilation to avoid pushing secretions into the lower airway.
  » Clarify the status of the patient's upper airway.
    › Are you able to bag-valve ventilate the patient with a mask? Is the patient intubatable?
  » Clarify what routine tracheostomy care looks like.
    › It is usually carried out every 12 hours or whenever necessary (PRN).
  » Determine the type of tracheostomy.
    › Is it cuffed or uncuffed?
    › Is the tube fenestrated or unfenestrated?
  » If the patient has oxygenation issues, consider the DOPE mnemonic:
    › **D**isplaced
    › **O**bstructed
    › **P**neumothorax
    › **E**quipment malfunction

- Ideally, a respiratory therapist should be present when the tracheostomy is being manipulated.

- If the patient is unstable, call otorhinolaryngology (ENT) immediately.

Indications

- A tracheostomy is indicated if a child has:
  - » Upper airway anomalies:
    - › Craniofacial anomalies
    - › Subglottic stenosis
  - » Prolonged ventilation requirements:
    - › Neurologic conditions
    - › Chronic lung disease

Complications

Respiratory Tract Infection

- Respiratory tract infection is the most common reason for hospital admission in children with a tracheostomy.
  - » The upper airway cannot carry out the important filtration function and natural cough mechanism.
- Bacterial colonization is common (often by gram-negative organisms such as *Pseudomonas*) and can be hard to differentiate from true infection.
  - » It is important to check previous culture results for earlier bacterial colonization.
- Treat a suspected bacterial respiratory infection with empiric antibiotics.
  - » Consider treatment for possible resistant organisms.

Bleeding

- Bleeding from suction trauma is common and is typically mild.
- It must be differentiated from the sentinel bleed that may occur with the formation of a tracheavascular fistula with a major (innominate) artery.

Accidental Decannulation

- If the tracheostomy tube is inadvertently removed (accidental decannulation/extubation), attempt to replace the tube.
- A tracheostomy tube that is one size smaller than their usual tube should be with the child at all times in case of accidental decannulation, as it can be difficult to reinsert the usual-sized tracheostomy tube.
  - » If the right size of (smaller) tracheal tube is unavailable, an endotracheal tube (ETT) can be used.
- If there are difficulties inserting the tube and the child is unstable, the stoma should be occluded and ventilation through the mouth with a mask or ETT should be performed.
  - » If this is not possible, obtain an urgent ENT referral.

ENTERAL FEEDING TUBES

Indications

- A feeding tube is indicated if a child cannot safely eat or drink or is unable to take in enough calories by mouth.

- The varying routes of enteral feeding tubes are:
  - » Nasogastric (NG)
  - » Nasojejunal (NJ)
  - » Gastrostomy tube (G-tube)
  - » Jejunostomy tube (J-tube)
  - » Gastro-jejunostomy tube (GJ-tube)

Complications

Displacement or Blockage

- If the feeding tube is blocked, attempt to flush it with water after aspirating the tube.
- For G-tubes, J-tubes, and GJ-tubes, replace the tube temporarily within an hour using a CORFLO tube or Foley catheter.
  - » Final tube replacement can then be performed by interventional radiology according to local protocols.

Feeding Intolerance

- Feeding intolerance is characterized by gagging, emesis, and abdominal pain.
- It can be caused by:
  - » Stomach filling too quickly / feed being too fast
  - » First morning feed (mucous swallowed at night)
  - » Excess air in the stomach
  - » Displaced tube
- It may also have non–tube-related causes (e.g., gastroenteritis).
- It is particularly a problem for J-tubes and GJ-tubes.
- A general approach to feeding intolerance includes:
  - » Checking tube placement (may require a contrast study), especially for J- and GJ-tubes
  - » Checking for signs of hydration
  - » Considering a trial of hydration solution (e.g., Pedialyte)

Erythema Around the Tube Site

- Mild erythema may be normal.
- If skin is wet from stomach fluids, either use a barrier wipe and foam dressing or expose the skin to air to keep the area dry.
- Assess tube stability:
  - » Confirm tube placement
  - » Ensure balloon is adequately filled (if applicable)
- Infection can be treated as cellulitis.
  - » Consider a topical fungal treatment if there is no improvement.

VENTRICULAR SHUNTS

Indications

- Ventricular shunts are used in the management of hydrocephalus (an accumulation of cerebrospinal fluid

[CSF] within the ventricular space at an inappropriate pressure).
  » The most common causes of hydrocephalus in pediatrics include:
    › Intraventricular hemorrhage
    › Spina bifida
    › Tumors
- The distal insertion site of a ventricular shunt is typically peritoneal (though it can be atrial or pleural).
- The components of a shunt include the proximal catheter, a valve, and a distal catheter.
  » Different types of valves exist:
    › Pressure-regulated
    › Flow-regulated
    › Antisiphon (prevents abrupt pressure changes with position)
    › On-off (for chemotherapy)
    › Programmable

Complications

Shunt failure

- Symptoms of shunt failure are:
  » Irritability
  » Nausea/vomiting
  » Headache
- Signs include:
  » Increased head circumference
  » Bulging fontanelle
  » Developmental concerns
- Investigations into and management of shunt failure include:
  » Imaging, including:
    › Shunt series (skull anteroposterior [AP] and lateral X-rays, chest X-ray [CXR], and abdominal AP and lateral X-ray)
    › CT head scan (noncontrast)
    › CT abdomen scan (noncontrast)
  - Neurosurgery consult
    › Shunt tap may be diagnostic or pressure alleviating.
    › Surgical replacement of the shunt may be required.

Shunt infection

- A shunt infection typically occurs in the early postoperative period.
- A general approach to shunt infection includes:
  » Consulting neurosurgery for possible externalization of shunt
  » Administering broad-spectrum antibiotics at meningitic doses

CENTRAL VENOUS ACCESS

Indications

- Central venous access may be necessary in patients requiring administration of prolonged IV therapy, frequent blood draws, hemodialysis, or total parenteral nutrition (TPN).
- Examples of central access include:
  » Peripherally inserted central catheter (PICC)
  » Indwelling central venous catheter (tunneled and nontunneled)
  » Implanted venous access device

Complications

Catheter Malposition

- Catheter malposition occurs frequently in children secondary to physical activity and loss of adhesion of dressing materials.
- It presents as lack of blood return.
  » The patient may have edema to the chest wall or neck, leaking at the insertion site, and arrhythmia.
- Order a CXR to confirm catheter placement.

Catheter Occlusion

- Potential causes of catheter occlusion include:
  » Kinking in the catheter
  » Improper tip placement
  » Catheter migration
  » Pinching of the catheter between the clavicle and first rib
- Occlusion may also be caused by precipitation or crystallization in the tubing.
  » Ensure appropriate flushing and infusion to prevent occlusion.
  » Consult pharmacy to determine whether a particular medication could be the culprit.
- Inspect the catheter site and tubing for evidence of occlusion.
- To relieve the occlusion:
  » Encourage deep breathing and coughing to alter intrathoracic pressure
  » Ask the patient to raise their arms and shrug their shoulders
  » Reposition the patient
  » For implanted venous access devices, verify needle placement and reaccess if necessary
- Thrombotic occlusions are another cause of difficulty with infusion or withdrawal from the line.
  » Rule out mechanical obstruction.
  » Consider local administration of tissue plasminogen activator (tPA) into the catheter lumen to restore patency.

» Follow local protocols and consult anticoagulation services if there are concerns with long-term anticoagulation needs.

Superior Vena Cava Syndrome

- Superior Vena Cava (SVC) syndrome is a caused by an obstruction of blood through the SVC due to mechanical compression or extensive venous thrombosis.
- It is characterized by:
  » Sudden onset edema of face, neck, and upper body
  » Shortness of breath
  » Cough/hoarseness
  » Dilation of neck veins
  » Chest pain
  » Decreased level of consciousness
- Obtain urgent imaging to determine etiology and management of symptoms.

Infection

- Localized infection can occur at the tube entrance or exit site.
- Infection is characterized by:
  » Erythema
  » Tenderness
  » Purulence
  » Positive cultures from swab
- Watch for signs of infection along the tunnel site.
- Take swabs and order blood cultures (from both the line and peripheral) prior to antibiotic initiation.
- Possible line removal should be the focus of treatment.
- Watch for signs of phlebitis.
  » Phlebitis may occur in the first week of insertion.
  » Symptoms of phlebitis include pain or swelling in addition to erythema.
  » Patient may have a red streak progressing along the affected vessel's path.

» Treatment includes:
  › Elevation of the affected limb
  › Warm compresses 4 times a day
  › Mild exercise of the limb to promote circulation

REFERENCES

Berry JG, Graham DA, Graham RJ, et al. Predictors of clinical outcomes and hospital resource use of children after tracheotomy. *Pediatrics.* 2009;124(2):563–572. https://doi.org/10.1542/peds.2008-3491. Medline:19596736

Berry JG, Hall DE, Kuo DZ, et al. Hospital utilization and characteristics of patients experiencing recurrent readmissions within children's hospitals. *JAMA.* 2011;305(7):682–690. https://doi.org/10.1001/jama.2011.122. Medline:21325184

Cohen A. *Pediatric neurosurgery: tricks of the trade.* New York: Thieme; 2016.

Gasco J, Nader R, editors. *The essential neurosurgery companion.* New York: Thieme; 2012. https://doi.org/10.1055/b-002-85480

Joffe AR, Grant M, Wong B, Gresiuk C. Validation of a blind transpyloric feeding tube placement technique in pediatric intensive care: rapid, simple, and highly successful. *Pediatr Crit Care Med.* 2000;1(2):151–155. https://doi.org/10.1097/00130478-200010000-00011. Medline:12813267

Kornbau C, Lee KC, Hughes GD, Firstenberg MS. Central line complications. *Int J Crit Illn Inj Sci.* 2015;5(3):170–178. https://doi.org/10.4103/2229-5151.164940. Medline:26557487

Mattox EA. Complications of peripheral venous access devices: prevention, detection, and recovery strategies. *Crit Care Nurse.* 2017;37(2):e1–e14. https://doi.org/10.4037/ccn2017657. Medline:28365664

Myers EN. *Operative otolaryngology: head and neck surgery.* 2nd ed. Saunders Elsevier; 2008. Chapter 68, Tracheostomy; p. 577.

Rusakow LS, Guaría M, Wegner CB, Rice TB, Mischler EH. Suspected respiratory tract infection in the tracheostomized child: the pediatric pulmonologist's approach. *Chest.* 1998;113(6):1549–1554. https://doi.org/10.1378/chest.113.6.1549. Medline:9631792

Sherman JM, Davis S, Albamonte-Petrick S, et al. Care of the child with a chronic tracheostomy. This official statement of the American Thoracic Society was adopted by the ATS Board of Directors, July 1999. *Am J Respir Crit Care Med.* 2000;161(1):297–308. Medline:10619835

Simon TD, Cawthon ML, Stanford S, et al; Center of Excellence on Quality of Care Measures for Children with Complex Needs (COE4CCN) Medical Complexity Working Group. Pediatric medical complexity algorithm: a new method to stratify children by medical complexity. *Pediatrics.* 2014;133(6):e1647–e1654. https://doi.org/10.1542/peds.2013-3875. Medline:24819580

1.7

Child Abuse

Carmen Coombs, David Warren

- Child abuse is defined as "any recent act or failure to act on the part of a parent or caretaker, which results in death, serious physical or emotional harm, sexual abuse or exploitation, or an act or failure to act which presents an imminent risk of serious harm" (CAPTA, 2010).
- Child abuse is often categorized into:
  » Physical abuse — nonaccidental physical contact that results in an injury and/or substantial pain
  » Sexual abuse — undesired or unconsented sexual activity
  » Neglect — failure to meet common basic needs
  » Emotional maltreatment — behavior that impairs psychological well-being
- Physical and sexual abuse are the forms most likely to be encountered in the emergency department (ED).
- The annual incidence of child abuse in Canada in 2008 was reported as 85 440 substantiated cases (14.19 per 1000 children).
- The annual incidence in the United States in 2014 was reported as:
  » 702 000 victims of child abuse (9.4 per 1000 children)
  » 1580 deaths due to child abuse (2.13 per 100 000 children)
- Perpetrators are usually well known to the child.
- Triggers for abuse are often normal elements of child development (e.g., crying in infancy, difficulty with potty training in toddlerhood).
- Multiple factors are involved in child abuse victims coming to the ED for care, including:
  » Acute nature of the injury
  » Lack of primary care
  » Proximity to an ED
  » Hours of operation of the ED
- The high prevalence and incidence of child abuse means emergency physicians will undoubtedly encounter these situations in their practice.

Risk Factors

- Child abuse affects children of all ages, races, and socioeconomic statuses.
- Because cases without obvious risk factors are more likely to be missed, a uniform approach to recognition is essential.

- Characteristics that place a child at increased risk of abuse can be divided into the following categories:
  » Child-related factors:
    › Young age
    › Developmental disability
    › Child of an unwanted pregnancy
    › Inability to report
  » Parent-related factors:
    › Substance abuse
    › Depression
    › Young age
  » Environmental factors:
    › Domestic violence
    › Social isolation
    › Poverty

Recognition and appropriate management of child abuse by ED providers is critical because the ED may be the first and/or only medical contact for the victim.

PHYSICAL CHILD ABUSE

- The most common abusive injuries include:
  » Bruises
  » Burns
  » Fractures
  » Head injuries
- 80% of child abuse fatalities occur in children < 4 years of age.
  » 60% of children who die from abuse have abusive head trauma.
  » Of all fatal head injuries in infants and young children, most are due to abuse.
- **20% to 30% of children who die from abuse and neglect have previously been evaluated by medical providers for abusive injuries that were not recognized as abuse.**
  » Many of these unrecognized injuries are minor injuries, such as bruises or intraoral injuries; these "minor" injuries, however, have major significance as they provide the opportunity to intervene before more serious injury occurs.

When to Suspect Physical Child Abuse

- Most injuries in children are accidental, but knowing

when to suspect abuse is critical because of the significant associated morbidity and mortality.

- A history of abuse is rarely disclosed initially, and no single injury or test is diagnostic of child abuse. Thus, suspecting child abuse requires the physician to interpret the child's injury or injuries in the context of the history provided and the developmental ability of the child.

Red Flags

- A child with a significant injury presents with an absent or vague history of the trauma.
- An injury is not consistent with the history provided.
  » Example: a 2-year-old reportedly spilled hot tea on herself but has immersion-pattern burns on both feet/ankles rather than the expected splash-pattern burns.
- The injury is not consistent with the developmental ability of the child.
  » Example: a 6-month-old (i.e., nonambulatory) infant with a femur fracture reportedly fell while playing.
- The history changes or evolves and/or different histories are provided by different people.
- There is a delay in seeking medical care.
- There is a history of past injuries in the child or unexplained injuries/deaths in siblings.

RED FLAG INJURIES

- Although almost any injury can be either abusive or accidental in nature, certain injuries should always raise concern for child abuse (see *Table 1.7.1*). The presence of more than 1 of these injuries greatly increases the level of concern.

Table 1.7.1. SPECIFIC INJURIES THAT SHOULD ALWAYS PROMPT CONSIDERATION OF CHILD ABUSE

Highly concerning injuries	Comments
Bruises	

• Any bruising in an infant, especially a premobile infant < 5 months of age
• Bruises in unusual/protected locations such as:
  » Face (cheeks, eyes/periorbital), ears, and/or neck
  » Trunk (abdomen, back)
  » Buttocks
  » Genital area (especially bruising on the penis)
• Multiple bruises in different stages of healing
• Patterned bruises, such as:
  » Handprints
  » Bite marks (adult size and pattern)
  » Looped cord markings
  » Linear belt marks
	• Bruising is the most common finding in abused children of all ages. The absence of bruising, however, does not rule out abuse.
	• Abusive bruises themselves are usually mild injuries but are extremely important. Bruising often precedes abuse fatalities and near-fatalities, and can present an opportunity to intervene before more serious injuries occur.
	• Half of infants with apparently isolated bruises have at least one other serious injury identified upon further investigation.
	• Most accidental bruising occurs over bony prominences and on the front of the body (e.g., knees, shins, forehead).

Highly concerning injuries	Comments
Burns	

• Immersion scald burns, especially:
  » Stocking and/or glove distribution
  » Symmetrically burned buttocks/genitals
• Contact burns, especially:
  » Cigarette burns (especially if multiple and/or in protected locations)
  » Well-demarcated patterned burns mirroring the hot object (e.g., clothing iron, cigarette lighter, curling iron, hair blow dryer, cooking items)
	• Most accidental scald burns in children occur due to spillage of hot liquids and are located on the anterior body surface, are asymmetric, and have obvious splash marks.
	• Most accidental contact burns occur when the hot object is touched or grasped (burning the palmar surface of the hand) or falls (causing multiple irregular burns as it falls).

Fractures	
• Any fracture in a nonambulatory infant or child • Rib fractures • Classical metaphyseal lesions • Femur fractures in infants < 18 months of age • Humerus fractures in infants < 18 months of age • Multiple fractures • Skull fractures, especially if bilateral and/or complex	• Most acute fractures are symptomatic but some abusive fractures (e.g., rib fractures, classical metaphyseal lesions) are often occult and only identified by imaging. • Fractures due to birth trauma are rare. The most common is a clavicle fracture and occurs in ~1% of births. • Acute rib fractures are difficult to visualize on X-ray. Healing rib fractures are easier to visualize due to callus formation. • A toddler's fracture (nondisplaced fracture of the distal tibia) is a common accidental injury that often happens in the context of normal toddler activity without a history of significant trauma.
Intracranial injury	
• Any intracranial injury in an infant or young child without a clear history of definite major trauma • Subdural hematoma • Cerebral edema • Hypoxic ischemic injury	• Most fatal head injuries in infants and young children are due to abuse rather than accidental injury. • Signs and symptoms of intracranial injury may be dramatic (e.g., seizure, apnea, altered mental status), subtle and nonspecific (e.g., sleepy, vomiting, irritability, macrocephaly), or absent. • Subdural hematomas are the most common form of abusive head injury, but any type of intracranial injury can be abusive in etiology. • Epidural hematomas are usually associated with accidental injuries. • Retinal hemorrhages are present in 60% to 65% of children with abusive head injuries and are rare in those with accidental head injuries.
Other concerning injuries	
• Oronasal bleeding and/or injured frenulum • Subconjunctival hemorrhage (should be thought of as a bruise to the eye, especially in infants) • Facial petechiae (due to strangulation) • Unexplained focal swelling • Unexplained abdominal trauma (e.g., duodenal hematoma, liver contusions/laceration) • Unexplained drowning • Any injury in an infant or child without an adequate explanation	

Management

- Stabilize, evaluate, and treat all injuries according to trauma protocols.

History

- Obtain and document the history.
  - » If possible, obtain the history from the patient as well as the caregiver(s) and/or witnesses; talking to older patients without their caregiver present may be helpful.
  - » Encourage an uninterrupted open narrative followed by clarifying questions.
  - » Avoid leading questions.
  - » If a history of an injury is provided, include:
    - › The events leading up to the injury
    - › The mechanism/location/timing of the incident
    - › The behavior of the child before and after the incident
    - › Any witnesses
  - » If a history of an injury is not provided, include:
    - › When the child was last observed acting normally
    - › When symptoms were first noted

Physical Exam

- Perform a complete physical exam.
  - » Document all pertinent positives and negatives.
  - » Always do a complete skin exam, paying close attention to high-risk areas such as the face, ears, neck, trunk, and genitals.
  - » Document findings in as much detail as possible, including measurements of findings and diagrams showing locations.
  - » Photograph all findings; include a measuring tape in photo for size, if possible.
  - » Examine the oral cavity to assess for frenulum and other intraoral injuries.
  - » Measure head circumference in all children < 2 years of age.

Investigations

- The following are useful studies to order when physical abuse is suspected; note that nonemergent studies are often obtained in coordination with a child abuse expert:
  - » Skeletal survey
    - › This is indicated in all children < 2 years of age.
    - › It assesses for occult acute and healing fractures.
    - › It includes special views of the skull, cervical spine, chest, ribs, pelvis, abdomen, spine, and long bones.
    - › A skeletal survey may be repeated 10 to 14 days after the initial presentation to improve diagnostic sensitivity and specificity.
  - » Intracranial imaging (CT and/or MRI)
    - › Emergent noncontrast head CT is indicated for all children with signs/symptoms of head injury to rapidly identify injuries requiring immediate intervention.
    - › Noncontrast head CT or brain MRI should be considered in asymptomatic infants < 1 to 2 years of age.
      - · MRI is more sensitive for subtle intracranial injuries and has the advantage of no radiation, but it often requires sedation and is not always readily available.
      - · Head CT scan is usually more readily available, does not typically require sedation, and is better at identifying associated skull fractures; it does, however, have associated radiation exposure and is not as sensitive as MRI for intracranial injury.
  - » Dilated eye exam (to identify retinal hemorrhages)
    - › This is indicated in all patients with suspected abusive head trauma.
    - › It should be performed by an ophthalmologist.
- Appropriate laboratory workups change in conjunction with each unique case of suspected child abuse.
  - » No one laboratory workup is routinely recommended for all cases of suspected child abuse.
  - » Trauma workups (e.g., Complete blood count [CBC], aspartate transaminase [AST], alanine transaminase [ALT], amylase, lipase, urinalysis) are helpful in many cases to identify associated visceral injuries.
  - » Additional workups may be helpful when the diagnosis is in question and organic etiologies need to be considered. These are best done in consultation with child abuse experts and not typically done in the ED setting. Such testing may include:
    - › Testing for underlying bone disease in patients with fractures:
      - · Calcium, phosphorus, alkaline phosphatase, 25-hydroxyvitamin D, parathyroid hormone (PTH), and/or testing for osteogenesis imperfecta
    - › Testing for underlying bleeding disorders in patients with bruising:
      - · CBC with platelets, prothrombin time (PT) / international normalized ratio (INR) / partial thromboplastin time (PTT), factor VIII level, factor IX level, and testing for von Willebrand disease
    - › Testing for underlying bleeding and/or metabolic disease in patients with intracranial hemorrhage:
      - · CBC with platelets, PT/INR/PTT, factor VIII level, factor IX level, fibrinogen, D-dimer
      - · Urine organic acids to screen for glutaric aciduria type I

SEXUAL CHILD ABUSE

- Sexual child abuse is defined as a child being engaged in sexual activities:
  - » That the child cannot comprehend

» For which the child is developmentally unprepared
» For which the child cannot give consent
» That violate the law or social taboos of society
- These activities may include:
  » All forms of fondling
  » Masturbation
  » Digital or object penetration of the anus, vagina, or oral areas
  » All genital contact
  » Exhibitionism, voyeurism, exposure, and production of pornography
- Sexual abuse occurs to 25% of females and 16% of males before the age of 18.
- Children are most frequently abused by someone they know and trust; this includes:
  » By adult authorities in 30% to 50% of cases
  » By teens in 25% to 35% of cases
- An ever-increasing number of children are solicited or exposed sexually online.
- The ED is far from the ideal setting to assess for sexual abuse.
  » It lacks appropriate space, equipment, an interdisciplinary interview team, specialized personnel for examination, and time to conduct an assessment; these all may lead to suboptimal care.
  » The most appropriate triage decision may be to defer examination to a specialized center.
  » At a minimum, all patients presenting must have a screening assessment to determine the safety for the child, the need for acute medical or psychiatric intervention, and acute forensic examination.

When to Suspect Sexual Child Abuse

- Sexual child abuse should be suspected when:
  » The child discloses intentionally or unintentionally to a parent, teacher, or other trusted adult or friend
  » Sexual abuse is witnessed by someone
  » The child exhibits sexualized behavior or other significant changes in behavior
  » The child complains of genital discomfort, genital bleeding, or other medical symptoms causing suspicion
  » The child is diagnosed with a sexually transmitted infection
- All of the above need evaluation/investigation. The child may be brought to the ED by children's aid/protection services (CAS) or police for medical evaluation, evidence collection, and crisis management.
- An emergency examination may be required in the ED.
  » Nonurgent examinations and follow-up can be conducted at appropriate local or regional specialized facilities.
- Indications for emergency evaluation include:
  » Medical, psychological, or safety concerns (e.g., bleeding, suicidal ideation)
  » History of anal, oral, or genital contact
  » Alleged assault within the previous 72 hours, necessitating forensic examination
  » Need for emergency contraception
  » Need for postencounter prophylaxis (PEP) for sexually transmitted infections (STIs) or HIV

History

- The diagnosis of pediatric sexual abuse is most dependent on the history provided by the child/adolescent.
- Investigative interviews are conducted by specially trained CAS and/or law enforcement officers.
- The ED interview is to ensure all medically relevant information is obtained to provide immediate care.
  » Obtain all information available from investigating authorities.
  » Interview the parents/caregivers separately from the child.
    › Ask about:
      · Their concerns / the situation / the incident
      · The what/who/when of disclosed events
      · Activities engaged in
      · Previous episodes, signs or symptoms, and behavioral changes
    › Reveal to caregivers that most (95%) examinations are normal.
- Interview patients > 3 years of age separately from the parents, if possible.
  » Interview patients in a comfortable setting and establish rapport with them prior to questions regarding event.
  » Use general to specific, nonleading questions.
  » Document quotations; do not paraphrase the child's answers.
  » Discuss the reasons for and process of the physical examination to allay fears and concerns.

Physical Exam

- The purpose and techniques to be used in the examination should be discussed in a developmentally appropriate manner (refer to Chapter 1.3, "Child Life").
  » The child should be offered a choice of an appropriate supportive person to be with him or her.
  » The child should be dressed in an appropriate examination gown and draped.
- Perform a complete head to toe examination, recognizing children may be victims of physical abuse as well.
  » Place special examination emphasis on the skin, mouth, breasts, and anogenital areas.
  » Forensic evidence may be present where sexual contact has occurred within 24 hours for prepubertal children and 72 hours for adolescents.
    › Recent DNA advances have expanded the collection window to 72 hours for prepubertal children and 5 days for adolescents, although local protocols may vary.

» Forensic evidence kits for adults may be adapted for children by excluding nonrelevant items.

» Forensic examinations require specific expertise that may be available by sexual assault nurse examiners, child abuse specialists, or emergency physicians with identified training.

- Genital examination should be performed with these considerations:
  » Examination position:
    › Supine frog leg or lithotomy
    › Prone knee-chest
  » Examination technique:
    › For female patients:
      · Labial separation and traction
      · Speculum (not indicated in children unless they are sedated, nor in adolescents unless they are > Tanner 3)
    › Prone knee-chest with gluteal lift
- Anal examination should be performed with these considerations:
  » Examination position:
    › Supine knee-chest
    › Prone knee-chest
    › Lateral decubitus
  » Examination technique:
    › Buttock separation
    › Prone knee-chest with gluteal lift

Table 1.7.2. MEDICAL ASSESSMENT OF CHILDREN WHO MAY HAVE BEEN SEXUALLY ABUSED

Findings in newborns or commonly seen in nonabused children	
Normal variants	**Comments**
• Normal variation in hymenal appearance: » Annular, crescentic, imperforate, septate, redundant	• Hymenal shape and dilatation should not be considered diagnostic.
• Anatomic variations: » Periurethral bands, intravaginal ridges or columns, linea vestibularis, diastasis ani, perianal skin tags, urethral dilatation, hyperpigmentation	• Various anatomic irregularities may be present. • Care should be exercised in regard to any findings in the midline as they may be developmental anomalies.
• Common childhood findings: » Genital tissue erythema, increased vascularity, labial adhesions, vaginal discharge, molluscum contagiosum, anal fissures, venous congestion in the anal area, anal dilatation with predisposing conditions (constipation, encopresis, sedation)	• The appearance of perineal findings changes significantly with age. • Consultation with personnel familiar with childhood examinations may be required.

Findings in newborns or commonly seen in nonabused children	
Conditions mistaken for abuse	**Comments**
• Anatomic: » Urethral prolapse, failure of midline fusion, rectal prolapse	
• Infectious/inflammatory findings: » Vulvar ulcers, lichen sclerosus et atrophicus	• Erythema and inflammatory changes of various nonsexually transmitted infections can be mistaken.
• Visualization difficulties: » Identifying pectinate/dentate line at anodermal rectal junction, partial dilatation of external anal sphincter with closed internal sphincter, postmortem color changes	• Postmortem changes should be confirmed by histologic examination.

Findings with no expert consensus	
Concerning findings	**Comments**
• Complete anal dilatation of the internal and external anal sphincters	• This is concerning when seen in the absence of predisposing factors.
• Notches or clefts at or below the 3 to 9 o'clock location	• Bumps and ridges are common and may be mistaken for complete tissue loss.
• Genital or anal condylomata acuminata in the absence of other concerns • Herpes 1 or 2 in genital area with no other concerns for abuse	• These infections, when presenting initially in children > 5 years of age, may warrant further follow-up from child protection services.
Findings caused by trauma	**Comments**
• Acute and healing trauma to external genital tissue: • Healed injuries are difficult to identify in the absence of previously documented trauma.	• Injuries could be accidental or inflicted. » Lacerations or bruising of labia, penis, scrotum, perineal tissues » Acute laceration of the posterior fourchette or vestibule » Perianal, posterior fourchette scars
• Injuries indicative of acute or healed trauma to genital tissue: » Bruising, petechiae, abrasions of hymen » Acute laceration of hymen or vagina » Perianal laceration with exposure of tissue below dermis » Healed hymenal transection/ cleft between 4 and 8 o'clock with absence of hymenal tissue » Defects in lower half of hymen extending to vaginal wall	

Findings caused by contact	
Diagnostic findings of abuse	**Comments**
• Genital, rectal, pharyngeal: » *Neisseria gonorrhoeae* » Syphilis » Genital or rectal Chlamydia trachomatis » *Trichomonas vaginalis*	• Findings indicate abuse unless there is evidence of perinatal transmission or clearly documented, but rare, nonsexual transmission.
• HIV	• HIV indicates abuse if transmission by blood transfusion has already been ruled out.
• Pregnancy • Semen in forensic specimens	

Investigations

- STIs are identified in < 5% of prepubescent children.
  - » Testing is recommended in adolescents because of the higher prevalence in this population.
  - » Considerations for testing include:
    - › Body fluid exposure
    - › Genital contact
    - › Presence of bleeding or discharge
    - › Genital or urinary symptoms
    - › Risk factors of perpetrator
    - › Family members with STIs
    - › The prevalence of STIs in the community
    - › Concerns about a possible STI in the child/family
- Urine nucleic acid amplification technology (NAAT) testing for prepubescent children should be confirmed by alternate tests.
- Postexposure prophylactic treatment is not recommended in prepubescent children because:
  - » Incidence is low
  - » Follow-up usually can be ensured
  - » There is low risk of ascending infection

Table 1.7.3. TESTING AND TREATMENT OF SUSPECTED SEXUALLY ABUSED CHILDREN

Organism or other concern	Testing	Treatment
Chlamydia trachomatis	• Vaginal: urine NAAT • Anus, throat: culture	• < 8 Azithromycin 15 mg/kg • > 8 Azithromycin 1 g PO
Neisseria gonorrheae	• Vaginal: urine NAAT • Anus, throat: culture	• Ceftriaxone 125 mg IM • Previous in nonresistant region, cefixime 8 mg/kg max 400 mg
Trichomonas vaginalis	• NAAT, culture • Wet mount: 55% sensitive	• Metronidazole 2 g PO once or 30 mg/kg divided and given twice daily for 1 week
HIV	• Rapid combined Ag/Ab test — or — • Antibody blood test	• 3 drug antiretroviral regimen; consult infectious disease specialist and/or Centers for Disease Control and Prevention (2016)
Hepatitis	• HBsAg testing if nonimmunized or unknown status	• HBIg: 0.06 mL/kg IM • Hepatitis B vaccine at 0, 1, 6 months
Toxicology	• Urine and serum testing in forensic kit	• Medical monitoring and management
Pregnancy	• Urine or serum test	• Pregnancy prophylaxis within 5 days with negative pregnancy test

Ag/Ab test combined antigen/antibody test. **HBIg** hepatitis B immunoglobulin. **HBsAg** hepatitis B surface antigen. **NAAT** nucleic acid amplification technology.

Reporting

- There is a legal and ethical obligation to **report any suspicion** for abuse to the appropriate child protection service.
  - » Medical professionals are mandated reporters.
  - » **Reporting is based on the suspicion that abuse is a possibility**. Reporting does not mean the case is definitively abuse.
- Involve social workers, child protection team, and other appropriate resources.
- Notify the child's primary care provider.
- Seek guidance on how other children who may be at risk for abuse from the same perpetrator (e.g., siblings, daycare attendees) should be evaluated and protected while the investigation takes place.

Documentation

- Include all history, physical examination, and laboratory findings.
- The results should be summarized in nonambiguous language that can be understood by nonmedical professionals.
- Photo documentation is recommended for all examinations with positive findings.

Disposition

- Admit patients to hospital (pediatric intensive care unit or inpatient pediatric floor) if medically indicated.
- Discharge patients from the ED only if the medical evaluation is complete and safe disposition can be arranged by child protection services from the ED.
- Admit patients to hospital if safe disposition cannot be arranged from the ED.

SEXUAL ASSAULT

- Sexual assault is defined as **any** involuntary sexual act in which a person is forced, threatened, or coerced to engage sexually against their will.
  - » This includes any sexual touching of a person who has not consented or cannot consent.
- Adolescents and young adults have the highest incidence of sexual assault of any age group.
  - » The 2009 Youth Risk Behavior Surveillance Survey found that 10.5% of female and 4.5% of male high school students had been forced to have sexual intercourse.
    - › Males were highest in the preadolescent age group; females were highest in the adolescent age group.
- Specific pediatric sexual assault protocols have been demonstrated to improve the ED investigation and management of this population.

» It is important that specifically trained personnel be available to support ED care.
» The initial investigation and management of cases of sexual assault is consistent with that of acute sexual abuse cases.

HUMAN TRAFFICKING OF MINORS

- Human trafficking is the recruitment, transfer, harboring, or receipt of persons by means of threat, use of force, coercion, fraud, deception, abuse of power, or the taking advantage of a position of vulnerability to achieve the consent of a person for the purpose of exploitation (most commonly prostitution, pornography, and sexual exploitation).
- Worldwide it is estimated 950 000 children are being trafficked.
  » The average age of entry into the commercial sex industry is 12 to 14 years.
  » Youth runaways and homeless adolescents are at high risk.
- An estimated 30% to 80% of victims will present for emergency care while in captivity.
  » Victims are unlikely to identify themselves due to fear, mistrust of authority, language difficulties, or a sense of shame.

When to Suspect Human Trafficking of Minors

- Helpful questions for taking a history when human trafficking is suspected include the following:
  » Can you come and go from your home whenever you please?
  » Has anyone at home ever physically harmed you?
  » Has anyone forced you to do things you didn't want to do?
  » Are there locks on your doors and windows?
  » Do you have to ask permission to eat, sleep, or use the bathroom?
  » Have you been denied food, water, sleep, or clothes?
  » Has anyone threatened your family?
  » Has anyone taken away your identification papers?

Red Flags

- A "friend" or "family member" doesn't allow the patient to answer questions or be alone with medical professionals.
- You get vague or inconsistent explanations of injuries or concerns.
- The patient has a lack of personal documentation or is unable to provide an address.
- The patient is anxious, nervous, avoids eye contact, or appears fearful.
- The patient or accompanying individual shows concern about contact with police or other authorities.

Physical Exam

- If you suspect trafficking, separate the patient from the accompanying individual for the physical examination.
  » One approach is to identify the separation as standard practice for a private physical examination.
- A general physical examination may show signs of:
  » Malnutrition and/or dehydration
  » Exhaustion
  » Untreated chronic disease
  » Skin injuries
  » Previous fractures
  » Tattoos
  » Signs of drug use or withdrawal
- The genitourinary examination may show signs of previous trauma, sexually transmitted disease, pelvic inflammatory disease, previous pregnancy, or abortion.
- Interactions with the child or adolescent may indicate psychiatric symptoms such as depression, anxiety, panic attacks, suicidal ideation, poor self-esteem, shame, or fear.

Management

- The priorities for medical management are as identified with any physically abused child or adolescent.
  » Identify and treat any acute, surgical, or medical issues such as hemorrhage, trauma, infection, or significant untreated disease.
- Patients should be considered at high risk for sexual exploitation and managed as protocols dictate for sexual assault/abuse victims.
- Trafficking victims often suffer from mental health concerns, and assessment and treatment may need to be initiated in the ED.
- If any member of the healthcare team suspects the patient is a victim of human trafficking, seek early involvement of a social worker or victim advocate.
  » If the patient is underage, immediate reporting to child protective services is mandated.
  » If you are concerned for the immediate safety of the patient, involve security or police as local protocols dictate.
  » For victims who are or have passed the age of consent, involve a patient advocate, inform the patient that services are available, and allow the patient access to and support for informing authorities.
- Hospital admission may facilitate ensuring safety and ongoing support for the child or adolescent.

REFERENCES

Adams J, Kellogg N, Farst K, et al. Updated guidelines for the medical assessment and care of children who may have been sexually abused. *J Pediatr Adolesc Gynecol.* 2016;29(2):81–87. Medline:26220352

Becker HJ, Bechtel K. Recognizing victims of human trafficking in the pediatric emergency department. *Pediatr Emerg Care.* 2015;31(2):144–147, quiz 148–150. https://doi.org/10.1097/PEC.0000000000000357. Medline:25651385

Centres for Disease Control and Prevention, U.S. Department of Health and Human Services. Updated guidelines for antiretroviral PEP after sexual, injection drug or other nonoccupational exposure to HIV—United States, 2016 [Internet]. Available from: http://stacks.cdc.gov/view/cdc/38856

Child Abuse Prevention and Treatment Act (CAPTA) Reauthorization Act of 2010, Public Law 111–320, (42, USC 5106a). 2010. Available from: www.acf.hhs.gov/programs/cb/laws_policies/cblaws/capta/capta2010.pdf

Children's Bureau, U.S. Department of Health and Human Services. Child maltreatment [Internet]. Available from: http://www.acf.hhs.gov/programs/cb/research-data-technology/statistics-research/child-maltreatment

Christian CW. Timing of the medical examination. *J Child Sex Abuse.* 2011;20(5):505–520. https://doi.org/10.1080/10538712.2011.607424. Medline:21970643

Christian CW; Committee on Child Abuse and Neglect, American Academy of Pediatrics. The evaluation of suspected child physical abuse. *Pediatrics.* 2015;135(5):e1337–e1354. https://doi.org/10.1542/peds.2015-0356. Medline:25917988

Crawford-Jakubiak JC; Committee on Child Abuse and Neglect; American Academy of Pediatrics Committee on Child Abuse. The evaluation of children in the primary care setting when sexual abuse is suspected. *Pediatrics.* 2013;132(2):e558–e567. Medline:23897912

Flaherty EG, Stirling J Jr; American Academy of Pediatrics, Committee on Child Abuse and Neglect. Clinical report: the pediatrician's role in child maltreatment prevention. *Pediatrics.* 2010;126(4):833–841. https://doi.org/10.1542/peds.2010-2087. Medline:20945525

Floyed RL, Hirsh DA, Greenbaum VJ, Simon HK. Development of a screening tool for pediatric sexual assault may reduce emergency-department visits. *Pediatrics.* 2011;128(2):221–226. https://doi.org/10.1542/peds.2010-3288. Medline:21788216

Government of Canada. Canadian guidelines on sexually transmitted infections [Internet]. Available from: www.phac-aspc.gc.ca/std-mts/sti-its/cgsti-ldcits/section-6-5-eng.php

Goyal MK, Mollen CJ, et al. Enhancing the emergency department approach to pediatric sexual assault care: implementation of a pediatric sexual assault response team program. *Pediatr Emerg Care.* 2013;29(9):969–973. https://doi.org/10.1097/PEC.0b013e3182a21a0d. Medline:23974714

Harper NS, Feldman KW, Sugar NF, Anderst JD, Lindberg DM; Examining Siblings to Recognize Abuse Investigators. Additional injuries in young infants with concern for abuse and apparently isolated bruises. *J Pediatr.* 2014;165(2):383–388.e1. https://doi.org/10.1016/j.jpeds.2014.04.004. Medline:24840754

International Labor Organization. 2012. Global estimate of forced labour: executive summary [Internet]. Available from: http://www.ilo.org/wcmsp5/groups/public/@ed_norm/@declaration/documents/publication/wcms_181953.pdf

Johnson CF. Sexual abuse in children. *Pediatr Rev.* 2006;27(1):17–27. https://doi.org/10.1542/pir.27-1-17. Medline:16387925

Kemp AM. Abusive head trauma: recognition and the essential investigation. *Arch Dis Child Educ Pract Ed.* 2011;96(6):202–208. https://doi.org/10.1136/adc.2009.170449. Medline:21954224

Lederer L, Wetzel C. The health consequences of sex trafficking and their implications for identifying victims in healthcare facilities. *Ann Health Law.* 2014;23:61–91.

Maguire S. Bruising as an indicator of child abuse: when should I be concerned? *Paediatr Child Health.* 2008;18(12):545–549. https://doi.org/10.1016/j.paed.2008.09.008

Maguire S, Cowley L, Mann M, Kemp A. What does the recent literature add to the identification and investigation of fractures in child abuse: an overview of review updates 2005–2013. *Evid Based Child Health.* 2013;8(5):2044–2057. https://doi.org/10.1002/ebch.1941

Maguire S, Okolie C, Kemp A. Burns as a consequence of child maltreatment. *Paediatr Child Health.* 2014;24(12):557–561. https://doi.org/10.1016/j.paed.2014.07.014

Pierce MC, Kaczor K, Aldridge S, O'Flynn J, Lorenz DJ. Bruising characteristics discriminating physical child abuse from accidental trauma. *Pediatrics.* 2010;125(1):67–74. https://doi.org/10.1542/peds.2008-3632. Medline:19969620

Pierce MC, Magana JN, Kaczor K, et al. The prevalence of bruising among infants in pediatric emergency departments. *Ann Emerg Med.* 2016;67(1):1–8. https://doi.org/10.1016/j.annemergmed.2015.06.021. Medline:26233923

Prevention CDC. Youth risk behavior surveillance-US, surveillance summaries, 2009. Morbidity and mortality weekly report. 2010;59(no. SS-5).

Public Health Agency of Canada. Canadian incidence study of reported child abuse and neglect 2008: major findings. Ottawa; 2010. Available from: http://www.phac-aspc.gc.ca/cm-vee/csca-ecve/2008/index-eng.php

Starling SP, Holden JR, Jenny C. Abusive head trauma: the relationship of perpetrators to their victims. *Pediatrics.* 1995;95(2):259–262. Medline:7838645

Tiyyagura G, Gawel M, Koziel JR, Asnes A, Bechtel K. Barriers and facilitators to detecting child abuse and neglect in general emergency departments. *Ann Emerg Med.* 2015;66(5):447–454. https://doi.org/10.1016/j.annemergmed.2015.06.020. Medline:26231409

U.S. Department of Justice, Office of Justice Programs, Office of Juvenile Justice and Delinquency Prevention. Burn injuries in child abuse. 2001. Available from: https://www.ncjrs.gov/pdffiles/91190-6.pdf

WHO World Report on Violence and Health 2002. Available from: http://www.who.int/violence_injury_prevention/violence/world_report/en/

1.8

Point-of-Care Ultrasound (POCUS)

Kirstin Weerdenburg

- Point-of-care ultrasound (POCUS) can be used for diagnostic or procedural applications.
- There is increased interest in its utility in the pediatric population, and it continues to evolve in pediatric emergency medicine (PEM) with specialized training programs and fellowship training.
- POCUS offers an attractive imaging modality because it:
  - » Is inexpensive and may direct further evaluation so that unnecessary and costly testing is avoided
  - » Is portable, so there is no need to transport the patient outside the emergency department
  - » Doesn't involve ionizing radiation exposure
  - » Is easily repeatable
  - » Is relatively painless

THE PHYSICS BEHIND ULTRASOUND

- A basic understanding of the terminology for and the physics underlying ultrasound (US) is essential to reliable image acquisition and accurate image interpretation.
- US machines generate US waves and receive the reflected echoes due to the properties of the crystal elements of the US probe (also called the transducer).
- Piezoelectric crystals are located on the probe surface, also known as the probe footprint. The crystals have different arrangements based on the type of probe.
  - » Piezoelectric crystals convert electrical energy to mechanical (sonographic) energy and vice versa.
  - » These crystals both generate the sound waves and receive them. When returning pressure waves that have been reflected from different mediums within the tissue deform the crystals, the resulting electrical energy is translated into a pixel on the screen.
    - › The specific shade of gray that the pixel has depends on the strength or amplitude of the returning echo — essentially, the electric current it generates.
- On the US screen, strong returning echoes become bright or white areas (hyperechoic), while weak returning echoes become gray or black areas (hypoechoic or anechoic).

- *Frequency* is the number of times per second a wave is repeated.
  - » High-frequency sound waves use more energy to produce more waves with returning echoes sent back at short distances to create high-resolution images of shallow depth.
  - » Low-frequency sound waves conserve energy and penetrate to deeper depths to create low-resolution images of deep depth.
- *Attenuation* is the diminishing intensity of a US wave as it travels over a distance and as it propagates through a particular medium due to absorption and scattering.
  - » US waves travel poorly through air and bone and better through fluid-containing mediums, such as blood vessels and urinary bladder.

PROBES

- There are several types of US probes used for POCUS, which provide diverse image formats because they operate at different frequencies and have assorted physical dimensions, footprints, and shapes.
- High-frequency probes penetrate less and provide higher-resolution images.
- Low-frequency probes penetrate more and provide lower-resolution images.
- There are four basic probes used for POCUS (see *Table 1.8.1*).

Table 1.8.1. POCUS PROBE COMPARISON

Type of probe	Frequencies (can vary)	Typical indications in PEM
Curvilinear/curved array	2 to 5 MHz	FAST/eFAST, renal, gallbladder, pregnancy, gynecologic, IVC
Linear array	5 to 15 MHz	Soft tissue, bone, skull, lung, intussusception, appendix, pyloric stenosis, testicular, ocular, vascular access, regional anesthesia
Phased array	1 to 5 MHz	Cardiac, IVC, FAST/eFAST
Endocavitary/intracavitary	8 to 15 MHz	Pregnancy, gynecologic

FAST/eFAST focused assessment with sonography for trauma / extended focused assessment with sonography for trauma. **IVC** inferior vena cava.

IMAGE ORIENTATION AND QUALITY

- Probe and screen marker, along with imaging planes, help with image orientation.
  - » Pay particular attention to image interpretation when using the phased array probe for the cardiac application, which on some US machines can change image orientation and the way the probe is held.
  - » Imaging planes include sagittal/longitudinal, transverse/axial, and coronal.
- Several scanning modes are used with POCUS:
  - » B-mode (brightness mode)
    - › This is the standard grayscale US; it is most commonly used.
  - » M-mode (motion mode)
    - › M-mode is often used simultaneously with B-mode scanning to assess lung sliding, cardiac scanning, and fetal heart rate measurement.
    - › M-mode provides a tracing of tissue movement over time relative to the probe's imaging plane (line through structure on screen).
  - » Color Doppler
    - › Color Doppler measures mean velocity and direction of flow overlaid on B-mode image.
    - › The color scale legend on the side of the screen represents directional color assignment with color superiorly representing flow toward the probe and color inferiorly representing flow away from the probe.
  - » Power Doppler
    - › This averages flow over several frames.
    - › It has greater sensitivity for low-flow states but does not demonstrate direction of flow.
  - » Spectral Doppler
    - › Spectral Doppler provides quantitative assessment of flow velocity at a single point with pulsed wave technology or along the entire line interrogated with continuous wave technology.
    - › It is helpful for distinguishing arterial and venous waveforms.
    - › It results in graphical or audible peaks to be interpreted.
- The most used knobs on the US machine with POCUS include:
  - » Gain
    - › Gain is the degree of amplification of returning signal.
    - › It increases or decreases the brightness of returning echoes on the US screen.
  - » Depth
    - › The depth knob adjusts the field of view to ensure the entire area of interest is optimally visible on the screen.
    - › The centimeter scale on side of screen indicates depth.
  - » Focus
    - › The focus knob improves image resolution or quality at a particular depth.
  - » Time-gain compensation
    - › Time-gain compensation allows for adjustment of gain at different levels.

SPECIFIC PEDIATRIC POCUS APPLICATIONS

EXTENDED FOCUSED ASSESSMENT WITH SONOGRAPHY FOR TRAUMA

- Extended focused assessment with sonography for trauma (eFAST) is useful for:
  - » Identifying the presence of free fluid in the abdomen
  - » Providing evidence of cardiac tamponade
  - » Identifying pneumothorax and hemothorax
- It is well-established in adult trauma care and is part of the advanced trauma life support (ATLS) protocol, but its utility in pediatric trauma is less definite due to imperfect test sensitivity and frequent use of nonoperative management for intraabdominal injury in children.
  - » The sensitivity of eFAST for identifying intraperitoneal free fluid has been reported to range widely (23% to 52%), with a specificity of 85% to 96% (negative predictive value of 48% to 54% and positive predictive value of 89% to 97%).
  - » While eFAST has been shown to detect free fluid in the abdomen, it has not been shown to help predict the need for laparotomy.
- Standard views include:
  - » Right upper quadrant (Morison's pouch, hepatorenal recess)
  - » Left upper quadrant (splenorenal recess)
  - » Pelvic
  - » Pericardial
  - » Thorax
- Fluid accumulated within any of the potential spaces appears as a black stripe outlining the adjacent structure (see *Image 1.8.1*).

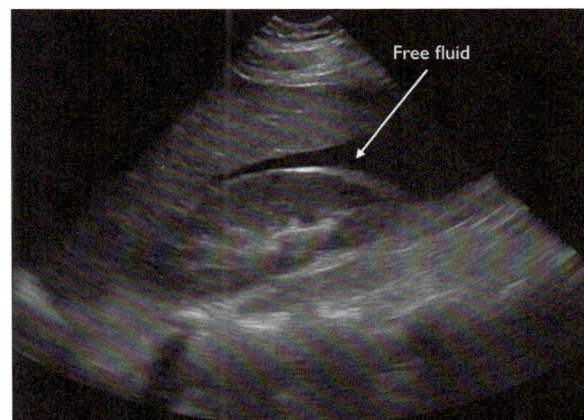

Image 1.8.1. Free fluid

» Ensure complete dynamic scanning of the hepatorenal and splenorenal spaces by fanning through these areas and not performing static views, as well as interrogating the area around the caudal tip of the liver.
- Presence of lung sliding and comet tails rules out pneumothorax.
  » Conversely, the absence of lung sliding and the presence of lung point suggests pneumothorax.

LUNG

- POCUS is useful in evaluating children for pneumonia, pleural effusion, pneumothorax, pulmonary contusion, and pulmonary edema.
- Several studies have found that POCUS lung application enables the diagnosis of community-acquired pneumonia in children with high accuracy (sensitivity and specificity both over 90%).
- Standard views depend on what is being evaluated for and include:
  » Bilateral midclavicular (anterior)
  » Bilateral midaxillary (lateral)
  » Bilateral posterior
- Lung consolidation with pneumonia has some distinctive findings:
  » Hepatization
  » Pleural shred sign
  » Tissue sign
  » B-lines
- Findings associated with pneumothorax are discussed above.

INTUSSUSCEPTION

- POCUS is an attractive modality to diagnose intussusception at the bedside and possibly expedite reduction.
  » Sensitivity of 85% and specificity of 97% has been reported with POCUS by novice PEM sonographers when compared with radiologists.
- Ileocolic intussusception appears as a "target" or "donut" sign on transverse view with a minimum diameter of 3 cm, and as a "pseudo kidney" or "sandwich sign" on oblique or longitudinal view (see *Image 1.8.2*).

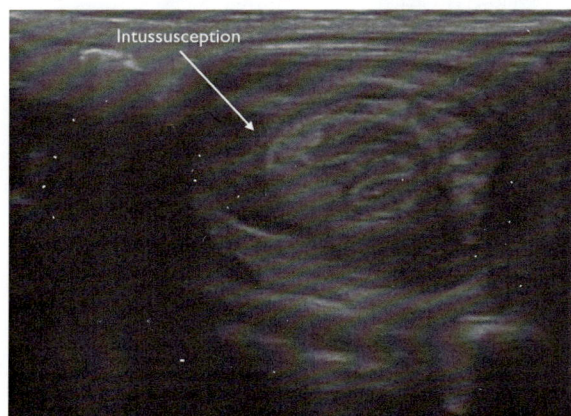

Image 1.8.2. Intussusception

APPENDICITIS

- Many have suggested a staged imaging approach to assess for appendicitis, with POCUS at the bedside as part of the initial assessment, then a comprehensive/diagnostic US for confirmation or indeterminate scans.
- Several prospective studies suggest that PEM sonographers using POCUS achieve similar sensitivities and specificities to radiologists.
  » PEM sonographers using POCUS report sensitivity of 85% and specificity of 93%.
- An inflamed appendix on US will be a blind-end tubular structure > 6 mm in diameter that is noncompressible and without peristalsis (see *Image 1.8.3*).
  » Secondary findings of appendicitis on US are:
    › Intraabdominal free fluid
    › Surrounding hyperechoic fat
    › Appendicolith
    › Appendix wall hyperemia

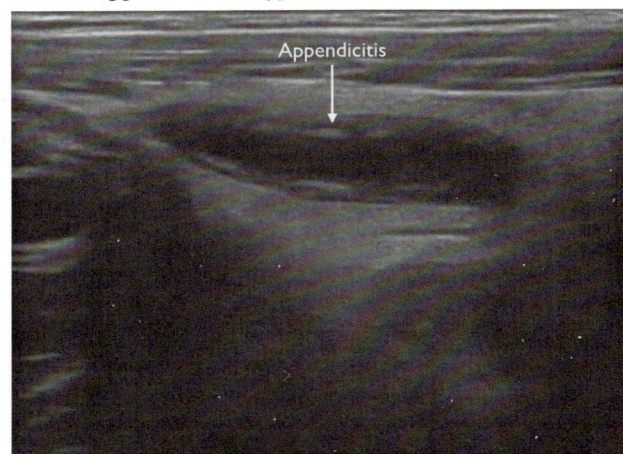

Image 1.8.3. Appendicitis

SOFT TISSUE FOREIGN BODY REMOVAL

- POCUS is useful for identifying the presence and location of a soft tissue foreign body, as well as to guide its removal.
- Studies to date have reported a high specificity and moderate sensitivity for the identification of foreign bodies, but studies have been highly heterogenic and with a high risk of bias.
- POCUS is superior to plain radiographs for the identification of radiolucent foreign bodies.
- Foreign bodies on US typically appear as hyperechoic (bright) objects with associated signs including halo sign, ring down artifact, posterior acoustic enhancement, and shadowing.
- POCUS can be used to locate the foreign body prior to removal without US guidance, or to guide the removal in real time.

LUMBAR PUNCTURE

- POCUS is useful to landmark the ideal needle insertion site and to identify surrounding anatomy, especially in those patients that may be more challenging, such as very young children, large body habitus, or those with distorted spinal anatomy (i.e., spina bifida, scoliosis, spinal surgery).

BLADDER CATHETERIZATION

- POCUS can assist healthcare providers in evaluating bladder volume prior to bladder catheterization in order to avoid an insufficient amount of urine being obtained for testing.

CENTRAL AND PERIPHERAL VENOUS ACCESS

- POCUS can assist healthcare providers in central or peripheral venous catheterization with several studies demonstrating significant increases in successful cannulation and significant decreases in associated complications when compared to traditional landmark techniques.
- POCUS can be used to locate the vein prior to cannulation without US guidance, or preferably can be used to guide cannulation in real time.

FUTURE OF POCUS

- Incorporation of POCUS at all levels of training (medical student, resident, fellow, faculty) has accelerated its progression into PEM, where physicians caring for children now routinely enhance their clinical examination and procedures by visualizing pertinent anatomy and pathology in real time.
- The number of indications/applications for POCUS continues to grow, allowing for new and innovative ways to utilize this technology.

ACKNOWLEDGEMENTS

All images from this chapter are provided by Dr. Jason Fischer, The Hospital for Sick Children, Toronto, Ontario.

REFERENCES

Abo A, Chen L, Johnston P, Santucci K. Positioning for lumbar puncture in children evaluated by bedside ultrasound. *Pediatrics.* 2010;125(5):e1149–e1153. https://doi.org/10.1542/peds.2009-0646. Medline:20403933

Atkinson P, Bowra J, Lambert M, Lamprecht H, Noble V, Jarman B. International Federation for Emergency Medicine point of care ultrasound curriculum. *CJEM.* 2015;17(2):161–170. https://doi.org/10.1017/cem.2015.8. Medline:26052968

Fox JC, Boysen M, Gharahbaghian L, et al. Test characteristics of focused assessment of sonography for trauma for clinically significant abdominal free fluid in pediatric blunt abdominal trauma. *Acad Emerg Med.* 2011;18(5):477–482. https://doi.org/10.1111/j.1553-2712.2011.01071.x. Medline:21569167

Mallin M, Dawson M. Introduction to bedside ultrasound: volume 1. Emergency ultrasound solutions. 2013. iBooks.

Marin JR, Lewiss RE; American Academy of Pediatrics, Committee on Pediatric Emergency Medicine, 2013–2014; Society for Academic Emergency Medicine (Reviewers); American College of Emergency Physicians, Pediatric Emergency Medicine Committee, 2013–2014; World Interactive Network Focused on Critical Ultrasound (Reviewers). Point-of-care ultrasonography by pediatric emergency medicine physicians. Policy statement. *Ann Emerg Med.* 2015;65(4):472–478. https://doi.org/10.1016/j.annemergmed.2015.01.028. Medline:25805037

Marin JR, Lewiss RE; American Academy of Pediatrics, Committee on Pediatric Emergency Medicine; Society for Academic Emergency Medicine; Academy of Emergency Ultrasound; American College of Emergency Physicians, Pediatric Emergency Medicine Committee; World Interactive Network Focused on Critical Ultrasound. Point-of-care ultrasonography by pediatric emergency medicine physicians. *Pediatrics.* 2015;135(4):e1113–e1122. https://doi.org/10.1542/peds.2015-0343. Medline:25825532

Marin JR, Zuckerbraun NS, Kahn JM. Use of emergency ultrasound in United States pediatric emergency medicine fellowship programs in 2011. *J Ultrasound Med.* 2012;31(9):1357–1363. https://doi.org/10.7863/jum.2012.31.9.1357. Medline:22922615

McLario DJ, Sivitz AB. Point-of-care ultrasound in pediatric clinical care. *JAMA Pediatr.* 2015;169(6):594–600. https://doi.org/10.1001/jamapediatrics.2015.22. Medline:25893571

Noble V, Nelson BP. *Manual of emergency and critical care ultrasound.* 2nd ed. New York, NY: Cambridge University Press; 2011. https://doi.org/10.1017/CBO9780511734281

Pereda MA, Chavez MA, Hooper-Miele CC, et al. Lung ultrasound for the diagnosis of pneumonia in children: a meta-analysis. *Pediatrics.* 2015;135(4):714–722. https://doi.org/10.1542/peds.2014-2833. Medline:25780071

Riera A, Hsiao AL, Langhan ML, Goodman TR, Chen L. Diagnosis of intussusception by physician novice sonographers in the emergency department. *Ann Emerg Med.* 2012;60(3):264–268. https://doi.org/10.1016/j.annemergmed.2012.02.007. Medline:22424652

Sivitz AB, Cohen SG, Tejani C. Evaluation of acute appendicitis by pediatric emergency physician sonography. *Ann Emerg Med.* 2014;64(4):358–364.e4. https://doi.org/10.1016/j.annemergmed.2014.03.028. Medline:24882665

Tseng HJ, Hanna TN, Shuaib W, Aized M, Khosa F, Linnau KF. Imaging foreign bodies: ingested, aspirated, and inserted. *Ann Emerg Med.* 2015;66(6):570–582.e5. https://doi.org/10.1016/j.annemergmed.2015.07.499. Medline:26320521

1.9

Transporting the Pediatric Patient

Laura Weingarten

PRINCIPLES OF PEDIATRIC TRANSPORT

- Ensure patient and team safety.
- Follow a structured and organized approach to patient assessment, such as Advanced Trauma Life Support (ATLS).
- Use checklists and protocols based on local practice standards.

SAFETY

- Between 1% and 61% of pediatric transports are complicated by adverse events.
- Children transported by specialized pediatric teams are less likely to experience adverse events and more likely to survive to hospital discharge.
- The referring and receiving physicians should agree on a defined treatment en route, with clear responsibilities as to who will follow up on any issues during transport.
  - » The referring/sending physician is usually responsible for patient care until arrival at the receiving facility.
- The referring physician should answer the following questions before a team departs:
  - » Does this child need a specialized transport team?
    - › Specialized teams are appropriate for transport of critically ill pediatric and neonatal patients.
  - » Does the team I am sending have adequate training, experience, and comfort with sick children?
  - » Does the team have advance directives or require additional orders?
- Critically ill children should be stabilized prior to transport, unless the risks of transport are outweighed by the benefits of time-sensitive treatment (e.g., epidural hematoma or bowel ischemia).

Table 1.9.1. QUESTION CHECKLIST FOR SAFE TRANSPORT OF THE PEDIATRIC PATIENT

Safety and documentation	• How will I secure the patient to the stretcher or incubator? • Are all monitors, pumps, and equipment well fastened? • Do I have a documentation form and medication record that meets local standards? • Do I have a mobile phone or other device to communicate changes in the patient's status to the receiving facility? • Has the patient's family received a written record to show where the patient is being transported? • Do I have the appropriate clothing, personal items, and food to keep myself safe during a long transport?
Monitoring and investigations	• Do I have the necessary and appropriately-sized cardiorespiratory and temperature monitors? • Would end-tidal CO_2 monitoring be beneficial? • Will I need to monitor glucose or perform any point-of-care testing before arriving at the receiving facility? • Can I see and hear all the alarm systems (low saturation, blocked infusions)?
Airway and breathing	• How will I manage a deterioration in the child's airway and respiratory status before arrival at the receiving facility? • Do I have necessary airway supplies, including an extra bag valve device, oropharyngeal and/or nasopharyngeal airways, and intubation equipment? • If this child requires support, do I have a backup plan if my noninvasive, high-flow oxygen or ventilator/circuit fails? • Do I have adequate oxygen and suction for the full duration of transport? • Does this child require cervical immobilization?
Circulation	• How will I manage a deterioration in the child's hemodynamic status before arrival at the receiving facility? • Is my IV/IO access adequate and appropriately secured? • What is my plan if access is lost en route to the receiving facility? • Do I need a backboard, defibrillator, infusion pump, or any special supplies?

MODE OF TRANSPORT

- Options include private vehicle, land ambulance, helicopter, or fixed-wing aircraft.
- The decision about which method of transport should be used depends on:
  » Patient acuity
  » Distance
  » Traffic
  » Weather
  » Availability of specialized teams for air/land transport

Table 1.9.2. PROS AND CONS OF LAND AND AIR TRANSPORT

	Land	Air
Examples	• Private vehicle • Ambulance	• Helicopter • Fixed-wing aircraft
Pros	• Fast dispatch • Able to stop for procedures • Able to accommodate extra team or family members	• Faster for longer distances • Helicopter can land on hospital helipad and at remote/austere scenes
Cons	• May be slower than flight for long-distance transport	• May require additional transport leg to/from airport
	• Traffic can be unpredictable	• Affected by weather or night visibility
	• Issues of pain or equipment dislodging with poor road conditions	• Small, noisy work area • Turbulence • Pressure at altitude may worsen some injuries/diseases • May not be able to accommodate family members

Management

Airway and Breathing Considerations

- Ensure the patient's airway is patent. Intubate prior to departure if there are any concerns about impending airway obstruction.
  » If the patient is intubated, secure the endotracheal tube (ETT) and confirm placement using multiple methods (e.g., direct visualization, end-tidal CO_2, auscultation, and/or imaging).
  » If the patient is intubated, place a gastric tube and leave it open to drainage.
- Ensure adequate suction and oxygen supply for duration of transport.
- Continuously monitor oxygen saturation and end-tidal CO_2.
  » For prolonged transport, consider point-of-care blood gas measurements to optimize oxygenation/ventilation.

- For trauma patients:
  » Ensure cervical spine immobilization based on mechanism of injury
  » Consider a tube thoracostomy prior to transport if there are signs of pneumothorax and depending on the mode and duration of transport
- For patients being transported by air:
  » Watch for hypoxia and provide supplemental oxygen as needed
  » Limit altitude or pressurize cabin to sea level in patients with proven or suspected pneumocephalus, ocular or dental injury, pneumothorax, bowel obstruction, or diving injury
  » Fill ETT cuff with saline, not air

Circulation Considerations

- Ensure adequate and/or ongoing volume resuscitation.
- Ensure sufficient fluids, blood products, and/or inotropic supports for duration of transport.
- Identify and control external hemorrhage with direct pressure, sutures, staples, or other hemostatic controls.
  » Identifying sources of internal hemorrhage may delay transport.
  » Relay significant bleeds to receiving facility if identified.
- Secure at least 1 and preferably 2 reliable IVs or IOs for transport.
  » Ensure cannula site is visible and ports are readily accessible.
- Consider using a catheter to monitor urine output in critically ill patients.
- If transporting by air, IV infusions will need to be by pump and not by gravity.

Disability Considerations

- Assess blood glucose prior to departure and as required.
- Check pupil size and reactivity.
- If signs of increased intracranial pressure (ICP) or herniation occur during transport:
  » Administer a dose of hypertonic saline (5 to 10 mL/kg) and/or mannitol (0.25 to 1.0 g/kg)
  » Hyperventilate until the child's clinical status improves (e.g., blown pupil becomes reactive or level of consciousness improves)
    › The target pCO_2 is less important than an improvement in the child's clinical status.
  » Notify the receiving hospital of the change in the child's clinical condition and ask for further medical advice

Exposure and Temperature Considerations

- Monitor temperature continuously for infants, small children, and unconscious patients.
- Maintain thermoregulation with hat and warm blankets, or by increasing ambient temperature as needed.
- Treat fever and hyperthermia with antipyretics.
- Perform a head-to-toe physical examination for rashes, unusual bruises, or skin marks.

REFERENCES

Barry P, Leslie A. *Paediatric and neonatal critical care transport.* London: BMJ Publishing Group; 2003.

Lorch SA, Myers S, Carr B. The regionalization of pediatric health care. *Pediatrics.* 2010;126(6):1182–1190. https://doi.org/10.1542/peds.2010-1119. Medline:21041285

Orr RA, Felmet KA, Han Y, et al. Pediatric specialized transport teams are associated with improved outcomes. *Pediatrics.* 2009;124(1):40–48. https://doi.org/10.1542/peds.2008-0515. Medline:19564281

Ramnarayan P, Thiru K, Parslow RC, Harrison DA, Draper ES, Rowan KM. Effect of specialist retrieval teams on outcomes in children admitted to paediatric intensive care units in England and Wales: a retrospective cohort study. *Lancet.* 2010;376(9742):698–704. https://doi.org/10.1016/S0140-6736(10)61113-0. Medline:20708255

Whyte HE, Jefferies AL; Canadian Paediatric Society, Fetus and Newborn Committee. The interfacility transport of critically ill newborns. *Paediatr Child Health.* 2015;20(5):265–275. Medline:26175564

Acute Presentations

2.1

Anaphylaxis

Waleed Alqurashi

- Anaphylaxis is a severe hypersensitivity reaction with rapid onset that can be fatal.
- The lifetime prevalence estimates range from 0.3% to 5.1%.
  - » Epidemiological studies indicate that the rate of anaphylaxis is increasing, especially in young people.
- The 3 main immunological triggers of anaphylaxis are:
  1. Food
     - › Food is the most common trigger of anaphylaxis in children.
     - › The most common foods that Canadian children are allergic to are:
       - · Milk
       - · Peanuts
       - · Tree nuts (e.g., almonds, cashews, and pistachios)
  2. Insect stings
     - › Hymenoptera venom — which is the venom associated with bee, wasp, and hornet stings — is the most common insect venom that causes severe allergy problems.
  3. Drugs
     - › Penicillin is the most common cause of anaphylaxis.

Immunology

- Anaphylaxis is thought to be mediated by 2 major pathways: immunologic and nonimmunologic.
  - » The **immunologic** pathway is complex, with 2 distinct mechanisms:
    1. Immunoglobulin E (IgE)-dependent reactions:
       - · IgE-dependent reactions primarily involve histamine release.
       - · They account for most anaphylactic reactions.
    2. IgE-independent reactions
       - · IgE-independent reactions are mainly mediated by either IgG or an immune complex/complement.
       - · They primarily involve the release of potent mediators such as platelet activating factor (PAF).
  - » The **nonimmunologic** pathway is caused by agents or events (e.g., cold air) that induce sudden, massive mast cell or basophil degranulation in the absence of immunoglobulins.

Risk Factors

- The severity of an anaphylactic reactions is increased by 4 factors:
  1. Augmenting factors
     - › Augmenting factors lower the reaction threshold or make symptoms more severe.
     - › They directly influence the immunological mechanism of an IgE-mediated allergy.
     - › Examples of augmenting factors include:
       - · Physical exercise
       - · Menstruation
       - · Alcohol
       - · Acute illness or infection
       - · Drugs (nonsteroidal anti-inflammatory drugs [NSAIDs], antacids, angiotensin-converting enzyme [ACE] inhibitors)
  2. Cofactors
     - › Cofactors potentiate the severity of the reaction through nonimmune mechanism.
     - › Examples of cofactors include:
       - · Adolescence (risk-taking behavior, poor recognition of the reaction severity, poor compliance with treatment)
       - · Psychiatric conditions and medications
       - · Drugs (beta-blockers)

3. Concurrent diseases
  › Concurrent diseases either lower the physiologic reserve or enhance the inflammatory process.
  › Examples of concurrent diseases include:
    · Chronic uncontrolled respiratory conditions (asthma, cystic fibrosis)
    · Cardiovascular diseases
    · Mastocytosis
4. Inappropriate treatment
  › Inappropriate treatment includes delayed or absent treatment of anaphylaxis with epinephrine.

Pathophysiology

- Respiratory and cardiovascular systems are the most common shock organs in human anaphylaxis.
- Respiratory effects include:
  » Asphyxia
  » Upper airway angioedema
  » Upper and lower airway inflammation
- Cardiovascular effects include:
  » Hypovolemia due to vascular extravasation (loss of up to 35% of effective blood volume within 10 minutes of the reaction) leading to hypotension
  » Early arteriolar dilation leading to hypotension and wide pulse pressure
  » Venodilation and blood pooling leading to lower venous return and cardiac output
  » Relative bradycardia and impaired myocardial contractility leading to lower cardiac output (and a potential for direct cardiac toxicity)

Diagnosis

- There are 3 diagnostic criteria for anaphylaxis, each reflecting a different clinical presentation (developed by the Second National Institute of Allergy and Infectious Disease/Food Allergy and Anaphylaxis Network Symposium). **Anaphylaxis is highly likely when any 1 of the following 3 criteria is fulfilled:**
  » Criterion 1:
    › Acute onset with involvement of the skin, mucosal tissue, or both
    — and —
    › At least 1 of:
      · Respiratory compromise
      · Hypotension or associated symptoms of end-organ dysfunction
  » Criterion 2:
    › 2 or more of the following after exposure to a **likely** allergen for that patient:
      · Involvement of the skin/mucosal tissue
      · Respiratory compromise
      · Reduced blood pressure (BP) or associated symptoms
      · Persistent gastrointestinal symptoms

» Criterion 3:
  › Hypotension after exposure to a **known** allergen for that patient:
    · Low systolic BP (see *Table 2.1.1*)

Table 2.1.1. DEFINITIONS OF LOW SYSTOLIC BLOOD PRESSURE

Age	Systolic BP
1 month to 1 year	< 70 mmHg
1 to 10 years	< (70 mmHg + [2 × age])
11 to 17 years	< 90 mmHg **or** > 30% decrease in systolic BP

Special Considerations

- Skin symptoms or signs are absent or unrecognized in up to 20% of anaphylactic episodes.
  » The absence of urticarial rash does not rule out anaphylaxis. There will be patients who do not meet any of the diagnostic criteria, but for whom the administration of epinephrine is appropriate.
- Anaphylaxis in infants and young children may present only with behavioral changes such as lethargy or hypotonia, excessive crying and fussiness, or abrupt cessation of activity or play.
- Anaphylaxis in a known asthmatic may be mistaken for an asthma exacerbation if accompanying skin symptoms and signs, or other signs suggestive of impending shock, are overlooked.
- Changes in BP may be undetected when measured very early during the episode, when the initial BP measurement is obtained after epinephrine administration, or when an inappropriately small BP cuff is used.

History

- The history taken for a patient with anaphylaxis should include:
  » Type of exposure
    › Was the patient exposed to a particular kind of food, insect bite, or medication?
  » Risk factors and triggers
  » Amount/duration of exposure
  » Location and time of the event
  » Duration of symptoms
  » Any treatment provided so far
  » Recurrence of symptoms if resolved initially
  » Details of treatment administered at the time of the reaction and during transport to hospital

Physical Exam

- Because anaphylaxis is a multisystem disease and the diagnosis is primarily clinical, it is crucial to perform a thorough clinical assessment to assess the extent of multisystem involvement (see *Table 2.1.2*).

Table 2.1.2. SYMPTOMS AND SIGNS OF ANAPHYLAXIS

Organ system	Signs and symptoms
Dermatological	• Urticaria • Erythema/flushing • Pruritus • Itching or tingling of tongue or palate • Rhinoconjunctivitis (runny nose or red eyes) • Facial swelling • Lip swelling • Tongue Swelling • Periorbital swelling
Respiratory	• Dyspnea • Wheeze • Cough • Throat swelling/tightness/itchiness • Stridor • Hoarseness • Bronchospasm • Accessory muscle use • Cyanosis • Drooling • Hypoxia (oxygen saturation < 92%)
Gastrointestinal	• Vomiting • Persistent abdominal pain • Loose stools • Dysphagia
Cardiovascular/neurologic	• Syncope • Dizziness/lightheadedness • Pale • Floppy • Altered level of consciousness • Hypotension • Incontinence of urine or stool

- Changes in vital signs such as hypotension, wide pulse pressure, and hypoxia (oxygen saturation < 92%) indicate severe anaphylaxis.
- The correct diagnosis of anaphylaxis has serious implications for immediate management and future prevention.

Management

- It is critical to treat anaphylaxis promptly.
- Death from respiratory or cardiac arrest can occur within minutes and is associated with delayed epinephrine treatment.
- Assess ABCs and ensure patient is appropriately monitored.
- Place patient in supine position, unless precluded by vomiting or respiratory distress.
- Fatality can occur within seconds if a patient stands or sits suddenly.

Epinephrine

- As soon as anaphylaxis is recognized, administer epinephrine 0.01 mg/kg IM to a maximum of 0.5 mg (use 1:1000 solution).
  - » This dose may be repeated at 5- to 15-minute intervals if there is no response or if response is inadequate.
  - » Up to 20% of patients may require a repeat dose.
- Refractory anaphylaxis protocol should be initiated for any anaphylactic shock that persists after a total of 3 doses of IM epinephrine.
- An IV bolus of epinephrine should be avoided because it is associated with significantly more dosing errors and serious adverse events such as myocardial infarction, malignant arrhythmia, and pulmonary edema.

Airway Management

- Intubate the patient if marked stridor or respiratory arrest is present.
- Failed attempts at intubation can lead to complete airway obstruction and fatality.
  - » Upper airway closure during anaphylaxis should be managed by the most skilled clinician available.

Breathing and Circulation Management

- Provide a Ventolin nebulizer for patients with wheeze/bronchospasm or asthma.
- Use a 0.9% normal saline bolus (20 to 40 mL/kg) for hypotensive or severe reactions.

Adjunctive Pharmacologic Therapies

- Agents that may be given as adjunctive therapies to epinephrine in the treatment of anaphylaxis include H_1 antihistamines, H_2 antihistamines, bronchodilators, and corticosteroids.
- None of these medications should be used as an initial treatment or as a sole treatment because they do not relieve upper or lower respiratory tract obstruction, hypotension, or shock and are not life-saving therapies.

H_1 ANTIHISTAMINES

- These agents relieve itching and urticarial rash.
- The use of H_1 antihistamines in anaphylaxis is extrapolated from studies of urticaria; however, there are no evidence-based studies to support their use in anaphylaxis.
- Pharmacologically, there are 2 generations of H_1 antihistamines:
  - » First-generation H_1 antihistamines
    - › Diphenhydramine is a classic example of a first-generation H_1 antihistamine.
      - · Dose at 1 mg/kg IV to a maximum dose of 50 mg.

> › First-generation H_1 antihistamines cross the blood-brain barrier and are associated with potentially harmful central nervous system effects, including somnolence and impairment of cognitive function.
>   · In susceptible patients, they could potentially induce fatal cardiac arrhythmias such as QT prolongation and torsade de pointes.
> › Given these serious safety concerns, in addition to their lower efficacy compared to the second-generation agents, their routine use in anaphylaxis is not recommended.
> » Second-generation H_1 antihistamines
>   › Cetirizine, loratadine, and rupatadine are examples of approved agents in Canada.
>   › Dosing for cetirizine:
>   · 6 months to 2 years of age: 2.5 mg PO
>   · 2 to 5 years of age: 2.5 to 5 mg PO
>   · > 5 years of age: 10 mg PO
>   › Advantages of second-generation over first-generation agents include:
>   · Faster onset and longer duration of action
>   · High safety profile
>   · No major cardiac side effects
>   · No sedative effect on children

H_2 ANTIHISTAMINES

- Systematic reviews have not identified any randomized, controlled trials that support the use of H_2 antihistamines — such as ranitidine — in anaphylaxis.

CORTICOSTEROIDS

- Because of the potential detrimental adverse effects of corticosteroids and lack of compelling evidence demonstrating an effective role in reducing anaphylaxis severity or preventing biphasic anaphylaxis, we do not advocate for their routine use in anaphylaxis.

Refractory Anaphylaxis

- If there is no improvement in anaphylactic shock after 3 doses of IM epinephrine and fluid resuscitation, then consider:
  » Epinephrine infusion
    › Dose at 0.05 to 0.1 mcg/kg per minute titrated to effect of symptoms and blood pressure.
  » Glucagon
    › Administer an IV bolus dose of 20 to 30 mcg/kg to a maximum of 1 mg.
    › Follow the bolus dose with an infusion of 5 to 15 mcg/kg per minute.
    › Consider glucagon in patients who remain hypotensive despite multiple doses of epinephrine, patients on beta-blockers, and pregnant adolescents.

» Methylene blue
  › Give 1 to 2 mg/kg per dose IV bolus over 5 minutes.
  › Methylene blue is contraindicated in patients with a glucose-6-phosphate dehydrogenase (G6PD) deficiency.

Disposition

- The pattern of an anaphylactic reaction can be uniphasic, biphasic, or refractory in nature.
- Previous literature reports a broad range in the reported incidence of biphasic reactions, from 3% to 23%.
- Most guidelines recommend a prolonged period of observation and monitoring after treating the initial reactions because of concerns about potentially fatal biphasic reactions.
- Risk factors for biphasic anaphylaxis include:
  » Delay in epinephrine administration or emergency department (ED) presentation for > 60 minutes from the onset of anaphylaxis
  » An anaphylactic reaction that requires > 1 injectable epinephrine therapy
  » Hypotension or wide pulse pressure at triage
  » Respiratory distress that requires treatment with inhaled bronchodilator in ED
- The following monitoring periods can be used as a guide.
  » The minimum observation period is 6 hours (timed from the onset of the reaction) for children with features of moderately severe anaphylaxis that resolve after epinephrine treatment.
  » Children who present to the ED with seemingly mild anaphylaxis need prolonged monitoring (4 to 6 hours) if epinephrine treatment is not administered or is delayed.
  » Children with mild anaphylaxis who are treated with timely epinephrine could be considered for early disposition from the ED (≤ 4 hours timed from the onset of the anaphylactic reaction).
- Children with refractory anaphylaxis and all patients with severe anaphylaxis should be admitted to hospital for at least 24 hours of monitoring.
  » Admission to an intensive care unit should be considered for patients who present with cardiovascular collapse or severe respiratory distress.
- The following factors should also be considered in decisions about a disposition plan:
  » Late evening and night ED presentations
  » Access to emergency care
  » Reliability of caregiver
  » History of severe asthma or biphasic reaction

Emergency Department Patient Discharge Instructions

- Inadequate discharge instructions and follow-up is one of the main gaps in anaphylaxis care in the ED.
- It is imperative that the following aspects of care are covered before discharge from the ED:
  - » Referral to an allergy specialist
    - › A single visit to an allergy clinic has been reported to improve parental knowledge of allergen avoidance, management of allergic reactions, and correct use of an autoinjector.
    - › Do not delegate the task of allergy specialist referral to the child's pediatrician or family physician. Establishing a diagnosis of food allergy has a significant impact on the lifestyle and quality of life of the whole family. It is imperative that this referral is done before discharge from ED.
  - » Anaphylaxis counseling
    - › Education for children and parents should include the following:
      - · Recognition of symptoms and signs of anaphylaxis
      - · Appropriate management steps, including the correct use of an epinephrine autoinjector (EAI), allergen avoidance, and prevention strategies
    - › The Canadian Society of Allergy and Clinical Immunology has a guide on pediatric anaphylaxis. See Anaphylaxis in School and Other Settings (2016) at www.aaia.ca.
    - › Provision of a written anaphylaxis action plan upon ED discharge may reduce the frequency and severity of future reactions, improve knowledge of allergen avoidance techniques, improve EAI use, and reduce anxiety.
  - » A prescription for an EAI
    - › Patients should be provided with a prescription for an EAI and advised to fill the prescription immediately.
    - › Instructions in the proper use of an EAI should be reviewed verbally, and patients should be given a trainer device to practice the correct steps of administering the prescribed device.
    - › A prescription for 2 EAIs should be considered for children with any of the following:
      - · Coexisting unstable or moderate-to-severe, persistent asthma and a food allergy
      - · Mast cell disease and/or elevated baseline tryptase
      - · Lack of rapid access to medical assistance
      - · Previous requirement for more than 1 dose of epinephrine before arrival to hospital
      - · Previous near-fatal anaphylaxis

REFERENCES

Alqurashi W, Alnaji F, Menon K. Refractory anaphylaxis: further considerations for emergency care providers. *Ann Allergy Asthma Immunol.* 2016;116(3):265–266. https://doi.org/10.1016/j.anai.2015.12.028. Medline:26945499

Alqurashi W, Ellis AK. Do corticosteroids prevent biphasic anaphylaxis? *J Allergy Clin Immunol Pract.* 2017;5(5):1194–1205. doi:10.1016/j.jaip.2017.05.022.

Alqurashi W, Stiell I, Chan K, Neto G, Alsadoon A, Wells G. Epidemiology and clinical predictors of biphasic reactions in children with anaphylaxis. *Ann Allergy Asthma Immunol.* 2015;115(3):217–223.e2. https://doi.org/10.1016/j.anai.2015.05.013. Medline:26112147

Alqurashi W, Stiell I, Neto G, Wells G. Diagnosis and management of children with anaphylaxis: a national survey of emergency physicians.CAEP/ACMU 2014 Scientific Abstracts, May 31 to June 4, 2014, Ottawa, Ontario. In: CJEM. Vol 16. Cambridge University Press; 2014:S19–S114.

Ben-Shoshan M, La Vieille S, Eisman H, et al. Anaphylaxis treated in a Canadian pediatric hospital: incidence, clinical characteristics, triggers, and management. *J Allergy Clin Immunol.* 2013;132(3):739–741.e3. https://doi.org/10.1016/j.jaci.2013.06.016. Medline:23900056

Campbell RL, Li JT, Nicklas RA, Sadosty AT. Emergency department diagnosis and treatment of anaphylaxis: a practice parameter. *Ann Allergy Asthma Immunol.* 2014;113(6):599–608. https://doi.org/10.1016/j.anai.2014.10.007. Medline:25466802

Canadian Society of Allergy and Clinical Immunology (CSACI). Anaphylaxis in school and other settings. 3rd rev. Canada: CSACI; 2016. Available from: http://www.aaia.ca/en/Anaphylaxis_3rd_EditionR.pdf

Choo KJ, Simons FE, Sheikh A. Glucocorticoids for the treatment of anaphylaxis. *Cochrane Database Syst Rev.* 2010;4(3):CD007596. Medline:20238355

Church MK, Maurer M, Simons FE, et al; Global Allergy and Asthma European Network. Risk of first-generation H$_1$-antihistamines: a GA(2)LEN position paper. *Allergy.* 2010;65(4):459–466. https://doi.org/10.1111/j.1398-9995.2009.02325.x. Medline:20146728

Cohen MB, Saunders SS, Wise SK, Nassif S, Platt MP. Pitfalls in the use of epinephrine for anaphylaxis: patient and provider opportunities for improvement. *Int Forum Allergy Rhinol.* 2017;7(3):276–286. doi:10.1002/alr.21884.

Dhami S, Panesar SS, Roberts G, et al; EAACI Food Allergy and Anaphylaxis Guidelines Group. Management of anaphylaxis: a systematic review. *Allergy.* 2014;69(2):168–175. https://doi.org/10.1111/all.12318. Medline:24251536

Institute for Safe Medication Practices Canada. Epinephrine use for anaphylaxis: a multi-incident analysis. June 2017;17(6):1–8. Available at: https://www.ismp-canada.org/download/safetyBulletins/2017/ISMPCSB2017-06-EpinephrineAnaphylaxis.pdf

Kastner M, Harada L, Waserman S. Gaps in anaphylaxis management at the level of physicians, patients, and the community: a systematic review of the literature. *Allergy.* 2010;65(4):435–444. https://doi.org/10.1111/j.1398-9995.2009.02294.x. Medline:20028373

Kemp SF. The post-anaphylaxis dilemma: how long is long enough to observe a patient after resolution of symptoms? *Curr Allergy Asthma Rep.* 2008;8(1):45–48. https://doi.org/10.1007/s11882-008-0009-7. Medline:18377774

Khan BQ, Kemp SF. Pathophysiology of anaphylaxis. *Curr Opin Allergy Clin Immunol.* 2011;11(4):319–325. https://doi.org/10.1097/ACI.0b013e3283481ab6. Medline:21659865

Lee S, Bellolio MF, Hess EP, Erwin P, Murad MH, Campbell RL. Time of onset and predictors of biphasic anaphylactic reactions: a systematic review and meta-analysis. *J Allergy Clin Immunol Pract.* 2015;3(3):408–16.e2. https://doi.org/10.1016/j.jaip.2014.12.010. Medline:25680923

Lee S, Sadosty AT, Campbell RL. Update on biphasic anaphylaxis. *Curr Opin Allergy Clin Immunol.* 2016;16(4):346–351. doi:https://doi.org/10.1097/ACI.0000000000000279.

Lieberman P. Treatment of patients who present after an episode of anaphylaxis. *Ann Allergy Asthma Immunol.* 2013;111(3):170–175. https://doi.org/10.1016/j.anai.2013.06.018. Medline:23987190

Lieberman P, Nicklas RA, Oppenheimer J, et al. The diagnosis and management of anaphylaxis practice parameter: 2010 update. *J Allergy Clin Immunol.* 2010;126(3):477–80.e42. https://doi.org/10.1016/j.jaci.2010.06.022. Medline:20692689

Lieberman P, Nicklas RA, Randolph C, et al. Anaphylaxis: a practice parameter update 2015. *Ann Allergy Asthma Immunol.* 2015;115(5):341–384. https://doi.org/10.1016/j.anai.2015.07.019. Medline:26505932

Muraro A, Roberts G, Worm M, et al; EAACI Food Allergy and Anaphylaxis Guidelines Group. Anaphylaxis: guidelines from the European Academy of Allergy and Clinical Immunology. *Allergy.* 2014;69(8):1026–1045. https://doi.org/10.1111/all.12437. Medline:24909803

Niggemann B, Beyer K. Factors augmenting allergic reactions. *Allergy.* 2014;69(12):1582–1587. https://doi.org/10.1111/all.12532. Medline:25306896

Nurmatov UB, Rhatigan E, Simons FE, Sheikh A. H2-antihistamines for the treatment of anaphylaxis with and without shock: a systematic review. *Ann Allergy Asthma Immunol.* 2014;112(2):126–131. https://doi.org/10.1016/j.anai.2013.11.010. Medline:24468252

Sampson HA, Muñoz-Furlong A, Campbell RL, et al. Second symposium on the definition and management of anaphylaxis: summary report—second National Institute of Allergy and Infectious Disease/Food Allergy and Anaphylaxis Network symposium. *Ann Emerg Med.* 2006;47(4):373–380. https://doi.org/10.1016/j.annemergmed.2006.01.018. Medline:16546624

Simons FE, Ardusso LR, Bilò MB, et al; World Allergy Organization. World allergy organization guidelines for the assessment and management of anaphylaxis. *World Allergy Organ J.* 2011;4(2):13–37. https://doi.org/10.1097/WOX.0b013e318211496c. Medline:23268454

Simons FE, Sheikh A. Anaphylaxis: the acute episode and beyond. *BMJ.* 2013 Feb 12;346:f602. https://doi.org/10.1136/bmj.f602. Medline:23403828

Smith PK, Hourihane JO, Lieberman P. Risk multipliers for severe food anaphylaxis. *World Allergy Organ J.* 2015;8(1):30. https://doi.org/10.1186/s40413-015-0081-0. Medline:26635908

Tejedor-Alonso MA, Moro-Moro M, Múgica García MV. Epidemiology of anaphylaxis. *Clin Exp Allergy.* 2015;45(6):1027–1039. https://doi.org/10.1111/cea.12418. Medline:25495512

Tejedor-Alonso MA, Moro-Moro M, Múgica-García MV. Epidemiology of anaphylaxis: contributions from the last 10 years. *J Investig Allergol Clin Immunol.* 2015;25(3):163–175, quiz 174–175. Medline:26182682

Wood RA, Camargo CA Jr, Lieberman P, et al. Anaphylaxis in America: the prevalence and characteristics of anaphylaxis in the United States. *J Allergy Clin Immunol.* 2014;133(2):461–467. https://doi.org/10.1016/j.jaci.2013.08.016. Medline:24144575

2.2

Altered Level of Consciousness

Tim Lynch

- Detecting an altered level of consciousness (ALOC) in an infant or child can be challenging as initial changes in behavior can be quite subtle.
- ALOC includes a spectrum of diagnoses that range in their presentation from confusion to coma.
- The following are definitions of different ALOCs:
  » Confusion — disorientation to time
  » Delirium — fluctuating disorientation to time, place, and person
  » Lethargy — severe drowsiness
  » Obtundation — slowed response to moderate stimulus
  » Stupor — vigorous stimuli required to arouse patient
  » Coma — state of unarousable unresponsiveness (Glasgow Coma Scale (GCS) of 8 or less; see *Table 18.1.1* on page 316)

Pathophysiology

- An ALOC can result from:
  » A depression of the cerebral cortex or reticular activating system in the brainstem and midbrain
  » A deficient substrate such as oxygen or glucose
  » A toxin — an endogenous substance such as ammonia or an exogenous substance such as drugs
  » A space-occupying lesion such as an infection, intracranial hemorrhage, or brain tumor

Differential Diagnosis

- On the differential diagnosis for ALOC, consider:
  » Hypoxia
  » Hypo- or hyperthermia
  » Metabolic disease — hypoglycemia, hyponatremia, inborn error of metabolism leading to elevated ammonia
  » Infection — sepsis, meningitis, encephalitis, brain abscess, myocarditis
  » Inflammation — acute demyelinating encephalitis
  » Trauma — concussion, epidural hematoma, subdural hematoma, intracerebral hemorrhage, subarachnoid hemorrhage, diffuse axonal injury, submersion injury
  » Suspected nonaccidental trauma (NAT; see Chapter 1.7, "Child Abuse")
  » Neoplasm — brain tumor
  » Arrhythmias
  » Hydrocephalus, ventriculoperitoneal (VP) shunt dysfunction

- » Seizure (consider nonconvulsive status epilepticus) and postictal state
- » Vascular disorder — stroke, subarachnoid hemorrhage, aneurysm, arteriovenous malformation
- » Liver or kidney failure
- » Intoxication
- » Psychiatric condition
- » Psychosomatic disorder — diagnosis of exclusion
- Based on age, common causes of ALOC to consider are listed in *Table 2.2.1*, below.

Table 2.2.1. COMMON CAUSES OF ALOC BASED ON AGE

Age category	Common causes to consider for altered level of consciousness at different ages
Newborn	• Hypoglycemia • Inborn error of metabolism — urea cycle defect, organic acidemia, congenital lactic acidosis, fatty acid oxidation disorder • Infection — sepsis
Infant	• Abuse, nonaccidental trauma • Infection — meningitis • Intussusception
Child	• DKA* • Poisoning — clonidine, opiate • Seizure • Infection — meningitis
Adolescent	• Overdose — ethanol, opiate, tricyclic antidepressant, anticholinergic • Toxic exposure — carbon monoxide • Trauma • DKA • Infection — Herpes encephalitis

DKA diabetic ketoacidosis.

* See Chapter 7.1, "Diabetic Ketoacidosis."

Management

- Evaluation should include the determination of the patient's level of consciousness and a detailed assessment to determine the cause of the ALOC.
- Obtain a history to understand:
  - » Timeline of the ALOC — rapid versus gradual onset
  - » Risk factors for infection — immunization status, recent febrile illness
  - » History of trauma
  - » History of headache or vomiting
  - » Seizure history
  - » Social situation — understand risk for NAT/abuse

Advanced Trauma Life Support (ATLS) Protocol

PRIMARY SURVEY

- Assess and ensure airway and breathing.
  - » Open airway using head-tilt/chin-lift maneuver (if there is no trauma) or jaw-thrust maneuver (if obstruction is present).
  - » Administer oxygen.
  - » Secure the airway if GCS < 8 (see *Table 18.1.1* on page 316).
  - » Assess respiratory rate, oxygen saturation, and breathing pattern, looking for abnormal patterns:
    - › Cerebral hemisphere dysfunction — posthyperventilation apnea (> 10 seconds apnea after 5 deep breaths) or Cheyne-Stokes respiration (rhythmic increase and decrease in respiratory amplitude)
    - › Midbrain and upper pons dysfunction — central reflex hyperpnea
    - › Pons dysfunction — apneustic respirations
    - › Medulla to C4 dysfunction — apnea
  - » Use C-spine precautions if there is trauma.
- Address circulation.
  - » Assess the following:
    - › Heart rate
    - › Pulses
    - › Capillary refill time
    - › Blood pressure
  - » Support circulation with normal saline 20 mL/kg if patient is hypotensive.
  - » Hypertension and bradycardia indicate raised intracranial pressure.
- Assess the patient for disability.
  - » Measure glucose at the bedside.
  - » Determine GCS.
  - » Assess pupils for:
    - › Size — evidence of miosis or mydriasis
    - › Pupillary light reflex — direct and consensual
    - › Evidence of anisocoria
    - › Extraocular movements as evidence of nerve palsies
- Assess the patient for exposure.
  - » Measure temperature.
  - » Assess skin for lesions or signs of trauma.

SECONDARY SURVEY

- Conduct a musculoskeletal assessment.
  - » Assess the patient's muscle tone and power and reflexes, looking for any focal or lateralizing neurologic signs.
- Assess the patient for abnormal postural reflexes with deep painful stimuli:
  - » Decorticate posturing — knee extension with elbow flexion
  - » Decerebrate posturing — knee extension with elbow extension
- Complete a head-to-toe exam with particular attention to:
  - » Scalp for signs of injury, and skull for depression or crepitus

- » Tympanic membranes for infection and hemotympanum
- » Presence or absence of papilledema or retinal hemorrhages
- If there are no concerns of trauma, check the patient's brainstem reflexes (such as oculocephalic response) by rotating the head from side to side.
  - » In a normal response, the eyes will move in the opposite direction of the head rotation.

Investigations

- Consider the following investigations to determine the cause of the ALOC:
  - » Bloodwork
    - › Glucose, electrolytes, calcium, magnesium, urea, creatinine
    - › Liver function tests — alanine transaminase (ALT), aspartate transaminase (AST), gamma-glutamyl transferase (GGT), international normalized ratio (INR), partial thromboplastin time (PTT), ammonia
    - › Complete blood count (CBC) with differential
    - › Blood culture if infectious etiology is suspected or if patient is febrile
    - › Blood gas, lactate
    - › Anticonvulsant levels
    - › For suspected metabolic abnormalities: ketone bodies, plasma free fatty acids, carnitine, pyruvate, serum amino acids
  - » Urine
    - › Culture
    - › Toxicology
    - › Ketones
    - › Organic acids and porphyrins
  - » Electrocardiogram (ECG)
  - » Lumbar puncture with measurement of opening pressure
    - › Look for evidence of infection.

- » Electroencephalogram (EEG) — if the patient has had a seizure
- » Imaging
  - › Chest X-ray (CXR)
  - › Diagnostic imaging — CT scan or MRI with or without head angiogram
    - · This is especially important for NAT and head and neck trauma.
  - › Ultrasound of abdomen if intussusception is suspected

Management

- Management of an ALOC depends on its etiology.
- Consider immediate therapy for:
  - » Hypoglycemia
  - » Hypoxia
  - » Opioid overdose
  - » Status epilepticus

Disposition

- Admit the patient to pediatric critical care for ongoing intensive care if the patient's clinical condition warrants it.

REFERENCES

American Heart Association. *Pediatric advanced life support provider manual.* First American Heart Association printing; 2016:23–114.

Avner JR. Altered states of consciousness. *Pediatr Rev.* 2006;27(9):331–338. https://doi.org/10.1542/pir.27-9-331. Medline:16950938

Fleisher GR, Ludwig S. *Textbook of pediatric emergency medicine.* 5th ed. Philadelphia, PA: Lippincott Williams and Wilkins; 2010. Chapter 12, Coma and Altered Level of Consciousness; p. 176–86.

MacNeill EC, Vashist S. Approach to syncope and altered mental status. *Pediatr Clin North Am.* 2013;60(5):1083–1106. https://doi.org/10.1016/j.pcl.2013.06.013. Medline:24093897

Trainor JL, Fuchs S, Isaacman DJ. *The pediatric emergency medicine resource.* 5th ed. Burlington, MA: Jones and Bartlett Learning; 2011. Chapter 5, Central nervous system; p. 168–97.

2.3

Apnea in Newborns and Infants

Rahim Valani

- Apnea is pathologic when there is either:
  » Cessation of respiratory effort or airflow for ≥ 20 seconds

  — **or** —

  » Cessation of respiration for < 20 seconds that is associated with:
    › Bradycardia
    › Cyanosis
    › Hypotonia
    › Oxygen desaturation
- Apnea is classified as central, obstructive, or mixed.
  » Central apnea
    › Impaired impulse from the brainstem leads to complete absence of respiratory effort.
  » Obstructive apnea
    › Respiratory effort is present, but there is no airflow due to obstruction of airway passages.
  » Mixed apnea
    › This is the most common type of apnea.
    › Both central and obstructive elements are present.
- The cause of apnea depends on the age of the patient. (See below for age-specific causes of apnea.)

History

- On history, ask:
  » What were the circumstances surrounding the event?
  » Where did the event occur (e.g., home, daycare)?
  » What was the duration of the episode?
  » Was the infant awake or asleep at the time of the episode?
  » Did the episode occurred during or shortly after feeding?
  » Was there cyanosis or pallor during the episode or shortly after?
  » Was the patient's muscle tone rigid or flaccid during the episode or slightly after?
  » Was CPR was performed by a parent, a caregiver, or medical personnel?
  » Did the patient experience a postictal state after the event?
  » Has the patient experienced recent illness or fever?
  » Is there a family history of unexplained deaths or brief resolved unexplained event (BRUE) in siblings?
- Review all the medications given to the infant (including herbal supplements), as well as any other medications that are present in the house.

UNDIFFERENTIATED APNEA

Management

- Assess the patient's ABCs.
- If there are signs of airway obstruction:
  » Ensure appropriate positioning of airway/neck
  » Note that bag valve mask (BVM) ventilation / continuous positive airway pressure (CPAP) may be required
    › CPAP has been shown to be beneficial for:
      · Apnea of prematurity (AOP)
      · Tracheomalacia

Investigations

- Obtain bloodwork:
  » Glucose
  » Complete blood count (CBC), electrolytes, liver enzymes, liver function, renal function
  » Calcium
  » Sepsis evaluation — blood, urine, cerebrospinal fluid (CSF) cultures
  » Blood gas
- Consider a urine toxicology screen.
- Consider imaging studies:
  » Electrocardiogram (ECG)
    › Look for arrhythmias or signs of channelopathies.
  » Chest X-ray (CXR)
- Other tests to consider depending on the clinical presentation, and include:
  » Cranial ultrasound, CT scan, or MRI
  » Cardiac echocardiogram
  » Electroencephalogram (EEG)
  » Esophageal pH probe
- Depending on the etiology, consultations with different subspecialties may be required, including:
  » Cardiology
  » Respirology
  » Neurology
  » Otorhinolaryngology (ENT)

- Admit all high-risk patients to hospital.
  - » If the patient is low risk, consider observation for 4 hours in the emergency department (ED).

APNEA IN THE DELIVERY ROOM

- Apnea in the delivery room can be due to:
  - » Brain injury / hypoxemic-ischemic event
  - » Intrapartum medications given to the mother
  - » Early onset sepsis
  - » Congenital malformations
  - » Metabolic causes
  - » Sudden unexplained postnatal collapse
    - › Sudden unexplained postnatal collapse is an unexplained collapse leading to death, NICU admission, or encephalopathy within the first 7 days of life in a full-term or late-preterm infant who appeared well at birth.

APNEA IN INFANTS 0 TO 3 DAYS OF AGE

- Apnea in infants 0 to 3 days of age may be caused by congenital central hypoventilation syndrome or apnea of prematurity.

CONGENITAL CENTRAL HYPOVENTILATION SYNDROME

- Congenital central hypoventilation syndrome is a severe respiratory and autonomic nervous system dysregulation involving multiple other organ systems, including:
  - » Cardiac
  - » Sudomotor
  - » Ophthalmic
  - » Neurologic
  - » Gastrointestinal
- The PHOX2B gene is helpful in defining the disease.

APNEA OF PREMATURITY

- Apnea of prematurity (AOP) is characterized by recurrent apneic episodes in premature infants (< 37 weeks gestational age) due to an immature central and autonomic nervous system.
- Incidence of AOP is inversely related to gestational age at birth.
  - » For infants of < 28 weeks gestational age, apnea frequently persists until term postmenstrual age.
  - » For infants of > 28 weeks gestational age, apnea resolves by 37 weeks postmenstrual age.
- AOP is defined by physiologic contributors including:
  - » Blunted response to oxygen and carbon dioxide
  - » Compromised lung volume
  - » Small airways prone to collapse and obstruction

- Infants with AOP cannot be discharged home safely and must be monitored in hospital.
- AOP may be treated with caffeine or theophylline.
  - » Resolution rates are similar with caffeine and theophylline; however, caffeine is dosed once daily and has more predictable absorption from the gut.
    - › Caffeine
      - · Give a loading dose of 20 mg/kg IV or PO, followed by 5 to 10 mg/kg maintenance daily.
      - · Caffeine is usually discontinued by 35 weeks postmenstrual age.
    - › Aminophylline
      - · Give a loading dose of 4 to 6 mg/kg IV or PO, followed by 2 to 6 mg/kg per day maintenance.

APNEA IN INFANTS 3 DAYS TO 1 YEAR OF AGE

- Maturation of the nervous and respiratory systems is ongoing in infants 3 days to 1 year of age.
- Apnea in infants 3 days to 1 year of age may be caused by periodic breathing or BRUE.

PERIODIC BREATHING

- Periodic breathing is a normal finding in term infants up to 6 months of age.
- It is a pattern of alternating breaths and brief respiratory pauses (5 to 10 seconds duration) usually lasting < 15 seconds per episode with no accompanying bradycardia.
- It is due to ongoing maturation of the nervous system.

BRIEF RESOLVED UNEXPLAINED EVENT (BRUE)

- BRUE is formerly known as apparent life-threatening event (ALTE).
- BRUE accounts for an estimated 0.6% to 1.7% of ED visits.
- BRUE occurs in infants < 1 year of age.
- It is characterized by:
  - » Apnea or decreased respirations
  - » Change in color (pallor or cyanosis)
  - » Change in muscle tone
  - » Altered level of responsiveness
- Infants are at low risk for BRUE if:
  - » They are > 60 days of age
  - » They are of gestational age ≥ 32 weeks and postconceptional age ≥ 45 weeks
  - » It is their first episode of apnea
  - » The event lasts < 1 minute
  - » No CPR was required by caregiver or trained medical providers
  - » There are no concerning features on history or physical exam

- If an explanation for the event is determined, then it is not considered BRUE.

Differential Diagnosis

- Consider the following on the differential diagnosis of BRUE:
  » Airway obstruction
    › Foreign body
    › Neck flexion
    › Structural abnormalities — tracheomalacia, vocal cord paralysis
  » Central nervous system (CNS) disorders
    › Intracranial bleed
    › Hypoxic ischemic injury
    › Congenital malformations — Arnold-Chiari malformation
  » Medications
    › Opioids
    › CNS depressants
    › Prostaglandin E1
  » Infection
    › Sepsis
    › Meningitis
    › Respiratory syncytial virus (RSV)
  » Metabolic disorders
    › Hypoglycemia
    › Hypercalcemia
    › Hypo- or hypernatremia
    › Inborn errors of metabolism
    › Kernicterus
  » Cardiovascular disorders
    › Structural cardiac diseases
    › Channelopathies
    › Arrhythmias
  » Other
    › Gastroesophageal reflux
    › Anemia
    › Nonaccidental injury (NAI)

Management

- For low-risk patients, educate parents and caregivers about BRUE and offer them resources for CPR training.
- Low-risk patients may be briefly monitored in the ER with continuous pulse oximetry.
- Depending on the presentation, it may be appropriate to order pertussis testing and an ECG.
- There should be no need to perform additional blood-work or investigations in the ED if BRUE is accompanied with a reassuring history and physical exam.

REFERENCES

Kondamudi NP, Virji M. Brief resolved unexplained event (BRUE). In: StatPearls [Internet]. Treasure Island, FL: StatPearls Publishing; 2017. https://www.ncbi.nlm.nih.gov/books/NBK441897/

Patrinos ME, Martin RJ. Apnea in the term infant. Semin Fetal Neonatal Med. 2017;22(4):240–244. https://doi.org/10.1016/j.siny.2017.04.003. Medline:28438477

Nafday SM, Long C. Respiratory distress and breathing disorders in the newborn. In: McInerny TK, Adam HM, Campbell DE, DeWitt TG, Foy JM, Kamat DM, editors. American Academy of Pediatrics textbook of pediatric care, 2nd ed. American Academy of Pediatrics; 2016.

2.4

Pediatric Fever

Vidushi Khatri, Rahim Valani

- 20% to 30% of pediatric emergency department (ED) and clinic visits are for fever.
- Fever is defined as a core (rectal) temperature of ≥ 38°C.
- Methods of measuring temperature are:
  » Rectal (the most accurate method)
    › Avoid taking rectal temperature in immunocompromised patients.
    › There is a risk of rectal perforation in neonates (less than 1 in 2 million measurements).
    › Measurements are affected by stool and depth of measurement.
  » Oral
    › Oral temperature is usually 0.6°C lower than rectal temperature due to respiration.
  » Axillary
    › Axillary temperature provides an inaccurate estimate of core temperature but is widely used as noninvasive.
    › The temperature sensor is often incorrectly placed; it should be placed over axillary artery.
  » Tympanic
    › Tympanic temperature is the estimate of thermal radiation emitted from tympanic membrane.

› Its reliability is highly dependent on thermometer brand and technology.

› When measuring for fever, children < 2 years of age may have a false negative due to a narrow meatus.

» Temporal artery

› Studies comparing temporal artery and rectal temperatures have had contradictory results.

› Temporal artery temperature is useful as a screening tool but should not be used to make clinical decisions.

- You may need to address fever phobia when parents present with their children.

» Fever is a symptom not a disease.

» The height of a fever is not predictive of serious bacterial infection in immunized patients.

» Febrile seizures occur when temperature increases rapidly, and not by the height of the fever alone.

» Seizures cannot be prevented with around-the-clock antipyretics.

Table 2.4.1. CANADIAN TASK FORCE ON PREVENTATIVE HEALTH — RECOMMENDED TEMPERATURE MEASURING TECHNIQUES

Age	Definitive measuring technique	Low-risk screening technique
Birth to 2 years	Rectal	Axillary (do not use in neonates)
2 to 5 years	Rectal	Axillary, tympanic, temporal artery
≥ 5 years	Oral	Axillary, tympanic, temporal artery

Management

- Keep the child comfortable and well-hydrated.
- Consider antipyretics:

» Acetaminophen 15 mg/kg PO or PR every 4 to 6 hours

› There is conflicting data regarding an increased risk of developing asthma linked with acetaminophen use in children.

» Ibuprofen 10 mg/kg PO every 6 hours

› Ibuprofen has an antiplatelet effect, so may be contraindicated in some children (oncology, bone marrow failure syndromes).

- There is some evidence that alternating or combined antipyretic therapy may be more effective at reducing temperature; however, there is a risk of dosing confusion and toxicity.

» There is no evidence that this improves child discomfort.

» There are no clear guidelines for whether alternating or combined therapy is a superior approach.

- Avoid cold baths and alcohol rubs.

FEVER AND INFECTION

- Infection is a common cause of fever.
- Serious bacterial infection risks being overlooked in patients with no focus of infection.

» For a well-appearing child, the incidence of occult bacteremia is 0.25% to 2.0%.

› Of these, 3% to 5% will end up with a serious bacterial infection (SBI).

Figure 2.4.1. INCIDENCE OF OCCULT BACTEREMIA AND SERIOUS BACTERIAL INFECTION IN A WELL-APPEARING CHILD

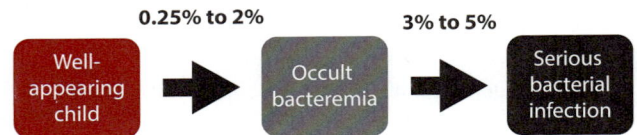

- The introduction of vaccines has resulted in a marked change in the incidence of bacteremia.

» *Haemophilus influenzae* B vaccine

› This vaccine reduced incidence of invasive *H. influenzae* by 95%.

» Pneumococcal conjugate vaccine (PCV)

› The vaccine efficacy for PCV-7 is 97%.

› PCV-7 lead to a 64% decrease in invasive disease.

› The introduction of PCV-13 lead to further decrease in invasive disease.

» Meningococcal vaccine

› The vaccine against serogroup C, Y, and W-135 has decreased the incidence of meningococcal infection to < 0.13 per 100 000.

Management

INFANT WITH FEVER (< 1 MONTH TO 2 MONTHS OF AGE)

- These infants are high risk due to an immature immune system and lack of vaccination; they must be investigated regardless of clinical appearance.
- Perform a full septic workup, including the following:

» Blood culture

» Urine culture

» Lumbar puncture

» Chest X-ray (CXR) and nasopharyngeal virology swab — consider if respiratory symptoms are present

- Treat with antibiotics and admit to hospital.

» Give:

› Ampicillin of 50 mg/kg every 6 hours

— **and** —

› Cefotaxime 50 mg/kg every 8 hours

» If herpes is a possibility, add:

› Acyclovir 20 mg/kg every 8 hours

INFANTS (1 TO 3 MONTHS)

- In a well-immunized community, this population is protected by herd immunity.
  » If there is no focus of infection and the infant is well appearing, consider a urinalysis and culture.
  » Ensure follow-up in 24 to 48 hours.
- Avoid routine blood cultures in immunized patients with no source of infection.
  » The rate of contaminated blood cultures is as high as 2%. This rate is higher than the rate of occult bacteremia, making the utility of routine blood cultures questionable.
- Note the following about other investigations:
  » White blood cell (WBC) count is not helpful; bandemia is a better predictor of bacterial infection.
  » Consider CXR only if respiratory symptoms are present.
- Infectious causes of fever include:
  » Viruses
    › 40% of infants with fever have positive virology.
    › Respiratory syncytial virus (RSV), enterovirus, and influenza are the most common.
  » Bacteria
    › *E. coli* and group B *Streptococcus* are most common.
    › 18% to 27% of cultures grow from more than one site (blood, urine, cerebrospinal fluid).

CHILD > 3 MONTHS

- In the postvaccine era, urinary tract infections (UTIs) are the most common cause of SBI (see "Urinary Tract Infections," below).
- If the child is well appearing, has no focus of infection, and has had ≥ 2 doses of *H. influenzae* and pneumococcal vaccines:
  » Do not order bloodwork
  » Consider urinalysis and send for culture
  » Ensure close follow-up

Investigations

- Initiate the following studies and tests:
  » Complete blood count (CBC)
    › A WBC count is not predictive of occult bacteremia; bandemia has higher predictive value.
  » C-reactive protein (CRP)
    › CRP is elevated within 4 to 6 hours of inflammation.
    › Notes on using different cut-offs:
      · CRP > 20: sensitivity of 88% and specificity of 61%
      · CRP > 40: sensitivity of 71% and specificity of 81%
    › CRP is useful for following the resolution of infection in admitted critical care patients.

» Erythrocyte sedimentation rate (ESR)
  › ESR is a nonspecific inflammatory marker.
  › It has low utility in the postvaccine era.
» Procalcitonin (PCT) as a biomarker
  › PCT is produced in the C-cells of the thyroid gland and neuroendocrine cells (intestines, lungs).
    · PCT is a precursor of calcitonin with a half-life of 24 hours.
  › For well appearing infants < 3 months, PCT performs better than CRP as a biomarker for ruling out occult bacteremia.
    · The optimal cut-off is > 0.6 ng/mL for patients < 3 years of age.
    · CRP rises more slowly than PCT and is less specific.

URINARY TRACT INFECTIONS

- UTIs are the most common SBI in infants and young children.
- They have a prevalence of 7% in patients < 2 years of age.
- Risk factors:
  » Female
  » Uncircumcised male < 1 year of age
  » Previous UTI
  » Suprapubic tenderness
  » Fever > 24 hours
  » Temperature > 39°C
  » Patient of non-African descent
- Sample collection, and collection method, is important.
  » Recommended collection methods include:
    › Bladder catheterization (sensitivity of 95% and specificity of 99%)
    › Suprapubic aspiration
    › Clean catch (false positives in uncircumcised male)
  » Avoid bag urine collection.
    › This has a specificity of 70% and high false positive rate of 85%.
- When interpreting urinalysis, it is important to consider that:
  » Nitrites indicate presence of gram-negative bacteria
    › The absence of nitrites may indicate gram-positive bacteria.
  » Frequent voiding in neonates and toddlers can cause false absence of leukocytes
  » A child with a negative urine dipstick (i.e., no nitrites, leukocytes) and no pyuria or bacteria on routine and microscopy (R+M) urinalysis has < 1% chance of having a UTI

- When interpreting a urine culture, it is important to:
  » Always send catheter samples or midstream samples for toilet-trained children
    › Bag urine culture rules out UTIs; however, positive culture on bagged specimen is likely contaminated.

Table 2.4.2. SENSITIVITY AND SPECIFICITY OF COMPONENTS OF URINALYSIS

Test	Sensitivity	Specificity
LKE positive	83	78
Nitrite positive	53	98
Either nitrite or LKE positive	93	72

LKE leukocyte esterase.

Management

- For patients < 6 months of age:
  » Admit to hospital
  » Give IV antibiotics: ampicillin and gentamicin
- For well-appearing patients > 6 months of age:
  » Commence outpatient management with close follow-up
  » Initiate first-line empirical management based on local susceptibility patterns; the Canadian Pediatric Society recommends:
    › Cefixime 8 mg/kg per day divided and given twice daily
    — **or** —
    › Cephalexin 25 to 50 mg/kg per day divided and given 3 or 4 times daily

OTHER CAUSES OF FEVER

- Consider these other possible causes of bacteria:
  » Occult bacterial infection:
    › Intraabdominal abscess, osteomyelitis, infective endocarditis
  » Autoimmune processes:
    › Inflammatory bowel disease, hyperthyroidism
  » Rheumatologic diseases:
    › Juvenile idiopathic arthritis, lupus, Kawasaki disease
  » Neoplastic disease:
    › Leukemia, lymphoma, hemophagocytic lymphohistiocytosis
  » Inflammatory disease:
    › Serum sickness, drug fever, periodic fever syndromes (i.e., familial Mediterranean fever)
  » Fever in the returning traveler:
    › See Chapter 10.1

REFERENCES

Greenhow TL, Hung YY, Herz AM, Losada E, Pantell RH. The changing epidemiology of serious bacterial infections in young infants. *Pediatr Infect Dis J.* 2014;33(6):595–599. https://doi.org/10.1097/INF.0000000000000225. Medline:24326416

Jhaveri R, Byington CL, Klein JO, Shapiro ED. Management of the non-toxic-appearing acutely febrile child: a 21st century approach. *J Pediatr.* 2011;159(2):181–185. https://doi.org/10.1016/j.jpeds.2011.03.047. Medline:21592518

Leduc D, Woods S; Canadian Pediatric Society. Temperature measurement in pediatrics [Internet]. 2017. Available from: https://www.cps.ca/en/documents/position/temperature-measurement

Mahajan P, Grzybowski M, Chen X, et al. Procalcitonin as a marker of serious bacterial infections in febrile children younger than 3 years old. *Acad Emerg Med.* 2014;21(2):171–179. https://doi.org/10.1111/acem.12316. Medline:24673673

Richardson M, Purssell E. Who's afraid of fever? *Arch Dis Child.* 2015;100(9):818–820. https://doi.org/10.1136/archdischild-2014-307483. Medline:25977564

Robinson JL, Finlay JC, Lang ME, Bortolussi R; Canadian Paediatric Society, Infectious Diseases and Immunization Committee, Community Paediatrics Committee. Urinary tract infections in infants and children: diagnosis and management. *Paediatr Child Health.* 2014;19(6):315–325. Medline:25332662

Sullivan JE, Farrar HC; Section on Clinical Pharmacology and Therapeutics, Committee on Drugs. Fever and antipyretic use in children. *Pediatrics.* 2011;127(3):580–587. https://doi.org/10.1542/peds.2010-3852. Medline:21357332

Trainor JL, Stamos JK. Fever without a localizing source. *Pediatr Ann.* 2011;40(1):21–25. https://doi.org/10.3928/00904481-20101214-06. Medline:21210596

Wong T, Stang AS, Ganshorn H, et al. Combined and alternating paracetamol and ibuprofen therapy for febrile children. *Evid Based Child Health.* 2014;9(3):675–729. https://doi.org/10.1002/ebch.1978. Medline:25236309

2.5

Chest Pain

Shabnam Minoosepehr

- Chest pain in children accounts for approximately 0.3% to 0.6% of visits to the emergency department (ED).
- The average age of presentation is 10 to 12 years.
  - » Younger children are more likely to have cardiorespiratory causes of chest pain.
  - » Adolescents are most likely to have a psychogenic etiology.
  - » Up to 30% of children miss school due to this symptom.
- Most often, chest pain in the pediatric population is benign and has a self-limited etiology; however, in the ED it is important to recognize when pediatric chest pain has life-threatening causes.

History

- When a patient presents to the ED with chest pain, the following information should be collected when taking the patient's history:
  - » Description and location of pain
  - » Duration of symptoms
  - » Family history of cardiorespiratory issues
  - » Sleep disturbances
  - » Pain associated with exertion or being syncopal
  - » Presence of fever
  - » Associated medical conditions (Marfan syndrome, asthma, lupus, Kawasaki disease, asthma)
  - » Dyspnea
  - » Any history of trauma
  - » Positional or pleuritic symptoms
  - » Drug / illicit substance use
  - » Presence of new rash

Red Flags

- Factors associated with organic causes of chest pain may present in the following ways:
  - » Exercise intolerance
  - » Pain worsening with exertion
  - » Palpitations
  - » Diaphoresis
  - » Syncope
  - » Pain radiating to the neck or arm
  - » Fever
  - » Past medical history:
    - › Kawasaki disease, sickle cell disease, connective tissue disorders, previous heart surgery, cocaine use, or diabetes
  - » Family history of sudden unexplained death, inherited thrombophilia, hypercoagulable state, bicuspid aortic valve

Physical Exam

- Take a complete set of vital signs.
- Pay attention to tachycardia, hypotension, and hypoxia.
- Listen for any adventitious breath sounds or lack of breath sounds.
- Look for any abnormal cardiovascular findings.
- Examine the patient for a new-onset murmur, gallop, irregular rhythm, cardiac rub, or distant heart sounds.

Differential Diagnosis

- The differential for pediatric chest pain is very broad.
- Based on a systematic review, the distribution of pediatric chest pain is as follows:
  - » Idiopathic (36%)
  - » Musculoskeletal (20%)
    - › Chest wall trauma, rib fracture, muscle strain, costochondritis, precordial catch syndrome, slipping rib syndrome
  - » Psychological (16%)
    - › Hyperventilation, anxiety
  - » Cardiac (10%)
    - › Anomalous coronary artery, Kawasaki disease, cocaine abuse, arrhythmia, pericarditis, myocarditis, hypertrophic cardiomyopathy, aortic or pulmonary stenosis, aortic dissection
  - » Gastrointestinal (10%)
    - › Gastroesophageal reflux, esophagitis, gastritis, foreign body ingestion
  - » Respiratory (8%)
    - › Asthma, pneumonia, pneumothorax, pneumomediastinum, pulmonary embolism, chronic cough

Investigations

- Investigations should be based on clinical presentation and physical examination.
  - » Patients with chest pain at rest, normal electrocardiogram (ECG), normal cardiac examination, and without risk factors (fever, family history, hypercoagulable state) do not have a cardiac etiology for their chest pain.

- Obtain an ECG for patients with:
  » Exertional chest pain
  » Suspected myocarditis or pericarditis
  » Abnormal findings on auscultation
  » Tachycardia
  » Syncope
  » Underlying medical conditions that predispose them to cardiac disease
- Obtain a chest X-ray (CXR) for patients with:
  » Unexplained pain of acute onset
  » Respiratory distress
  » A new finding on auscultation (e.g., murmur, gallop, wheeze, crackles, friction rub)
  » Fever
  » Significant cough
  » Trauma
  » A history of drooling or foreign body ingestion
  » An underlying medical condition (e.g., sickle cell anemia)
- An echocardiogram is useful in patients with:
  » An abnormal physical exam
  » An abnormal ECG
  » A concerning family history (e.g., hypertrophic cardiomyopathy)
  » Exertional chest pain
- Troponin assays are useful for screening / narrowing down the differential diagnosis but are not conclusive for myocarditis.
  » An abnormal troponin assay is suggestive of myocarditis (89% specificity and 34% sensitivity).
  » Normal or high laboratory workup results cannot predict ejection fraction.

Management

- The initial management of pediatric chest pain is dependent on the broad differential (see "Differential Diagnosis," above) and patient stability.

- If the patient is unstable, start with stabilization of airway, breathing, and circulation; then, follow the pediatric advance life support (PALS) guidelines.
- Consider consulting cardiology or the pediatric intensive care unit early.
- If the patient is stable, treat chest pain based on its etiology.

REFERENCES

Cava JR, Sayger PL. Chest pain in children and adolescents. *Pediatr Clin North Am.* 2004;51(6):1553–1568, viii. https://doi.org/10.1016/j.pcl.2004.07.002. Medline:15561173

Drossner D, Hirsh D, Sturm J, et al. Cardiac disease in pediatric patients presenting to a pediatric ED with chest pain. *Am J Emerg Med.* 2011;29:632–638. https://doi.org/10.1016/j.ajem.2010.01.011. Medline:20627219

Eslick GD. Epidemiology and risk factors of pediatric chest pain: a systematic review. *Pediatr Clin North Am.* 2010;57(6):1211–1219. https://doi.org/10.1016/j.pcl.2010.09.013. Medline:21111114

Friedman KG, Alexander ME. Chest pain and syncope in children: a practical approach to the diagnosis of cardiac disease. *J Pediatr.* 2013;163(3):896–901.e3. https://doi.org/10.1016/j.jpeds.2013.05.001. Medline:23769502

Friedman KG, Kane DA, Rathod RH, et al. Management of pediatric chest pain using a standardized assessment and management plan. *Pediatrics.* 2011;128(2):239–245. https://doi.org/10.1542/peds.2011-0141. Medline:21746719

Jindal A, Singhi S. Acute chest pain. *Indian J Pediatr.* 2011;78(10):1262–1267. https://doi.org/10.1007/s12098-011-0413-1. Medline:21541647

Kane DA, Fulton DR, Saleeb S, Zhou J, Lock JE, Geggel RL. Needles in hay: chest pain as the presenting symptom in children with serious underlying cardiac pathology. *Congenit Heart Dis.* 2010;5(4):366–373. https://doi.org/10.1111/j.1747-0803.2010.00436.x. Medline:20653703

Selbst SM. Approach to the child with chest pain. *Pediatr Clin North Am.* 2010;57(6):1221–1234. https://doi.org/10.1016/j.pcl.2010.09.003. Medline:21111115

Thull-Freedman J. Evaluation of chest pain in the pediatric patient. *Med Clin North Am.* 2010;94(2):327–347. https://doi.org/10.1016/j.mcna.2010.01.004. Medline:20380959

Yeh TK, Yeh J. Chest pain in pediatrics. *Pediatr Ann.* 2015;44(12):e274–e278. https://doi.org/10.3928/00904481-20151110-01. Medline:26678235

Cardiac Emergencies

3.1

Cardiogenic Shock

Jan Hanot, Jonathan Duff

- Cardiogenic shock is defined as inadequate heart function causing insufficient oxygen delivery to tissues relative to the oxygen demand and leading to tissue hypoxia.
- Cardiogenic shock represents 5% to 13% of diagnosed shock cases in pediatric patients.
- The most common causes of cardiogenic shock are:
  » Cardiomyopathy (primary or secondary)
  » Myocarditis
  » Arrhythmia
  » Congenital heart disease
- Rare causes of cardiogenic shock are:
  » Endocarditis
  » Kawasaki disease (See Chapter 9.1)
  » Takotsubo cardiomyopathy
    › Takotsubo cardiomyopathy is stress-induced cardiomyopathy that results in left ventricle (LV) systolic dysfunction, characterized by:
      · Normal coronaries and ballooning of the LV apex
      · Possible transient bump in cardiac enzymes
  » Rheumatic fever
  » Chordae tendineae rupture
    › This can be primary or secondary to bacterial endocarditis.
  » Drug or toxin ingestion (beta-blockers, calcium channel blockers, and anti-arrhythmics)
- Noncardiac causes of cardiogenic shock are:
  » Sepsis
  » Pulmonary embolus
  » Pneumothorax
  » Tamponade

Diagnosis

- Patients may present with any of the following:
  » Tachycardia
  » Tachypnea
  » Dyspnea (crackles on auscultation)
  » Hepatomegaly
  » Signs of poor perfusion, such as:
    › Pallor
    › Cold extremities
    › Mottled skin
    › Prolonged capillary refill
    › Weak pulses
    › Diaphoresis
    › Cyanosis
- In infants, always ask about issues related to feeding and growth, as feeding mimics a cardiac stress test in pediatric patients. Watch for the following:
  » History of poor feeding
  » Diaphoresis and/or dyspnea during feeding
  » Failure to thrive

Investigations

- The laboratory workup for cardiogenic shock should include:
  » Cardiac indicators:
    › Troponin
    › N-terminal pro b-type natriuretic peptide (NT-proBNP)
      · Levels of NT-proBNP can be elevated for the first few days after birth.
      · Increased levels of NT-proBNP are seen in the presence of high intraventricular pressures and can indicate heart failure.
      · Elevated levels of NT-proBNP correlate with level of functional capacity.
  » Indicators of shock and end-organ perfusion:
    › pH, lactate, and $ScvO_2$ (when available)
    › Blood urea nitrogen (BUN) and creatinine (indicating renal function)

- Aspartate transaminase (AST), alanine transaminase (ALT), gamma-glutamyl transferase (GGT), alkaline phosphatase, and bilirubin (indicating liver enzymes and function)
  - Clotting parameters (international normalized ratio [INR], partial thromboplastin time [PTT], glucose)
  - Complete blood count (CBC)
    · Ensure the patient is not anemic and hematocrit is normal.
  » Electrolytes
    › Sodium, potassium, calcium, magnesium, phosphate
- Consider these imaging studies:
  » Electrocardiogram (ECG)
    › Look for possible arrhythmias, ST-changes, and QT-interval prolongation.
  » Chest X-ray (CXR)
    › Check for signs of cardiomegaly or pulmonary edema.
  » Transthoracic echocardiogram
    › Check for left ventricle (LV) and right ventricle (RV) function, valvular disease, and congenital anatomical heart disease.

Management
- Involve specialists early, including pediatric cardiology, pediatric intensive care, pediatric cardiac surgery, pediatric anesthesia.
- If necessary, contact other centers with more expertise.

Initial Management
- Restore adequate oxygen delivery to tissues.
  » Follow pediatric advanced life support (PALS) guidelines on resuscitation.
  » Aim for oxygen supplementation $SaO_2 > 95\%$ (or normal baseline in case of cyanotic congenital heart disease).
  » Optimize ventricular preload.
    › Administer a very careful fluid titration of 2.5 ml/kg crystalloid bolus.
      · Aggressive fluid boluses have been shown to increase mortality.
    › Reassess the patient after each bolus for worsening heart failure and/or pulmonary edema.
    › In case of heart failure, consider diuretics only if there are no clinical signs of shock (furosemide 1 mg/kg IV bolus).
  » Consider inotropes early (central access is not required; in emergency department [ED], IO or IV are acceptable). These include:

    › Epinephrine infusion 0.05 to 0.1 mcg/kg per minute IV (if signs of shock are present)
    › Milrinone infusion 0.2 to 0.75 mcg/kg per minute IV
    › Dobutamine 5 to 20 mcg/kg per minute IV
  » Use positive pressure ventilation (PPV) to reduce LV afterload.
    › Noninvasive ventilation (such as continuous positive airway pressure [CPAP]) is preferable to invasive ventilation to avoid risk of cardiac arrest during intubation.
  » Discontinue cardiodepressive medications (i.e., beta-blockers, etc.).
  » Transfuse packed red blood cells (RBCs) if hemoglobin level is insufficient for adequate oxygen delivery.
    › A higher hemoglobin level may be required in cases of congenital cyanotic heart disease.
  » Consider venoarterial extracorporeal membrane oxygenation (ECMO) if the patient is refractory to conventional therapy.
- Correct the underlying cause:
  » Arrhythmia (avoid giving beta-blockers or calcium channel blockers)
  » Electrolyte disturbance
  » Thromboembolic disorder
  » Pneumothorax
  » Tamponade
  » Infection
  » Duct dependent congenital cardiac lesion
- Minimize cardiac oxygen demand (requires PICU admission).
  » Use sedation as tolerated by patient; be aware that sedation can lead to significant deterioration.
  » Prevent fever.

Hospital Admission
- Admit to a PICU with expertise in pediatric cardiac care.
- For long-distance transport, a team with expertise in cardiac critical care and transport should be found.

REFERENCES

Bronicki RA, Taylor M, Baden H. Critical heart failure and shock. *Pediatr Crit Care Med.* 2016;17(8 Suppl 1):S124–S130. https://doi.org/10.1097/PCC.0000000000000777. Medline:27490590

Epstein D, Wetzel RC. Cardiovascular physiology and shock. In: Nichols DG, Ungerleider RM, Spevak PJ, et al. editors. *Critical heart disease in infants and children.* 2nd ed. Philadelphia, PA: Mosby Elsevier; 2006:17–72.

3.2

Supraventricular Tachycardia

Tim Lynch

- Supraventricular tachycardia (SVT) is the most common pediatric arrhythmia requiring treatment in the emergency department (ED).
- SVT has an estimated incidence of 1 per 250 well-appearing children.
- Its presentation and heart rates vary based on age.

Table 3.2.1. SVT HEART RATES AND SYMPTOMS BY AGE

	Infant	Child
Heart rate (bpm)	≥ 220	≥ 180
Presenting symptoms	• Nonspecific • Vomiting • Irritability • Diaphoresis • Grunting • Cyanosis • Poor feeding	• Cardiorespiratory • Palpitations • Chest pain • Syncope • Dizziness • Shortness of breath

- Complications are rare but may include:
  » Congestive heart failure
  » Shock

Pathophysiology

- SVT is most commonly caused by a reentry mechanism involving an accessory atrioventricular (AV) pathway.
  » AV nodal reentry tachycardia (AVNRT) is the most common.
    › Depending on pathway and circuit, conduction through AV node may be antegrade or retrograde.
    › There are two distinct pathways with different rates of conduction and different refractory periods:
      · α pathway — slow conduction with short refractory period
      · β pathway — fast conduction with long refractory period
  » AV reentry tachycardia (AVRT) is less common.
    › AVRT involves the Wolff-Parkinson-White (WPW) pathway.

Risk Factors

- Risk factors for SVP include:
  » Underlying cardiac lesion:
    › Abnormal electrophysiology — WPW syndrome
    › Structural lesion 20% — Ebstein anomaly, repaired transposition of the great arteries, single ventricle lesions
  » Drugs:
    › Sympathomimetics — cold medications, cocaine
    › Energy drinks with high levels of caffeine

Diagnosis

- Electrocardiogram (ECG) findings associated with SVP include:
  » Heart rate ≥ 220 bpm in infants and ≥ 180 bpm in children and adolescents
  » No identifiable P-waves due to increased heart rate
  » Inability to measure PR interval and QRS < 0.09 seconds (narrow complex)
- Note that:
  » SVT with aberrant conduction may be due to WPW or a bundle branch block
    · Treat as ventricular tachycardia until proven otherwise.
  » Brugada syndrome criteria have not been validated in pediatric patients
- Beat-to-beat variability with activity is **not** associated with SVT.

Management

- Ensure the patient is monitored, with oxygen and vascular access (IV or IO).
  » Monitor and record ECG continuously during any vagal maneuver or any pharmacologic or electrical therapy.
- Start with vagal maneuvers to slow conduction through the AV node.
  » Carotid massage is contraindicated in infants and young children, and ocular pressure is potentially harmful and should be avoided.

- In infants:
  - › Apply ice to face to take advantage of the diving reflex (use crushed ice in a bag with water and apply to the forehead and bridge of nose for 20 seconds).
  - › Do not cover the nose or mouth.
- In children:
  - › Ask them to blow into a straw to inflate an attached glove to create a Valsalva maneuver
  — **or** —
  - › Ask them to bear down like they are trying to have a bowel movement

STABLE PATIENT WITH ADEQUATE PERFUSION

- Treat stable patients with adequate perfusion with adenosine.
  - » Adenosine blocks conduction through the AV node.
  - » Adenosine has a short half-life of 10 seconds, so either administer as an IV/IO push followed by a bolus of normal saline or use a double syringe setup.
  - » Give first dose as a 0.1 mg/kg (maximum 6 mg) IV push.
    - › For repeat doses, give 0.2 mg/kg (maximum 12 mg).
  - » Adenosine can cause chest pain and a short period of asystole.
  - » It is safe to use in pregnancy.
- Alternative agents:
  - » Amiodarone 5 mg/kg over 10 minutes
    - › Amiodarone is a class III antiarrhythmic.
    - › It increases refractoriness.
    - › Watch for signs of hypotension.
  - » Procainamide 15 mg/kg over 15 minutes
    - › Procainamide is a class Ia antiarrhythmic.
    - › It slows conduction and increases refractoriness.
    - › Do not use with amiodarone due to QT interval prolongation.
    - › Watch for signs of hypotension and QT prolongation.
- Verapamil is contraindicated in infants because of the possibility of cardiac arrest and shock-refractory hypotension due to its negative inotropic effect.
- Consider synchronized cardioversion.
  - » If patient is stable, consider procedural sedation (See Chapter 1.5).
  - » Give an initial dose of 0.5 to 1.0 J/kg.
  - » For subsequent doses, give 2.0 J/kg.

UNSTABLE PATIENT WITH POOR PERFUSION

- Consider vagal maneuvers while preparing adenosine and electrical cardioversion.
  - » If IV is already present, administer adenosine.
  - » If adenosine is ineffective, then initiate synchronized cardioversion at 0.5 to 1.0 J/kg.
    - › If this is unsuccessful, then initiate synchronized cardioversion at 2.0 J/kg.

POSTCARDIOVERSION

- Postcardioversion, repeat ECG to look for any signs of preexcitation.
  - » WPW findings include:
    - › Short PR interval
    - › Delta wave — slurred upstroke of QRS complex
    - › Widened QRS
    - › Possible ST- and T-wave discordant changes
- Investigate the cause of SVT.
  - » Look for risk factors on history.
  - » Order bloodwork:
    - › Hemoglobin — check to rule out anemia
    - › Electrolytes
    - › Blood gas and lactate
    - › Thyroid-stimulating hormone (TSH)
  - » Order a chest X-ray (CXR).
  - » Check 4 limb blood pressure.

Disposition

- Unstable patients with inadequate perfusion should be admitted to hospital postcardioversion.
- For stable patients with adequate perfusion:
  - » Admit infants for monitoring and cardiology assessment
  - » Discuss child and adolescent cases with on-call cardiologist and outpatient consultation
- Prognosis is excellent if there are no cardiac structural lesions present.

REFERENCES

American Heart Association. *Pediatric advanced life support provider manual.* First American Heart Association printing; 2016:259–275.

Fleisher GR, Ludwig S. *Textbook of pediatric emergency medicine.* 5th ed. Baltimore: Williams and Wilkins; 2010:596–600, 706–11.

Salerno JC, Seslar SP. Supraventricular tachycardia. *Arch Pediatr Adolesc Med.* 2009;163(3):268–274. https://doi.org/10.1001/archpediatrics.2008.547. Medline:19255396

Sanatani S, Potts JE, Reed JH, et al. The study of antiarrhythmic medications in infancy (SAMIS): a multicenter, randomized controlled trial comparing the efficacy and safety of digoxin versus propranolol for prophylaxis of supraventricular tachycardia in infants. *Circ Arrhythm Electrophysiol.* 2012;5(5):984–991. https://doi.org/10.1161/CIRCEP.112.972620. Medline:22962431

3.3

Acute Pericarditis

Melissa Chan

- Acute pericarditis is the inflammation of the pericardial sac with or without pericardial effusion.
- It accounts for 1% to 5% of children who present to the emergency department (ED) with chest pain.
- Idiopathic and viral pericarditis are the most common causes of acute pericarditis in North America.
- Adolescent males are the most commonly affected.

Pathophysiology

- In most cases, infiltration of pericardial tissue by granulocytes and lymphocytes results in a fibrous reaction, creating exudate and adhesions.
- Etiologies may be:
  - » Infectious
    - › Viral infection is more common than bacterial in developed world.
    - › Tuberculosis (TB) is the most common infectious cause of acute pericarditis worldwide.
  - » Autoimmune (e.g., systemic lupus erythematosus, rheumatic fever, rheumatoid arthritis)
  - » Metabolic and endocrine (e.g., uremia, thyroid disease)
  - » Oncologic
  - » Postcardiotomy
  - » Idiopathic (40% to 70%)
- Inflammation can be contiguous to the myocardium, resulting in myopericarditis.
- Inflammation can result in a pericardial effusion.

Diagnosis

Based on criteria from the European Society of Cardiology.

- Acute pericarditis is an inflammatory pericardial syndrome that can be diagnosed with at least 2 of the 4 following criteria:
  1. Pericarditic chest pain (> 85% to 90% of cases)
  2. Pericardial rubs (≤ 33% of cases)
  3. New widespread ST elevation or PR depression on electrocardiogram (ECG) (up to 60% of cases)
  4. Pericardial effusion (new or worsening, up to 60% of cases)
- Additional supporting findings include:
  - » Elevated markers of inflammation such as:
    - › C-reactive protein (CRP)

- › Erythrocyte sedimentation rate (ESR)
- › White blood cell (WBC) count
- » Evidence of pericardial inflammation seen with specialized imaging technique (i.e., cardiac CT or MRI)

History

- The patient history should include information about:
  - » Chest pain (usually pleuritic) that improves by sitting up or leaning forward
  - » Travel history
  - » History of cardiac surgery
  - » Autoimmune or metabolic conditions
  - » Cancer
    - › Is the child currently a cancer patient currently on active chemotherapy?

Physical Exam

- The physical exam should check for:
  - » Vital signs
    - › Fever
    - › Tachycardia
    - › Tachypnea
  - » Presence of a pericardial rub

Investigations

- Initiate laboratory workup for:
  - » Recommended inflammatory markers: WBC, ESR, CRP
  - » Electrolytes — to rule out other causes of electrocardiogram (ECG) changes
  - » Troponins — may be elevated
  - » Blood cultures — often negative but should be drawn if fever or other signs of sepsis
- Chest X-ray (CXR) is recommended to rule out pulmonary pathology; however, it is generally normal unless there is a large pericardial effusion.
- Look for classic stages for acute pericarditis on ECG:
  - » Stage 1: diffuse ST elevation
  - » Stage 2: normalization of ST elevations, start of PR depressions: flattening of the T-waves
  - » Stage 3: T-wave inversion
  - » Stage 4: normalization of the ECG
- Echocardiogram is recommended for all acute cases of pericarditis, with urgent assessment if pericardial effusion/tamponade suspected.

Management

- Any hemodynamically unstable patient or any patient with a large effusion or tamponade requires emergent consultation and admission.
  » Request a cardiology / surgical / intensive care consult and possible pericardiocentesis.
- If the patient appears ill and you suspect a bacterial cause, cover with broad spectrum antibiotics.
  » *Staphylococcus* and *Streptococcus* are the most common bacterial pathogens.
- Consider admission if the patient has high-risk features (see "Prognosis," below).
- A surgical consultation may be required for patients with constrictive, recurrent, or purulent pericarditis.
- Treat the underlying cause, if known.
- For uncomplicated, well-appearing patients with no risk factors, supportive care is the mainstay of treatment. This may include:
  » Nonpharmacologic measures
    › Patients should limit physical activity and abstain from competitive activities until symptoms and tests normalize.
  » Nonsteroidal anti-inflammatory drugs (NSAIDs)
    › NSAIDs are first-line treatment for viral and idiopathic causes.
    › No studies currently exist that compare types of NSAIDs.
    › Dosing:
      · 30 to 50 mg/kg per 24 hours divided every 8 hours
      · Maximum of 2.4 g per day
  » Colchicine
    › Colchicine can be considered as an adjunct to NSAIDs for recurrent pericarditis.
    › Dosing:
      · For children ≤ 5 years, give 0.5 mg per day

- For children > 5 years, give 1.0 to 1.5 mg per day in 2 or 3 divided doses
    › Few pediatric studies and limited evidence exist for colchicine use in cases of pericarditis.
  » Steroids
    › Steroids are not routinely recommended unless pericarditis has an autoimmune cause.
    › Evidence is limited for steroid use; steroids may increase chances of recurrence.
    › If used, low-dose steroids are recommended (e.g., prednisone 0.2 to 0.5 mg/kg per day).

Prognosis

- High-risk factors for a poor prognosis include:
  » Fever > 38°C
  » Subacute course
  » Large pericardial effusion or cardiac tamponade
  » Failure to respond to NSAIDs within 7 days

REFERENCES

Adler Y, Charron P, Imazio M, et al; European Society of Cardiology (ESC). 2015 ESC guidelines for the diagnosis and management of pericardial diseases: the Task Force for the Diagnosis and Management of Pericardial Diseases of the European Society of Cardiology (ESC). *Eur Heart J.* 2015;36(42):2921–2964. https://doi.org/10.1093/eurheartj/ehv318. Medline:26320112

Bergmann KR, Kharbanda A, Haveman L. Myocarditis and pericarditis in the pediatric patient: validated management strategies. *Pediatr Emerg Med Pract.* 2015;12(7):1–22, quiz 23. Medline:26197653

Imazio M, Brucato A, Cemin R, et al; ICAP Investigators. A randomized trial of colchicine for acute pericarditis. *N Engl J Med.* 2013;369(16):1522–1528. https://doi.org/10.1056/NEJMoa1208536. Medline:23992557

Imazio M, Gaita F, LeWinter M. Evaluation and treatment of pericarditis: a systematic review. *JAMA.* 2015;314(14):1498–1506. https://doi.org/10.1001/jama.2015.12763. Medline:26461998

Lilly LS. Treatment of acute and recurrent idiopathic pericarditis. *Circulation.* 2013;127(16):1723–1726. https://doi.org/10.1161/CIRCULATIONAHA.111.066365. Medline:23609551

3.4

Syncope and Breath-holding Episodes

Andrew Dixon

SYNCOPE

- Syncope is the temporary loss of consciousness from reversible disruption of cerebral functioning due to inadequate cardiac output with resultant cerebral hypoperfusion.
- Syncope is a presenting symptom in 1% to 3% of pediatric emergency department (ED) visits.
  - » It accounts for 6% of hospital admissions.
  - » It is more common in adolescents than in younger children.
    - › 15% to 25% of adolescents experience at least 1 episode of syncope.
- 10% to 15% of patients who present to the pediatric ED for evaluation of syncope are ultimately diagnosed with a serious illness.
- About 80% of pediatric fainting is neurocardiogenic syncope (also known as vasovagal or reflex syncope).
  - » Neurologic disorders — mostly seizures — account for about 10% of episodes of transient loss of consciousness.
  - » 2% to 3% of these are due to cardiac pathology.

Pathophysiology

Neurocardiogenic syncope is from a stimulus (pain, fear, anxiety, or other stimulus) that causes venous pooling in the legs (increased capacitance)

Leading to:

- » A decrease in ventricular preload
  — **and** —
- » A compensatory increase in heart rate and contractility with the relatively empty left ventricle

Triggering:

- » An exaggerated Bezold-Jarisch reflex, which both decreases sympathetic drive and increases vagal tone, leading to bradycardia, hypotension, or both

History

- History should include the following pertinent items:
  - » Hydration status
  - » Last meal
  - » Environmental conditions
    - › Where and when did the syncopal event take place?
  - » Activity preceding the event
    - › Syncope related to exertion is more worrisome.
  - » Use of drugs
  - » Medications that the patient is taking, and those other members of the family are taking
  - » Position of the child at the time of the event
  - » Family history of structural cardiac disease, dysrhythmias, sudden death, migraines, or seizures
  - » Prodromes
    - › Sensation of warmth, nausea, lightheadedness, and a visual gray-out or tunneling of vision are indicative of benign neurocardiogenic syncope.
- Statements by witnesses that the patient appeared dead and required CPR must be taken seriously and should be comprehensively evaluated.
- Loss of consciousness occurs *with* the onset of movements in seizures, but loss of consciousness *precedes* movements in most cases of true syncope.

Table 3.4.1. EVENTS EASILY MISTAKEN FOR CARDIOVASCULAR SYNCOPE

Condition	Distinguishing characteristics
Basilar migraine	Headache, loss of consciousness (rare), other neurologic symptoms
Seizure	Loss of consciousness simultaneous with motor event; may have a prolonged postictal phase
Vertigo	Rotation or spinning sensation without loss of consciousness
Hyperventilation	Inciting event, paresthesias or carpopedal spasm, and tachypnea
Hysteria	No loss of consciousness, and patient may be indifferent to the event
Hypoglycemia	Confusion progressing to loss of consciousness; patient requires glucose administration to recover

Risk Factors

- Risk factors for a serious cause of syncope include:
  - » Episode occurred mid–exertional event
  - » Patient is < 6 years old
  - » Patient has a history of cardiac disease or pathologic heart murmur
  - » Patient's family has a history of sudden death, long QT syndrome, sensorineural hearing loss, or cardiac disease
  - » Recurrent episodes of syncope
  - » Episode occurred while sitting or lying down
  - » Patient experienced prolonged loss of consciousness
  - » Premonitory symptoms and physical precipitating factors were absent
  - » Patient uses medications that can alter cardiac conduction

Physical Exam

- Complete cardiovascular, neurologic, and pulmonary examinations are important.
  - » Findings are usually normal, regardless of the seriousness of the cause.
- Assess the patient's postural vital signs.
- Any abnormal findings in the cardiovascular assessment require an in-depth cardiac evaluation.

Investigations

- An electrocardiogram (ECG) should be done for all children presenting with syncope in whom any risk factors for cardiac disease are present.
  - » A detailed history, physical exam, and ECG have a 96% sensitivity for detecting cardiac syncope.
  - » Review the ECG for signs of:
    - › Conduction abnormalities:
      - · Tachyarrhythmias — supraventricular tachycardia (SVT), Wolff-Parkinson-White (WPW) syndrome, congenital prolonged QT syndrome
      - · Bradyarrhythmias — atrioventricular (AV) blocks
    - › Structural abnormalities:
      - · Left ventricular hypertrophy (LVH) — high voltage
      - · Arrhythmogenic right ventricular dysplasia — epsilon wave
    - › Drugs/toxins:
      - · Tricyclic antidepressant (TCA) toxicity; medications that can increase QT
- Consider performing a chest X-ray (CXR) and capillary blood glucose test.
- Routine laboratory studies are not needed in a child with a clear episode of vasovagal syncope.
- Only consider laboratory workups in patients with an atypical presentation; persistent, decreased level of consciousness in the ED; or other worrisome associated symptoms.
  - » A serum chemistry panel, hematocrit, thyroid function test, or chest radiograph may be warranted in the ED if indicated by history.
- An electroencephalogram (EEG) has a very low diagnostic yield in syncope and should not be used routinely.

Note: For the majority of patients, a careful history for red flags, a complete cardiac and neurologic exam, postural vital signs, and an ECG constitute an appropriate emergency workup. If all of these are normal, a diagnosis of neurocardiogenic syncope is likely and no further testing is required in the ED.

Management

- Most children who experience syncope are already fully recovered upon arrival at the ED.
- A continued altered level of consciousness should prompt an evaluation for continued neurologic, cardiovascular, or psychological derangements.
- Treatment of neurocardiogenic syncope includes reassurance, increased water intake (1.5 to 2.5 L per day or until urine is consistently clear) and salt intake (2 to 5 g per day), and isometric counterpressure maneuvers.

Disposition

- If, after an appropriately thorough history taking, a physical examination, and an ECG, no concerning features are elicited, the child may be discharged home with follow-up by the child's primary physician.
- Children with cardiac histories or risk factors may require admission or follow-up with pediatric cardiology.
  - » Consider referring the patient for an echocardiogram.

BREATH-HOLDING EPISODES

- Breath-holding episodes are most commonly seen in children 6 to 18 months of age, but can be seen as late as 4 years old.
- The event usually occurs when the child experiences an emotional or minor physical trauma.
- Usually the child cries excessively for about a minute, resulting in a breath-holding episode and brief loss of consciousness.
- A breath-holding episode often occurs with facial cyanosis or pallor with an appearance of being dazed, and can involve involuntary muscle twitching, all of which can be quite dramatic to the observer.

- Episodes are categorized as:
  - » Cyanotic — more common (about 55% to 85% of cases)
  - » Pallid — commonly associated with myoclonic jerks that can be confused with a seizure

History

- Get a good history of the events surrounding the episode.
- Ask about the need for CPR or blowing on the face.
- Ask whether there was a seizure-like episode.

Physical Exam

- Conduct physical exam as with syncope, above.

Investigations

- Consider an ECG to rule out prolonged QT syndrome.
- Breath-holding episodes can be associated with iron deficiency anemia.
  - » Consider testing iron and ferritin levels.

Management

- These are benign, self-limited episodes and do not require further investigation or treatment.

REFERENCES

DiMario FJ. Prospective study of children with cyanotic and pallid breath-holding spells. *Pediatrics*. 2001;107(2):265–269. https://doi.org/10.1542/peds.107.2.265. Medline:11158456

Goldman RD. Breath-holding spells in infants. *Can Fam Physician*. 2015;61(2):149–150. Medline:25676645

Ikiz MA, Cetin II, Ekici F, Güven A, Değerliyurt A, Köse G. Pediatric syncope: is detailed medical history the key point for differential diagnosis? *Pediatr Emerg Care*. 2014;30(5):331–334. https://doi.org/10.1097/PEC.0000000000000123. Medline:24759488

Manolis AS. Evaluation of patients with syncope: focus of age-related differences. *Am Coll Cardiol Curr J Rev*. 1994;3(13).

Massin MM, Bourguignont A, Coremans C, Comté L, Lepage P, Gérard P. Syncope in pediatric patients presenting to an emergency department. *J Pediatr*. 2004;145(2):223–228. https://doi.org/10.1016/j.jpeds.2004.01.048. Medline:15289772

McHarg ML, Shinnar S, Rascoff H, Walsh CA. Syncope in childhood. *Pediatr Cardiol*. 1997;18(5):367–371. https://doi.org/10.1007/s002469900202. Medline:9270107

Moodley M. Clinical approach to syncope in children. *Semin Pediatr Neurol*. 2013;20(1):12–17. https://doi.org/10.1016/j.spen.2012.12.003. Medline:23465769

Prodinger RJ, Reisdorff EJ. Syncope in children. *Emerg Med Clin North Am*. 1998;16(3):617–626, ix. https://doi.org/10.1016/S0733-8627(05)70021-3. Medline:9739778

Ritter S, Tani LY, Etheridge SP, Williams RV, Craig JE, Minich LL. What is the yield of screening echocardiography in pediatric syncope? *Pediatrics*. 2000;105(5):e58. https://doi.org/10.1542/peds.105.5.e58. Medline:10799622

Yilmaz U, Doksoz O, Celik T, Akinci G, Mese T, Sevim Yilmaz T. The value of neurologic and cardiologic assessment in breath holding spells. *Pak J Med Sci*. 2014;30(1):59–64. Medline:24639832

3.5

Congenital Heart Disease

Eman Loubani

- The incidence of congenital heart disease (CHD) is 12 to 14 per 1000 live births.
  - » Incidence has increased due to improved detection of milder cases through echocardiography and other advanced technologies.
- The vast majority of CHD is of unknown etiology; most cases are assumed to be multifactorial involving both environmental and genetic factors. These may include:
  - » Genetic predisposition
    - › Trisomy 21
    - › Turner syndrome
    - › DiGeorge syndrome
  - » Environmental association
    - › Toxins
    - › Drugs
    - › Infections

- Rarely, CHD is linked to a single gene defect.
- CHD can be classified as acyanotic or cyanotic.

ACYANOTIC CONGENITAL HEART DEFECTS

- Acyanotic congenital heart defects account for approximately 65% of CHD.
  - » This category of CHD is further subdivided into:
    - › Left-to-right shunting acyanotic lesions
      - · These are defects in the division between the left and right cardiac structures.
      - · Shunting of oxygenated blood occurs from left (high pressure) to right (lower pressure) sides of the heart.

· Clinical manifestations are due to fluid overload.

· Lesions include atrial septal defects, ventricular septal defects, and patent ductus arteriosus (PDA).

› Obstructive acyanotic lesions

· These lesions are characterized by significant narrowing of valve or blood vessel.

· The pressure proximal to the obstruction is greater than the pressure distal to the obstruction.

· Obstructive acyanotic lesions may result in hypertrophy of cardiac chamber proximal to site of obstruction.

· Lesions include aortic coarctation and aortic stenosis.

ATRIAL SEPTAL DEFECT (ASD)

- ASD accounts for 13% of CHD.
- ASD is caused by a deficiency of tissue in the region of the fossa ovalis.
- There are 4 types of ASD (all with essentially the same clinical presentation):
  1. Ostium secundum (fossa ovalis defect) — 50% to 80% of ASD cases
  2. Ostium primum — 30% of ASD cases
  3. Sinus venosus defect — 10% of ASD cases
  4. Coronary sinus ASD

Physical Exam

- Patients are usually asymptomatic.
- Auscultation shows wide split S2 or fixed split S2 with no variation with respiration.
- Listen for a pulmonary systolic ejection murmur in the left upper sternal border (due to increased flow across pulmonary valve) and soft middiastolic flow murmur at the left lower sternal border (secondary to large volume flow across tricuspid valve).
- Patients with a large defect may present with symptoms of congestive heart failure; this is rare.

Investigations

- Chest X-ray (CXR) findings include:
  » Cardiomegaly (if ASD is significant enough to result in congestive heart failure)
  » A prominent main pulmonary artery
  » Increased pulmonary vascular markings
- Electrocardiogram (ECG) findings:
  » May be normal in children with small ASD
  » May show right ventricular (RV) hypertrophy and rSR[1] in right chest leads

Management

- Employ conservative management in mild to moderate cases.
  » 80% of small defects spontaneously close by 2 years of age.
- Use surgical closure in severe cases that include right heart enlargement, pulmonary overcirculation, and/or substantial left-to-right shunting through the ASD.

VENTRICULAR SEPTAL DEFECT (VSD)

- VSD is the most common congenital heart defect.
  » It is found in up to 2% to 5% of newborns on echocardiography, but most defects close spontaneously and are never symptomatic.
- VSD is associated with:
  » Down syndrome
  » Parental use of marijuana and cocaine
- VSD is classified based on size and location:
  » Size
    › Very small
    › Small — pulmonary to systemic flow ratio < 2
    › Moderate — pulmonary to systemic flow ratio > 2
    › Large — the same size as aortic root
  » Location
    › Perimembranous (70% of all VSDs)
      · In upper region of ventricular septum (beneath tricuspid valve)
    › Muscular/trabecular (20%)
      · In muscular wall between the right and left ventricles
    › Outlet/infundibular/conal (5%)
      · Between left and right ventricular outflow tracts
      · Just below pulmonary valve
    › Inlet (5%)
      · In the posterior portion of ventricular septum
      · Behind tricuspid valve

Physical Exam

- The clinical presentation depends on the size and location of the VSD.
  » In cases of very small / small VSD:
    › The defect often presents with asymptomatic cardiac murmur (grade 3/6 systolic murmur best heard at the left lower sternal border)
  » In cases of moderate/large VSD:
    › A murmur is usually detected later (> 6 weeks old)
    › The defect presents with signs and symptoms of congestive heart failure, including tachypnea, poor feeding, poor weight gain, and hepatomegaly

Investigations

- CXR findings:
  » Are normal for small defects
  » For large defects, may include:
    › Signs of congestive heart failure, including cardiomegaly and increased pulmonary vascular markings
    › Enlarged left atrium, left ventricle, and pulmonary artery
- An ECG can show electrical evidence of left and/or right ventricular hypertrophy.

Management

- For very small / small VSDs:
  » Follow and monitor; these often close spontaneously
- For moderate/large VSDs:
  » Provide nutritional support to optimize weight gain. This may include fortification of breast milk / formula
  » Commence medical management of congestive heart failure, including use of diuretics
  » Consider surgical closure
    › Surgical closure is undertaken in symptomatic patients who are not responding to medical management.

PATENT DUCTUS ARTERIOSUS

- The ductus arteriosus is a connection between the main pulmonary artery and descending aorta that is normally present during fetal development to allow passage of deoxygenated blood from the pulmonary artery to the descending aorta, where it travels to the placenta for oxygenation.
- Normally, there is functional closure of the ductus arteriosus within 12 hours of birth and anatomic closure by 3 weeks of age.
- The incidence of isolated PDA is 6% to 11%.
  » PDA can be associated with other congenital heart defects.
  » There is an increased incidence of PDA in preterm infants.

Physical Exam

- Findings depend on the size of the PDA:
  » Small PDA — asymptomatic murmur
  » Moderate to large PDA — symptoms of congestive heart failure (dyspnea, diaphoresis, poor weight gain)
- Auscultatory findings:
  » Left upper sternal border has a continuous murmur (through both systole and diastole)
    › This is termed a "machinery murmur" due to its rumbling sound and variation between beats.
  » Bounding arterial pulses (found in all but very small PDA)

Investigations

- CXR findings
  » In cases of small PDA, are normal
  » In cases of moderate to large PDA, include cardiomegaly and increased pulmonary vascular markings
- ECG findings are usually normal but may show left atrial and left ventricular enlargement.

Management

- Closure (surgical or transcatheter) is recommended in all cases of PDA to prevent endocarditis.
- If PDA is asymptomatic, closure can be delayed until 6 to 12 months of age.

AORTIC STENOSIS

- Aortic stenosis is categorized as valvular, subvalvular, or supravalvular.
- Valvular aortic stenosis is most common.
  » It is most often secondary to bicuspid aortic valve (fusion of the thickened, nonpliable valve leaflets).

Physical Exam

- Most aortic stenosis is asymptomatic with incidental findings of systolic ejection murmur best heard at the right upper sternal border with radiation to the carotids.
- There may be increased left ventricular (LV) impulse.

Investigations

- CXR findings:
  » In most cases show no cardiomegaly
  » May show cardiomegaly in neonates or if progression to heart failure occurs
  » May show dilated ascending aorta
- ECG findings:
  » May be normal or may show LV hypertrophy
  » In severe aortic stenosis, show inverted T-waves in the left sided chest leads

Management

- Treat aortic stenosis with balloon aortic valvuloplasty.

COARCTATION OF THE AORTA

- Coarctation of the aorta accounts for 4% to 6% of CHD.
- It is juxtaductal, occurring around the site of the insertion of the ductus arteriosus into the aorta, distal to the left subclavian artery.
- It is most commonly in the thoracic aorta, though (rarely) it can occur in the abdominal aorta.
- It is commonly associated with other CHDs:
  » PDA, ASD, aortic stenosis, bicuspid aortic valve

Physical Exam

Neonates

- Coarctation of the aorta presenting in the neonatal period is usually more severe.
- Neonates may present with:
  » Absent/delayed femoral pulses (compared with brachial pulse)
  » Symptoms of congestive heart failure and shock:
    › Diaphoresis
    › Dyspnea
    › Pallor
    › Irritability

Older Infant or Child

- Findings are subtle; most patients are asymptomatic.
- Four-limb blood pressures (BPs) show lower systolic BP in lower extremities versus upper extremities.
- Patients may present with:
  » Brachial-femoral delay
  » Hypertension

Adult

- Most patients are asymptomatic.
- Patients may present with:
  » Hypertension
  » Symptoms of claudication of lower extremities, especially with exercise

Investigations

- CXR findings include:
  » In neonates, cardiomegaly and increased pulmonary vasculature (secondary to congestive heart failure)
  » In older children and adults, rib notching (may be seen)
    › If present, rib notching will be found in posterior third of ribs 3 to 8 due to erosion of the ribs by collateral vessels
- ECG findings may be normal, but:
  » In cases of severe defect (presenting in the neonatal period), ECG may show RV hypertrophy
  » In older children and adults, ECG is usually normal but may show signs of LV hypertrophy (increased voltage, ST- and T-wave changes in the left precordial leads).

Management

Neonates

- In cases of congestive heart failure, administer diuretics or digitalis.
- For shock, administer a prostaglandin E1 (PGE1) infusion to reopen PDA.
  » This stabilizes the patient until definitive management can be instituted.

Older Children / Adults

- For hypertension, the only effective treatment is to relieve obstruction immediately with:
  » Surgical correction
    › Resection with end-to-end anastomosis.
    › This is preferred for long segment coarctations.
  » Balloon angioplasty of narrowed segment
    › This can be used in smaller segment involvement.

CYANOTIC CONGENITAL HEART DEFECTS

- Cyanotic congenital heart defects can be classified as:
  » Ductal dependent
    › Tetralogy of Fallot
    › Tricuspid atresia
    › Pulmonary atresia or stenosis
  » Ductal independent
    › Truncus arteriosus
    › Transposition of the great arteries
    › Total anomalous pulmonary venous return
    › Hypoplastic left heart syndrome

TETRALOGY OF FALLOT

- Tetralogy of Fallot accounts for 10% of all CHDs; it is the most common cause of cyanosis in children > 1 year of age.
- The condition consists of 4 cardiac abnormalities:
  1. Large ventricular septal defect (VSD)
  2. Pulmonary stenosis (PS) — varies in severity
  3. RV hypertrophy
  4. Overriding aorta — aorta displaced to the right over the VSD rather than over the left ventricle

Note: Pentalogy of Fallot includes the 4 cardiac abnormalities of Tetralogy of Fallot plus atrial septal defect (ASD).

- 15% of cases are associated with syndromes:
  » Trisomy 21
  » DiGeorge syndrome
  » Alagille syndrome
- 40% of cases are associated with other cardiac anomalies:
  » Right-sided aortic arch
  » Coronary artery anomalies
  » Aorticopulmonary collateral vessels
  » PDA, complete atrioventricular septal defect (AVSD)
  » Aortic valve regurgitation (uncommon)

Physical Exam

- The clinical presentation depends on the degree of PS.
  » Cases with mild PS usually present later in childhood.
  » Cases with severe PS usually present in infancy; cyanosis usually develops between 2 and 6 months of age.

- Presenting symptoms include cyanosis, exercise intolerance, and hypercyanotic ("Tet") spells.
- Clubbing occurs after the first few months of life.
- Auscultatory findings include:
  » Harsh, crescendo-decrescendo systolic ejection murmur best heard at the left upper sternal border
  » Single S2

Investigations

- CXR findings include:
  » A "boot-shaped heart" — upturned apex, concave main pulmonary artery
  » Normal or decreased pulmonary vasculature
- ECG findings include:
  » Right atrial and ventricular enlargement
  » Right axis deviation
  » Prominent R-waves in anterior leads with prominent S-waves in posterior leads
  » May have upright T-waves in V1 after 2 days of life

Management

- Manage via surgical correction.
- Administer antibiotic endocarditis prophylaxis until complete surgical repair is undertaken.

Hypercyanotic Spells (Tet Spells)

- The goal of management is to increase systemic vascular resistance.
- Manage via:
  » Knee to chest position
  » Oxygen
  » Morphine 0.1 mg/kg IV per dose
  » IV fluid bolus 10 to 20 mL/kg normal saline
  » Beta-blockers
    › Beta-blockers are used if the above measures fail to abort the spell.
      · IV propranolol 0.1 mg/kg per dose
      · IV esmolol 0.1 mg/kg per dose

PULMONARY STENOSIS (PS)

- PS may be valvular, subvalvular, or supravalvular.
  » Valvular stenosis is the most common form.

Physical Exam

- PS usually presents with asymptomatic systolic ejection murmur.
- Most cases also have systolic ejection click.
- The splitting of S2 varies, depending on the severity of the stenosis.
  » The greater the severity, the more widely split the S2.

Investigations

- CXR findings include:

  » No cardiomegaly
  » Dilated main pulmonary artery
- ECG findings include:
  » RV hypertrophy
  » Possible right atrial enlargement

Management

- For mild PS:
  » There are no exercise restrictions; follow-up by cardiology for monitoring
  » Condition often remains mild and some cases resolve spontaneously
- For moderate to severe PS:
  » Condition often progresses
  » Manage via balloon pulmonary valvuloplasty; this is the treatment of choice

TRANSPOSITION OF THE GREAT ARTERIES (TGA)

- Transposition of the great arteries (TGA) is the most common cyanotic CHD presenting in neonates (5% of all CHD).
- With TGA, the aorta arises from the right ventricle and the pulmonary artery arises from the left ventricle.

Physical Exam

TGA WITH INTACT SEPTUM

- Cyanosis develops as the ductus arteriosus closes within the first week of life.
- Patients present with progressive tachypnea, lethargy, and poor feeding.

TGA WITH VSD

- TGA with VSD presents with symptoms of congestive heart failure (dyspnea, diaphoresis, poor feeding) at 4 to 8 weeks of age.
- Minimal cyanosis is present.

TGA WITH VSD AND PS

- Presentation depends on the severity of PS.
  » Cases with mild to moderate PS present with congestive heart failure and a later presentation (similar to patients with VSD alone).
  » Cases with severe PS have a similar presentation to patients with Tetralogy of Fallot.

Investigations

- CXR findings include:
  » An "egg-shaped" heart — a classic CXR finding
  » If VSD is present, cardiomegaly and increased pulmonary vascular markings.
  » If VSD and PS are present, cardiomegaly in mild to moderate PS

›   In severe PS, findings may show normal, increased, or decreased pulmonary vascular markings.

- ECG findings:
  »   Is normal in cases of TGA with intact septum
  »   Shows LV hypertrophy, RV hypertrophy, and left atrial enlargement in cases of TGA with VSD
  »   Shows RV hypertrophy with or without LV hypertrophy in cases of TGA with VSD and PS.

Management

- Initial stabilization of the patient involves:
  »   PGE1 infusion (0.05 mcg/kg per minute) to maintain patency of the ductus arteriosus and allow mixing of the parallel circulations
    ›   Complications of PGE1 infusion are:
      ·   Apnea
      ·   Hypotension
      ·   Fever
      ·   Arrhythmias
      ·   Seizure
  »   Balloon atrial septostomy
- For definitive management, an arterial switch operation is the most commonly used procedure at present.

TRICUSPID ATRESIA

- Tricuspid atresia is the third most common cyanotic congenital heart defect, accounting for 1.4% of all CHDs.
- Tricuspid atresia is caused by the absence of the tricuspid valve, leading to a lack of connection between right atrium and right ventricle.
- There must be a connection (atrial septal defect) between right and left atria in order for tricuspid atresia to be survivable in fetal life (this connection is usually in the form of a large patent foramen ovale).
- Tricuspid atresia leads to an enlarged right atrium, an enlarged left atrium, a hypertrophic left ventricle, and a hypoplastic right ventricle.
- Tricuspid atresia is classified as follows:
  »   Type I
    ›   Type I accounts for 70% to 80% of all tricuspid atresia cases.
    ›   Anatomy of the great arteries is normal.
    ›   Type I tricuspid atresia may present with or without ventricular septal defect (VSD).
  »   Type II
    ›   Type II accounts for 12% to 25% of all cases of tricuspid atresia.
    ›   It is characterized by D-transposition of the great arteries (D-TGA).
    ›   All cases have associated VSD.

›   Type III
  ›   Type III accounts for 3% to 6% of all tricuspid atresia.
  ›   It is characterized by malposition of the great arteries other than D-TGA.

Physical Exam

- Half of cases with tricuspid atresia present within 24 hours of birth; most present within the first month of life.
- Patients may present with:
  »   Cyanosis
  »   Cardiac murmur

Investigations

- CXR findings are dependent on the presence or absence of VSD.
  »   With absent or small VSD:
    ›   CXR findings are normal or show decreased pulmonary blood flow, leading to decreased pulmonary vascular markings
    ›   Heart size is normal
  »   With large VSD:
    ›   CXR shows increased pulmonary blood flow, leading to increased pulmonary vascular markings
    ›   CXR shows cardiomegaly.
- ECG may show:
  »   Tall P-waves, left axis deviation, LV hypertrophy, decreased RV forces

Management

- For initial management, maintain patency of ductus arteriosus with PGE1 infusion.
- Management surgically via staged surgical palliation.

REFERENCES

Agrawala B, Bacha E, Cao Q, Hijazi Z. Clinical manifestations & diagnosis of coarctation of the aorta. In: UpToDate. Wolters Kluwer. (Topic updated: Sept 21, 2016). Available from: https://www.uptodate.com/contents/clinical-manifestations-and-diagnosis-of-coarctation-of-the-aorta

Doyle T, Kavanaugh-McHugh A. Pathophysiology, clinical features, and diagnosis of tetralogy of Fallot. In: UpToDate. Wolters Kluwer. (Topic updated: May 6, 2015). Available from: https://www.uptodate.com/contents/pathophysiology-clinical-features-and-diagnosis-of-tetralogy-of-fallot

Hoffman JI. Natural history of congenital heart disease: problems in its assessment with special reference to ventricular septal defects. *Circulation*. 1968;37:97–125.

Hoffman JI. Incidence of congenital heart disease: I. postnatal incidence. *Pediatr Cardiol*. 1995;16(3):103–113.

McDaniel NL. Ventricular and atrial septal defects. *Pediatr Rev*. 2001;22(8):265–270. https://doi.org/10.1542/pir.22-8-265. Medline:11483852

Mitchell SC, Korones SB, Berendes HW. Congenital heart disease in 56,109 births. Incidence and natural history. *Circulation*. 1971;43(3):323–332. https://doi.org/10.1161/01.CIR.43.3.323. Medline:5102136

Syamasundar RP, editor. *Congenital heart disease: selected aspects*. InTech. 2012. Available from: https://www.intechopen.com/books/congenital-heart-disease-selected-aspects

4.1

Seizures

Sasha Litwin, Shelly Weiss

- Seizures account for 1% of pediatric emergency department (ED) visits.
- 4% to 10% of children will experience a seizure in the first 16 years of life.
  » Less than half of this group will have a second seizure.
- The incidence of epilepsy in children ranges from 41 to 187 per 100 000.
  » The prevalence of epilepsy in children is consistently higher than the incidence and ranges from 3.2 to 5.5 per 1000 in developed countries, and 3.6 to 44 per 1000 in underdeveloped countries
- Most seizures are brief; one study showed that, of patients who presented to the pediatric ED, seizures lasted:
  » < 5 minutes in 76%
  » 5 to 30 minutes in 20%
  » 30 to 60 minutes in 2%
  » > 60 minutes in 2%
- Febrile seizures are the most common type of seizure in children presenting to the ED.

Classification

- Seizures can be classified as:
  » Focal onset (previously called partial)
    › Focal onset seizures can be aware (previously called simple) or impaired awareness (previously called complex).
    › Focal onset seizures may be:
      · Motor (e.g., automatisms, atonic, clonic, epileptic spasms)
      · Nonmotor (e.g., autonomic, behavior arrest, cognitive, sensory)
      · Focal to bilateral tonic–clonic

  » Generalized onset
    › Generalized onset seizures always have impaired awareness.
    › Generalized onset seizures may be:
      · Motor (e.g., tonic, clonic, myoclonic, atonic)
      · Nonmotor (absence) (e.g., typical, atypical)
  » Unknown onset
  » Unclassified
- Seizures can also be classified as:
  » Febrile or afebrile
  » Provoked or unprovoked
- Epilepsy is defined as:
  » At least 2 unprovoked seizures occurring more than 24 hours apart
  — **or** —
  » One unprovoked seizure and a high probability of further seizures
  — **or** —
  » The diagnosis of an epileptic syndrome
- Multiple unprovoked seizures within a 24-hour period are considered a single event, so they would not establish the diagnosis of epilepsy.
- It is important to take a careful history in the ED to determine whether there have been previous unrecognized seizures.

History

- Obtain a description of the seizure, including:
  » Events leading up to the seizure
  » Activity at the time of the seizure
  » Any preceding sensations/aura or mood/behavior changes
  » Presence of fever at or around the time of seizure onset

» The duration of the seizure
» Whether the seizure ended spontaneously or whether medication was required
» Postictal state (e.g., lethargy, confusion, headache, or postictal focal changes)
» Further details: laterality (unilateral or bilateral), loss of consciousness, posture, body parts involved, head turning, eye deviation, mouth movements, problems with swallowing (e.g., sialorrhea [drooling]), changes or pauses in breathing, pallor or cyanosis, vocalizations, automatisms, bladder incontinence, lip or tongue biting, other injuries

- Collect a history of possible provoking factors:
  » Trauma (accidental or nonaccidental)
  » Ingestion (e.g., overdose of regular medications, new medications, over the counter medications/supplements, household chemicals, nonprescription drugs, or alcohol use or withdrawal)
  » Metabolic problems (e.g., hypoglycemia, hyperglycemia, hypocalcemia, or hyponatremia)
  » Central nervous system (CNS) neoplasm (e.g., fevers; night sweats; weight loss; vomiting; headaches; or neurologic, behaviour, or personality changes noticed by the family)
  » Genetic diseases or inborn error of metabolism (e.g., coarse facies, previous decompensation with a viral illness, consanguinity)
  » Presence of fever, known infection, or intercurrent illness
    › If fever is present, consider CNS infections such as meningitis and encephalitis.
    › Consider other sources of fever (e.g., viral infection, otitis media, pneumonia, pharyngitis, soft tissue infection, gastroenteritis, urinary tract infection, sepsis).
  » Lifestyle changes (e.g., sleep deprivation, stress)
  » Change in or noncompliance with antiepileptic medications
  » Previous hyper/hypotension or cardiac disease (e.g., syncope or arrhythmias)
  » Pregnancy in adolescents (e.g., eclampsia)
- Other pertinent history includes:
  » Past medical history, including previous seizures, febrile seizures, epilepsy, developmental delay, learning disabilities, genetic or metabolic diseases
  » Medications, over the counter medications or supplements, immunizations
  » Recent travel or contact with visitors from abroad with infectious symptoms
  » Family history of febrile seizures, afebrile seizures, seizure disorders, developmental delay, genetic or metabolic syndromes
  » Consanguinity
  » Previously unrecognized seizures

Red Flags on History

- Red flags on history include:
  » Recent changes in behaviour, learning, or memory
  » Unexplained daytime fatigue
  » New onset nocturnal enuresis
  » New headaches or unexplained emesis

Physical Exam

- For patients who are postictal in the ED, assess:
  » ABCs
  » Level of consciousness
  » Vital signs, including temperature
  » Growth parameters (height, weight, and head circumference)
  » Signs of active infection (e.g., conjunctivitis, bulging tympanic membranes, swollen/exudative oropharynx, rhinorrhea or nasal congestion, respiratory findings, rashes)
  » Signs of meningitis/encephalitis (e.g., decreased level of consciousness, nuchal rigidity, irritability, petechial rash)
  » Signs of raised intracranial pressure (e.g., decreased level of consciousness, dilated pupils, bradycardia, hypertension, abnormal respiration)
  » Signs of trauma (e.g., bruising or bleeding)
  » Neurocutaneous skin findings (e.g., hypopigmented lesions, café au lait spots)
  » Focal neurological signs (e.g., asymmetric pupillary response, unilateral hyper/hypotonicity, clonus or hyper/hyporeflexia, asymmetric plantar response, asymmetric sensory examination, abnormal gait, abnormal cerebellar signs)

Red Flags on Physical Exam

- Red flags on physical exam include:
  » Evidence of acute infection, especially meningitis (e.g., nuchal rigidity, lethargy, irritability)
  » Petechiae/bruising
  » Trauma
  » Change in growth parameters (e.g., change in weight or head circumference if previous growth parameters are available)
  » Evidence of neurocutaneous syndrome
  » Focal neurologic signs

FEBRILE SEIZURES

- Febrile seizures are defined as seizures in children 6 months to 3 years of age with fever over 38ºC that do not result from a metabolic problem, trauma, or CNS infection.
- Febrile seizures are very common, occurring in 2% to 5% of all children and up to 10% of children from some Asian populations.
  » They are equally common in males and females.

» They most commonly occur between 18 and 24 months of age but can occur in children up to 5 years of age.
» In children under 6 months of age, consider a full septic workup, including lumbar puncture for cerebrospinal fluid (CSF) analysis.
- A family history of seizures will be found in 25% to 40% of patients with febrile seizures (multifactorial or autosomal dominant due to sodium and gamma-aminobutyric acid [GABA] channelopathies).
- The incidence of febrile seizure follows a seasonal pattern of viral infections.
- The source of fever is usually undetermined, but if a source is found, it is most commonly acute otitis media.
- Febrile seizures can be classified as:
  » Simple/typical febrile seizures
    › A single event in 24 hours
    › Duration < 15 minutes
    › Nonfocal
    › Generalized tonic–clonic seizure
  » Complex/atypical febrile seizures
    › More than one event in 24 hours
    › Duration > 15 minutes
      · Focal symptomatology
      · Postictal neurological abnormalities (e.g., Todd's paresis)
- Complex/atypical febrile seizures account for one third of all febrile seizures.
- Febrile status epilepticus is a febrile seizure lasting more than 30 minutes.
  » Febrile status epilepticus accounts for 5% of febrile seizures.

Investigations

- For a simple febrile seizure in a well-appearing child, no investigations are required.
  » Consider investigating capillary blood sugar.
  » There is no role for electroencephalogram (EEG) in the acute setting; up to 30% of patients will have transient postictal changes that do not affect management.
  » There is no role for outpatient EEG.
  » Targeted investigations based on clinical history and physical exam may be helpful to determine the cause of the fever (e.g., chest X-ray [CXR] or urinalysis).
- For a complex febrile seizure in a well-appearing child:
  » There are no evidence-based recommendations to guide investigations
  » Incidence of bacteremia, urinary tract infection, and pneumonia are similar in well-appearing children with complex febrile seizures and children with fevers without seizures, so the indications for blood cultures, urinalysis, or imaging is the same in both groups

» Neuroimaging is not routinely recommended but should be considered if the child had a focal seizure or has prolonged postictal focal abnormalities.
» There is no clear role for outpatient EEG.
» A lumbar puncture is necessary if CNS infection is suspected; however:
  › Routine lumbar puncture among children with febrile seizures has been shown to be of limited value for both simple and complex febrile seizures
  › Risk of bacterial meningitis is extremely low without other clinical signs and symptoms
  › A higher level of suspicion is needed if the patient is already on antibiotics or is not vaccinated
- For either type of febrile seizure in an unwell-appearing child, investigations including bloodwork, lumbar puncture, and/or neuroimaging should be guided by the clinical scenario.

Management

- Observe the child in the ED until they are back to baseline activity without focal deficits.
- Counseling plays a major role in the management of these patients. Helpful information to relay to the family includes the following:
  » Febrile seizures are not classified as a type of epilepsy.
  » The risk of developing epilepsy after a febrile seizure is 2% to 5%, which is slightly higher than the risk in the general population.
  » Patients have a 20% or higher risk of having a subsequent febrile seizure.
  » Brain damage from seizure activity is unlikely before at least 45 minutes of continuous seizure activity (according to research in animal models).
  » There is no increased risk of behavioral, developmental, or learning difficulties from simple febrile seizures.
  » There is no evidence that antipyretic medications prevent febrile seizures.
  » There is no evidence that intermittent use of antiepileptic medications during febrile illnesses will prevent febrile seizures.
  » Caregivers should call their local EMS if a seizure lasts for > 3 to 4 minutes; the EMS team may give medication for a seizure lasting more than 5 minutes.

FIRST UNPROVOKED AFEBRILE SEIZURE

- The lifetime incidence of an unprovoked afebrile seizures is 5% in the general population.
- The literature reports that between 30% and 50% of children experience subsequent seizures after a first unprovoked afebrile seizure.
  » About half of seizures recur within 6 months and 88% within 2 years.
  » Very few (3%) recur after 5 years.

Classification

- A fist seizure may be classified as:
  - » A provoked seizure (e.g., caused by medication, metabolic abnormality, toxin)
  - » An acute symptomatic seizure (e.g., trauma, stroke, intracranial infection)
  - » A remote symptomatic seizure (e.g., due to a preexisting brain injury)
  - » A seizure associated with an epileptic syndrome

Investigations

- There is no role for routine laboratory investigations in well-appearing children.
  - » Consider testing sodium, magnesium, calcium, phosphorous, and glucose levels if patient has ongoing seizures in the ED.
  - » Investigations in neonates are guided by clinical scenario.
- Consider screening patients for toxic ingestions if clinically indicated.
- There is no role for routine lumbar puncture in an afebrile, well-appearing patient with no signs or symptoms of meningitis or encephalitis.
- Emergent neuroimaging is recommended for patients with:
  - » Focal seizures
  - » Focal neurologic deficits
  - » Prolonged postictal focal deficits
  - » Persistent altered mental status
  - » Suspected head trauma, especially if the child is on anticoagulants
- Clinically relevant intracranial abnormalities occur in 11% of children with first, unprovoked seizures, but abnormalities requiring ED management occur in < 1%, suggesting that most children do not require neuroimaging in the ED.
  - » Consider CT scan for emergent imaging.
  - » If outpatient neuroimaging is arranged, MRI is the preferred modality.
- There is no role for EEG in the acute setting, but an EEG should be arranged in the outpatient setting.
  - » Using EEG to diagnose epilepsy after a first unprovoked seizure has a sensitivity of 58% and a specificity of 70% in pediatric patients.

Management

- If the seizure has stopped, observe the patient in the ED until the child is back to baseline activity and without focal deficits.
- Consult a pediatrician or pediatric neurologist in the ED or admit for urgent consultation if there are any concerns that the child is not back to baseline or has ongoing focal deficits.

- Antiepileptic medications are not indicated for a first unprovoked afebrile seizure.
- Refer the child to a pediatrician or pediatric neurologist for an EEG and assessment as an outpatient.
  - » EEG as an outpatient can help determine seizure type, epilepsy syndrome, and likelihood of recurrence.
  - » No recommendations exist for postseizure EEG timing.
- Counseling the family is important. Let the family know that:
  - » Referral will be made to a pediatrician or pediatric neurologist for assessment and ongoing care
  - » The consultant physician will arrange for an EEG and determine if there is a need for brain imaging
  - » There is usually no indication for antiepileptic medications after a first afebrile, unprovoked seizure
  - » There are some issues around child safety to be aware of
    - › For adolescents, parents must be aware of local laws regarding driving or the ability to obtain driver's licenses for people with seizures.
    - › Parents should consider taking a CPR course.
    - › Parents should call EMS if a seizure lasts for > 3 to 4 minutes.
    - › Parents should use common sense precautions for a child who has had any seizure (e.g., a responsible adult should always watch the child during any activity in water, such as swimming or bathing, and should decide if the child should participate in active sports).

STATUS EPILEPTICUS

- Status epilepticus is defined as continuous or recurrent seizure activity lasting more than 30 minutes; however, once the seizure lasts more than 5 minutes, it is likely to be prolonged.
  - » The longer seizures continue, the more difficult they are to abort with medications, so early treatment is essential.
- Approximately 10% to 12% of children and adults with a first unprovoked seizure will present with status epilepticus as their first seizure.
- Status epilepticus is more common in children with epilepsy and in infants < 1 year of age.
- The annual incidence of status epilepticus in children is reported as 10 to 73 episodes per 100 000 children and is highest in children < 2 years of age (135 to 156 per 100 000 children).
- Mortality from status epilepticus in children is between 3% to 8%.
- The recurrence rate is 17%.
- The most common cause of status epilepticus is febrile status epilepticus.

Investigations

- There is no clear evidence for or against laboratory testing in status epilepticus; however, glucose and electrolyte abnormalities are easily treated, so testing for them is recommended.
  - » Electrolytes (sodium, calcium) and glucose were abnormal in approximately 6% of children with status epilepticus in one study.
- Check levels of antiepileptic medications for patients regularly taking these medications; interpret findings with caution if you are not evaluating a trough level.
- Maintain a high suspicion for a CNS infection and consider empiric antibiotics and antiviral medication until the patient is stable enough to do a lumbar puncture.
- Blood cultures should be obtained and antibiotics should be given if there is suspicion of infection/sepsis.
- Consider a toxicology screening if it is clinically indicated or if the etiology of the seizure is unknown.
- If clinically indicated, screen for inborn errors of metabolism.
- Neuroimaging is recommended after the patient is stabilized and the seizure has stopped.
  - » MRI is more sensitive than CT scan and is recommended, if available, for first-time status epilepticus.
  - » If MRI is unavailable or trauma is suspected, a CT scan is recommended.
- An EEG should be considered in the acute setting to assess for nonconvulsive status epilepticus and to determine the location and type of seizure.

Management

- The first priority is to stabilize ABCs.
  - » Ensure the patient is in a safe position — lateral decubitus if they are actively vomiting, otherwise supine.
  - » Apply oxygen, position the airway with a chin lift or jaw thrust, suction, and secure the airway if needed.
  - » Assist ventilation as needed.
  - » Obtain IV access or, if unable, insert an IO line.
  - » Check patient's pupillary reactivity, temperature, and point-of-care glucose.

Note: Continuous cardiorespiratory monitoring is essential. Anticonvulsant medications may cause loss of airway reflexes and respiratory depression, hypotension, and cardiac arrhythmias.

- First-line medications:
  - » Benzodiazepines (lorazepam, diazepam, or midazolam)
    - › Initial dose may be repeated once after 5 minutes if the seizure continues.
    - › The second dose of benzodiazepines will be less effective than the first.
    - › If there is no IV access available, intranasal (IN) or buccal midazolam, or sublingual lorazepam, are superior to rectal diazepam.
    - › IV, IN, or IO medications are more effective than IM medications.
- Second-line medications:
  - » Fosphenytoin (if not available, use phenytoin)
    - › Fosphenytoin is the standard first-line treatment for benzodiazepine-resistant seizures in children > 1 year of age; however, this is not evidence based.
    - › Dosing is the same as phenytoin equivalents.
    - › It can be given more quickly than phenytoin and has fewer side effects.
      - · Side effects include hypotension, bradycardia, arrhythmias, severe vascular irritation with extravasation.
    - › Avoid sodium channel blockers such as fosphenytoin in patients with known sodium channelopathies.
    - › If the patient is on phenytoin maintenance, consider phenobarbital for the initial loading dose.
  - » Phenobarbital
    - › Phenobarbital is recommended for infants < 1 year of age.
      - · Side effects include respiratory depression (especially if benzodiazepine has been used), hypotension, sedation.

Note: Levetiracetam or valproate may be considered for children with medically refractory status epilepticus. Further research on the use and efficacy of levetiracetam and valproate in status epilepticus is ongoing for both of these medications.

- If the seizure continues after first- and second-line medications, there is no clear evidence to guide therapy.
  - » Treatment may include escalating therapy with thiopental, pentobarbital, or intravenous midazolam.
- If the patient is unresponsive to second-line agents or if there is any issue of airway compromise, then consider endotracheal intubation, alert the pediatric intensive care unit, and consult pediatric neurology.
  - » Nonconvulsive status epilepticus may continue undetected if paralytics are used for intubation.
- In addition to acute treatment of status epilepticus, identify and treat possible etiologies.
  - » Correct glucose and electrolyte abnormalities if necessary.
  - » Consider that febrile status epilepticus may be caused by a CNS infection, so have a low threshold for giving empiric IV antibiotics/antiviral medications.

Figure 4.1.1. CURRENT TREATMENT GUIDELINES FOR STATUS EPILEPTICUS AT THE HOSPITAL FOR SICK CHILDREN, TORONTO, ONTARIO, AS OF MARCH 2017

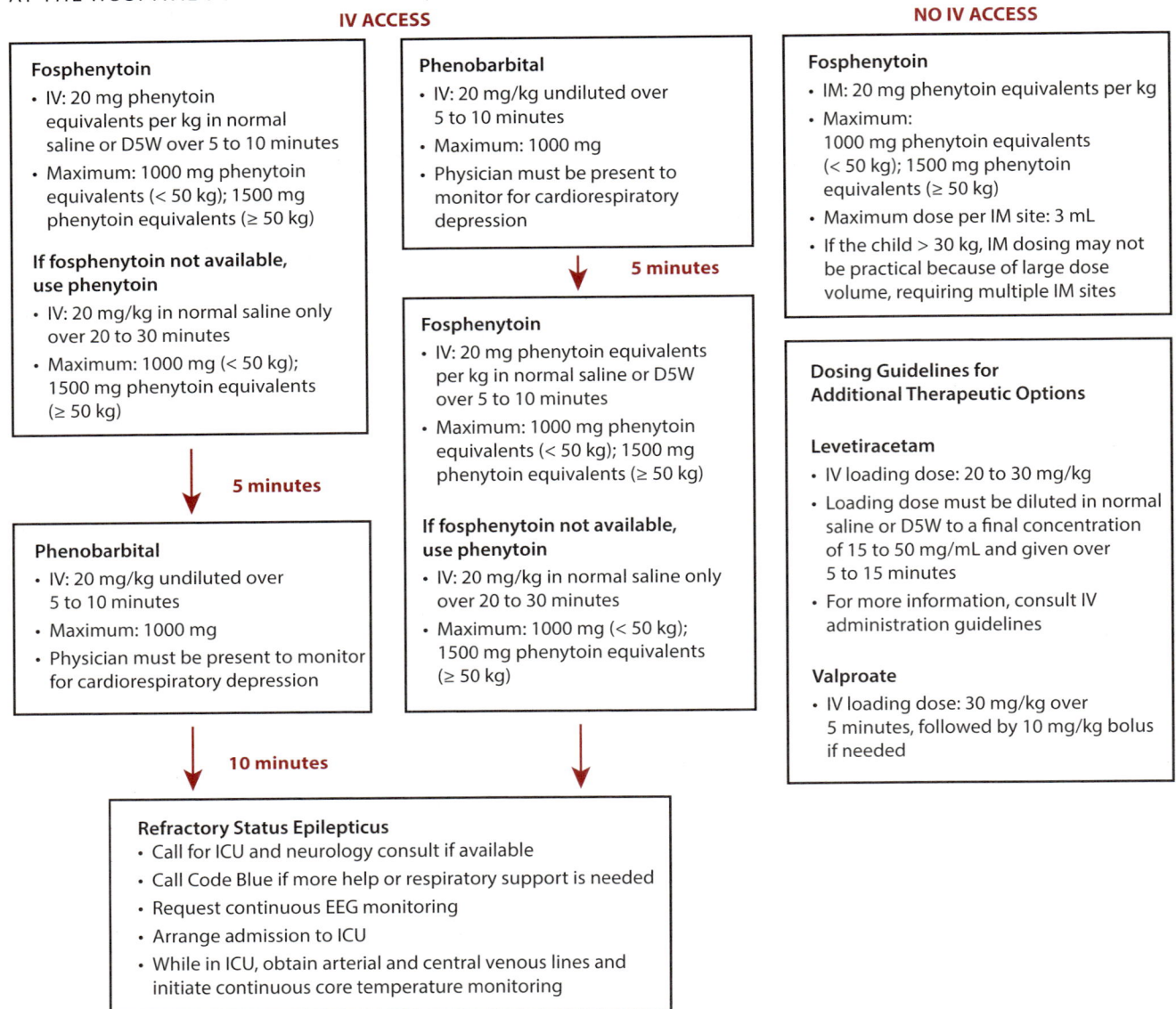

IV ACCESS

NO IV ACCESS

Fosphenytoin
- IV: 20 mg phenytoin equivalents per kg in normal saline or D5W over 5 to 10 minutes
- Maximum: 1000 mg phenytoin equivalents (< 50 kg); 1500 mg phenytoin equivalents (≥ 50 kg)

If fosphenytoin not available, use phenytoin
- IV: 20 mg/kg in normal saline only over 20 to 30 minutes
- Maximum: 1000 mg (< 50 kg); 1500 mg phenytoin equivalents (≥ 50 kg)

5 minutes

Phenobarbital
- IV: 20 mg/kg undiluted over 5 to 10 minutes
- Maximum: 1000 mg
- Physician must be present to monitor for cardiorespiratory depression

10 minutes

Phenobarbital
- IV: 20 mg/kg undiluted over 5 to 10 minutes
- Maximum: 1000 mg
- Physician must be present to monitor for cardiorespiratory depression

5 minutes

Fosphenytoin
- IV: 20 mg phenytoin equivalents per kg in normal saline or D5W over 5 to 10 minutes
- Maximum: 1000 mg phenytoin equivalents (< 50 kg); 1500 mg phenytoin equivalents (≥ 50 kg)

If fosphenytoin not available, use phenytoin
- IV: 20 mg/kg in normal saline only over 20 to 30 minutes
- Maximum: 1000 mg (< 50 kg); 1500 mg phenytoin equivalents (≥ 50 kg)

Fosphenytoin
- IM: 20 mg phenytoin equivalents per kg
- Maximum: 1000 mg phenytoin equivalents (< 50 kg); 1500 mg phenytoin equivalents (≥ 50 kg)
- Maximum dose per IM site: 3 mL
- If the child > 30 kg, IM dosing may not be practical because of large dose volume, requiring multiple IM sites

Dosing Guidelines for Additional Therapeutic Options

Levetiracetam
- IV loading dose: 20 to 30 mg/kg
- Loading dose must be diluted in normal saline or D5W to a final concentration of 15 to 50 mg/mL and given over 5 to 15 minutes
- For more information, consult IV administration guidelines

Valproate
- IV loading dose: 30 mg/kg over 5 minutes, followed by 10 mg/kg bolus if needed

Refractory Status Epilepticus
- Call for ICU and neurology consult if available
- Call Code Blue if more help or respiratory support is needed
- Request continuous EEG monitoring
- Arrange admission to ICU
- While in ICU, obtain arterial and central venous lines and initiate continuous core temperature monitoring

Note: If IV access is not available, then other routes such as intranasal, buccal, sublingual, rectal, or intramuscular should be used. The IN and IM routes have faster onset compared to the buccal/sublingual route. The PR route is a last resort as absorption can be erratic.

SEIZURE MIMICS IN THE EMERGENCY DEPARTMENT

- It can be challenging to differentiate seizures from seizure mimics.
- The preferred term for seizure mimic events are *nonepileptic events*. (This a better term than *pseudoseizures* or *nonepileptic seizures,* as using the word *seizure* in the term can be confusing for parents).
- Symptoms and signs of nonepileptic events are:
  » Abnormal movements start or stop on command
  » Pelvic thrusting
  » Eyes closed during event
  » No change in vital signs
  » No postictal period (although focal onset seizures with awareness may not have a postictal period)
- Common seizure mimics include:
  » Tics and other movement disorders
  » Breath holding episodes
  » Sandifer syndrome and gastrointestinal reflux disease
  » Syncope from all causes
    › It is important to consider arrhythmias or structural cardiac defects.
  » Migraine headaches
  » Shuddering attacks
  » Masturbation or other self-stimulation
  » Sleep disorders (e.g., restless leg syndrome, benign sleep myoclonus, myoclonus with falling asleep or waking up, cataplexy as symptom of narcolepsy)
- If the ED diagnosis is a nonepileptic event, upon discharge ask caregivers to take a video of the episodes to show to their healthcare team.

COMPLEX EPILEPSY

- Patients with epilepsy, especially those with medically refractory seizures, can come to the ED with breakthrough or increased seizure activity.
- Patients with epilepsy are more likely to have status epilepticus.
- In some cases, antiepileptic medications can be adjusted by the ED physician, but in children with more complex epilepsy, or those who have been on multiple antiepileptic medications, a consult with a pediatrician or pediatric neurologist is indicated.
- With some antiepileptic medications, serum levels can help determine compliance with medication or improper use of medication.
  » It is important to consider the time of antiepileptic medications serum level in relation to dosing (e.g., trough vs random serum level) in determining compliance and efficacy.
  » Serum levels are not helpful with all antiepileptic medications; your hospital pharmacist or formulary can guide the utility of checking antiepileptic serum levels.
- Each antiepileptic medication has specific adverse effects, from simple to life-threatening.
  » It is beyond the scope of this chapter to include all side effects of antiepileptic medications.
  » Information from the formulary, hospital pharmacist, or pediatric neurology team can guide management.
  » If you are obtaining bloodwork for a child on antiepileptic medications, it is generally a good idea to evaluate hematologic, hepatic, and renal function.
- Other treatments for children with complex epilepsy include vagal nerve stimulation, ketogenic diet, and, more recently, the use of cannabinoids.
  » None of these treatments are options for acute management in the ED.
- It is appropriate to consult a pediatric neurologist for evaluation of these complex patients in the ED.

REFERENCES

Bergamo S, Parata F, Nosadini M, et al. Children with convulsive epileptic seizures presenting to Padua Pediatric Emergency Department: the first retrospective population-based descriptive study in an Italian Health District. *J Child Neurol.* 2015;30(3):289–295. https://doi.org/10.1177/0883073814538670. Medline:25008906

Bergey GK. Management of a first seizure. *Continuum (Minneap Minn).* 2016;22(1 Epilepsy):38–50. Medline:26844729

Bouma HK, Labos C, Gore GC, Wolfson C, Keezer MR. The diagnostic accuracy of routine electroencephalography after a first unprovoked seizure. *Eur J Neurol.* 2016;23(3):455–463. https://doi.org/10.1111/ene.12739. Medline:26073548

Camfield P, Camfield C. Incidence, prevalence and aetiology of seizures and epilepsy in children. *Epileptic Disord.* 2015;17(2):117–123. Medline:25895502

Chen J, Lau E, editors. Status epilepticus guidelines. In: *SickKids drug handbook and formulary.* 35th ed. Toronto, ON: Wolters Kluwer Clinical Drug Information, Inc; 2017.

Dayan PS, Lillis K, Bennett J, et al. Prevalence of and risk factors for intracranial abnormalities in unprovoked seizures. *Pediatrics.* 2015;136(2):e351–e360. https://doi.org/10.1542/peds.2014-3550. Medline:26195538

Fiest KM, Suaro KM, Wiebe S, et al. Prevalence and incidence of epilepsy: a systematic review and meta-analysis of international studies. *Neurology.* 2017;88(3):296–303. Medline:27986877

Fisher RS, Acevedo C, Arzimanoglou A, et al. ILAE official report: a practical clinical definition of epilepsy. *Epilepsia.* 2014;55(4):475–482. https://doi.org/10.1111/epi.12550. Medline:24730690

Guedj R, Chappuy H, Titomanlio L, et al. Risk of bacterial meningitis in children 6 to 11 months of age with a first simple febrile seizure: a retrospective, cross-sectional, observational study. *Acad Emerg Med.* 2015;22(11):1290–1297. https://doi.org/10.1111/acem.12798. Medline:26468690

Hirtz D, Ashwal S, Berg A, et al. Practice parameter: evaluating a first nonfebrile seizure in children: report of the quality standards subcommittee of the American Academy of Neurology, The Child Neurology Society, and The American Epilepsy Society. *Neurology.* 2000;55(5):616–623. https://doi.org/10.1212/WNL.55.5.616. Medline:10980722

Kimia AA, Bachur RG, Torres A, Harper MB. Febrile seizures: emergency medicine perspective. *Curr Opin Pediatr.* 2015;27(3):292–297. https://doi.org/10.1097/MOP.0000000000000220. Medline:25944308

NEUROLOGIC EMERGENCIES

Lux AL. Treatment of febrile seizures: historical perspective, current opinions, and potential future directions. *Brain Dev.* 2010;32(1):42–50. https://doi.org/10.1016/j.braindev.2009.09.016. Medline:19854599

Offringa M, Newton R. Prophylactic drug management for febrile seizures in children. *Cochrane Database Syst Rev.* 2012;(4):CD003031. Medline:22513908

Pallin DJ, Goldstein JN, Moussally JS, Pelletier AJ, Green AR, Camargo CA. Seizure visits in US emergency departments: epidemiology and potential disparities in care. *Int J Emerg Med.* 2008;1(2):97–105. https://doi.org/10.1007/s12245-008-0024-4. Medline:19384659

Rosenbloom E, Finkelstein Y, Adams-Webber T, Kozer E. Do antipyretics prevent the recurrence of febrile seizures in children? A systematic review of randomized controlled trials and meta-analysis. *Eur J Paediatr Neurol.* 2013;17(6):585–588. https://doi.org/10.1016/j.ejpn.2013.04.008. Medline:23702315

Santillanes G, Luc Q. Emergency department management of seizures in pediatric patients. *Pediatr Emerg Med Pract.* 2015;12(3):1–25, *quiz 26–27.* Medline:25799698

Shinnar S, Berg AT, Moshe SL, et al. The risk of seizure recurrence after a first unprovoked afebrile seizure in childhood: an extended follow-up. *Pediatrics.* 1996;98(2 Pt 1):216–225. Medline:8692621

Shinnar S, Maytal J, Krasnoff L, Moshe SL. Recurrent status epilepticus in children. *Ann Neurol.* 1992;31(6):598–604. https://doi.org/10.1002/ana.410310606. Medline:1514772

Sofou K, Kristjánsdóttir R, Papachatzakis NE, Ahmadzadeh A, Uvebrant P. Management of prolonged seizures and status epilepticus in childhood: a systematic review. *J Child Neurol.* 2009;24(8):918–926. https://doi.org/10.1177/0883073809332768. Medline:19332572

Steering Committee on Quality Improvement and Management, Subcommittee on Febrile Seizures, American Academy of Pediatrics. Febrile seizures: clinical practice guideline for the long-term management of the child with simple febrile seizures. *Pediatrics.* 2008;121(6):1281–1286. https://doi.org/10.1542/peds.2008-0939. Medline:18519501

Strobel AM, Gill VS, Witting MD, Teshome G. Emergent diagnostic testing for pediatric nonfebrile seizures. *Am J Emerg Med.* 2015;33(9):1261–1264. https://doi.org/10.1016/j.ajem.2015.06.004. Medline:26152916

Subcommittee on Febrile Seizures, American Academy of Pediatrics. Neurodiagnostic evaluation of the child with a simple febrile seizure. *Pediatrics.* 2011;127(2):389–394. https://doi.org/10.1542/peds.2010-3318. Medline:21285335

Teach SJ, Geil PA. Incidence of bacteremia, urinary tract infections, and unsuspected bacterial meningitis in children with febrile seizures. *Pediatr Emerg Care.* 1999;15(1):9–12. https://doi.org/10.1097/00006565-199902000-00003. Medline:10069303

Whelan H, Harmelink M, Chou E, et al. Complex febrile seizures: a systematic review. *Dis Mon.* 2017;63(1):5–23. https://doi.org/10.1016/j.disamonth.2016.12.001. Medline:28089358

4.2

Pediatric Stroke

Amita Misir

- The incidence of stroke in children 1 month to 19 years of age is estimated at 2 to 3 per 100 000 per year.
  - » Some studies report as high as 13 per 100 000 per year.
- The peak age for both ischemic stroke and intraparenchymal brain hemorrhage is in the first year of life.
  - » Males appear to be at higher risk than females.
- Perinatal stroke is defined as cerebrovascular lesions occurring from 28 weeks gestational age through the first 7 days of life.
  - » Recent estimates suggest that ischemic stroke occurs in ~1 per 4000 live births.
  - » Perinatal stroke accounts for 25% of all cases of pediatric stroke, making it 17 times more likely to occur during this period than any other time in childhood.
  - » Eighty percent of perinatal strokes are ischemic, with the remainder resulting from cerebral sinovenous thrombosis or hemorrhage.
- A transient ischemic attack (TIA) is a transient episode (typically lasting < 1 hour) of neurologic dysfunction caused by focal brain, spinal cord, or retinal ischemia without acute infarction.
  - » This diagnosis can only be made retrospectively.
  - » A TIA may actually represent a stroke in evolution with a stuttering or "waxing/waning" course.

Pathophysiology

ARTERIAL ISCHEMIC STROKE

- Pediatric arterial ischemic stroke can be defined as a "clinical presentation consistent with stroke combined with radiographic evidence of ischemia or infarction in a known arterial distribution" (Bernard et al, 2008).
- The zone of ischemic injury has 3 distinct areas based on CT/MRI perfusion studies:
  1. Ischemic "core" — where neurons are irreversibly injured
  2. "Penumbra" surrounding the "core" — where neurons are injured, but injuries are quickly reversible if the metabolic demands are replenished quickly
  3. Outer "oligemic area" — where neurons have decreased blood supply, but are still intact and at risk if reduced perfusion persists
- A cascade of inflammatory changes ensues after an

arterial occlusion at a cellular level, leading to further neuronal injury:

- » Hydrogen and lactic acid accumulation
- » Release of free radicals, arachidonic acid, nitric oxide, and cytokines

- Three general mechanisms cause arterial ischemic stroke:
  1. Thrombotic — in situ obstruction of an artery; can be due to disease of arterial wall
  2. Embolic — particles of debris or embolism originating elsewhere that are dislodged and block arterial access to a particular brain region
  3. Systemic hypoperfusion — lack of adequate perfusion to part(s) of the brain

HEMORRHAGIC STROKE

- The types of hemorrhagic stroke are:
  - » Intracerebral hemorrhage
    - › Arterioles or small arteries bleed directly into brain, forming localized hematoma that gradually enlarge.
  - » Subarachnoid hemorrhage
    - › High-pressure blood is released directly into cerebrospinal fluid (CSF).
    - › There is a resultant rapid increase in intracranial pressure (ICP).
    - › Etiology includes:
      · Rupture of arterial aneurysm (most common cause)
      · Vascular malformations
      · Bleeding diatheses
      · Trauma

CEREBRAL SINOVENOUS THROMBOSIS

- The pathophysiology of cerebral sinovenous thrombosis is incompletely understood.
  - » It likely involves at least 2 different mechanisms:
    1. Thrombosis of cerebral veins or dural sinus, leading to cerebral parenchymal lesions or dysfunction
    2. Occlusion of dural sinus, resulting in decreased CSF absorption and elevated intracranial pressure
- Obstruction of the venous structures results in increased venous pressure, decreased capillary perfusion pressure, and increased cerebral blood volume.
  - » This leads to disruption in the blood-brain barrier, which causes vasogenic edema with leakage of blood plasma into interstitial space.
- As intravenous pressure continues to increase, mild parenchymal changes, severe cerebral edema, and

venous hemorrhage may occur due to venous or capillary ruptures.

- See *Table 4.2.1* for risk factors associated with stroke.

Table 4.2.1. RISK FACTORS ASSOCIATED WITH THE TYPES OF PEDIATRIC STROKE

Type of stroke	Selected common risk factors (in pediatric population)
Arterial ischemic stroke	• SCD • Congenital and acquired heart disease (various types; uncorrected complex congenital heart disease is highest risk) • Moyamoya disease and Moyamoya syndrome; can be associated with Neurofibromatosis type 1, Down syndrome, cranial radiotherapy, and/or Asian heritage; stroke often provoked by hyperventilation (i.e., crying) with subsequent decrease in cerebral blood flow • Cervicocephalic arterial dissection, either traumatic or spontaneous • Focal cerebral arteriopathy of childhood, also known as transient cerebral arteriopathy of childhood: a clinical syndrome characterized by unilateral focal or segmental stenosis of distal carotid arteries and middle, anterior, and posterior cerebral arteries; often improves or self-resolves in 6 months; may be associated with preceding varicella infection • Fibromuscular dysplasia • Vasculitis (can be associated with intracranial infections such as meningitis, tuberculosis, and varicella, also inflammatory disease such as systemic lupus erythematosus, or Kawasaki disease) • Hypercoagulable states
Hemorrhagic stroke	• Intracranial arterial aneurysms; often associated with coarctation of the aorta, autosomal dominant polycystic kidney disease, Ehlers-Danlos syndrome type IV, family history of intracranial aneurysms • Arteriovenous malformations or cavernous malformations • Bleeding diatheses and/or platelet count < 20 000
Cerebral sinovenous thrombosis	• Dehydration, hypoxia (i.e., poststrangulation), post–lumbar puncture • Anemia (iron deficiency, SCD, thalassemia, autoimmune hemolytic) • OCP, pregnancy, and puerperium • Malignancy • Cardiac disease (cyanotic or postoperative/postcatheterization) • Renal disease (nephrotic syndrome) • Down syndrome • Head and neck infections (meningitis, mastoiditis, ear infections, tonsillitis, sinusitis)

OCP oral contraceptive pill. **SCD** sickle cell disease.

Figure 4.2.1. PATHOPHYSIOLOGY OF CEREBRAL SINOVENOUS THROMBOSIS

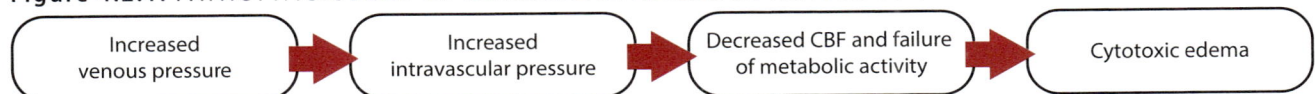

Increased venous pressure → Increased intravascular pressure → Decreased CBF and failure of metabolic activity → Cytotoxic edema

CBF cerebral blood flow.

NEUROLOGIC EMERGENCIES

» Up to 50% of patients will not have an identifiable risk factor at the time of presentation.

History

- Consider typical signs and symptoms either by age or by anatomic/physical mechanism (see *Tables 4.2.2* and *4.2.3*).

Table 4.2.2. CLINICAL FEATURES BY AGE

Age	Clinical features
Neonates and infants	• Acute focal motor seizures, usually after first 12 hours of life • Unexplained apneas and/or cyanosis • Altered mental status • Asymptomatic • Early "hand preference" on developmental follow-up (for presumed perinatal arterial ischemic stroke)
Children and adolescents	• Abrupt onset of acute focal neurological deficit, sometimes with self-resolving and "stuttering" course • Headache (regardless of whether ischemic or hemorrhagic mechanism) • Speech or language changes

- Cerebral sinovenous thrombosis and vertebral-basilar distribution arterial ischemic stroke can present with vague and nonspecific symptoms that can make recognition challenging, often leading to delays in diagnosis.

Note: Arterial ischemic stroke can present with a stuttering course over several hours with periods of recovery and even periods of normal function during the acute period of stroke evolution. Do not rule out stroke on the basis of apparent improvement/resolution of neurologic function.

Investigations

- Urgent neuroimaging is essential.
- Given that the diagnosis is not known a priori, the following provides a reasonable guideline for investigations.
  » Urgent MRI with diffusion-weighted imaging (DWI) and MR angiography (MRA) and/or MR venography (MRV) of the head and neck is highly recommended as the initial study.
  › CT with CT angiography (CTA) of the head and

Table 4.2.3. CLINICAL FEATURES BY ANATOMIC/PHYSICAL MECHANISM

Stroke type	Anatomy involved	Clinical features
Arterial ischemic stroke	ACA	• Contralateral leg weakness and somatosensory loss • Executive function abnormalities (inability to focus on task, apathy, confusion, poor judgment, difficulty problem solving, repetition of a single thought)
	MCA	• Contralateral arm and face weakness • Dysarthria • Hemianesthesia • Aphasia if dominant hemisphere is affected • Apraxia and sensory hemineglect if nondominant hemisphere is affected
	PCA	• Contralateral visual field loss (homonymous hemianopia) • Unilateral cortical blindness • Memory loss
	Vertebrobasilar artery	• Headache, nausea, vomiting, dizziness • Cranial nerve deficits: diplopia, dysconjugate gaze, gaze preference, nystagmus, vertigo • Gait and coordination: staggering gait, intermittent rhythmic movements (may be confused for seizures) • Depressed level of consciousness • Crossed symptoms (one side of face and other side of body)
	ICA	• Ipsilateral neck, scalp, or head pain in cervicocephalic arterial dissection (with potentially minor or no trauma) • Ipsilateral partial Horner syndrome (decreased pupil size, drooping eyelid, decreased sweating on affected side) • Ipsilateral cranial nerve palsies • Audible bruit • Features of ACA/PCA stroke, depending on location
Hemorrhagic stroke	Parenchymal hemorrhage or subarachnoid space	• Acute-onset severe headache, vomiting, and rapid deterioration of neurological function (older children) • Irritability (younger children) • Focal or generalized seizures
Cerebral sinovenous thrombosis	Cerebral vein or dural sinuses	• Headache (generally gradual onset, increasing over several days, severe dull generalized head pain) • Signs of increased intracranial pressure (i.e., headache worsens with recumbency; may be associated with nausea, vomiting, papilledema, peripheral visual field loss) • Focal or generalized seizures • Motor weakness with monoparesis or hemiparesis • Variable and subtle clinical presentation

ACA anterior cerebral artery. **ICA** internal carotid artery. **MCA** middle cerebral artery. **PCA** posterior cerebral artery.

neck can be substituted, depending on availability, local expertise, and clinical situation.

> › Ultrasound and CT can easily miss cerebral sinovenous thrombosis and early arterial ischemic stroke.

- » If clinical suspicion is specifically for cerebral sinovenous thrombosis, a CT followed by a CT venogram (CTV) has excellent sensitivity and specificity for cerebral sinovenous thrombosis.

- Cerebral angiography is generally considered when an MRI/MRA is inconclusive or negative and clinical suspicion remains, or if invasive treatment (i.e., mechanical thrombectomy, medical thrombolysis) is being considered.

- The initial laboratory workup should include:
  - » International normalized ratio (INR), partial thromboplastin time (PTT), type and screen
  - » Complete blood count (CBC)
  - » Fibrinogen
  - » Glucose and electrolytes
  - » D-dimer
    - › An elevated D-dimer supports the diagnosis of cerebral sinovenous thrombosis, but a normal D-dimer does not exclude the diagnosis of cerebral sinovenous thrombosis in patients with other suggestive symptoms.
      - · In adult recommendations, individual assays of D-dimer may vary, but it is reasonable to use the same threshold levels used in diagnostic protocols for deep venous thrombosis (i.e., D-dimer > 500 ng/mL of fibrinogen equivalent units).
      - · Adult data suggests the sensitivity of D-dimer is 82% to 94% for cerebral sinovenous thrombosis; the sensitivity in adult patients with cerebral sinovenous thrombosis appears to be lower in those with isolated headache and subacute or chronic presentations and in those with a single affected venous sinus.

- All patients suspected of having stroke should ultimately undergo a full diagnostic evaluation for:
  - » Hypercoagulable states
    - › Antithrombin, protein C, protein S, factor V Leiden deficiencies
  - » Hypocoagulable states, done in consultation with or by a hematologist or stroke specialist

- Follow-up imaging for embolic strokes should also include an echocardiogram and carotid artery imaging to identify potential sources of embolic stroke.

Management

General Measures

- General supportive care and neuroprotective strategies are indicated for all stroke types. This includes:

- » Positioning
  - › Keep the head of the bed between 0° and 15° **unless** increased ICP is suspected, in which case raise the head of the bed to 30° with patient's head placed in midline position.
- » Normotension
  - › The target systolic blood pressure (SBP) is between the 50th and 90th percentile for the patient's age group; treat low blood pressure (BP) with normal saline with or without pressors.
  - › Treat significant hypertension with labetalol to lower BP by 25% over 24 hours, unless you suspect a hemorrhage with obvious ICP, in which case allow permissive hypertension to maintain cerebral perfusion pressure (CPP).
- » Normovolemia
  - › Continue to keep the patient on maintenance fluid, and bolus whenever necessary (PRN) if there are any signs of hypotension or inadequate fluid resuscitation.
- » Normoglycemia:
  - › For patients ≥ 2 years of age, do no give glucose in IV fluids unless the patient is hypoglycemic.
  - › For patients < 2 years of a.ge, use glucose-containing isotonic fluids (i.e., D5W added to 0.9% saline).
- » Normothermia
  - › Treat patients with fever with acetaminophen.
- » Seizure control
  - › Treat patients with any suspected seizure activity with antiepileptics as soon as possible (see Chapter 4.1).
- » Normoxemia
  - › Maintain oxygen saturation > 95%.

- If there are signs and symptoms of increased ICP, consider:
  - » Elevating the head of the bed to 30°
  - » Placing patient's head in midline position
  - » Administering 3% normal saline 5 to 10 mL/kg over 5 to 10 minutes
  - » Giving mannitol 0.25 to 1.0 g/kg over 10 minutes
  - » Hyperventilating (aim for end-tidal CO_2 between 25 and 30), particularly if there are signs of brain herniation (i.e., unilateral enlarged pupil, sudden decrease in level of consciousness, respiratory arrest)
  - » Consulting neurosurgery

Emergent Treatment With Thrombolytics

- There is ongoing research looking at the effectiveness of tissue plasminogen activator (tPA) in pediatric arterial ischemic stroke; consult the nearest pediatric center for advice.

- Thrombolytics may be considered in certain situations for cerebral sinovenous thrombosis and arterial ischemic stroke in children > 12 years of age (some centers use > 2 years of age).

- If considered, intravenous tPA must be given within 4.5 hours of stroke onset; intraarterial tPA must be given within 6 hours of stroke onset.
  - » Exclusion criteria are:
    - › Major surgery or hemorrhage within the past 2 weeks
    - › Invasive procedure in the last 3 days
    - › Central nervous system (CNS) hemorrhage/ trauma/surgery in the past 2 months
    - › Current CNS pathology (aneurysm, neoplasm, or vascular malformation)
    - › Premature (< 32 weeks gestational age)
    - › Active bleeding at the time of therapy
    - › Inability to maintain platelets > 50 000 or fibrinogen > 100 mg/dL using transfusion support
    - › Uncontrolled hypertension
    - › Witnessed seizure at stroke onset
- Use of thrombolytics requires a multidisciplinary team that has the institutional capacity and should only be done in consultation with an experienced pediatric neurologist.
- Stroke screening questions to rapidly assess a patient with potential arterial ischemic stroke that may be eligible for thrombolysis include:
  - » Is there a focal neurological deficit?
    - › Unilateral weakness or sensory change
    - › Vision loss or double vision
    - › Speech difficulty
    - › Dizziness or trouble walking
  - » Did the problem begin or get worse suddenly?
  - » Has the problem been present for less than 5 hours?
    - › When was the child last seen well?

Specific Treatment

- Specific treatment options for pediatric stroke includes:
  - » Antiplatelet agents (e.g., ASA)
  - » Anticoagulation (e.g., unfractionated heparin, low–molecular weight heparin [LMWH], oral anticoagulation)
  - » Surgical treatments (e.g., mechanical thrombectomy, decompressive craniotomy, vascular bypass)
- Specific treatment for stroke varies depending on the nature and location of the stroke as well as patient characteristics.
  - » In general, perinatal stroke management consists of supportive therapy only.
  - » Intravenous hydration and exchange transfusion to target HbS < 30% is recommended for strokes due to sickle cell disease (SCD).
  - » Anticoagulation (initially with unfractionated heparin or LMWH followed by warfarin) for 3 to 6 months is generally recommended for pediatric cerebral sinovenous thrombosis beyond the neonatal period.

- » There is some variation of consensus in guidelines for initial antithrombotic treatment for pediatric arterial ischemic stroke beyond the neonatal period.
  - › The American College of Chest Physicians (ACCP) recommends either unfractionated heparin, LMWH, or ASA as initial therapy until dissection and embolic causes have been excluded.
  - › The American Heart Association (AHA) Stroke Council guidelines state that it may be reasonable to initiate anticoagulation with LMWH or unfractionated heparin (1 mg/kg every 12 hours) for up to 1 week pending completion of the diagnostic evaluation.
  - › The Royal College of Physicians and Surgeons of Canada recommends initial therapy with ASA (5 mg/kg).
- Any specific treatment is best initiated in consultation with a pediatric neurologist, neurosurgeon, and/or hematologist.

REFERENCES

Andrade A, Yau I, Moharir M. Current concepts in pediatric stroke. *Indian J Pediatr.* 2015;82(2):179–188. https://doi.org/10.1007/s12098-014-1604-3. Medline:25416087

Bernard TJ, Goldenberg NA. Pediatric arterial ischemic stroke. [viii.]. *Pediatr Clin North Am.* 2008;55(2):323–338, viii. https://doi.org/10.1016/j.pcl.2008.01.002. Medline:18381089

DeVeber G, Kirkham F. Guidelines for the treatment and prevention of stroke in children. *Lancet Neurol.* 2008;7(11):983–985. https://doi.org/10.1016/S1474-4422(08)70231-X. Medline:18940691

Ferro J, Canhao P. Etiology, clinical features and diagnosis of cerebral venous thrombosis. In: UpToDate, Wolters Kluwer. (Accessed on Oct 23, 2016). Available from: http://www.uptodate.com

Hartman AL, Lunney KM, Serena JE. Pediatric stroke: do clinical factors predict delays in presentation? *J Pediatr.* 2009;154(5):727–732.e1. https://doi.org/10.1016/j.jpeds.2008.11.011. Medline:19111319

Mackay MT, Prabhu SP, Coleman L. Childhood posterior circulation arterial ischemic stroke. *Stroke.* 2010;41(10):2201–2209. https://doi.org/10.1161/STROKEAHA.110.583831. Medline:20829517

Rafay MF, Pontigon AM, Chiang J, et al. Delay to diagnosis in acute pediatric arterial ischemic stroke. *Stroke.* 2009;40(1):58–64. https://doi.org/10.1161/STROKEAHA.108.519066. Medline:18802206

Rivkin MJ, Bernard TJ, Dowling MM, Amlie-Lefond C. Guidelines for urgent management of stroke in children. *Pediatr Neurol.* 2016;56:8–17. https://doi.org/10.1016/j.pediatrneurol.2016.01.016. Medline:26969237

Roach ES, Golomb MR, Adams R, et al; American Heart Association Stroke Council; Council on Cardiovascular Disease in the Young. Management of stroke in infants and children: a scientific statement from a special writing group of the American Heart Association Stroke Council and the Council on Cardiovascular Disease in the Young. *Stroke.* 2008;39(9):2644–2691. https://doi.org/10.1161/STROKEAHA.108.189696. Medline:18635845

Rollins N, Pride GL, Plumb PA, Dowling MM. Brainstem strokes in children: an 11-year series from a tertiary pediatric center. *Pediatr Neurol.* 2013;49(6):458–464. https://doi.org/10.1016/j.pediatrneurol.2013.07.007. Medline:24080274

Shellhaas RA, Smith SE, O'Tool E, Licht DJ, Ichord RN. Mimics of childhood stroke: characteristics of a prospective cohort. *Pediatrics.* 2006;118(2):704–709. https://doi.org/10.1542/peds.2005-2676. Medline:16882826

Smith S, Fox C. Ischemic stroke in children and young adults: etiology and clinical features. In: UpToDate. Wolters Kluwer. (Accessed on Oct 23, 2016). Available from: http://www.uptodate.com

Smith S, Fox C. Ischemic stroke in children: evaluation, initial management and prognosis. In: UpToDate. Wolters Kluwer. (Accessed on Oct 23, 2016). Available from: http://www.uptodate.com

Steinlin M, Pfister I, Pavlovic J, et al; Swiss Societies of Paediatric Neurology and Neonatology. The first three years of the Swiss Neuropaediatric Stroke Registry (SNPSR): a population-based study of incidence, symptoms and risk factors. *Neuropediatrics*.

2005;36*(2)*:90–97. https://doi.org/10.1055/s-2005-837658. Medline:15822021

Zimmer JA, Garg BP, Williams LS, Golomb MR. Age-related variation in presenting signs of childhood arterial ischemic stroke. *Pediatr Neurol*. 2007;37*(3)*:171–175. https://doi.org/10.1016/j.pediatrneurol.2007.05.010. Medline:17765804

4.3

Meningitis and Encephalitis

Shruti Mehrotra

BACTERIAL MENINGITIS

- Bacterial meningitis continues to be associated with considerable mortality and morbidity if not treated early.
- In all age groups, the common bacterial pathogens to consider are:
  » *Neisseria meningitides*
  » *Streptococcus pneumoniae*
    › *S. pneumoniae* remains the most common cause of bacterial meningitis in children > 1 month of age.
  » *Hemophilus influenzae* type b (Hib)
- Overall, the incidence of acute bacterial meningitis has significantly decreased since the introduction of conjugated vaccines against *N. meningitidis*, *S. pneumoniae*, and Hib in Canada and United States.
- The incidence of bacterial meningitis per 100 000 persons, based on age, is:
  » < 2 months of age — 80.7
  » 2 to 23 months of age — 6.9
  » 2 to 10 years of age — 0.56
  » 11 to 17 years of age — 0.43

Risk Factors

- Risk factors in children include:
  » Immunocompromised states — HIV, asplenic
  » Sickle cell disease (SCD)
  » Central nervous system (CNS) hardware: ventriculo-peritoneal (VP) shunt, cochlear implant
  » Unimmunized
  » Exposure: daycare, exposure to another case

Note:

- In unimmunized or incompletely immunized children, a higher index of suspicion is needed for bacterial meningitis due to the above pathogens.
- There are increasing concerns about penicillin-resistant *S. pneumoniae* (varies by region), along with cross-resistance to cephalosporins.

Table 4.3.1. PATHOGENS TO CONSIDER BY AGE OF CHILD AND IMMUNE STATUS

All age groups / unimmunized or incompletely immunized individuals	Neonates (0 to 1 month)	Immunocompromised
• *Streptococcus pneumoniae* • Hib • *Neisseria meningitidis*	• GBS (also known as *Streptococcus agalactiae*) • *Listeria monocytogenes* • *Escherichia coli* • *Klebsiella pneumoniae* • *Enterococcus* spp. • *Salmonella* spp.	• *Listeria monocytogenes* • Gram-negative bacteria: » *E. coli* » *Klebsiella pneumoniae* » *Citrobacter koseri* » *Serratia marcescens*

GBS group B *Streptococcus*.

History

- Ask about the following on history:
  » Immunization status
  » Travel history
  » Contact with another case
  » Presence of rash

» Headache or stiff neck
» Exposure to high-density / crowded areas (dormitories, gyms)
» Impaired immune status — diabetes, SCD

Physical Exam

- Signs and symptoms can be very nonspecific, especially in younger children.
- In any pediatric patient, consider meningitis in the differential diagnosis if the patient presents with:
  » Fever
  » Irritability
  » Lethargy
  » Poor feeding
  » Vomiting
  » Upper respiratory tract infectious symptoms
- Signs in infants include unwellness, irritability or lethargy, seizures, apnea, bulging fontanelle, and purpuric or petechial rash.
- Signs in children 18 months of age and older include headache, neck stiffness, photophobia, rash, and seizures.
  » Kernig sign has a sensitivity of 53% and a specificity of 85%.
  » Brudzinski sign has a sensitivity of 66% and a specificity of 74%.
    › Neither test is reliable, especially in children < 1 year of age.

Investigations

- Order bloodwork: complete blood count (CBC), differential, electrolytes, urea, creatinine, glucose, international normalized ratio (INR), partial thromboplastin time (PTT).
- Blood cultures may be positive in 80% to 90% of Hib and *S. pneumoniae* cases and in up to 50% of meningococcal disease or neonatal disease cases.
- Urine cultures are recommended especially in infants < 2 months of age or immunocompromised children.
- Chest X-rays (CXRs) are recommended in infants < 2 months of age with respiratory symptoms.
- Order a lumbar puncture (LP) once the patient is stable.
  » If antimicrobial therapy has been given, cerebrospinal fluid (CSF) is still useful for culture within 2 hours and cell count within 2 days — see *Table 4.3.2.*
    › Contraindications for performing LP are:
      · Focal neurological signs
      · Glasgow coma scale (GCS) < 8 (see *Table 18.1.1* on page 316).
      · Cardiorespiratory compromise
      · Signs of cerebral herniation

Table 4.3.2. CEREBROSPINAL FLUID RESULTS INDICATING BACTERIAL MENINGITIS

CSF marker	Neonates	Infants & children
WBC	• > 0.03 × 10⁹/L — greater than 60% polymorphonuclear cells	• Very young infants: » > 0.01 × 10⁹/L • Older children with typical WBC 0.50 × 10⁹/L, mainly polymorphonuclear cells: » > 0.005 × 10⁹/L
Protein	• > 1.7 g/L	• > 0.6 g/L
CSF/blood glucose ratio	• < 0.5 to 0.6	• < 0.4
Gram stain	• Microorganisms seen	• Microorganisms seen
Other	• Latex agglutination for GBS	• Cell count and protein/glucose changes remain for 2 days after start of antibiotics • Send PCR for *N. meningitidis* and *S. pneumoniae*

CSF cerebral spinal fluid. GBS group B *Streptococcus*. PCR polymerase chain reaction. WBC white blood cell.

· Coagulopathy
· Signs of purpura fulminans
- A CT head scan should be considered in certain circumstances prior to an LP; however, do not delay antibiotics while waiting for a CT.
  » A CT should be done when considering:
    › Other causes for presenting symptoms (intracranial mass or bleed)
    › Complications of meningitis (cerebral abscess)
    › Presence of focal neurological findings
    › Papilledema
    › Prior neurosurgery (trauma, shunt, mass)

Management

- For all patients with suspected meningitis, ensure droplet and respiratory precautions.

Toxic and Unstable Patients

- Assess and stabilize the ABCs.
- Assess patients using the GCS.
- Provide supplemental oxygen, establish an IV, and place the patient on full cardiorespiratory monitoring.
- Provide antibiotics immediately (see *Table 4.3.3*).
- If the patient has associated septic shock, then fluid resuscitate aggressively in the first hour.
  » Give normal saline 20 mL/kg and reassess.
  » Monitor for signs of increased intracranial pressure.
  » Consider vasopressors after 2 or 3 boluses of normal saline:
    › Epinephrine at 0.05 to 0.1 mcg/kg per minute
- Normalize glucose:
  » Dextrose 10% solution 5 mL/kg if hypoglycemic

Table 4.3.3. INITIAL EMPIRIC ANTIBIOTICS BY AGE AND PATHOGENS

Adapted from Le Saux (2014; reaffirmed January 2017).

Age	Common bacterial pathogens	Antibiotic regimen
Neonates (0 to 4 weeks)	• GBS • E. coli • Listeria monocytogenes	• ≤ 0 to 7 days of age, > 2 kg: » Ampicillin 150 mg/kg per day IV divided every 8 hours — and — » Cefotaxime 100 to 150 mg/kg per day divided every 8 to 12 hours • > 7 days of age, > 2 kg: » Ampicillin 200 mg/kg per day IV divided every 6 hours — and — » Cefotaxime 100 to 150 mg/kg per day divided every 6 to 8 hours
4 to 12 weeks	• GBS • E. coli • L. monocytogenes • H. influenzae • S. pneumoniae • N. meningitidis	• Vancomycin 60 mg/kg per day IV divided every 6 hours – and – • Cefotaxime 300 mg/kg per day divided every 6 hours (to a maximum of 8 to 12 g per day) • If patient is immunocompromised or if listeria risk factors are present, add: » Ampicillin 300 mg/kg per day IV divided every 6 hours (to a maximum of 12 g per day)
12 weeks and older	• H. influenzae • S. pneumoniae • N. meningitidis	• Vancomycin 60 mg/kg per day IV divided every 6 hours – and – • Ceftriaxone 100 mg/kg per dose at 0, 12, and 24 hours; then 100 mg/kg per dose every 24 hours (to a maximum of 2 g per dose and 4 g per day)

For penicillin-resistant strains of *S. pneumoniae*: IV meropenem 120 mg/kg per day in divided doses administered every 6 to 8 hours to a maximum dose 6 g per day.

GBS group B *Streptococcus*.

- Treat fever with antipyretics:
  - » Acetaminophen 15 mg/kg PO or 20 mg/kg PR
- Treat any seizure activity.
  - » Benzodiazepines are first line treatment:
    - › Lorazepam 0.1 mg/kg
    - › Diazepam 0.2 mg/kg
- Watch for signs of cerebral herniation:
  - » Level of consciousness — GCS < 8
  - » Pupillary response to light — poor unilateral or bilateral, or fixed
  - » Papilledema
  - » Posturing — decerebrate or decorticate
  - » Muscle tone — flaccid or tonic
  - » Respiratory abnormalities — apnea, arrest, Cheyne-Stokes, hyperventilation
- LP can be delayed until patient is stable.

Stable Patients

- Perform a full examination:
  - » Respiratory/cardiovascular status
  - » Assessment of level of consciousness
  - » Detailed neurological examinations to detect focal neurological signs, posturing, cranial nerve abnormalities
  - » Dermatological exam for purpuric or petechial rash
- Establish IV access and cardiac and oximetry monitoring.
- Begin fluid therapy based on the patient's hydration status.
- Antimicrobial therapy should not be delayed.
  - » It is ideally administered after the LP is completed (see *Table 4.3.3*).

DEXAMETHASONE

- Use of dexamethasone is controversial.
  - » Dexamethasone is indicated if Hib meningitis is suspected.
    - › Consider dexamethasone also for *S. pneumoniae* meningitis.
  - » Relative contraindications for dexamethasone are:
    - › Aseptic meningitis
    - › Partially treated meningitis
    - › Infants < 6 weeks of age
  - » Dexamethasone comes with the risk of gastrointestinal (GI) bleed.
- Give dexamethasone 0.6 mg/kg per day in 4 divided doses administered every 6 hours, and give 20 minutes before or with the first dose of antibiotics.
  - » Continue for 2 days of Hib or *S. pneumoniae*.

ASEPTIC MENINGITIS

- Consider aseptic meningitis in the patient who presents with meningitis-like symptoms, but whose Gram stain / CSF cultures are negative.
- The most common causes of aseptic meningitis are viruses, specifically enteroviruses.

History

- The patient may have nonspecific symptoms, including fever, headache, vomiting, irritability, and signs of meningeal irritation.
- Kernig and Brudzinsky signs may be positive in a patient > 18 months of age.

Investigations

- CSF studies may show:
  - » White blood cells (WBCs) 0.02 to 2 × 10^9/L; < 30% polymorphonuclear cells
  - » Glucose normal or slightly decreased

» Protein slightly elevated — 0.3–0.8 g/L
» Gram stain and CSF cultures negative

Management

- Administer antibiotics as per meningitis until cultures come back negative.
- Provide supportive treatment with fluids and electrolyte management.
- Arrange for a neurology consult.

ENCEPHALITIS

- Encephalitis is a syndrome of neurological dysfunction caused by inflammation of the brain parenchyma.
- Encephalitis may have infectious or noninfectious causes (see *Table 4.3.4*).

Table 4.3.4. CAUSES* OF ACUTE ENCEPHALITIS IN CHILDREN

Viruses	Other infectious causes	Noninfectious causes
Common causes of acute encephalitis (Herpes family)	• Mycoplasma • Pneumoniae • *Bartonella henselae* (Cat-scratch disease) • *Rickettsia* spp. (Rocky Mountain spotted fever) • Lyme disease • Syphilis	• SLE • Antibody-mediated (NMDA receptor) • HLH syndrome • Paraneoplastic • Hashimoto disease (thyrotoxicosis) • Toxins
• HSV type 1 (most common) • HSV type 2 (immunocompromised) • *Varicella zoster* (postinfectious cerebellitis) • EBV (immunocompromised) • CMV (immunocompromised) • Human herpes virus 6 & 7 (immunocompromised)		
Causes of aseptic meningitis	**Postinfectious causes**	

• Enteroviruses:
  » Enterovirus 70, 71 (also myelitis)
  » Coxsackievirus
  » Echoviruses
• Respiratory viruses (influenza, adenovirus)
	• ADEM
	• Acute hemorrhagic leukoencephalopathy	

Very rare causes of acute encephalitis		
• Parvovirus • Measles virus • Mumps virus • West Nile virus (arboviruses) • Chikungunya virus • Rabies virus • Zika virus		

ADEM acute disseminated encephalomyelitis. **CMV** cytomegalovirus. **EBV** Epstein-Barr virus. **HLH** hemophagocytic lymphohistiocytosis. **HSV** herpes simplex virus. **NMDA** N-methyl-D-aspartate. **SLE** systemic lupus erythematosus.

*This is not an exhaustive list, but rather a list of the more common pathogens/diseases to consider.

- The most commonly diagnosed encephalitis is herpes simplex virus (HSV) encephalitis (majority HSV type 1).

History

- Items to ask for specifically on history are:
  » Travel history
    › Camping
    › Visiting farms
  » Mosquito or tick bites
  » Contact with animals

Physical Exam

- Look for the following on physical exam:
  » Fever, headache, vomiting, irritability, poor appetite, rash, recent upper respiratory tract infection (URTI) symptoms
  » Altered level of consciousness: disorientation, confusion, somnolence
  » Aggressive or apathetic behaviour
  » Ataxia
  » Focal neurological deficits
  » Seizures or status epilepticus

Investigations

- Consider the following studies:
  » Bloodwork:
    › CBC, differential, acute and convalescent serum for pathogens
    › Enteroviruses, HSV, *Bartonella*, mycoplasma, varicella, measles, Epstein-Barr virus (EBV), cytomegalovirus (CMV), human herpesvirus 6, parvovirus, respiratory viruses
  » CSF:
    › May show normal or elevated WBC, mildly elevated protein, variable glucose
    › Should be sent for PCR and culture
  » Nasopharyngeal swab:
    › Respiratory viruses
  » Viral throat swab:
    › Adenovirus, enterovirus, HSV
  » Bacterial throat swab:
    › Mycoplasma PCR
  » Viral stool cultures:
    › Adenovirus, enterovirus
  » CT head scan:
    › May be normal initially
  » MRI head:
    › Is more sensitive than CT for acute encephalitic changes
    › May show temporal lobe edema and hemorrhage with HSV
  » Electroencephalogram (EEG):
    › Helps in localizing encephalitic area of brain
- Consider blood cultures and purified protein derivative (PPD) skin test to show other causes of encephalopathy.

Management

- Stabilize patients if they have a low GCS score, are in status epilepticus, or are seizing.
- Monitor GCS score, treat seizure activity, and look for signs of raised intracranial pressure or progression of disease.
- Consider acyclovir empirically for infectious encephalitis.
- Consult infectious diseases and neurology for more specific treatments.

REFERENCES

Allen UD, Robinson JL; Canadian Paediatric Society, Infectious Diseases and Immunization Committee. Prevention and management of neonatal herpes simplex virus infections. *Paediatr Child Health.* 2014;19(4):201–206. https://doi.org/10.1093/pch/19.4.201. Medline:24855418

Canadian Paediatric Society, Infectious Diseases and Immunization Committee. Zika virus: what does a physician caring for children in Canada need to know? [cited 2016 Dec 19]. Practice Point. www.cps.ca

Curtis S, Stobart K, Vandermeer B, Simel DL, Klassen T. Clinical features suggestive of meningitis in children: a systematic review of prospective data. *Pediatrics.* 2010;126(5):952–960. https://doi.org/10.1542/peds.2010-0277. Medline:20974781

Kneen R, Michael BD, Menson E, et al; National Encephalitis Guidelines Development and Stakeholder Groups. Management of suspected viral encephalitis in children: Association of British Neurologists and British Paediatric Allergy, Immunology and Infection Group national guidelines. *J Infect.* 2012;64(5):449–477. https://doi.org/10.1016/j.jinf.2011.11.013. Medline:22120594

Le Saux N; Canadian Paediatric Society, Infectious Diseases and Immunization Committee. Guidelines for the management of suspected and confirmed bacterial meningitis in Canadian children older than one month of age. *Paediatr Child Health.* 2014;19(3):141–146. https://doi.org/10.1093/pch/19.3.141. Medline:24665226

Maconochie IK, Bhaumik S. Fluid therapy for acute bacterial meningitis. *Cochrane Database Syst Rev.* 2016;11:CD004786. Medline:27813057

Swanson D. Meningitis. *Pediatrics in review.* 2015;36(12):514.

Thigpen MC, Whitney CG, Messonnier NE, et al; Emerging Infections Programs Network. Bacterial meningitis in the United States, 1998–2007. *N Engl J Med.* 2011;364(21):2016–2025. https://doi.org/10.1056/NEJMoa1005384. Medline:21612470

NEUROLOGIC EMERGENCIES

4.4

Idiopathic Intracranial Hypertension (Pseudotumor Cerebri)

Anna Kempinska

- Idiopathic intracranial hypertension is a syndrome of increased intracranial pressure (ICP) with normal cerebrospinal fluid (CSF) content and no evidence of structural lesions on neuroimaging.
- The condition is also known as primary intracranial hypertension.
  - » It was formerly called benign intracranial hypertension but this name was retracted due to the potential for visual complications.
- There is no recognized cause.
- The rate of incidence in the pediatric population is 1 in 100 000.
- The female-to-male ratio in pediatric patients is:
  - » Prepubertal 1:1
  - » Postpubertal 2:1
- Children are less likely to be overweight compared to adults.
- The condition is unlikely in children < 10 years of age and very rare in children < 3 years of age.
- Characteristic symptoms and findings are headache and papilledema.

Pathogenesis

- The actual mechanism of idiopathic intracranial hypertension is unclear; however, proposed mechanisms include:
  - » Possible cerebral venous outflow abnormality
    - › It is uncertain whether this is the cause or result of increased ICP.
  - » Increased CSF outflow resistance
  - » Impaired CSF reabsorption by arachnoid villi
  - » Increased abdominal and intracranial venous pressure
  - » Altered sodium and water retention
  - » Abnormality of vitamin A metabolism

History

- Items to collect on the history include:
  - » Headache (in > 90% of patients, though less common in young children), which:
    - › Is usually severe
    - › Is throbbing or pulsatile
    - › Possibly causes nausea or vomiting
    - › Worsens with position change and is relieved

by rest / nonsteroidal anti-inflammatory drugs (NSAIDs)
- » Vision change/loss, which:
  - › May be monocular or binocular
  - › Is usually transient; sustained loss can occur but is rare
  - › Is sometimes evoked by position change or bright lights
- Pulsatile tinnitus
- Photopsia (flashes of light)
- Retrobulbar pain (sometimes in trigeminal nerve root distribution)
- Irritability (infants)
- Back pain and neck stiffness

Risk Factors

- Factors that put patients at higher risk for idiopathic intracranial hypertension include:
  - » Weight:
    - › Obesity or significant recent weight gain
  - » Medications:
    - › Growth hormone (usually within 1 year of therapy)
    - › Tetracycline (usually within a few weeks to months of therapy)
    - › Retinoids
    - › Others (limited evidence): lithium, thyroid replacement, nitrofurantoin, oral contraceptive use, withdrawal from corticosteroids
  - » Excess dietary vitamin A intake (may be a factor)
- There may be a possible genetic link.
- The condition is associated with multiple systemic illnesses causing secondary intracranial hypertension:
  - » Iron deficiency anemia
  - » Polycystic ovary syndrome (PCOS)
  - » Rheumatologic and endocrine conditions
    - › Addison disease, hypothyroidism

Physical Exam

- Findings on physical exam include:
  - » Generally normal neurologic exam
  - » Papilledema (usually bilateral but can be unilateral)
  - » Visual field loss
    - › This occurs before loss of visual acuity.
  - » Cranial nerve VI palsy
    - › This is caused by the effect of elevated ICP on the abducens nerve.
    - › Other cranial nerve palsies have been reported.

Diagnosis

- Idiopathic intracranial hypertension is a diagnosis of exclusion and should be considered for any child with headache and papilledema.
  - » Strongly consider idiopathic intracranial

hypertension if papilledema is not present but the patient's history is strongly suggestive.
- Diagnostic criteria for prepubertal primary intracranial hypertension criteria can be found in *Table 4.4.1*.

Table 4.4.1. CRITERIA FOR DIAGNOSIS OF PRIMARY INTRACRANIAL HYPERTENSION

	1.	CSF opening pressure of: » 18 cm H2O in children < 8 years of age — or — » 25 cm H2O in children > 8 years of age — or — » 25 cm H2O in children < 8 years of age without optic edema
	2.	No focal neurologic signs (with the exception of cranial nerve IV or VI palsy)
	3.	Normal CSF composition
	4.	Exclusion of recognized secondary causes
	5.	Bilateral optic disc edema
	6.	Symptoms suggestive of elevated intracranial pressure (headache, nausea, vomiting, transient visual obscurations, tinnitus) that improve following CSF drainage
Definitive diagnosis		Patient meets criteria 1 to 6
Probable diagnosis		Patient meets criteria 1 to 4 and either 5 or 6

Reproduced from Aylward Pediatric Neurology (2013) with permission.

Investigations

- Obtain urgent neuroimaging to exclude a secondary cause of intracranial hypertension (i.e., mass lesion, venous thrombosis).
  - » MRI with MR venography is the recommended test of choice.
    - › Possible findings:
      - · Tortuosity / enlargement of optic nerve
      - · Empty sella
      - · Flattening of posterior aspect of globe
      - · Transverse venous sinus stenosis
  - » CT scan is helpful in cases where MRI is difficult to obtain or delayed.
    - › Findings:
      - · Absence of mass/tumor
      - · Slit-like ventricles
    - › CT venography may show transverse venous sinus stenosis with no sign of thrombus.
- A lumbar puncture (LP) must be performed if no structural cause for increased ICP is identified on neuroimaging.
  - » The opening pressure must be documented. Intracranial pressure is considered elevated if:
    - › Pressure is > 18 cm H_2O in patients < 8 years of age (>25 cm H_2O if optic edema is absent)
    - › Pressure is > 25 cm H_2O in patients ≥ 8 years of age.

- CSF should be sent for cell count and culture as well to ensure there is no infection.
  - › Normal cell count, protein, and glucose are seen with pseudotumor cerebri.
- Involve ophthalmology to:
  - » Confirm papilledema
  - » Monitor treatment response

Management

- Acute management is based on the severity of symptoms.

Management in the ED

- Use LP to drain CSF.
- First-line medical therapy:
  - » Acetazolamide (carbonic anhydrase inhibitor)
    - › Acetazolamide reduces the rate of CSF production.
    - › Start at a dose of 20 mg/kg per day PO divided and given twice daily.
      - · This may be increased up to 100 mg/kg per day.
    - › For adolescents, use 500 mg PO twice daily
      - · This may be increased up to 4000 mg/day
- Alternative medical therapies:
  - » Furosemide 1 to 2 mg/kg per day divided and given twice daily
    - › Consider adding to acetazolamide if there is no improvement.
  - » Topiramate 1 to 3 mg/kg per day divided and given twice daily to a maximum of 200 mg per day
- Emergent treatment of severe symptoms and/or visual dysfunction is:
  - » Lumboperitoneal or ventriculoperitoneal shunt

Management on Discharge

- Continue medical therapy as above.
- Stop medications that risk causing pseudotumor cerebri.
- Suggest weight loss for patients with a high body mass index.

Complications

- Complications may include:
  - » Visual loss (up to 10%)
  - » Cranial nerve deficit

- Chronic symptoms may require a CSF shunt or optic nerve fenestration.
- Recurrence is common.

Disposition

- Consider admission to hospital if the patient has severe symptoms, persistent vomiting, and visual changes.
- Follow up with neurology and ophthalmology.

REFERENCES

Aylward SC. Pediatric idiopathic intracranial hypertension: a need for clarification. *Pediatr Neurol.* 2013;49(5):303–304. https://doi.org/10.1016/j.pediatrneurol.2013.05.019. Medline:23958286

Aylward SC, Aronowitz C, Reem R, Rogers D, Roach ES. Intracranial hypertension without headache in children. *J Child Neurol.* 2015;30(6):703–706. https://doi.org/10.1177/0883073814540522. Medline:25038131

Bidot S, Saindane AM, Peragallo JH, Bruce BB, Newman NJ, Biousse V. Brain imaging in idiopathic intracranial hypertension. *J Neuroophthalmol.* 2015;35(4):400–411. https://doi.org/10.1097/WNO.0000000000000303. Medline:26457687

Biousse V, Bruce BB, Newman NJ. Update on the pathophysiology and management of idiopathic intracranial hypertension. *J Neurol Neurosurg Psychiatry.* 2012;83(5):488–494. https://doi.org/10.1136/jnnp-2011-302029. Medline:22423118

Chern JJ, Tubbs RS, Gordon AS, Donnithorne KJ, Oakes WJ. Management of pediatric patients with pseudotumor cerebri. *Childs Nerv Syst.* 2012;28(4):575–578. https://doi.org/10.1007/s00381-011-1657-9. Medline:22258754

Dwyer CM, Prelog K, Owler BK. The role of venous sinus outflow obstruction in pediatric idiopathic intracranial hypertension. *J Neurosurg Pediatr.* 2013;11(2):144–149. https://doi.org/10.3171/2012.10.PEDS1299. Medline:23176141

Fleisher GR. *Textbook of pediatric emergency medicine.* Philadelphia: Lippincott Williams & Wilkins; 2010.

Friedman DI, Liu GT, Digre KB. Revised diagnostic criteria for the pseudotumor cerebri syndrome in adults and children. *Neurology.* 2013;81(13):1159–1165. https://doi.org/10.1212/WNL.0b013e3182a55f17. Medline:23966248

Glatstein MM, Oren A, Amarilyio G, et al. Clinical characterization of idiopathic intracranial hypertension in children presenting to the emergency department: the experience of a large tertiary care pediatric hospital. *Pediatr Emerg Care.* 2015;31(1):6–9. https://doi.org/10.1097/PEC.0000000000000177. Medline:25207755

Soiberman U, Stolovitch C, Balcer LJ, Regenbogen M, Constantini S, Kesler A. Idiopathic intracranial hypertension in children: visual outcome and risk of recurrence. *Childs Nerv Syst.* 2011;27(11):1913–1918. https://doi.org/10.1007/s00381-011-1470-5. Medline:21538129

4.5

Ataxia

Rahim Valani

- Ataxia is defined as a disorder of intentional movement that is characterized by unsteadiness or shakiness.
- Motor coordination requires:
  » Proprioception input from joint and muscles
  » A motor pathway from the cerebral cortex and basal ganglia to the lower motor neuron
  » Cerebellar control
  » Vestibular system input
- Being unable to walk or having poor coordination can be due to various causes, including:
  » Pain
  » Weakness
  » Cerebellar issues
  » Dystonia
  » Myoclonus
  » Vertigo
- Most causes of ataxia affect the cerebellar system.
  » Cerebellar dysfunction can result in:
    › Gait or limb ataxia
    › Dysmetria
    › Tremors
    › Nystagmus
    › Dysarthria
- Ataxia can be categorized based on duration:
  » Acute cerebellar ataxia
  » Subacute cerebellar ataxia
  » Intermittent cerebellar ataxia
  » Chronic cerebellar ataxia — progressive or nonprogressive

History

- When obtaining the patient's history, consider the following clinical features:
  » Problems with walking or balance
  » Frequent falls
  » Other neurologic symptoms — visual, motor, sensory
  » Duration of symptoms
  » Recent or intercurrent illnesses
  » Any level of altered sensorium
  » Headache
  » Vomiting
  » Presence of rash — either current or recent
  » Recent head injury
  » Medications — both prescribed and those that patient can access
  » Recreational drug use

Physical Exam

- Assess the patient for altered level of consciousness / altered sensorium
- General findings are:
  » Rash
  » Mental status exam
  » Signs of head injury
  » Speech — evidence of slurred speech, difficulty in word finding, or incomprehensible words
- Conduct a neurologic exam, with particular attention to:
  » Cranial nerve exam, with assessment of:
    › Presence of nystagmus
    › Funduscopy
    › Visual fields
    › Visual acuity
  » Cerebellar testing:
    › Gait
    › Stance
    › Romberg test
    › Finger-nose test
    › Diadochokinesia (rapid alternating movement)
    › Tremor
  » Motor exam:
    › Muscle tone
    › Muscle strength
  » Sensory exam:
    › Proprioception
    › Vibration
  » Deep tendon reflexes

Investigations

- Investigations should include:
  » Bloodwork
    › Complete blood count (CBC)
    › Electrolytes and renal function
  » Lumbar puncture for cerebrospinal fluid (CSF) analysis and opening pressures
    › Cell count
    › Protein, glucose
    › Bacterial and viral cultures

- » Urine toxicology screen
- » Imaging
  - › CT scan of head
  - › MRI
- » Electroencephalogram (EEG)
- Other tests to consider:
  - » Thyroid stimulating hormone (TSH), free T_4
  - » Ethanol level
  - » Antiepileptic medication levels (phenytoin, carbamazepine)

ATAXIA CAUSED BY DRUGS OR TOXINS

- Ataxia may be caused by:
  - » Intoxication / substance abuse:
    - › Alcohol or any of the toxic alcohols (see Chapter 19.4)
    - › Dextromethorphan
    - › Marijuana (see Chapter 19.7)
  - » Medication:
    - › Antiepileptic medications:
      - · Benzodiazepines
      - · Dilantin
      - · Carbamazepine
      - · Lamotrigine
      - · Phenobarbital
    - › Antineoplastic agents and immunosuppressants:
      - · Cyclosporin
      - · Tacrolimus
      - · Cytosine arabinoside
  - » Other toxins:
    - › Lead
    - › Mercury
    - › Thallium

Management

- Initiate symptomatic management for most causes.
- For toxins, call the regional Poison Control Centre to discuss the role of specific antidotes, dialysis, or other considerations.

ACUTE POSTINFECTIOUS CEREBELLAR ATAXIA

- Acute postinfectious cerebellar ataxia is the most common cause of acute ataxia in children (30% to 50% of cases).
- The condition is usually seen in children 1 to 4 years of age, 1 to 3 weeks after a viral infection.
- The most common etiologies are:
  - » Varicella (chickenpox)
    - › Ataxia occurs in 1 per 4000 cases of varicella; in the postvaccinal era, for those receiving the

varicella vaccine, the estimated incidence is 1.5 per 100 000 vaccine doses.
  - » Mumps
  - » Parvovirus
  - » Epstein-Barr virus (EBV)
- Acute postinfectious cerebellar ataxia is a self-limiting condition.

Investigations

- CSF may show pleocytosis but is usually normal.
- EEG can show slowing but is otherwise normal.
- Neuroimaging is normal; if no abnormalities are detected, consider other causes.

Management

- Management is symptomatic.
- Some studies recommend deferring neuroimaging and CSF analysis if the patient has a normal mental status exam, no focal neurologic findings, and no history of recent infection.
  - » A neurology follow-up must be done.

ACUTE DISSEMINATING ENCEPHALOMYELITIS

- Acute disseminating encephalomyelitis (ADEM) is an inflammatory demyelinating disorder that usually follows a recent infection.
- It affects white matter tracts of the CNS.
- Incidence is estimated to be 0.4 per 100 000, with a mean age of 6.5 years.
  - » 64% of patients present between 2 to 10 years of age.

Diagnosis

- Diagnosis is based on the following findings:
  - » Polyfocal immune-mediated demyelinating lesions of the CNS
  - » Presence of encephalopathy not explained by fever
  - » Characteristic demyelinating lesions on MRI:
    - › Multiple, asymmetrically distributed, hyperintense areas on T2 and FLAIR images
    - › Poorly marginated lesions
    - › Infratentorial involvement — seen in 50% of cases

Management

- Consult the neurology team regarding management.
  - » Options include:
    - › High-dose steroids
    - › Intravenous immunoglobulin
    - › Cyclosporin
    - › Plasma exchange

CEREBROVASCULAR EVENTS

- Cerebrovascular events include:
  - » Hemorrhagic or nonhemorrhagic strokes (see Chapter 4.2).
  - » Venous sinus thrombosis
  - » CNS vasculitis

LABYRINTHITIS

- Most children present with severe nausea and vomiting as they cannot articulate the sensation of vertigo.
- Management involves the symptomatic treatment of vestibular neuritis and labyrinthitis with antinausea medications.
- Symptoms usually resolve within a few weeks.

OPSOCLONUS-MYOCLONUS SYNDROME (KINSBOURNE SYNDROME)

- Opsoclonus-myoclonus syndrome can be associated with neuroblastoma.
  - » Always exclude neuroblastoma as the etiology.
    - › 50% of cases have neuroblastoma.
    - › Only 2% to 4% of children with neuroblastoma have opsoclonus-myoclonus syndrome.
    - › Urine catecholamines have only a 24% sensitivity in diagnosing neuroblastoma.

Management

- Consult oncology if neuroblastoma is present.
  - » The decision between surgical versus medical therapy is made based on the stage of the neuroblastoma.
- Consult neurology if there is no tumor.

GLUTEN ATAXIA

- Gluten ataxia presents with gait ataxia, nystagmus, peripheral neuropathy, and MRI-depicted brain changes.
- Symptoms begin with gluten ingestion, which is considered the trigger.

Management

- Gluten ataxia improves with a gluten-free diet.
- Refer the patient to gastroenterology for gluten-sensitivity testing.

BASILAR MIGRAINE

- For more information on basilar migraine, see Chapter 4.6.

MILLER-FISHER VARIANT OF GUILLAIN-BARRÉ SYNDROME

- The Miller-Fisher variant is associated with the clinical triad of ataxia, areflexia, and ophthalmoplegia.
- The presence of serum anti-GQ1b antibodies is suggestive.
- For more information on the Miller-Fisher variant of Guillain-Barré syndrome, see Chapter 4.8.

NUTRITIONAL DEFICIENCY

- Assess the patient for deficiencies in thiamine, cobalamin, vitamin E, zinc, or folate.
- The condition may be subacute or chronic.
- Management depends on the specific deficiency.

REFERENCES

Caffarelli M, Kimia AA, Torres AR. Acute ataxia in children: a review of the differential diagnosis and evaluation in the emergency department. *Pediatr Neurol.* 2016;65:14–30. https://doi.org/10.1016/j.pediatrneurol.2016.08.025. Medline:27789117

Maria BL. *Current management of child neurology.* 3rd ed. Hamilton: BC Decker Inc; 2005.

Pavone P, Praticò AD, Pavone V, et al. Ataxia in children: early recognition and clinical evaluation. *Ital J Pediatr.* 2017;43(1):6. https://doi.org/10.1186/s13052-016-0325-9. Medline:28257643

Rossi A, Martinetti C, Morana G, Severino M, Tortora D. Neuroimaging of infectious and inflammatory diseases of the pediatric cerebellum and brainstem. *Neuroimaging Clin N Am.* 2016;26(3):471–487. https://doi.org/10.1016/j.nic.2016.03.011. Medline:27423804

4.6

Migraine

Shabnam Minoosepehr

- Headache is a common pediatric complaint in the emergency department (ED) and can have many causes.
- Primary headache disorders are those with no other cause:
  » Migraines
  » Tension-type headaches
  » Cluster headaches
- Pediatric migraines are prevalent:
  » Ages 3 to 7 years — 1.2% to 3.2%
  » Ages 7 to 11 years — 4% to 11%
  » ≥ 15 years — 8% to 23%
- About 60% of children with migraines are prepubertal males; after puberty, females outnumber males 3:1.
- Migraine headache is usually frontotemporal. Occipital headache in children is rare and calls for diagnostic caution.

Classification

- The International Headache Society (2013) gives classification and variations of pediatric migraine headaches.
- Migraines can be classified as:
  » Migraine with aura
    › A migraine with aura may be visual, sensory, speech, motor, brainstem, or retinal.
  » Migraine without aura
    › A migraine without aura lasts 4 to 72 hours if untreated or unsuccessfully treated.
    › It is usually bilateral; unilateral symptoms usually occur in late adolescence.
    › It is pulsatile in quality.
    › It is moderate to severe on the pain scale.
    › It is aggravated by or causes avoidance of routine physical activity.
    › It is accompanied by nausea and/or vomiting.
    › It is associated with photophobia and phonophobia.
- Migraine variants include:
  » Hemiplegic migraine
    › Hemiplegic migraine is characterized by abrupt onset of hemiparesis, usually followed by headache.
  » Basilar artery migraine
    › Basilar artery migraine is more common in females.
    › It is defined as migraine with aura with at least 2 of the following:
      · Dysarthria
      · Tinnitus
      · Hypacusia
      · Diplopia
      · Decreased level of consciousness
      · Vertigo
      · Ataxia
      · Visual disturbances in both hemifields
      · Bilateral sensory symptoms
  » Retinal migraine
    › A retinal migraine is brief (a few seconds to 1 minute) and involves sudden monocular blackouts or bright, blinding episodes of visual disturbance during or after headache.
  » Alice in Wonderland syndrome
    › This syndrome is characterized by unusual visual illusions and spatial distortions that precede headaches; visual distortions include:
      · Micropsia (objects appear smaller)
      · Macropsia (objects appear larger)
      · Metamorphopsia (objects appear abnormally shaped)
      · Teleopsia (objects appear farther away)
  » Acute confusional migraine
    › Acute confusional migraine lasts 4 to 24 hours.
    › It is associated with agitation, lethargy, and impaired sensorium.
    › It may be accompanied by neurological deficits such as aphasia, anisocoria, and memory deficits.
  » Ophthalmoplegic migraine
    › Ophthalmoplegic migraine is defined as 2 or more headache episodes accompanied by paresis of 1 or more of the third, fourth, and sixth cranial nerves.
  » Episodic syndromes
    › Episodic syndromes are previously known as childhood periodic syndromes, cyclic vomiting syndrome, abdominal migraine, benign paroxysmal vertigo of childhood, and benign paroxysmal torticollis.
    › Episodic syndromes are considered migraine precursors.

Pathophysiology

- The pathophysiology of migraine headaches is not fully understood.

- It is believed that migraines are primarily a neuronal process associated with an underlying genetic predisposition that causes a hyperexcitable cerebral cortex, which in turn causes headaches.

Differential Diagnosis

- On the differential diagnosis, consider:
  » Carbon monoxide poisoning
  » Drug toxicity
  » Cerebrovascular abnormality
  » Encephalitis / meningitis / brain abscess
  » Head injury / contusion
  » Dental infection / sinus infection
  » Aneurysm / subarachnoid hemorrhage
  » Glaucoma
  » Primary and metastatic disease
  » Hydrocephalus
  » Hypoglycemia
  » Malignant hypertension

History

- Assess the onset, severity, quality, radiation, and temporal profile of the headache.
- Determine the treatment used so far.
- Look for any associated neurologic or ocular symptoms.
- Ask about specific precipitants:
  » Stress/anxiety
  » Hunger
  » Menstruation
  » Foods/beverages that are cold or contain nitrates, glutamine, caffeine, or tyramine (cheese, nuts)
  » Oral contraceptives
  » Lack of sleep
  » Physical exertion / fatigue
  » Reading / refractive error
  » Sunlight / screen glare
  » Barometric pressure change
  » Infection
  » Traumatic injury

Investigations

- Brain imaging in migraines is not useful for diagnosis; only 1% yield significant findings.
- A history representative of migraine and normal physical examination is the most effective way of making the diagnosis.
- The American College of Radiology suggests considering an MRI (if available) to rule out structural lesions in the following cases:
  » Migraine with neurologic deficit
  » Ophthalmologic migraine with unilateral ptosis or complete third nerve palsy
  » Basilar artery migraine syndrome
  » Acute confusional migraine syndrome that persists
  » Progressive chronic headache
  » Hemiplegic migraine
  » Seizure and postictal headache
- Laboratory studies such as bloodwork and lumbar puncture are only helpful if you are trying to rule out other causes of headache such as infection or increased intracranial pressure.

Management

- Consider a bolus of 20 mL/kg 0.9% normal saline for migraine patients.

Nonsteroidal Anti-inflammatory Drugs and Acetaminophen

- Nonsteroidal anti-inflammatory drugs (NSAIDs) are first-line management for acute migraines without significant nausea or vomiting. Consider:
  » Ibuprofen 10 mg/kg
  » Ketorolac 0.5 mg/kg with maximum 30 mg intravenously if the patient is experiencing severe nausea/vomiting or if IV bolus of fluids is already being given
- Acetaminophen is also a good first-line option, although NSAIDs have been proven more effective.

Dopamine Receptor Antagonists

- Consider the following dopamine receptor antagonists:
  » Prochlorperazine 0.15 mg/kg, to a maximum 10 mg
    › Prochlorperazine has the best evidence for treatment of acute migraine in children.
    › Its side effects include agitation, dystonic reactions, akathisia, and possible prolongation of QT.
    › If the patient develops acute dystonic reaction / extrapyramidal reaction, treat them with diphenhydramine.
  » Metoclopramide 0.15 to 2 mg/kg, to a maximum 10 mg

Triptans

- Triptans are serotonin agonists for 5-HT receptors.
- They inhibit the release of vasoactive peptides and promote vasoconstriction.
- Consider sumatriptan nasal spray 5 to 20 mg for patients aged 12 to 17 years.

Antiepileptics

- Consider a sodium valproate bolus of 15 to 20 mg/kg IV over 5 minutes followed by 15 to 20 mg/kg PO 4 hours later.

Dihydroergotamine (DHE)

- Dihydroergotamine is a 5-HT receptor agonist.
- It is considered because of its vasoconstriction effect.

- For patients > 30 kg or > 9 years of age:
  - » Give 1 mg IV over 5 to 15 minutes
    - › A 2.5 mg dose may be repeated in 1 hour if needed.
- For patients < 30 kg or < 9 years of age:
  - » Give 0.5 mg IV over 5 to 15 minutes
    - › This dose can be repeated in 1 hour.

Dexamethasone

- Treatment of migraine with dexamethasone in combination with any of the above treatments has been shown to decrease the rate of return to the ED in the adult population.
- Consider dexamethasone in teenagers.

REFERENCES

Alfonzo MJ, Bechtel K, Babineau S. Management of headache in the pediatric emergency department. *Pediatr Emerg Med Pract.* 2013;10(1):1–25. Medline:26505695

American College of Radiology. ACR appropriateness criteria: headache child [PDF]. 2017 [cited 2016 Feb 12]. Available from: https://www.guideline.gov/summaries/summary/37921

Bigal ME, Lipton RB. The prognosis of migraine. *Curr Opin Neurol.* 2008;21(3):301–308. https://doi.org/10.1097/WCO.0b013e328300c6f5. Medline:18451714

Headache Classification Committee of the International Headache Society (HIS). The international classification of headache disorders, 3rd edition (beta version). *Cephalagia.* 2013;33(9):629–808.

Kabbouche M. Management of pediatric migraine headache in the emergency room and infusion center. *Headache.* 2015;55(10):1365–1370. https://doi.org/10.1111/head.12694. Medline:26486800

Lewis D, Ashwal S, Hershey A, Hirtz D, Yonker M, Silberstein S; American Academy of Neurology Quality Standards Subcommittee; Practice Committee of the Child Neurology Society. Practice parameter: pharmacological treatment of migraine headache in children and adolescents: report of the American Academy of Neurology Quality Standards Subcommittee and the Practice Committee of the Child Neurology Society. *Neurology.* 2004;63(12):2215–2224. https://doi.org/10.1212/01.WNL.0000147332.41993.90. Medline:15623677

Lewis DW. Pediatric migraine. *Pediatr Rev.* 2007;28(2):43–53. https://doi.org/10.1542/pir.28-2-43. Medline:17272520

Schwedt TJ, Guo Y, Rothner AD. "Benign" imaging abnormalities in children and adolescents with headache. *Headache.* 2006;46(3):387–398. https://doi.org/10.1111/j.1526-4610.2006.00371.x. Medline:16618255

Tarantino S, Capuano A, Torriero R, et al. Migraine equivalents as part of migraine syndrome in childhood. *Pediatr Neurol.* 2014;51(5):645–649. https://doi.org/10.1016/j.pediatrneurol.2014.07.018. Medline:25155656

NEUROLOGIC EMERGENCIES

4.7

Myasthenia Gravis

Vidushi Khatri, Rahim Valani

- Myasthenia gravis is the most common disorder of neuromuscular junction.
- Incidence of myasthenia gravis is estimated to be 1 to 10 per 1 million per year.
- Myasthenia gravis is an autoimmune disorder characterized by fatigable skeletal muscle.
- The muscle weakness is due to autoantibodies that attack acetylcholine receptors (AChRs) at the neuromuscular junction (NMJ).
- Patients with myasthenia gravis have **only** motor manifestations of the disease.
- **Pupils are always spared in myasthenia gravis**, helping to differentiate it from other disorders.

Classification

- There are 5 classifications of myasthenia gravis:
  1. Minimal manifestation status
     - › Patients have no symptoms or functional limitations.
     - › Some weakness may be apparent on clinical exam.
  2. Remission
     - › Patients have no symptoms or signs of the disease.
       - · Weakness of eyelid closure is allowed under this classification.
     - › Patients are on active treatment.
  3. Ocular myasthenia gravis
     - › Patients with any weakness of the ocular muscles fall under this classification.
     - › Strength is intact in limbs, facial, and bulbar muscles.
  4. Impending myasthenic crisis (see "Myasthenic Crisis," below)
     - › This is characterized by rapid clinical deterioration eventually resulting in crisis.
  5. Refractory myasthenia gravis
     - › Patients have worsening or no improvement of symptoms after being on treatment.

Pathophysiology

Normal Muscle Contraction of a Healthy Patient

- Presynaptic terminals contain vesicles filled with acetylcholine (ACh).
- An action potential stimulates terminal motor neurons, causing a calcium influx and ACh exocytosis.
- ACh binds to AChR, causing the Na/K influx that stimulates muscle contraction.

Myasthenia Gravis Pathogenesis

- Autoantibodies target AChRs, leading to the complement-mediated destruction of AChRs.
- Muscle fatigability in myasthenia gravis is explained by acetylcholine overwhelming the reduced numbers of AChRs.

History

- Questions to ask on history are:
  » Does the patient have any sensory symptoms?
  » Does the patient have fluctuating muscle weakness that worsens at the end of the day or in other circumstances? — For instance:
    › Exercise / physical stress
    › Infection
    › Fever
    › Recent use of medication that precipitates/exacerbates myasthenia gravis (aminoglycosides, fluoroquinolones, beta-blockers, procainamide)
  » Does the patient have improved strength after resting?
  » Does the patient have ocular symptoms? — For example:
    › Diplopia
    › Blurry vision
    › Worsening ptosis over the course of day
- Prepubertal myasthenia gravis is more likely to present with purely ocular symptoms.
  » Ptosis can be unilateral and cause amblyopia.
  » Generalized muscle weakness is rare in prepubertal cases.
- Postpubertal patients present with symptoms similar to adults.
  » Ocular symptoms commence at onset with 80% developing generalized muscle weakness during the course of the disease.
- Facial muscle weakness in the patient results in expressionlessness and a "myasthenic sneer," in which only the midlip rises.

Physical Exam

- Weakness may involve any component of the skeletal muscle system:
  » Ocular
    › Asymmetric and bilateral ptosis and ophthalmoplegia
    › Normal pupillary reaction to light and accommodation
  » Bulbar (considered life-threatening due to inability to protect airway)
    › Poor gag reflex and palate elevation
    › Possible weak mastication
  » Facial
    › "Myasthenic sneer" from involvement of orbicularis oris muscle
  » Respiratory (known as a myasthenic crisis; see "Myasthenic Crisis," below)
    › Respiratory muscle weakness from diaphragmatic and intercostal muscle involvement
    › Possible stridor due to adduction of vocal cords
  » Periphery muscles
    › Typically, proximal muscle involvement (i.e., arms weaker than legs)
- Deep tendon reflexes are normal.

Investigations

- It is important to image the thymus, as myasthenia gravis is associated with thymic hyperplasia.
- Screen for thyroid abnormalities (seen in up to 25% of adult cases of myasthenia gravis).
- Consider the following investigations:
  » Assays for AChR-Ab, MuSK-Ab, or titin
    › Seropositive myasthenia gravis patients will have positive assays.
  » Electromyography (EMG)
    › EMG is recommended for diagnosis.
    › Sensitivity is increased if both facial and peripheral muscles are investigated.
  » Repetitive nerve stimulation
    › Look for compound motor action potential amplitude decrement of above 10% in response to 3Hz repetitive supramaximal nerve stimulation.
  » Edrophonium (Tensilon test)
    › Edrophonium is a rapid-acting reversible acetylcholinergic inhibitor, used to differentiate myasthenia gravis from cholinergic crisis.
    › A positive test shows reduced ptosis or ophthalmoparesis upon administration of edrophonium.
    › Tensilon tests are usually performed in an intensive care setting due to risk of bradycardia and bronchospasm.
    › A positive test is also seen with:
      · Lambert-Eaton myasthenic syndrome (inadequate release of ACh from nerve terminals)
      · Motor neuron disease
      · Cavernous sinus tumors
      · Brain stem lesions
      · End stage renal disease
    › For dosing, see Table 4.7.1.

Table 4.7.1. DOSING OF EDROPHONIUM FOR TENSILON TEST

Age and/or weight	Initial dose	Repeat dosing
Newborns and infants	0.15 mg/kg	• Begin with test dose of 0.01 mg/kg • Can repeat 0.15 mg/kg to a maximum of 0.6 mg
> 1 year and weight < 34 kg	0.5 to 1.0 mg	• Can repeat 1.0 mg doses to a maximum of 5 mg
> 34 kg	2.0 mg	• Repeat 2.0 mg to a maximum of 10.0 mg

Diagnosis

- Consider alternative diagnoses if the history includes nonmotor neurologic symptoms.
- Consider concurrent autoimmune diseases, such as rheumatoid arthritis and systemic lupus erythematosus (SLE).

Differential Diagnosis

- *Table 4.7.2* shows indicators for differentiating between myasthenia gravis, Guillain-Barré syndrome, and botulism.

Management

- Depending on clinical presentation, management may include:
  » First-line medication:

› Acetylcholine-esterase inhibitors (Pyridostigmine)
  · Administer an initial dose of 0.5 to 1.0 mg/kg per day divided every 6 hours.
  · This is less useful in MuSK-Ab positive patients, as they respond better to corticosteroids, plasma exchange, and immunosuppressants.
» Nonsteroidal immunosuppressive agents:
  › Azathioprine (0.5 to 1.0 mg per day)
  › Cyclosporine
  › Methotrexate
  › Tacrolimus
  › Mycophenolate mofetil
» Glucocorticoids (tuberculosis [TB] skin test and/ or chest X-ray [CXR] must be completed prior to initiating steroid therapy):
  › Prednisone or prednisolone 0.5 to 1 mg/kg
» Intravenous immunoglobulin (IVIG) and plasma exchange therapy
  › IVIG is appropriate for short-term treatment in patients with respiratory compromise or dysphagia.
  › Maintenance therapy using IVIG is an alternative to immunosuppressive agents.
» Thymectomy:
  › Thymectomy is a long-term treatment option in pre- or postpubertal children.
  › It is useful only if patients are AChR-Ab positive.
  › It helps minimize the use of or reduce duration of immunotherapy.

NEUROLOGIC EMERGENCIES

Table 4.7.2. DISTINGUISHING MYASTHENIA GRAVIS, GUILLAIN-BARRÉ SYNDROME, AND BOTULISM

	Myasthenia gravis	Guillain-Barré syndrome	Botulism
Pathophysiology	• Auto-antibodies attack acetylcholine receptor at neuromuscular junction	• Antecedent infection causes immune response towards peripheral nerve	• Neurotoxin caused by *Clostridium botulinum*
Motor symptoms	• **Fatigable, asymmetric** weakness • Presents in smaller muscle groups first (i.e., extraocular muscles)	• **Ascending, symmetric** limb weakness	• **Descending, symmetric** weakness • Cranial nerves → trunk → extremities → diaphragm
Sensory involvement	• None	• Fine paresthesia/neuropathic pain as presenting symptom	• None
Bulbar involvement	• Dysarthria, dysphagia • Facial, neck muscle involvement possible	• Rare, but can occur	• Common
Respiratory involvement	• Myasthenic crisis • Rare, precipitated by surgery/infection	• Uncommon (13%)	• Will progress if treatment is delayed
Ocular symptoms	• Often first presentation • Ptosis, diplopia, oculomotor palsy	• Miller-Fisher variant	• Diplopia from extraocular muscle paralysis
Deep tendon reflexes	• Normal	• Decreased or absent	• Decreased or absent
Autonomic dysfunction	• None	• 50% progression • Orthostatic hypotension • Bradycardia • Loss of sweating	• Present • Paralytic ileus • Urinary retention • Orthostatic hypotension • Reduced salivation
Treatment	• Acetylcholine esterase inhibitor	• Supportive	• < 1 year of age: botulism immunoglobulin • > 1 year of age: botulism antitoxin

> › It may also be considered if the patient has failed to respond to immunotherapy or develops severe side effects from current treatment.

Prognosis

- Children with myasthenia gravis experience higher rates of remission than adults.
- Prepubertal Caucasian children have the highest rates of spontaneous remission.

MYASTHENIC CRISIS

- A myasthenic crisis is respiratory muscle weakness that may require mechanical ventilation.
- A crisis can be precipitated by:
  - » A change in medications
  - » An underlying stressor, such as infection
  - » The inability to clear secretions, resulting in aspiration

Management

- Implement supportive care with ABCs.
- Monitor respiratory function with negative inspiratory force (NIF) and forced vital capacity (FVC).
- Indications for intubation are:
  - » Worsening NIF over time
  - » NIF < 20 cm H_2O
  - » FVC < 10 to 15 mL/kg
  - » 10% decrease in FVC from upright to supine position
- If intubation is required, a rapid-onset nondepolarizing paralytic agent (rocuronium) is recommended.
- IVIG and plasmapheresis are first-line treatments for myasthenic crisis.
- A myasthenic crisis must be distinguished from a cholinergic crisis, as they can clinically mimic each other but have opposing treatments (see *Table 4.7.3*).

Table 4.7.3. CHARACTERISTICS TO DIFFERENTIATE CHOLINERGIC AND MYASTHENIC CRISES

Cholinergic crisis	Myasthenic crisis
Overdose of acetylcholine-esterase inhibitor	Decreased number of functional AChRs
Increased secretions	Normal secretions
Bradycardia	Tachycardia
Constricted pupils	Normal pupils
Tensilon test: symptoms are exaggerated	Symptoms relieved

NEONATAL MYASTHENIA GRAVIS

- Neonatal myasthenia gravis is found in 10% to 20% of infants or children born to mothers with myasthenia gravis.
  - » It is caused by placental transfer of maternal AChR antibodies.

Physical Exam

- Common symptoms in newborns are generalized muscle weakness, hypotonia, poor suck, and weak cry.
- Symptoms usually present by day 3 of life.
- The infant's deep tendon reflexes are intact.
- Additional findings include:
  - » Scoliosis
  - » Joint contractures
  - » Apnea, especially during febrile infections

Diagnosis

- A clinical diagnosis is possible when the maternal diagnosis is known.

Management

- Provide supportive care with small, frequent feedings via nasogastric tube and with respiratory support if needed.
- Administer acetylcholine-esterase inhibitor (neostigmine).
  - » This results in improvement of clinical symptoms over 2 to 3 hours.
  - » Give neostigmine 30 minutes before each feed.

Prognosis

- 90% of patients recover fully by 2 months of life.

REFERENCES

Berezovsky DE, Sitko KR. Pediatric myasthenia gravis: a review. *J Pediatr Neurol*. 2017;16(1):62–69.

Della Marina A, Trippe H, Lutz S, Schara U. Juvenile myasthenia gravis: recommendations for diagnostic approaches and treatment. *Neuropediatrics*. 2014;45(2):75–83. https://doi.org/10.1055/s-0033-1364181. Medline:24470240

Finnis MF, Jayawant S. Juvenile myasthenia gravis: a paediatric perspective. *Autoimmune Dis*. 2011; *Article ID 404101*. http://dx.doi.org/10.4061/2011/404101

Grob D, Brunner N, Namba T, Pagala M. Lifetime course of myasthenia gravis. *Muscle Nerve*. 2008;37(2):141–149. https://doi.org/10.1002/mus.20950. Medline:18059039

Kubiszewska J, Szyluk B, Szczudlik P, et al. Prevalence and impact of autoimmune thyroid disease on myasthenia gravis course. *Brain Behav*. 2016;6(10):e00537. https://doi.org/10.1002/brb3.537. Medline:27781146

Liew WKM, Kang PB. Update on juvenile myasthenia gravis. *Curr Opin Pediatr*. 2013;25(6):694–700. https://doi.org/10.1097/MOP.0b013e328365ad16. Medline:24141560

Sanders DB, Wolfe GI, Benatar M, et al. International consensus guidance for management of myasthenia gravis. *Neurology*. 2016;87(4):419–425. https://doi.org/10.1212/WNL.0000000000002790. Medline:27358333

4.8

Guillain-Barré Syndrome

Vidushi Khatri, Rahim Valani

- Guillain-Barré syndrome (GBS) is the most common cause of acute flaccid paralysis in infants and children.
  » The estimated incidence of GBS is 1.34 cases per 100 000 children < 15 years of age.
- Acute inflammatory demyelinating polyneuropathy is the most common variant of GBS (90% of GBS cases in North America).
  » Acute inflammatory demyelinating polyneuropathy is an idiopathic, autoimmune symmetrical ascending polyneuropathy.
  » It usually causes weakness, areflexia, and paresthesias.
  » It may cause autonomic dysfunction.
- Other variants include:
  » Miller-Fisher syndrome (10% of cases)
    › Miller-Fisher syndrome is characterized by oph-thalmoplegia, ataxia, and areflexia.
    › Weakness appears later.
  » Polyneuritis cranialis
    › Polyneuritis is characterized by multiple cranial nerve palsies and peripheral sensory loss.
- The prognosis for GBS is generally very favorable in children.

Pathophysiology

- The proposed pathophysiology consists of a preceding respiratory or gastrointestinal infection causing an immune response directed towards the myelin and axons of peripheral nerves.
- Infections associated with GBS include:
  » Bacterial: *Campylobacter jejuni* enteritis, mycoplasma
  » Viral: cytomegalovirus (CMV), Epstein-Barr virus (EBV), influenza-like illness
- There is a small risk of GBS associated with the influenza and rabies vaccines.

History

- Patients develop symptoms 2 to 4 weeks after infection resolution.
- Classic symptoms are:
  » Fine paresthesia in toes/fingertips, followed by symmetric ascending weakness
  » Visual symptoms (diplopia, decreased visual acuity)
  » Neuropathic pain (a usual presenting sign in children)
  » Gait unsteadiness

Physical Exam

- Look for the following on physical exam:
  » Symmetric weakness
  » Diminished/absent reflexes
  » Sensory symptoms: pain, paresthesia rather than loss of sensation
  » Autonomic dysfunction (develops in 51% of cases)
    › Cardiac dysrhythmia
    › Orthostatic hypotension
    › Transient/persistent hypertension
    › Bladder dysfunction
    › Ileus
  » Respiratory muscle involvement (mechanical ventilation is required in 13% of cases)

Note:
- Some variants of GBS have unusual presentation — for example, the Miller-Fisher variant, unlike other variants, has bulbar/facial involvement characterized by external ophthalmoplegia and ataxia.
- Be careful about sampling cerebrospinal fluid (CSF) too early in the disease's course — up to one-half of patients will have normal CSF protein when sampled within 1 week of symptom onset.

Diagnosis

- Presence of fever, incontinence, or constitutional symptoms should lead to alternative diagnosis (see *Table 4.8.1*).

Table 4.8.1. SAMPLE DIFFERENTIAL DIAGNOSIS BY SYMPTOM

Symptom	Differential diagnosis
Lower limb paresthesias	• Nutrient deficiency (i.e., vitamin B_{12}), hypothyroidism, hypocalcemia, vasculitis
Muscle weakness	• Spinal cord lesion, peripheral nerve vasculitis, critical illness myopathy, transverse myelitis
Gait unsteadiness	• Posterior fossa structural lesion, toxin ingestion, neuroblastoma
Isolated muscle weakness	• Neuromuscular junction disorder (myasthenia gravis, botulism)

» See *Table 4.7.2* (page 95) to differentiate between myasthenia gravis, GBS, and botulism.

- Conversion disorder can present with any subset of symptoms and should be included in every differential diagnosis.

- Hyperreflexia, spasticity, and ataxia indicate a central cause (intracranial or upper motor neuron process).

Investigations

- No single investigation can confirm or exclude a diagnosis of GBS.
- The following are recommended investigations:
  » CSF analysis
    › CSF analysis may show elevated CSF protein (> 0.45 g/L) with normal CSF white count (i.e., albuminocytologic dissociation).
    › It has a high specificity but low sensitivity.
  » Electromyography (EMG)
    › EMG will establish underlying pathophysiology as demyelinating or axonal.
    › Findings on EMG include:
      · Reduced motor conduction velocity
      · Partial conduction block or abnormal temporal dispersion
      · Prolonged motor distal latency
      · Prolonged or absent F-wave latencies
  » MRI
    › Spinal MRI can show nonspecific nerve root enhancement and cauda equina.

Management

- Serial pulmonary function testing showing a vital capacity of < 20 mL/kg is consideration for ICU admission.
  » Peak inspiratory/expiratory pressure is the preferred mode of monitoring.

- Management of GBS includes:
  » IVIG dose: 1 g/kg × 2 days
  » Plasma exchange
  » Gabapentin — consider for neuropathic pain
- Newer modalities still under investigation:
  » Interferon beta-1 alpha
  » Cyclophosphamide
  » Rituximab

Prognosis

- The majority of patients reach nadir of function in 2 to 4 weeks.
- 80% to 90% of pediatric cases are completely clinically resolved within 6 months to 1 year.
- Prognosis is less favorable for children < 2 years of age, who may require ventilator support or become quadriplegic on day 10.
- Up to 20% of cases may result in residual disability.

REFERENCES

Bordini BJ, Monrad P. Differentiating familial neurpathies from Guillain-Barré syndrome. *Pediatr Clin North Am.* 2017;64(1):231–252. https://doi.org/10.1016/j.pcl.2016.08.015. Medline:27894447

Esposito S, Longo MR. Guillain-Barré syndrome. *Autoimmun Rev.* 2017;16(1):96–101. https://doi.org/10.1016/j.autrev.2016.09.022. Medline:27666816

Korinthenberg R, Schessl J, Kirschner J. Clinical presentation and course of childhood Guillain-Barré syndrome: a prospective multicentre study. *Neuropediatrics.* 2007;38(1):10–17. https://doi.org/10.1055/s-2007-981686. Medline:17607598• A laryngeal mask airway (LMA) can be used as an alternative for airway management.

Respiratory Emergencies

5.1

Stridor

Iwona Baran

- Stridor is a high-pitched, musical, monophonic sound made when breathing.
  » It is caused by turbulent airflow through a partially obstructed airway.
- It is not a diagnosis, but rather a sign that requires immediate attention.

Pathophysiology

- The pressure exerted on a partially closed/obstructed tube by a gas is equal in all directions, except during the linear movement created by breathing.
- If the partially obstructed tube is flexible, linear airflow through it will cause its wall to collapse.
- The phase of stridor can indicate the level of airflow obstruction/narrowing.
  » If the obstruction is in the supraglottic airway above the vocal cords (a flexible tube), then it causes inspiratory stridor.
  » If the obstruction is in the glottic and subglottic airway, it usually produces a biphasic stridor.
  » If the obstruction is in the intrathoracic airway, it causes expiratory stridor.

Management

- Assess the degree of airway obstruction and respiratory distress, level of consciousness, color, and perfusion.
- Initiate resuscitative measures as necessary.
- If the patient is stable, proceed to history and examination.
- If the patient is unstable, perform emergency airway evaluation in the emergency department (ED) or operating room (OR) with appropriately trained personnel.

History

- History should include:
  » Presence of fever
  » Time and speed of onset of stridor
  » Stridor quality (e.g., inspiratory, expiratory, biphasic, change with position or activity)
  » Any cyanosis, apnea, or increased respiratory effort
  » Feeding and growth
  » History of choking
  » Past medical history (especially perinatal issues, previous surgery, presence of any congenital anomalies, history of prior airway instrumentation)

Physical Exam

- Look for:
  » Hypoxia
  » Signs of respiratory distress or airway compromise
  » Dysphagia or drooling
  » Hemangiomas
  » Syndromic abnormalities

Etiology

- The causes of stridor can be organized in many different ways: acute versus chronic, congenital versus acquired, infectious versus noninfectious, or by location of the narrowed airway (as done below).

Supraglottic Airway

- The supraglottic airway includes the airway from the nose to just above the vocal cords.
  » It is easily distensible and collapsible because of lack of cartilage.
  » It has multiple tissue planes, so localized infections can spread and form abscesses.
- Important diagnoses at this level include:
  » Epiglottitis
  » Retropharyngeal abscess
  » Diphtheria
  » Peritonsillar abscesses
  » Anaphylaxis
  » Burn

- » Hereditary angioedema
- » Foreign body
- Presentation includes:
  - » Inspiratory stridor
  - » Drooling (because obstruction is above the level of the esophagus and patients may be unable to swallow)
  - » Muffled / "hot-potato" voice
- Obstruction in the supraglottic airway can quickly progress to full obstruction of the airway.

Glottic and Subglottic Airway

- The glottic and subglottic airway extends from the vocal cords to the trachea before entering the thoracic cavity.
- It is not as collapsible as the supraglottic airway because cartilage (cricoid cartilage and incomplete tracheal cartilaginous rings) surrounds the majority of its length.
- Most common acquired diagnoses at this level:
  - » Laryngotracheobronchitis (croup)
  - » Foreign body aspiration
- Other diagnoses include:
  - » Bacterial tracheitis (it is important not to miss this diagnosis)
  - » Laryngomalacia
  - » Tracheomalacia
  - » Vocal cord paralysis
  - » Subglottic hemangioma
  - » Subglottic stenosis
  - » Recurrent respiratory papillomatosis
  - » Laryngeal web
- Presentation includes:
  - » Inspiratory or biphasic stridor
  - » Hoarse-sounding voice (if vocal cords are involved)
  - » Possible drooling, depending of severity of obstruction

Intrathoracic Airway

- The intrathoracic airway includes the trachea that lies within the thoracic cavity and the mainstem bronchi.
- Some diagnoses at this level include:
  - » Vascular rings
  - » Foreign body aspiration
- Presentation includes:
  - » Stridor that is loudest on expiration (since intrathoracic pressure rises on expiration and tends to cause airway collapse).

SPECIFIC CAUSES OF STRIDOR

CROUP

- Croup is the most common infectious cause of acute stridor.
- Croup is seen especially in children under 2 or 3 years of age.
- It is caused by viruses, including parainfluenza, respiratory syncytial virus, influenza A and B, and rhinoviruses.

Physical Exam

- Patients have a viral prodrome of several days, consisting of rhinorrhea, cough, and other upper respiratory tract infection (URTI) symptoms.
- Patients present with:
  - » Cough (similar to seal bark)
  - » Stridor (inspiratory and sometimes biphasic)
  - » Hoarse voice
- Patients may present with fever.
- Patients do not usually have toxic appearance.

Diagnosis

- The diagnosis of croup is clinical.
  - » Other, more life-threatening diseases (i.e., anaphylaxis, epiglottitis, abscesses, foreign bodies) need to be ruled out.
  - » There is no role for radiographs, except to rule out other possible causes.
  - » There is no role for routine bloodwork.

Management

- No studies with positive results prove the efficacy of humidified mist.
  - » Give humidified oxygen as needed.
- Provide systemic steroids (dexamethasone dose ranges from 0.15 to 0.6 mg/kg).
- Administer nebulized racemic epinephrine for moderate/severe cases (i.e., stridor at rest).
  - » If epinephrine is administered, monitor the patient in the ED for up to 2 hours to ensure there is no rebound of stridor or work of breathing once medication wears off.
- Admit patients if they:
  - » Are toxic
  - » Are dehydrated
  - » Show significant work of breathing or stridor
  - » Show no improvement with epinephrine
  - » Require multiple doses of epinephrine

BACTERIAL TRACHEITIS

- Bacterial tracheitis is a rare cause of stridor in children.
- It is seen especially in children 4 to 6 years of age.
- It is caused by an invasive exudative bacterial infection of the soft tissues of the trachea (most commonly *Staphylococcus aureus*).

Physical Exam

- Patients present with:
  » Viral URTI prodrome
  » Croup-like symptoms of rhinorrhea, cough, possible fever, stridor
  » Progressive airway obstruction and respiratory distress (as the trachea gets superinfected with bacteria, purulent exudate obstructs airway)

Diagnosis

- Consider this diagnosis in a child with possible croup who is not responding to therapy or who has returned to the ED with worsening symptoms and a toxic appearance.
- A lateral neck X-ray may be helpful if considering other diagnoses.
  » Look for irregularity of the margins of the tracheal mucosa below the subglottis or shadows within the tracheal lumen.
  » A definitive diagnosis requires an endoscopy and direct visualization of the trachea.

Management

- Treat bacterial tracheitis with ceftriaxone 75 to 100 mg/kg.
  » If there is a high incidence of methicillin-resistant *Staphylococcus aureus* (MRSA) in the community, consider:
    › Clindamycin 40 mg/kg per day divided every 8 hours
    — or —
    › Vancomycin 45 mg/kg per day divided every 8 hours
- Provide oxygen as needed.
- In severe cases, consider intubation and frequent airway suctioning.

FOREIGN BODY ASPIRATION

- This cause of stridor is seen most often in toddlers (1 to 3 years of age) due to their developmental stage.
- Most foreign bodies lodge in a bronchial tree; they are less likely to lodge within or above the larynx, and least likely to lodge within the trachea.

Physical Exam

- Laryngotracheal foreign body presentation involves:
  » Acute stridor or respiratory arrest
  » No fever
  » Possible history of choking or witnessed foreign body aspiration
- Bronchial foreign body presentation involves:
  » Subacute presentation
  » Recurrent cough, wheezing
  » Possible fever

Diagnosis

- A radiograph is indicated, but only 10% of aspirated foreign bodies are radio-opaque.
- Hypoinflation on inspiration and hyperinflation on expiration films are indicative of a foreign body in the airway.
- Diagnosis may require direct laryngoscopy or bronchoscopy.

Management

- Remove foreign body (in the ED or OR).
- If the patient is in respiratory failure:
  » Give back blows or abdominal thrusts
  » Directly inspect the oropharynx and remove foreign body
    › If these methods are unsuccessful, directly inspect hypopharynx and then larynx with laryngoscopy, and remove foreign body with Magill forceps.
      · If this is unsuccessful, consider intubation (possibly selective bronchus intubation).

REFERENCES

Boudewyns A, Claes J, Van de Heyning P. Clinical practice: an approach to stridor in infants and children. Eur J Pediatr. 2010;169(2):135–141. https://doi.org/10.1007/s00431-009-1044-7. Medline:19763619<

Majumdar S, Bateman NJ, Bull PD. Paediatric stridor. Arch Dis Child Educ Pract Ed. 2006;91(4):ep101–ep105. https://doi.org/10.1136/adc.2004.066902.

Pfleger A, Eber E. Assessment and causes of stridor. Paediatr Respir Rev. 2016;18:64–72. Medline:26707546

Rothrock SG, Perkin R. Stridor in children: a review, update, and current management recommendations. Emergency Medicine Reports; 1997; Available from: https://www.ahcmedia.com/articles/37287-stridor-in-children-a-review-update-and-current-management-recommendations

5.2

Bronchiolitis

Iwona Baran

- Bronchiolitis is viral-induced acute bronchiolar inflammation with signs and symptoms of upper and lower airway obstruction.
- The most common cause of bronchiolitis is respiratory syncytial virus (RSV). Other causes include:
  » Influenza
  » Parainfluenza
  » Human metapneumovirus
  » Rhinovirus
  » Coronavirus
  » Adenovirus
- Incidence peaks in winter months due to the prevalence of causative viruses (especially RSV).
- It affects mainly children < 2 years of age.
- Bronchiolitis is a self-limited illness lasting 1 to 2 weeks; it requires supportive management.

Pathophysiology

- The virus invades the epithelial cells of the nasopharynx and spreads to the mucosa of the lower respiratory tract.
  » As the cells lining the bronchi die, they slough into the bronchial lumen.
  » This causes an increase in mucus production which, along with the sloughed-off cells, leads to plugging of the smaller airways, atelectasis, and turbulent airflow.

Risk Factors

- Risk factors for severe illness include:
  » Prematurity
  » Age < 2 months
  » Apnea
  » Underlying cardiopulmonary disease
  » Airway abnormalities
  » Neuromuscular disorders
  » Immunodeficiency

Physical Exam

- Signs and symptoms of bronchiolitis include:
  » Fever
  » Decreased appetite
  » Rhinorrhea
  » Dry, wheezy cough
- On examination, there are fine inspiratory crackles, high-pitched expiratory wheeze, and increased respiratory effort.

Diagnosis

- Diagnosis of bronchiolitis is largely clinical.
  » Patients have histories of upper respiratory infection with cough and coryza.
  » Symptoms progressively worsen over 2 to 5 days.
  » Wheeze and respiratory distress changes from minute to minute.
  » Patients may or may not have fever.
- There is no need for bloodwork or virology testing for diagnosis.
- There is no evidence to support obtaining a chest X-ray (CXR) except if there is suspicion of a different pathology.

Management

- As bronchiolitis is self-limiting, it only requires supportive management. The following are recommended means of supportive management in hospital:
  » Small frequent feeds
  » Nasal suctioning as needed
  » Intermittent oxygen saturation monitoring
  » Supplemental oxygen as needed for oxygen saturations < 90%
  » High-flow nasal cannula — may be considered, especially in infants
- There is no evidence for use of steroids (inhaled or oral).
- There is no evidence for bronchodilators (Ventolin or epinephrine) in the emergency department (ED).
  » A trial may be considered in severe cases.
- There is no evidence for hypertonic saline in the ED.
  » It may shorten length of stay when used for inpatients.
- There is no need for antibiotics.

Complications

- Complications of bronchiolitis include:
  » Dehydration
  » Apnea
  » Respiratory failure
  » Aspiration pneumonia
  » Secondary bacterial infection

Prevention

- Bronchiolitis may be prevented by:
  » Routine infection control measures
  » Good hand hygiene
  » Breastfeeding
  » Palivizumab (brand name: Synagis) for high-risk children, given monthly during RSV season

Disposition

- Determine whether outpatient or inpatient management is appropriate.
- Admit to hospital if:
  » Patient is toxic appearing
  » Patient is lethargic
  » Patient is feeding poorly or is dehydrated
  » Patient is in moderate to severe respiratory distress
  » Patient is apneic
  » Caregivers not able to continue care at home

- If the patient is to be discharged home, anticipatory guidance should be given. Advise caregivers about:
  » Small frequent feeds
  » Nasal suctioning
  » Monitoring fluid intake and urine output
  » Watching for signs of deterioration

REFERENCES

Bourke T, Shields M. Bronchiolitis. *BMJ Clin Evid.* 2011;2011(308):1–43. Medline:21486501

Hartling L, Fernandes RM, Bialy L, et al. Steroids and bronchodilators for acute bronchiolitis in the first two years of life: systematic review and meta-analysis. *BMJ.* 2011;342(Apr 6):d1714. https://doi.org/10.1136/bmj.d1714. Medline:21471175

Principi T, Coates AL, Parkin PC, Stephens D, DaSilva Z, Schuh S. Effect of oxygen desaturations on subsequent medical visits in infants discharged from the emergency department with bronchiolitis. *JAMA Pediatr.* 2016;170(6):602–608. https://doi.org/10.1001/jamapediatrics.2016.0114. Medline:26928704

Ralston SL, Lieberthal AS, Meissner HC, et al; American Academy of Pediatrics. Clinical practice guideline: the diagnosis, management, and prevention of bronchiolitis. *Pediatrics.* 2014;134(5):e1474–e1502. https://doi.org/10.1542/peds.2014-2742. Medline:25349312

5.3

Asthma

Rahim Valani

- Asthma is a reversible, diffuse lower airway obstruction that has 3 overlapping causes:
  1. Airway inflammation and edema
  2. Bronchial smooth muscle constriction
  3. Mucus plugging
- It has a lifetime prevalence of 11% to 16%.
  » Asthma exacerbations account for 3% to 7% of all pediatric emergency department (ED) visits, with > 50% being preschoolers.
- Triggers for asthma include:
  » Allergen exposure
  » Change in weather
  » Exercise
  » Respiratory tract infections

Diagnosis

- Diagnosis in children > 6 years of age is based on clinical presentation and objective measurements, including:
  » Spirometry with reversible obstruction
  » FEV_1/FVC (forced expiratory volume in 1 sec / forced vital capacity) < 0.8 to 0.9

  » FEV_1 improvement by ≥ 12% when treated with a beta agonist
  » Peak expiratory flow (PEF) variability
  » Increase in PEF by ≥ 20% when treated with a beta agonist
  » Positive challenge test (methacholine or exercise)
- Diagnosis in children < 6 years of age is difficult due to their inability to reliably perform pulmonary function testing. Thus, the diagnosis is more clinical.
  » Patient has a history of documented wheezing.
  » Signs of airflow obstruction improve with use of a short-acting beta agonist (SABA), usually salbutamol.
  » There is no clinical suspicion of an alternate diagnosis.
- The majority of cases that present to the ED are mild.
  » Severe cases constitute 2% to 3% of asthmatics presenting to the ED.
    › Severe asthma is defined as failure to improve after 2 hours of treatment in the ED and moderate hypoxemia.
    › Severe asthma is formerly known as status asthmaticus.

Physical Exam

- On physical exam, attend to:
  - » Cough
  - » Dyspnea
  - » Wheezing
  - » Sputum production
  - » Increased work of breathing
  - » Prolonged expiratory phase
  - » Clinical features suggestive of severe symptoms:
    - › Altered mental status
    - › Decreased activity/feeding
    - › Limited ability to speak with each breath
    - › Use of accessory muscles and nasal flaring
    - › Audible wheezing
    - › Hypoxia (oxygen saturation < 92%)
      - · An oxygen saturation ≤ 92% pretreatment is associated with higher morbidity and increased risk of hospitalization.

Severity Classification

- Asthma severity can be classified according to the Pediatric Respiratory Assessment Score (PRAM):
  - » Mild — PRAM 0 to 3 and FEV_1 > 70% predicted
  - » Moderate — PRAM 4 to 7 and FEV_1 50% to 70% predicted
  - » Severe — PRAM 8 to 12 and FEV_1 < 50% predicted

Table 5.3.1. PEDIATRIC RESPIRATORY ASSESSMENT SCORE (PRAM)

Adapted from Ducharme, Chalut, Plotnick, et al. (2008)

Respiratory sign	0	1	2	3
Suprasternal retractions	Absent	–	Present	–
Scalene retractions	Absent	–	Present	–
Air entry*	Normal	Decreased at bases	Widespread decrease	Absent/minimal
Wheezing*	Absent	Expiratory only	Inspiratory and expiratory	Audible without stethoscope
SpO_2 (without O_2 supplementation)	≥ 95%	92% to 94%	≤ 92%	

*In cases of asymmetry, use the most severely affected lung zone for rating.

History

- Items to consider on history include:
  - » Onset of symptoms (e.g., timing, rapidity, season)
  - » Triggers, including recent respiratory illnesses
  - » Response to treatment at home/school
  - » Severity of symptoms
  - » Use of metered dose inhaler (MDI) and management of asthma
  - » Poor control of asthma symptoms, which include:
    - › Daytime symptoms > 4 times per week
    - › Nighttime symptoms > 1 time a week
    - › Need for SABA > 4 times a week
  - » Prior ED visits, ICU visits, or hospitalizations in the past 12 months
  - » Prior intubation for asthma
  - » High risk of destabilization and relapse, indicated by:
    - › Hospital admission or an ED visit in the past 12 months
    - › Recent corticosteroid use
    - › Use of multiple medications for asthma control
    - › Maximal use of asthma medications
    - › Prior ICU admission
    - › Frequent use of SABA
    - › Presence of environmental triggers

Risk Factors

- Risk factors for asthma can be either endogenous or environmental.
  - » Endogenous risk factors:
    - › Atopy
    - › Ethnicity — African and Hispanic ancestry
    - › Male gender
    - › Genetic predisposition
  - » Environmental factors:
    - › Allergens
    - › Obesity
    - › Respiratory infection
    - › Lower socioeconomic status
    - › Smoking exposure

Management

- Management of asthma depends on its severity (see *Table 5.3.1*, above).

MILD ASTHMA

- Treat mild asthma (PRAM 0 to 3 and FEV1 > 70% predicted) with SABA via MDI

MODERATE ASTHMA

- For moderate asthma (PRAM 4 to 7 and FEV1 50% to 70% predicted):
  - » Treat with supplemental oxygen (to keep oxygen saturation > 92%) and SABA via MDI. Give 3 times at 20-minute intervals
  - » Consider ipratropium via MDI
  - » Consider oral corticosteroids

SEVERE ASTHMA

- For severe asthma (PRAM 8 to 12 and FEV_1 < 50% predicted):
  - » Provide patient with 100% oxygen via a nonrebreather mask (keep oxygen saturation > 92%).
  - » Treat with SABA and ipratropium via MDI or nebulized
  - » Consider systemic corticosteroids
  - » Consider IM epinephrine 1:1000
  - » Obtain IV access and start IV fluids
  - » Administer continuous salbutamol (nebulized, IV)

- Consider blood gases
- Contact the PICU
- Avoid intubation unless absolutely necessary
  › Up to 26% of patients have associated complications:
    · Pneumothorax
    · Impaired venous return
    · Cardiovascular collapse

IMPENDING RESPIRATORY FAILURE

- For impending respiratory failure (lethargy, cyanosis, decreased respiratory effort, rising pCO_2):
  » Treat with 100% oxygen and support ventilation as needed, and continuous SABA and ipratropium via nebulizer
  » Consider systemic corticosteroids
  » Consider IV salbutamol and IV magnesium sulfate
  » Order chest X-ray and emergent ICU consultation
  » Patient may need intubation (ketamine is the agent of choice due to its bronchodilator properties)

ACUTE EXACERBATION

- Treat hypoxemia by administering supplemental oxygen.
  » Maintain oxygen saturation > 92%.
- Administer a SABA via MDI, as this:
  » Is more efficient in drug delivery than nebulized treatment
  » Can limit ED stay
  » Has fewer side effects, with less medication deposition in the oropharynx
  » Carries less risk of infection transmission in the ED
- SABA dosing can be weight based or age based.
  » Weight-based dosing:
    › < 20 kg: 5 puffs (0.1 mg/puff)
    › > 20 kg: 10 puffs
  » Age-based dosing:
    › 1 to 3 years old: 4 puffs
    › 4 to 6 years old: 6 puffs
    › 7 years and older: 8 puffs
  » Nebulized treatment dosing (weight-based):
    › < 10 kg: 1.25 mg
    › 10 to 20 kg: 2.5 mg
    › > 20 kg: 5 mg
- Watch for side effects, including:
  » Tachycardia (sinus tachycardia, supraventricular tachycardia)
  » Hypokalemia
  » Hyperglycemia
- Consider an IV salbutamol infusion for patients with severe asthma who do not respond to conventional treatment.
  » This requires continuous cardiac monitoring.
  » Administer a 7.5 to 10 mcg/kg (maximum 0.5 mg) loading dose over 2 minutes.

- If this bolus results in inadequate therapy, then:
  › 5 to 10 mcg/kg per minute for 1 hour, then reduce to 1 to 2 mcg/kg per minute (ramp down)
  — or —
  › 1 mcg/kg per minute and titrate up in increments of 1 mcg/kg per minute to a maximum of 5 mcg/kg per minute (ramp up)
- Administer corticosteroids.
  » Start the first dose as soon as possible.
  » For mild to moderate symptoms, patient can be discharged home and given:
    › Prednisone 1 to 2 mg/kg loading dose (maximum of 50 mg), followed by 1 mg/kg for a minimum of 3 days
    — or —
    › Dexamethasone 0.15 to 0.3 mg/kg per day (maximum of 10 mg) for 2 to 3 days
  » For moderate to severe symptoms, give:
    › Methylprednisolone 1 mg/kg per dose (maximum 125 mg) IV
    — or —
    › Hydrocortisone 4 to 5 mg/kg IV
- Consider anticholinergic agents for patients 18 months of age and older.
  » The real benefit of these agents is only shown in severe asthmatic patients; however, it is worth considering in moderate asthmatics as well.
  » Anticholinergic agents improve lung function and reduces admission rates by 30%.
  » There is no evidence for use beyond the first hour of treatment.
  » Use these agents with caution in children who are allergic to soy.
  » Ipratropium dosing (20 mcg/puff) is weight based, repeated every 20 minutes to a maximum of 3 doses:
    › < 20 kg: 3 puffs
    › > 20 kg: 6 puffs
- Consider treating with magnesium sulfate.
  » Magnesium sulfate is an adjuvant therapy (SABA and corticosteroids are the first-line acute management agents).
  » It reduces the likelihood of hospital admission.
  » It is not associated with significant side effects when used in the ED.
    › Side effects may include:
      · Muscle weakness
      · Potential vasodilation with hypotension
      · Pain at site of infusion
      · Paresthesias
  » The mechanism of action of magnesium sulfate is as follows:
    › It effects a transient block of NMDA-receptor smooth muscles resulting in bronchodilation
    › It inhibits histamine release from mast cells
    › It decreases mucus production from secretory glands

- » Magnesium sulfate has a half-life of 2 to 2.5 hours.
- » Give magnesium sulfate 25 to 50 mg/kg IV bolus to a maximum of 2 g IV.
- » Inhaled magnesium sulfate is not recommended as it has shown inconsistent benefits.
- Chest X-ray is rarely indicated unless:
  - » An alternative diagnosis is suspected
  - » The patient fails to improve with maximal conventional therapy

Disposition

- The patient should be admitted to hospital for:
  - » Ongoing need for supplemental oxygen
  - » Ongoing respiratory effort with increased work of breathing
  - » Requirement of SABA more frequently than every 4 hours
  - » Deteriorating condition while on systemic steroid therapy
- Prior to discharging a patient home:
  - » Prepare a written asthma action plan
  - » Review the technique for using inhaled asthma medications and maintaining the device with patient and caregivers
  - » Advise the family to start a symptom diary over next 2 weeks to identify asthma triggers
  - » Consider starting the patient on an inhaled corticosteroid, with close follow-up by the primary care provider

REFERENCES

Alberta Medical Association. Guidelines for the management of acute asthma in adults and children. Available from: http://www.pemdatabase.org/files/Acute_asthma.pdf

BCGuidelines.ca, Guidelines & Protocols Advisory Committee. Asthma in children: diagnosis and management.. 2015. Available from: https://www2.gov.bc.ca/gov/content/health/practitioner-professional-resources/bc-guidelines/asthma-children

Chalut DS, Ducharme FM, Davis GM. The Preschool Respiratory Assessment Measure (PRAM): a responsive index of acute asthma severity. J Pediatr. 2000;137(6):762–768. https://doi.org/10.1067/mpd.2000.110121. Medline:11113831

Ducharme FM, Chalut D, Plotnick L, et al. The Pediatric Respiratory Assessment Measure: a valid clinical score for assessing acute asthma severity from toddlers to teenagers. J Pediatr. 2008;152(4):476–480.e1. https://doi.org/10.1016/j.jpeds.2007.08.034. Medline:18346499

Ducharme FM, Dell SD, Radhakrishnan D, et al. Diagnosis and management of asthma in preschoolers: a Canadian Thoracic Society and Canadian Paediatric Society position paper. Can Respir J. 2015;22(3):135–143. https://doi.org/10.1155/2015/101572. Medline:25893310

Irazuzta JE, Chiriboga N. Magensium sulfate infusion for acute asthma in the emergency department. J Pediatr. 2017; 93(Suppl 1):19–25. https://doi.org/10.1016/j.jped.2017.06.002.

Lougheed MD, Leniere C, Ducharme FM, et al; Canadian Thoracic Society Asthma Clinical Assembly. Canadian Thoracic Society 2012 guideline update: diagnosis and management of asthma in preschoolers, children and adults: executive summary. Can Respir J. 2012;19(6):e81–e88. https://doi.org/10.1155/2012/214129. Medline:23248807

Lung Association Ontario. Pediatric emergency department asthma clinical pathway. 2014. Available from: https://lungontario.ca/wp-content/uploads/2017/10/pedacp-information-package-september-2014.pdf

Oritz-Alvarez O, Mikrogianakis A; Canadian Paediatric Society, Acute Care Committee. Managing the pediatric patient with an acute asthma exacerbation. Paediatr Child Health. 2012;17(5):251–255. https://doi.org/10.1093/pch/17.5.251. Medline:23633900

Usmani OS, Barnes PJ, Grippi MA, et al, editors. Fishman's pulmonary diseases and disorders. 5th ed. New York: McGraw-Hill; 2015. Asthma: clinical presentation and management.

5.4

Pneumonia

Jo-Anna Hudson, Kevin Chan

- Pneumonia is the leading infectious cause of death in children globally.
- Yearly there are more than 150 million cases of pneumonia in children under the age of 5 years.
  - » This accounts for 16% of all deaths in children under the age of 5.
- It is most prevalent in South Asia and sub-Saharan Africa.
- Pneumonia is caused by bacteria, viruses, or both.

- There is a mixed viral and bacterial picture in 30% to 50% of cases.
- The prevalence of viral etiology decreases after the age of 2 years.
- The most common viral agents causing pneumonia (see also *Table 5.4.1*) are:
  - » Respiratory syncytial virus (RSV)
    - › 20% to 30% of RSV cases cause lower respiratory tract infections.

› Annual epidemics of RSV occur during winter and early spring.
» Influenza A
» Parainfluenza types 1 through 3

Table 5.4.1. COMMON INFECTIOUS AGENTS OF PNEUMONIA BY AGE GROUP IN CHILDREN

Age	Common bacterial agents	Common viral agents
Birth to 3 weeks	• Group B *Streptococcus* • Gram-negative bacteria • *Listeria monocytogenes*	
3 weeks to 3 months	• *Streptococcus pneumoniae* • *Chlamydia trachomatis*	• Respiratory syncytial virus • Human metapneumovirus • Parainfluenza viruses • Influenza A and B • Rhinovirus • Adenovirus • Enterovirus
3 months to preschool age	• *Streptococcus pneumoniae* • *Mycoplasma pneumoniae* • *Hemophilus influenzae* type B • *Staphylococcus aureus*	• Respiratory syncytial virus • Human metapneumovirus • Parainfluenza viruses • Influenza A and B • Rhinovirus • Adenovirus • Enterovirus
School-aged children and adolescents	• *Mycoplasma pneumoniae* • *Streptococcus pneumoniae* • *Chlamydophila pneumoniae*	• Rhinovirus • Adenovirus • Influenza A and B

- Common bacterial agents causing pneumonia (see also *Table 5.4.1*) are:
  » *Streptococcus pneumoniae*
    › This is the most common bacterial cause of pneumonia.
    › The pneumococcal vaccine has decreased the rate of invasive disease.
    › Children in daycare are at a higher risk of infection.
    › Breastfeeding is protective against *Streptococcus pneumoniae*.
  » *Staphylococcus aureus*
    › This accounts for 3% to 5% of pneumonia cases.
  » *Mycoplasma*
    › Its small size allows it to be spread as a droplet from person to person.
    › Immunity against *Mycoplasma* is not long lasting, allowing for repeat infections.

History

- Neonates can present with nonspecific symptoms.
  » They rarely have a cough.
  » Symptoms can include:
    › Fever
    › Irritability
    › Poor feeding
    › Hypoxemia
    › Respiratory distress
- Common symptoms for children include:
  » Fever
  » Cough
  » Difficulty breathing
  » Poor feeding / decreased intake
  » Vomiting
  » Lack of interest in regular activities
  » Headache
  » Abdominal pain
  » Chest pain
- The sudden onset of rigors suggests a bacterial etiology.
- Mycoplasma pneumonia usually presents with mild symptoms for about 10 days, followed by onset of fever and cough.
- Influenza typically presents with sudden onset of generalized myalgias, fever, then cough and sore throat.

Physical Exam

- Tachypnea is the most significant clinical sign.
  » In a febrile child, tachypnea has a high negative predictive value for pneumonia and a low positive predictive value.
- Common physical findings include:
  » Fever
  » Tachypnea
  » Increased work of breathing (chest retractions, grunting, nasal flaring, crepitation)
  » Rhonchi
  » Crackles
  » Wheezing
- Signs of a consolidation include:
  » Dullness to percussion
  » Increased tactile fremitus
  » Increased bronchial breathing
- Signs of an effusion include:
  » Dullness to percussion
  » Decreased tactile fremitus
  » Decreased breath sounds
- Wheezing with hypoxia is suggestive of bronchiolitis or asthma.
- All children should also be assessed for signs of dehydration and sepsis.

Investigations

- All children should have their pulse oximetry checked to assess hypoxemia.
- In resource-limited areas where radiography is not available, the World Health Organization criteria for diagnosis of pneumonia is tachypnea plus cough.

RESPIRATORY EMERGENCIES

Imaging

- Chest X-ray (CXR) is recommended.
  - » This is the standard for diagnosing pneumonia in the emergency department.
  - » It is recommended for a febrile child with respiratory distress with hypoxemia.
  - » CXR lacks the specificity to distinguish between pneumonia etiologies.
  - » It is not proven to change management or outcomes.
  - » It is best used when history and physical exam are not consistent.
  - » Bacterial pneumonia will show alveolar disease, typically with lobar consolidation with air bronchograms.
  - » Viral pneumonia shows patchy infiltrates.
  - » Mycoplasma pneumonia shows either bilateral focal or interstitial infiltrates.
- Ultrasonography has a higher sensitivity than chest radiography.

Bloodwork

- Patients with minor disease do not require any bloodwork for disease management.
- For those with more serious disease, bloodwork, including the following, can help determine response to treatment:
  - » A complete blood count (CBC)
    - › Higher white blood cell (WBC) count is associated with bacterial pneumonia.
  - » Acute phase reactants such as erythrocyte sedimentation rate, C-reactive protein, or serum procalcitonin concentration.
- Blood cultures should be performed if the patient has systemic inflammatory response syndrome (SIRS), with suspicion of sepsis, or when the patient is being hospitalized.

Pathogen Detection

- If sputum is available, it should be sent for Gram staining and culture.
- Children admitted during the influenza season should have their nasopharyngeal secretions tested for viral etiology for cohorting purposes.

Management

- Most cases of pneumonia can be treated as outpatients.
- Considerations for hospitalization are:
  - » Hydration status
  - » Overall appearance
  - » Age
    - › Neonates should be admitted.
    - › Maintain a low threshold for admission in children < 6 months of age.
  - » Severity of illness (e.g., complicated pneumonia)
  - » Comorbidity

Prevention

- Recommendations to help prevent spread of the infection include:
  - » Frequent handwashing
  - » Avoiding tobacco smoke
  - » Breastfeeding
  - » Reducing exposure to other children
  - » Immunizations
- There are several vaccines available to protect against some of the common infectious agents that can cause pneumonia, including:
  - » Pneumococcal conjugate vaccine 10 and 13
  - » Hemophilus influenzae type B conjugate vaccines
  - » Influenza virus vaccines
    - › These are available but not widely used in low- and middle-income countries.
- There is no vaccine against RSV, but palivizumab is a human monoclonal antibody against RSV that can be given to high-risk infants to prevent severe lung disease.

Viral Therapy

- Consider treating patients promptly with neuraminidase inhibitors (within the first 48 hours) if influenza is detected or suspected.
  - » Oseltamivir
    - › Oseltamivir is used in children > 1 year of age.
    - › Dosing is weight-based (duration of therapy is for 5 days):
      - · ≤ 15 kg: 30 mg PO twice daily
      - · 15 to 23 kg: 45 mg PO twice daily
      - · 23.1 to 40 kg: 60 mg PO twice daily
      - · ≥ 40 kg: 75 mg PO twice daily
  - » Zanamivir
    - › Zanamivir is used in children > 7 years of age.
    - › Dosing is 2 inhalations (5 mg/inhalation) every 12 hours for 5 days.
- Supportive care measures are recommended when a virus is detected or is suggested by the clinical picture and CXR; these include:
  - » Supplemental oxygen
  - » IV hydration
  - » Antipyretics and analgesics for fever and pain relief
  - » Bronchodilators as indicated, depending on the history
- Avoid using antibiotics unless a secondary bacterial infection is suspected.

Antimicrobial Therapy

- When treating uncomplicated pneumonia, the goal is to provide good coverage for Streptococcus pneumoniae.
  - » Amoxicillin is first-line treatment when the patient's condition is not life threatening.
    - › Give amoxicillin 80 to 90 mg/kg per day divided and given three times daily for 10 days.

- When treating pneumonia with respiratory distress or sepsis:
  - » Give third generation cephalosporin for broader coverage:
    - › Ceftriaxone 50 to 75 mg/kg per day IV or IM
  - » Consider vancomycin or clindamycin for coverage against rare occurrences of methicillin-resistant *Staphylococcus aureus* (MRSA):
    - › Vancomycin 40 to 60 mg/kg per day divided every 6 to 8 hours
    - › Clindamycin 30 to 40 mg/kg per day divided every 6 to 8 hours
  - » Transition to ampicillin and then amoxicillin when appropriate
  - » Treat for 10 days total
- When treating pneumonia with empyema:
  - » Treatment is similar to that for pneumonia with respiratory distress, with modifications such as chest tube placement and culturing of the obtained pleural fluid
  - » Treat for 2 to 4 weeks
- For atypical agents (*Mycoplasma pneumoniae* and *Chlamydia pneumoniae*):
  - » Treat with:
    - › Clarithromycin 15 mg/kg per day divided and given twice daily for 7 to 10 days
    — or —
    - › Azithromycin 10 mg/kg on day 1, and 5 mg/kg on days 2 to 5
  - » Note that resistance to macrolides is becoming increasingly common
- If aspiration is suspected, anaerobic coverage should be added.

Follow-up

- Improvement should occur within 48 to 72 hours of starting antibiotics.
- If there is no improvement, repeat CXR to reassess for complications.

REFERENCES

Aoki FY, Allen UD, Stiver HG, Laverdière M, Evans GA. The use of antiviral drugs for influenza: a foundation document for practitioners. *Can J Infect Dis Med Microbiol.* 2013;24(suppl c):1C–15C. https://doi.org/10.1155/2013/130913.

Le Saux N, Robinson JL; Canadian Paediatric Society, Infectious Diseases and Immunization Committee. Uncomplicated pneumonia in healthy Canadian children and youth: practice points for management. *Paediatr Child Health.* 2015;20(8):441–445. https://doi.org/10.1093/pch/20.8.441. Medline:26744558

Leung DT, Chisti MJ, Pavia AT. Prevention and control of childhood pneumonia and diarrhea. *Pediatr Clin North Am.* 2016;63(1):67–79. https://doi.org/10.1016/j.pcl.2015.08.003. Medline:26613689

Parrott GL, Kinjo T, Fujita J. A compendium for *Mycoplasma pneumoniae. Front Microbiol.* 2016;7:513. https://doi.org/10.3389/fmicb.2016.00513. Medline:27148202

Principi N, Esposito S. Biomarkers in pediatric community-acquired pneumonia. *Int J Mol Sci.* 2017;18(2):447. https://doi.org/10.3390/ijms18020447. Medline:28218726

Rey-Jurado E, Kalergis AM. Immunological features of respiratory syncytial virus-caused pneumonia—implications for vaccine design. *Int J Mol Sci.* 2017;18(3):556. https://doi.org/10.3390/ijms18030556. Medline:28273842

Richards AM. Pediatric respiratory emergencies. *Emerg Med Clin North Am.* 2016;34(1):77–96. https://doi.org/10.1016/j.emc.2015.08.006. Medline:26614243

Stuckey-Schrock K, Hayes BL, George CM. Community-acquired pneumonia in children. *Am Fam Physician.* 2012;86(7):661–667. Medline:23062094

World Health Organization (WHO). Pneumonia. [cited 2017 Mar 10]. Available from: http://www.who.int/mediacentre/factsheets/fs331/en/

5.5

Pulmonary Embolus

Iwona Baran

- Pulmonary embolus (PE) is a partial or complete obstruction of the pulmonary artery or its branches caused by the detachment of a thrombus (partial or complete) within the systemic venous system.
- The estimated incidence is 0.7 to 0.9 per 10 000 children per year.
- The age distribution for PE is bimodal, with peaks seen in neonates and adolescents.
- The mortality rate is 8.9% to 10%, which is higher than in adults.

Pathophysiology

- The development of venous thromboembolism (VTE) is associated with Virchow's triad.
  - » Virchow's triad is a set of 3 conditions that predispose an individual to thrombus formation:
    1. Stasis of blood flow
    2. Hypercoagulability
    3. Endothelial injury
  - » Stasis is the main reason for VTE in adults, but in

children, the condition is more commonly due to injury to veins and hypercoagulability.

- Unless there is a coexisting cardiopulmonary disorder, a clot obstructing < 50% of pulmonary circulation is usually silent.
- The effects of clot obstruction (i.e., clots that obstruct > 50% of pulmonary circulation) include:
  » Hemodynamics, which are characterized by:
    › Increased right ventricular afterload (due to increased pulmonary vascular resistance)
    › Right ventricle dilation and hypertrophy
    › Possible cardiac ischemia from compression of the right coronary artery
    › Tricuspid regurgitation
    › Right-sided heart failure
    › Decreased left ventricular filling (due to leftward shift of the interventricular septum from right ventricular hypertrophy)
    › Decreased cardiac output, hypotension, cardiogenic shock
  » Lung physiology, which is characterized by:
    › Increased physiologic dead space
    › Decreased perfusion of alveoli distal to clot obstruction with normal ventilation resulting in V/Q mismatch
    › Compensatory increase in minute ventilation and hyperventilation
    › Decreased blood CO_2, initially resulting in respiratory alkalosis
    › Decreased surfactant production and subsequent atelectasis
    › Increased pulmonary vascular resistance due to release of vasoactive and bronchoactive agents (thromboxane, histamine, serotonin)

History

- A high degree of suspicion is required for PE in pediatric patients as it is an infrequent diagnosis with nonspecific signs and symptoms.
- Symptoms include:
  » Dyspnea
  » Pleuritic chest pain
  » Cough
  » Hemoptysis
  » Fever
  » Palpitations
- Signs include:
  » Unexplained persistent tachypnea
  » Acute right heart failure
  » Cyanosis
  » Hypotension
  » Dysrhythmia
  » Pallor
  » Syncope
  » Sudden death

Risk Factors

- Pediatric patients are much less likely than adults to have idiopathic PE.
- Underlying medical conditions that predispose patients to VTE are:
  » Central venous lines — most common risk factor in pediatric patients
  » Oral contraceptive pill
  » Malignancy — especially acute lymphoblastic leukemia (ALL)
  » Congenital heart disease
  » Collagen vascular disease
  » Significant trauma or surgery
  » Severe infection / sepsis
  » Nephrotic syndrome
  » Inflammatory bowel disease
  » Steroid therapy
  » Sickle cell disease (SCD)
  » Obesity
  » Thrombophilia
  » Previous thrombus without pulmonary embolus
- Typical adult risk factors, such as the following, also may play a smaller role:
  » Abortion
  » Prolonged immobilization
  » IV drug use
  » Rheumatic heart disease
  » Smoking

Diagnosis

- **Adult clinical prediction rules cannot be used in pediatric cases.**
  » There are no validated rules for the pediatric population.
- Initial tests should include electrocardiogram (ECG), chest X-ray (CXR), and arterial blood gas (ABG) to rule out other causes of similar symptoms, though these tests are nonspecific for PE.
- Typical findings on ECG are:
  » Sinus tachycardia (most common finding)
  » Right axis deviation
  » Right bundle branch block
  » "S1Q3T3" of acute cor pulmonale
    › This is characterized by a large S wave in lead I, Q wave in lead III, and inverted T wave in lead III.
    › It indicates acute right heart strain.
    › It is usually seen with massive PE.
  » ST segment and T wave abnormalities
- CXR may be normal, but may show:
  » Cardiac enlargement
  » Pleural effusion
  » Elevated hemidiaphragm
  » Atelectasis
  » Parenchymal opacity

» Westermark sign — a sharp cutoff of pulmonary vessels with distal hypoperfusion in a segmental distribution within the lung

» Hampton hump — a shallow, hump-shaped opacity in the periphery of the lung, with its base against the pleural surface and the hump toward the hilum

» Fleischner sign — a prominent central pulmonary artery

- ABG shows hypoxemia, hypocapnia, and respiratory alkalosis.

- D-dimer is a useful test in adults to rule out PE if they have normal D-dimer and there is low clinical suspicion.

  » This test is **not** useful in pediatric patients.

- Other imaging modalities that may be useful include:

  » Ventilation-perfusion scanning

    › A normal perfusion scan rules out clinically relevant PE.

  » Helical CT scan

    › Consider this as a first-line test.

    › It is reliable, relatively fast, and noninvasive.

    › The main risk is related to radiation exposure.

  » MRI angiography

    › MRI has no associated radiation risk.

    › Consider the issue of availability.

    › MRI takes longer and may require sedation.

  » Echocardiography

    › This allows direct visualization of thrombi or provides indirect signs of PE:

      · Right ventricle dilatation

      · Hypokinesis

      · Abnormal motion of interventricular septum

      · Tricuspid valve regurgitation

      · Lack of collapse of the inferior vena cava (IVC) during inspiration

    › Echocardiography has poor sensitivity, specificity, and accuracy.

  » Ultrasonography

    › Ultrasonography can help diagnosis a deep vein thrombosis (DVT) as indirect evidence of PE.

Management

High-Risk Patients

- Management of high-risk patients (i.e., massive PE, hemodynamically unstable) involves:

  » Thrombolytic therapy — tissue plasminogen activator (tPA)

    › Give tPA 0.03 to 0.06 mg/kg per hour over 24 to 96 hours.

      · Alternatively, give a high dose of 0.1 to 0.5 mg/kg per hour over 6 hours.

    › Contraindications to thrombolytic therapy are:

      · Major surgery or hemorrhage within the past 2 weeks

      · Invasive procedure in the last 3 days

      · CNS hemorrhage/trauma/surgery in the past 2 months

      · Current CNS pathology (aneurysm, neoplasm, or vascular malformation)

      · Premature infant (< 32 weeks gestational age)

      · Active bleeding at the time of therapy

      · Inability to maintain platelets > 50 x 10^9/L or fibrinogen > 1 g/L using transfusion support

  » Embolectomy (surgical vs via catheter)

    › Embolectomy is used if thrombolytic therapy is contraindicated or has failed.

  » IVC filter to prevent PE

    › IVC filter is used if the patient has acute proximal DVT and contraindication to anticoagulation.

Non–High-risk and Stable Patients

- Non–high risk and stable patients receive anticoagulation for several months, via one of two methods.

  » Option 1: Unfractionated heparin (UFH) for 5 to 10 days followed by warfarin therapy for 3 to 6 months.

    › Heparin bolus is usually 50 to 75 IU/kg over 10 minutes, then a maintenance dose of 20 to 28 IU/kg per hour.

    › Heparin is titrated to achieve a target antifactor Xa range of 0.35 to 0.7 IU/mL, or a partial thromboplastin time (PTT) of 60 to 85 seconds.

    › There are issues with monitoring, venous access, and adverse events, including:

      · Bleeding

      · Osteoporosis

      · Heparin-induced thrombocytopenia (HIT)

    › Warfarin is titrated to achieve an international normalized ratio (INR) range of 2.0 to 3.0.

    › Warfarin dosing is as follows:

      · Day 1 loading dose is 0.2 mg/kg PO one time to a maximum of 5 mg

      · After loading dose, dosing is titrated to achieve desired INR range

  » Option 2: Low–molecular weight heparin (LMWH)

    › Age- and weight-based LMWH dosing nomograms should be used.

      · Enoxaparin dosing is 1 to 1.5 mg/kg per dose SC every 12 hours, then titrate to effect.

      · Dalteparin dosing is 100 to 150 IU/kg SC every 12 hours to a maximum of 18 000 IU SC, then titrate to effect.

      · Tinzaparin dosing is 175 to 275 IU/kg SC daily, then titrate to effect.

    › Titrate to achieve a peak antifactor Xa range of 0.5 to 1.0 IU/mL.

    › The advantages of LWMH are that:

      · It requires less monitoring

      · There is no need for venous access

      · It doesn't interfere with drugs or diet

      · It carries a lower risk of HIT

REFERENCES

Agha BS, Sturm JJ, Simon HK, Hirsh DA. Pulmonary embolism in the pediatric emergency department. Pediatrics. 2013;132(4):663–667. https://doi.org/10.1542/peds.2013-0126. Medline:23999960

Brandão LR, Labarque V, Diab Y, Williams S, Manson DE. Pulmonary embolism in children. Semin Thromb Hemost. 2011;37(7):772–785. https://doi.org/10.1055/s-0031-1297168. Medline:22187400

Dijk FN, Curtin J, Lord D, Fitzgerald DA. Pulmonary embolism in children. Paediatr Respir Rev. 2012;13(2):112–122. Medline:22475258

Greene LA, Goldenberg NA. Deep vein thrombosis: thrombolysis in the pediatric population. Semin Intervent Radiol. 2012;29(1):36–43. https://doi.org/10.1055/s-0032-1302450. Medline:23449161

Lilje C, Chauhan A, Turner JP, et al. Pediatric pulmonary embolism: diagnostic and management challenges. World J Pediatr Congenit Heart Surg. 2018;9(1):110–113. Medline:27619327

Parasuraman S, Goldhaber SZ. Venous thromboembolism in children. Circulation. 2006;113(2):e12–e16. https://doi.org/10.1161/CIRCULATIONAHA.105.583773. Medline:16418440

Patocka C, Nemeth J. Pulmonary embolism in pediatrics. J Emerg Med. 2012;42(1):105–116. https://doi.org/10.1016/j.jemermed.2011.03.006. Medline:21530139

Place RC. Pulmonary embolism in the paediatric emergency department. Clin Pediatr Emerg Med. 2005;6(4):244–252. https://doi.org/10.1016/j.cpem.2005.09.003

Thacker PG, Lee EY. Pulmonary embolism in children. AJR Am J Roentgenol. 2015;204(6):1278–1288. https://doi.org/10.2214/AJR.14.13869. Medline:26001239

5.6

Pneumothorax

Rahim Valani

- A pneumothorax is a collection of air in the pleural space.
- Pneumothorax can be classified as:
  » Primary — occurs in patients without underlying lung pathology
  » Secondary — occurs in patients with underlying lung pathology
  » Spontaneous
  » Traumatic
  » Iatrogenic

PRIMARY SPONTANEOUS PNEUMOTHORAX

- The rate of incidence of primary spontaneous pneumothorax is difficult to estimate in the pediatric population. The following best estimates are age adjusted for the pediatric population:
  » 7.4 to 18 cases per 100 000 per year for males
  » 1.2 to 6 cases per 100 000 per year for females
- Most cases occur in adolescents and young adults.
- The exact etiology of primary spontaneous pneumothorax is unknown.
  » There is a high correlation with the rupture of blebs.
- Other proposed mechanisms include:
  » Pleural porosity after inflammation
  » Peripheral air trapping
  » Hereditary predisposition
  » Connective tissue abnormalities
  » Peripheral ischemia
  » Low body mass index (BMI)

- The recurrence rate of primary spontaneous pneumothorax is 50%.
  » Risk factors for primary spontaneous pneumothorax recurrence are:
    › Pulmonary fibrosis
    › History of smoking or second-hand smoke exposure
    › Asthenic habitus
    › Younger age

SECONDARY SPONTANEOUS PNEUMOTHORAX

- Secondary spontaneous pneumothorax is most commonly due to:
  » Asthma
  » Cystic fibrosis
  » Marfan syndrome
  » Bronchiolitis obliterans
  » Foreign body
  » Congenital lobar emphysema
  » Catamenial pneumothorax
  » Pulmonary infections
  » Pulmonary metastases — osteogenic sarcoma

Physical Exam

- Clinical presentation can vary depending on the size of the pneumothorax, the rate of expansion, and the patient's cardiorespiratory reserve.
- Presenting symptoms include:
  » Chest pain (87%) — most common complaint
  » Dyspnea (43%)

» Cough

» Valsalva maneuver (heavy lifting / straining)

- Other symptoms are:
  » Tachycardia
  » Tachypnea
  » Decreased breath sounds
  » Hyperresonance to percussion
  » Hypoxia and hypotension — usually with large pneumothorax or impending tension pneumothorax

Investigations

- A diagnosis can be made clinically; however, imaging is required to the determine size of the pneumothorax and guide management.
  » Chest X-ray (CXR) is the most common imaging modality.
    › Ideally, an erect PA film is taken.
    › Inspiration/expiration films can help identify smaller pneumothoraces.
    › Estimating the size of the pneumothorax based on adult formulas/rules is not as reliable in pediatric patients.
  » Ultrasound is increasingly being used at the bedside (see Chapter 1.8).
    › Ultrasound can help guide needle aspiration.
    › Findings on ultrasound for pneumothorax include:
      · Absence of lung sliding
      · Absence of B-lines
      · Absence of lung pulse
      · Presence of lung point
    › Ultrasound may detect secondary causes of pneumothorax.
    › It is useful in guiding surgical management.
  » Transillumination has been used in neonates.
  » CT scan is used to detect small pneumothoraces if there is a high clinical suspicion, though the clinical significance of this is unclear.

Management

- Tension pneumothorax should be treated immediately with needle decompression followed by a tube thoracostomy.
- For **primary spontaneous pneumothorax**, if the pneumothorax is small, observe the patient in the emergency department (ED) for 3 to 6 hours.
  » Provide supplemental oxygen.
  » If there is no progression, the patient can be discharged home.

- Consider:
  » Needle aspiration.
    › Needle aspiration has a variable success rate in the pediatric population.
  » Chest tube
  » Small bore (pigtail) catheter
- Consider surgical management options:
  » Blebectomy or wedge resection
  » Pleurectomy
  » Pleural abrasion
  » Pleurodesis
  » Staple line covering

REFERENCES

Cattarossi L, Copetti R, Brusa G, Pintaldi S. Lung ultrasound diagnostic accuracy in neonatal pneumothorax. *Can Respir J.* 2016;2016:6515069. https://doi.org/10.1155/2016/6515069. Medline:27445558

Dotson K, Johnson LH. Pediatric spontaneous pneumothorax. *Pediatr Emerg Care.* 2012;28(7):715–720, quiz 721–723. https://doi.org/10.1097/PEC.0b013e31825d2dd5. Medline:22766594

Johnson NN, Toledo A, Endom EE. Pneumothorax, pneumomediastinum, and pulmonary embolism. *Pediatr Clin North Am.* 2010;57(6):1357–1383. https://doi.org/10.1016/j.pcl.2010.09.009. Medline:21111122

Maconochie IK, Howell A, Walton E. Spontaneous pneumothorax in children: the problem with rare presentations. *Arch Dis Child.* 2015;100(10):903–904. https://doi.org/10.1136/archdischild-2015-308309. Medline:26141540

Matuszczak E, Dębek W, Hermanowicz A, Tylicka M. Spontaneous pneumothorax in children: management, results, and review of the literature. *Kardiochir Torakochirurgia Pol.* 2015;12(4):322–327. https://doi.org/10.5114/kitp.2015.56782. Medline:26855648

Ng C, Tsung JW. Point-of-care ultrasound for assisting in needle aspiration of spontaneous pneumothorax in the pediatric ED: a case series. *Am J Emerg Med.* 2014;32(5):488.e3–488.e8. https://doi.org/10.1016/j.ajem.2013.11.011. Medline:24360316

Robinson PD, Blackburn C, Babl FE, et al; Paediatric Emergency Departments International Collaborative (PREDICT) research network. Management of paediatric spontaneous pneumothorax: a multicentre retrospective case series. *Arch Dis Child.* 2015;100(10):918–923. https://doi.org/10.1136/archdischild-2014-306696. Medline:25670402

Robinson PD, Cooper P, Ranganathan SC. Evidence-based management of paediatric primary spontaneous pneumothorax. *Paediatr Respir Rev.* 2009;10(3):110–117, quiz 117. https://doi.org/10.1016/j.prrv.2008.12.003. Medline:19651381

Soccorso G, Anbarasan R, Singh M, Lindley RM, Marven SS, Parikh DH. Management of large primary spontaneous pneumothorax in children: radiological guidance, surgical intervention and proposed guideline. *Pediatr Surg Int.* 2015;31(12):1139–1144. https://doi.org/10.1007/s00383-015-3787-8. Medline:26306420

Sudduth CL, Shinnick JK, Geng Z, McCracken CE, Clifton MS, Raval MV. Optimal surgical technique in spontaneous pneumothorax: a systematic review and meta-analysis. *J Surg Res.* 2017;210:32–46. https://doi.org/10.1016/j.jss.2016.10.024. Medline:28457339

5.7

Cystic Fibrosis

Rahim Valani

- Cystic fibrosis (CF) is a chronic and progressive disease that affects many organ systems.
- CF is an autosomal recessive disorder caused by mutation of the cystic fibrosis transmembrane conductance regulator (CFTR) gene.
  - » Over 2000 mutations are known. These can be categorized into 6 distinct classes (see *Table 5.7.1*).

Table 5.7.1. CLASSIFICATION OF MUTATION TYPES FOR CFTR GENE

Type	Mutation effects
I	Absence of CFTR protein
II	CFTR trafficking defect
III	Defective channel regulation
IV	Decreased channel conductance
V	Decreased quantity of CFTR
VI	Decreased stability of the CFTR protein with high turnover

- The rate of incidence of CF is 1 in 3000 to 4000 among live Caucasian births.
  - » The majority of cases among individuals of northern European Caucasian ancestry is from the mutation of codon 508 (termed F508del), which is a Class II mutation.
  - » 40% to 45% of patients are homozygous for this mutation.
- The consequences of a CFTR gene mutation are:
  - » Decreased open time for chloride passage
  - » Premature pleocytosis of the cell

Diagnosis

- Screening and diagnosis can be done with newborns or when CF is suspected.
  - » Newborn screening is done by measuring the amount of immunoreactive trypsinogen.
  - » Diagnosis is made by sweat test (abnormal results) and/or the presence of 2 disease-causing mutations (see *Table 5.7.1*, above).
    - › Sweat test measures sweat chloride concentration.
    - › Abnormal sweat test results:
      - · For children < 6 months of age: 30 to 59 mmol/L chloride concentration
      - · For children > 6 months: > 60 mmol/L chloride concentration

History

- Signs and symptoms of CF are usually seen at an earlier age.
- Signs and symptoms can vary:
  - » Failure to thrive
  - » Meconium ileus
    - › Meconium ileus is seen in 15% of CF patients.
  - » Severe and recurrent respiratory infections
  - » Reactive airway disease
  - » Prolonged neonatal jaundice
  - » Vitamin K deficiency
  - » Steatorrhea
  - » Nasal polyps and sinusitis

Management

- Goals of therapy are to:
  - » Optimize respiratory function and prevent disease progression and complications
    - › Respiratory complications and failure are the most common causes of morbidity and mortality.
  - » Attain age-appropriate growth
  - » Optimize nutritional status
- Novel targeted therapies are emerging that have potential benefits for children with CF:
  - » Lumacaftor — improves abnormal CFTR trafficking
  - » Ivacaftor — activates defective CFTR at the surface caused by class II CFTR mutation
  - » Combination lumacaftor and ivacaftor — approved in the United States for children > 12 years of age with 2 F508del mutations

Management of Severe Cases Requiring Hospital Admission

- Management of severe cases involves:
  - » Bronchodilators:
    - › Salbutamol
      - · Salbutamol may be nebulized or delivered via metered dose inhaler (MDI) — route depends on severity and infection precautions.
  - » Aggressive airway clearance:
    - › Mucolytic agents
      - · Mucolytic agents can trigger bronchospasm, so consider pretreating with a bronchodilator.
    - › Dornase alpha or 7% hypertonic saline

» Antibiotics
› Double coverage for known *Pseudomonas* infection:
· Tobramycin 9 mg/kg per day divided and given every 8 hours or 10 mg/kg per day every 24 hours
— **and** —
· Ceftazidime 150 mg/kg per day divided and given every 8 hours
— **or** —
· Piperacillin-tazobactam 300 mg/kg per day (piperacillin component) divided and given every 8 hours
» Noninvasive positive pressure ventilation
- Steroids are not recommended in the absence of asthma or wheezing.

Complications

SELECTED NONRESPIRATORY COMPLICATIONS

- Pancreatic insufficiency affects 85% of the CF population.
  » This is treated with oral pancreatic enzyme supplementation and fat-soluble vitamin supplementation.
  » Patients may also have diabetes mellitus (DM).
- Liver disease affects 15% to 30% of CF patients.
  » Live disease is characterized by abnormalities of intra- and extrahepatic biliary tracts.
  » The end result is biliary fibrosis, which results in liver cirrhosis and eventually portal hypertension.
- Chronic sinusitis is seen in 30% of CF patients.
  » Chronic sinusitis presents with purulent nasal drainage, nasal congestion, and facial pain.
  » Patients may also have decreased sense of smell.
  » Management of chronic sinusitis involves:
    › Saline irrigation
    › Topical steroids
    › Irrigation with 3% hypertonic saline

RESPIRATORY COMPLICATIONS

- The progression of the CF leads to worsening respiratory function:
  » Mucous plugging, inflammation, and bacterial infections lead to progressive small airway obstruction and bronchiectasis
  » Chronic *Staphylococcus aureus,* methicillin-resistant *S. aureus* (MRSA), and/or *Pseudomonas aeruginosa* infections
    › It is impossible to eradicate mucoid *Pseudomonas* once a patient is infected.
- The progression of the disease is tracked by measuring the patient's forced expiratory volume in 1 second (FEV_1).

- Respiratory progression is of chronic symptoms with exacerbations.
  » Respiratory exacerbations result from:
    › Impaired mucociliary clearance
    › Chronic bacterial colonization
    › Underlying airway inflammation and destruction
  » Presenting symptoms of respiratory exacerbations include:
    › Increased cough
    › Change in sputum quantity and quality
    › Shortness of breath
    › Increased work of breathing
    › Fatigue
    › Fever
    › Desaturation
    › Hemoptysis
- Other possible respiratory complications include:
  » Hemoptysis
    › Hemoptysis affects 9.1% of CF patients.
    › Chronic infection and inflammation lead to bronchial artery hypertrophy.
      · Thin wall increases risk of arterial rupture.
    › Risk factors for hemoptysis are:
      · *S. aureus* growth
      · Diabetes mellitus
    › Mortality is estimated at 35% within the first year of a massive hemorrhage (> 240 mL in 24 hours or > 100 mL per day over several days).
  » Pneumothorax (see Chapter 5.6)
    › The annual incidence of pneumothorax is 0.64% among CF patients.
    › There is increased incidence among:
      · Older patients
      · Patients with *Pseudomonas aeruginosa, Burkholderia cepacia,* or *Aspergillus* growth
      · Patients with $FEV_1 < 40\%$ predicted

Investigations

- The following are useful in detecting/tracking respiratory exacerbation:
  » Complete vital signs
    › Always check oxygen saturation.
  » Auscultation for new crackles or wheezing
  » Chest X-ray (CXR)
  » Bloodwork
    › Complete blood count (CBC)
    › Electrolytes, renal function, liver enzymes
    › Calcium, magnesium, phosphate
    › C-reactive protein (CRP)
    › Blood and sputum cultures
    › Venous blood gas and lactate

Management

- For chronic airway infection (MRSA or *P. aeruginosa*):
  - » Inhaled tobramycin reduces exacerbations in children > 6 years old with persistent growth of *P. aeruginosa*
  - » Some evidence that giving regular antibiotics to children < 6 years of age leads to fewer *S. aureus* infections
- Manage airway secretions with:
  - » Airway clearance therapies
  - » Mucolytic therapy
- Treat chronic airway inflammation with:
  - » Deoxyribonuclease I (Dornase alpha) and inhaled 7% hypertonic saline (recommended for patients > 6 years of age)
  - » Oral azithromycin and high-dose ibuprofen
- For pneumothorax:
  - » Management depends on size of the pneumothorax (see Chapter 5.6)
    - › For nontension pneumothorax, manage via:
      - · Observation / conservative management (for small pneumothoraces)

- · Needle aspiration
- · Pigtail catheter
- · Tube thoracostomy

REFERENCES

Fajac I, De Boeck K. New horizons for cystic fibrosis treatment. *Pharmacol Ther.* 2017;170:205–211. https://doi.org/10.1016/j.pharmthera.2016.11.009. Medline:27916649

Goetz DM, Singh S. Respiratory system disease. *Pediatr Clin North Am.* 2016;63(4):637–659. https://doi.org/10.1016/j.pcl.2016.04.007. Medline:27469180

Lahiri T, Hempstead SE, Brady C, et al. Clinical practice guidelines from the Cystic Fibrosis Foundation for preschoolers with cystic fibrosis. *Pediatrics.* 2016;137(4):e20151784. https://doi.org/10.1542/peds.2015-1784. Medline:27009033

Paranjape SM, Mogayzel PJ. Cystic fibrosis in the era of precision medicine. *Paediatr Respir Rev.* 2017;S1526-0542(17)30024-6. Medline:28372929

Sanders DB, Fink AK. Background and epidemiology. *Pediatr Clin North Am.* 2016;63(4):567–584. https://doi.org/10.1016/j.pcl.2016.04.001. Medline:27469176

Smyth AR, Rosenfeld M. Prophylactic anti-staphylococcal antibiotics for cystic fibrosis. *Cochrane Database Syst Rev.* 2017;4(4):CD001912. Medline:28417451

Waters V, Ratjen F. Pulmonary exacerbations in children with cystic fibrosis. *Ann Am Thorac Soc.* 2015;12(2 Suppl 2):S200–S206. Medline:26595740

Musculoskeletal Emergencies

6.1

Compartment Syndrome

Hanyang Liu, Matthew Choi

- Acute compartment syndrome is a surgical emergency and can be limb or life threatening.
- It must be recognized and treated before irreversible ischemic damage occurs.
- It can result from any condition that increases compartmental content without a compensatory increase in size of the myofascial envelope; the most common cause is trauma.

Table 6.1.1. ETIOLOGY OF COMPARTMENT SYNDROME

Traumatic (most common)	• Fracture or dislocation 　» High-risk fractures are: 　　› Supracondylar humerus 　　› Carpometacarpal fracture–dislocation 　　› Distal radius or ulna • Crush injuries • Burn (thermal and chemical) 　» Especially circumferential, full-thickness burn • Electrocution / electrical injuries 　» May be deceptive due to innocuous-appearing entry and exit wounds, but may be masking deep muscle injury • Snakebite envenomation • Iatrogenic injury 　» Hematoma following vein/arterial puncture 　» IV fluid extravasation 　» Fracture manipulation
Nontraumatic	• Tightly applied cast or splint, circumferential dressing • External compression from prolonged positioning of a limb • Bleeding • Reperfusion injury after prolonged ischemia (e.g., arterial repair) • Infection • Spontaneous hemorrhage • Postviral rhabdomyolysis

Pathophysiology

- Interstitial tissue pressure increases to above physiologic levels within a myofascial envelope, resulting in reduced end-capillary perfusion pressure and restricted perfusion.
- Ischemic tissue injury is initially reversible but becomes irreversible as time progresses.
  - » Muscle damage begins after 3 hours and is nearly complete at 6 hours.
- Necrosis causes a further increase in interstitial pressure, creating a positive feedback loop that can only be reversed with compartment decompression.
- Extensive rhabdomyolysis can cause:
  - » Hyperkalemia (cardiac arrhythmias)
  - » Myoglobin precipitation that can result in renal failure

Compartments in the Body

- Compartment syndrome can affect any compartment of the body. These compartments are:
  - » Upper extremity:
    - › Arm
      - · 2 compartments: anterior and posterior
    - › Forearm
      - · 3 compartments: flexor, extensor, and mobile extensor wad (lateral)
    - › Hand — multiple small compartments (10 in total)
      - · Thenar
      - · Hypothenar
      - · Interossei (4 dorsal and 3 volar)
      - · Adductor pollicis
  - » Abdomen
  - » Buttocks
  - » Lower extremity:
    - › Thigh
      - · 3 compartments: anterior, posterior, and medial

> › Leg
>   - 4 compartments: anterior, lateral, deep posterior, and superficial posterior
> › Foot — 9 compartments:
>   - Medial
>   - Lateral
>   - Interossei (4)
>   - Central (3)

Physical Exam

- Compartment syndrome presents as a **tense**, swollen compartment.
- Watch for the 6 Ps:
  1. **P**ain:
     › Pain **out of proportion** to nature of injury is an early finding.
     › Look also for pain with **passive stretching** of compartmental contents.
  2. **P**aresthesia:
     › The typical sequence of progression is: paresthesia, decreased light touch, decreased sensation, anesthesia.
  3. **P**aresis/paralysis:
     › This presents as progressive motor weakness, usually preceded by sensory changes.
  4. **P**allor
  5. **P**oikilothermia (cool or cold; a late finding)
  6. **P**ulselessness (a very late finding)
     › Presence of pulses does not exclude compartment syndrome.
     › Irreversible tissue damage can occur even in the presence of palpable pulses.
- Children who lack cognitive or language ability to verbalize symptoms may present with the following:
  » Restlessness
  » Agitation
  » Anxiety
  » Increasing analgesic requirements (dosage and/or frequency)

Diagnosis

- Compartment syndrome is predominantly a clinical diagnosis.
- Interstitial tissue pressure can be used for confirmation.
- Pertinent information to collect on history includes:
  » Mechanism of injury (high vs low energy)
  » Concomitant injuries (altered mental status or neurological compromise)
  » Medical comorbidities (abnormal bleeding diatheses)
  » Medications being taken by the patient (anticoagulation or antiplatelet)

Investigations

- Interstitial tissue pressure is useful when history and examination are unreliable (i.e., in cases of patients who have altered mental status or are very young).
  » Use a Stryker Intracompartmental Pressure Monitor (Stryker needle), or a 16- or 18-gauge angiocatheter connected to an arterial line transducer.
    › Normal pressure is 0 to 15 mmHg.
    › The threshold for acute compartment syndrome is:
      - 30 to 50 mmHg to absolute
      — **or** —
      - 30 mmHg within mean arterial pressure
      — **or** —
      - 20 mmHg within diastolic blood pressure
- Bloodwork is often normal, but check:
  » Electrolytes — possible hyperkalemia (rhabdomyolysis)
  » Lactate — may be elevated
  » Creatine kinase — may be increased (rhabdomyolysis)
- Urinalysis may show possible presence of myoglobinuria (rhabdomyolysis).

Management

- Loosen or remove any constrictive dressing, splint, or cast.
- Elevate affected extremities to the level of the heart.
  » Do not elevate them above level of heart, as this may exacerbate ischemia.
- Use supportive noncircumferential splinting to immobilize the affected area for comfort.
- Ensure frequent (hourly) reevaluation if the diagnosis is uncertain but there is concern about acute compartment syndrome.
- In case of elevated creatine kinase (CK) or myoglobinuria, consider crystalloid resuscitation.

Hyperkalemia

- Watch for signs and symptoms of hyperkalemia; obtain an urgent electrocardiogram (ECG) to see if any ECG abnormalities are present, such as:
  » Peaked T-waves, shortened QT interval, prolonged PR interval, ST segment changes, and widening of the QRS complex
- If ECG abnormalities are present, then consider:
  » IV Calcium gluconate 60 mg/kg
    › If using a 10% gluconate solution, this would be equivalent to 0.6 mL/kg.
  » Salbutamol (nebulized) starting with 2.5 mg and repeating as needed while other medications are being drawn and started
  » Insulin/glucose combination: insulin 0.1 U/kg with 400 mg/kg of glucose, both given IV
  » Kayexalate 1 g/kg PO
- Consider hemodialysis in severe refractory cases.

Surgical Management

- Request surgical consultation for definitive management (fasciotomy).
- In anticipation of possible fasciotomy:
  - » Give nothing by mouth
  - » Order bloodwork: complete blood count (CBC), electrolytes, international normalized ratio (INR), partial thromboplastin time (PTT), group and screen

REFERENCES

Bae DS, Kadiyala RK, Waters PM. Acute compartment syndrome in children: contemporary diagnosis, treatment, and outcome. *J Pediatr Orthop.* 2001;21(5):680–688. https://doi.org/10.1097/01241398-200109000-00025. Medline:11521042

Blaisdell FW. The pathophysiology of skeletal muscle ischemia and the reperfusion syndrome: a review. *Cardiovasc Surg.* 2002;10(6):620–630.

Colohan S, Saint-Cyr M. Management of lower extremity trauma. In: Neligan PC, Song DH, editors. *Plastic surgery.* 3rd ed., vol. 4. London: Elsevier; 2013. P. 63–91.

Donaldson J, Haddad B, Khan WS. The pathophysiology, diagnosis and current management of acute compartment syndrome. *Open Orthop J.* 2014;8(1):185–193. https://doi.org/10.2174/1874325001408010185. Medline:25067973

Hessmann MH, Ingelfinger P, Rommens PM. Compartment syndrome of the lower extremity. *Eur J Trauma Emerg Surg.* 2007;33(6):589–599. https://doi.org/10.1007/s00068-007-7161-y. Medline:26815086

Leversedge FJ, Moore TJ, Peterson BC, Seiler JG III. Compartment syndrome of the upper extremity. *J Hand Surg Am.* 2011;36(3):544–559, quiz 560. https://doi.org/10.1016/j.jhsa.2010.12.008. Medline:21371631

Talbot SG, Rogers GF. Pediatric compartment syndrome caused by intravenous infiltration. *Ann Plast Surg.* 2011;67(5):531–533. https://doi.org/10.1097/SAP.0b013e3182085915. Medline:21301289

6.2

Necrotizing Fasciitis

Hanyang Liu, Matthew Choi

- Necrotizing fasciitis (NF) refers to the spread of infection beneath the superficial fascia and is the most common subtype of necrotizing soft-tissue infection.
  - » Necrotizing soft-tissue infections are rare, but potentially fatal.
  - » Necrotizing soft-tissue infections affect skin, subcutaneous tissue, superficial fascia, and sometimes muscle.
- NF is a rare condition in the pediatric population (0.8 cases per million children per year).
  - » It has a pediatric mortality rate of ~5% (much lower than in adults).
- It is important to distinguish NF from nonnecrotizing soft-tissue infections (cellulitis or erysipelas).
- The management principles for all necrotizing soft-tissue infections are the same.

Classification

- The classification of NF is based on the causative organisms (see *Table 6.2.1*).
- Types I and II account for the vast majority of cases.

Pathophysiology

- Bacteria are introduced to subcutaneous tissue by direct inoculation (abrasions, laceration, needle punctures, or recent varicella infection) or hematogenous spread.
  - » Sometimes trauma cannot be identified.
- Bacteria multiply and produce enzymes (collagenase, hyaluronidase, lipase, streptokinase) and toxins, resulting in tissue necrosis and vessel thrombosis.
- Vessel thrombosis results in:
  - » Poor perfusion of affected area
  - » Infarction of overlying skin
- There is rapid spread of the infecting organism along fascial planes.
  - » Cytokines from tissue necrosis and bacterial toxins lead to septic shock.

Streptococcus Toxic Shock Syndrome

- *Streptococcus* toxic shock syndrome (STSS) may occur in type II NF.
- Group A beta-hemolytic streptococci (GAS) superantigens cause profound activation of T cells, leading to massive cytokine release and capillary leak, resulting in hypotension, disseminated intravascular coagulation (DIC), hypoalbuminemia, and acute respiratory distress syndrome (ARDS).
- STSS significantly increases mortality.

Risk Factors

- Risk factors for necrotizing fasciitis are:
  - » Recent trauma, surgery, or varicella infection (usually 4 to 6 days after onset of rash)

MUSCULOSKELETAL EMERGENCIES

Table 6.2.1. CLASSIFICATION OF NECROTIZING FASCIITIS (NF) BASED ON ITS CAUSATIVE ORGANISMS

Causative organisms	Typical body region affected	Patient population	Remarks
Type I — Polymicrobial			
Broad variety, including: • Non-GAS • *Staphylococcus aureus* • CoNS • *Bacteroides* spp. • *Peptostreptococcus* spp. • *Escherichia coli* • *Pseudomonas aeruginosa* • *Klebsiella* spp. • *Enterobacter* spp. • *Proteus* spp. • *Clostridium* spp. • *Serratia* spp. • *Salmonella* spp. • Mucorales family fungi	• Head, neck, trunk, and perineum (Fournier gangrene)	• Presence of medical commodities, recent trauma, or recent surgery • Neonatal period: possible complication of omphalitis, circumcision, placement of scalp electrodes, and necrotizing enterocolitis	• Responsible for majority of mortalities in pediatric population
Type II — GAS			
• GAS, also called *Streptococcus pyogenes* • Occasionally with concomitant *Staphylococcus aureus* • May be MRSA (prevalence increasing)	• Extremities	• Immunocompetent • Risk factor: recent varicella infection	• Commonly referred to as "flesh-eating disease" • More common than type I in pediatric population (unlike adult population)
Type III — Monomicrobial			
• Marine *Vibrio* spp. • *Clostridium* spp. (anaerobic) • *Aeromonas hydrophila*	• All	• Marine *Vibrio* spp.: immunocompetent patients; entry portal is puncture from fish or marine insects, or ingestion • *Clostridium* spp.: GI and obstetric surgical wounds, intravenous drug user • *Aeromonas hydrophila*: recent freshwater and soil exposure	• Rapidly progressing (*Vibrio* spp. And and *Clostridium* spp.) • *Clostridium perfringens* causes "gas gangrene"
Type IV — Fungal			
• *Candida* spp. • Zygomycetes	• All	• *Candida* spp: immunocompromised patients • Zygomycetes: immunocompetent patients	• *Candida* spp: very rare, aggressive • Zygomycetes: after trauma or burns

CoNS coagulase-negative staphylococci. **GAS** group A beta-hemolytic streptococci. **GI** gastrointestinal. **MRSA** methicillin-resistant *Staphylococcus aureus*. **Non-GAS** non–group A beta-hemolytic streptococci.

» Presence of skin lesions (e.g., atopic dermatitis, venous leg ulcers)
» Presence of comorbidities:
   › Diabetes mellitus
   › Cardiovascular disease
   › Malnutrition
   › Obesity
   › Intravenous drug use
   › Immunosuppression

Physical Exam

• NF may be nonspecific and similar to cellulitis early in its course.
• Distinguishing features of NF are:
   » Localized pain but normal overlying skin
   » Patient is often hemodynamically unstable with altered mental status

» Systemic manifestations: fevers, chills, vomiting, sore throat (more common in type II NF), flu-like symptoms

Note: Immunocompromised patients have blunted systemic response and may lack systemic symptoms initially.

» Excruciating pain out of proportion to size and appearance of lesion
» Tenderness extends beyond apparent area of involvement
» Erythema
   › Mark borders with date and time.
   › The rate of progression can be rapid.
» Crepitus
» Tense swelling and "woody" induration
» Skin discoloration (violaceous, dusky, or black) or necrosis

» Hemorrhagic vesicles or bullae
» Noncontinuous "skip" lesions of skin abnormality
» Numbness
» "Dishwater" discharge if skin and subcutaneous tissue are not intact

Investigations

- The gold standard investigative procedure for NF is fascial biopsy.
  » In practice, NF is a **clinical diagnosis.**
  » The laboratory scoring systems proposed for NF diagnosis are not clinically validated.
  » Imaging is not necessary for diagnosis.
    › If there is a high index of clinical suspicion, **do not delay consultation for surgical assessment while waiting for imaging studies**.
  » Rapid diagnosis is critical to improve outcome.
- Bloodwork demonstrates nonspecific findings.
  » Usually leukocytosis is seen; otherwise, bloodwork is often normal.

Table 6.2.2. LABORATORY INVESTIGATIONS FOR NECROTIZING FASCIITIS

Blood test	Comments
CBC	• Leukocytosis with left shift (but can be normal)
Electrolytes, creatinine, and BUN	• Often normal • Possible hyponatremia and elevated creatinine and BUN
Extended electrolytes	• Often normal • Possible hypocalcemia (indicates extensive fatty necrosis; sign of increased severity)
Lactate	• May be elevated
ABG or VBG	• Possible metabolic acidosis
CRP	• May be elevated
CK	• Normal CK does not rule out NF • Elevated with myonecrosis

ABG arterial blood gas. **BUN** blood urea nitrogen. blood gas. **CBC** complete blood count. **CK** creatine kinase. **CRP** C-reactive protein. **VBG** venous blood gas.

- Order blood culture.
  » Gram stain and culture of wound exudate may provide a clue as to causative organisms and help guide subsequent antibiotic choice.
    › Likely organisms based on Gram stain:
      · Gram-positive cocci in pairs and chain: GAS
      · Gram-positive bacilli and spores: *C. perfringens*
      · Gram-negative bacilli: polymicrobial

Note: The presence of organisms does not diagnose NF and their absence does not exclude NF.

- Consider imaging.
  » Imaging has limited utility as the diagnosis is primarily clinical, but it can help differentiate NF from an abscess.
    › Plain radiograph may show gas in soft tissue; it has poor sensitivity but high specificity.
    › CT scan has moderate (~80%) sensitivity.
    › MRI has high (90% to 100%) sensitivity, but poor specificity.
    › Ultrasonography has poor sensitivity and specificity.

Management

- Aggressively manage ABCs.
  » IV crystalloid resuscitation
- Give antibiotics early; do not delay antibiotic administration if blood cultures cannot be obtained expediently.
  » Early empiric broad spectrum antibiotics are used to slow systemic sepsis and bacterial spread.
    › Note, however, that due to thrombosed vessels and necrotic tissue, antibiotics cannot penetrate infected tissue; therefore, antibiotics alone are inadequate treatment.
  » Consider the following antibiotic treatments:
    › Piperacillin/tazobactam or meropenem
      · For patients > 9 months of age give piperacillin/tazobactam 60 to 75 mg/kg every 6 hours.
      · For patients > 3 months of age give meropenem 20 mg/kg every 8 hours.
    › Vancomycin 10 to 13 mg/kg every 8 hours
    › Clindamycin 10 to 13 mg/kg every 8 hours
      · Clindamycin reduces exotoxin production by GAS.
- In anticipation of possible surgical debridement:
  » Give nothing by mouth
  » Initiate studies:
    › CBC, electrolytes, international normalized ratio (INR), partial thromboplastin time (PTT), group and screen, fibrinogen level
- Consider calling blood bank to have blood products and clotting factors available.
- Arrange surgical consultation for definitive management.
  » Depending on the level of clinical suspicion, the surgeon may perform bedside fascial biopsy, or take the patient directly to the operating room (OR) for debridement.
  » Patients may require multiple debridements and/or amputation.
- Arrange infectious disease consultation.
- Consider chemoprophylaxis (penicillin, first-generation cephalosporin, clindamycin, or erythromycin for 10 days) for parents and other close household contacts of patients with type II NF.

REFERENCES

Anaya DA, Dellinger EP. Necrotizing soft-tissue infection: diagnosis and management. *Clin Infect Dis.* 2007;44(5):705–710. https://doi.org/10.1086/511638. Medline:17278065

Angoules AG, Kontakis G, Drakoulakis E, Vrentzos G, Granick MS, Giannoudis PV. Necrotising fasciitis of upper and lower limb: a systematic review. *Injury. Int J Care Injured.* 2007;38(5):S18–S25. https://doi.org/10.1016/j.injury.2007.10.030.

Bidic SM, Schaub T. Infections of the hand. In: Neligan PC, Chang J, editors. *Plastic Surgery.* 3rd ed., vol. 6. London: Elsevier; 2013. p. 333–44.

Laupland KB, Davies HD, Low DE, Schwartz B, Green K, McGeer A; Ontario Group A Streptococcal Study Group. Invasive group A streptococcal disease in children and association with varicella-zoster virus infection. *Pediatrics.* 2000;105(5):e60. https://doi.org/10.1542/peds.105.5.e60. Medline:10799624

Leung AKC, Eneli I, Davies HD. Necrotizing fasciitis in children. *Pediatr Ann.* 2008;37(10):704–710. https://doi.org/10.3928/00904481-20081001-03. Medline:18972853

Morgan MS. Diagnosis and management of necrotising fasciitis: a multiparametric approach. *J Hosp Infect.* 2010;75(4):249–257. https://doi.org/10.1016/j.jhin.2010.01.028. Medline:20542593

Sarani B, Strong M, Pascual J, Schwab CW. Necrotizing fasciitis: current concepts and review of the literature. *J Am Coll Surg.* 2009;208(2):279–288. https://doi.org/10.1016/j.jamcollsurg.2008.10.032. Medline:19228540

Stevens DL, Bisno AL, Chambers HF, et al; Infectious Diseases Society of America. Practice guidelines for the diagnosis and management of skin and soft tissue infections: 2014 update by the Infectious Diseases Society of America. *Clin Infect Dis.* 2014;59(2):e10–e52. https://doi.org/10.1093/cid/ciu296. Medline:24973422

6.3

Hand Infections

Jouseph Osama Barkho, Matthew Choi

Diagnosis

- Clinical diagnosis of hand infections is made based on clinical signs and symptoms:
  » Erythema
  » Swelling
  » Purulence
  » Pain
  » Heat
  » Loss of function

Differential Diagnosis

- Always consider infection mimics in the differential diagnosis:
  » Juvenile gout and pseudogout (history of recurrent attacks in predictable joint patterns)
  » Pyogenic granuloma
  » Retained foreign body with inflammatory reaction
  » Metastatic tumors

Physical Exam

- Expose and examine the entire affected extremity.

Investigations

- Radiographs are a useful adjunct to rule out foreign bodies and free air.
- Ultrasonography is helpful to better define a deep abscess or if the pathology lies close to neurovascular structures.
- Obtain cultures.
  » Staphylococcal, streptococcal, and anaerobic species are most commonly cultured:
    › *Staphylococcus*: abscess phenotype
    › *Streptococcus*: cellulitic phenotype
  » In immunocompromised patients, consider gram-negative, anaerobic, and fungal species.

Management

- Use principles of infection management.
  » Obtain cultures **before** initiating antibiotic therapy.
  » Give empiric antibiotics for most common pathogens; tailor antibiotics to culture results.
  » Control the infection source with incision and drainage of purulent collections.
  » Remove foreign bodies.
  » Commence tetanus prophylaxis.
  » Admit the patient with IV antibiotics if they appear toxic.
- Conditions associated with methicillin-resistant *Staphylococcus aureus* (MRSA), which should prompt appropriate empiric antibiotic coverage, are:
  » Recent hospitalization
  » IV drug use
  » Recent antibiotic use
  » Compromised immunity (diabetes, organ disease, malignancy, chemotherapy)
  » Parent(s) working in a healthcare field

- Oral antibiotic options for methicillin-resistant *Staphylococcus aureus* (MRSA) coverage include trimethoprim-sulfamethoxazole or clindamycin.

PARONYCHIA

- Paronychia is the most common infection of the hand.
- It can be acute or chronic.
- It involves cellulitis with or without abscess surrounding the nail plate.
- Etiology:
  » Finger sucking
  » Nail biting
  » Hang nail
  » Dishwashing
- Treatment:
  » Examine the hand for drainable abscess.
    › Manage abscess via incision and drainage, antibiotics, and finger splint for comfort and protection
  » If only cellulitis exists, treat with antibiotics, warm compresses, a finger splint, and elevation.
  » Remove nail plate if there is deep purulence.

FELON

- Felon is an abscess of the volar fingertip pulp, trapped by anatomical septations in the fat.
- Etiology:
  » Inoculation by puncture wound
- Management:
  » Incision and drainage, antibiotics, and splint

FLEXOR (SUPPURATIVE) TENOSYNOVITIS

- Flexor tenosynovitis is an infection with purulence in the closed anatomical space of the flexor tendon sheath.
  » It only occurs on the surface of the flexor.
- Flexor tenosynovitis is a surgical emergency with risk of finger or hand loss, sepsis, and death if left untreated.
- Etiology:
  » A minor event that inoculates the nutrient-rich flexor tendon sheath
  » Possible local extension of a neglected cellulitis
- Look for Kanavel's 4 cardinal diagnostic signs of flexor tenosynovitis:
  1. Fusiform swelling of the affected digit
  2. Resting flexed posture
  3. Exquisite pain with passive extension of the digit
  4. Tenderness with palpation along the entire flexor tendon sheath (most reliable sign)
- Kanavel's signs are less obvious in children, and lack of patient cooperation can lower their diagnostic accuracy; therefore, always have a high index of suspicion.

Note: The flexor tendon sheath extends from the A1 pulley overlying the volar metacarpal head to the terminal insertion of the flexor digitorum profundus at the volar base of the distal phalanx. Therefore, true flexor tenosynovitis causes tenderness on the volar surface of the digit, from the metacarpal head all the way to the distal interphalangeal joint.

REFERENCES

Bae, DS. Hand, wrist and forearm fractures in children. In: Wolfe SW, Hotchkiss RN, Pederson WC, Kozin SH, Cohen MS, editors. *Green's operative hand surgery*. 7th ed. Philadelphia: Elsevier; 2017.

Chung MT, Wilson P, Rinker B. Community-acquired methicillin-resistant *Staphylococcus aureus* hand infections in the pediatric population. *J Hand Surg Am*. 2012;37(2):326–331. https://doi.org/10.1016/j.jhsa.2011.10.048. Medline:22192163

Harness N, Blazar PE. Causative microorganisms in surgically treated pediatric hand infections. *J Hand Surg Am*. 2005;30(6):1294–1297. https://doi.org/10.1016/j.jhsa.2005.06.018. Medline:16344191

MUSCULOSKELETAL EMERGENCIES

6.4

Hand Injuries

Jouseph Osama Barkho, Matthew Choi

- In the case of hand injuries, as with any trauma, rule out concomitant injuries.
- History, examination, and radiographs are paramount to diagnosis.
- Absorbable suture materials are ideal for pediatric lacerations as they avoid the trauma of removal.
  » Consider chromic, plain gut, or Vicryl Rapide.
- Note that some injuries in this chapter are classified according to the Salter-Harris classification system. See *Table 18.6.1* (page 330) for details on this system.

History

- The following should be noted to better understand the specifics of the injury:
  » Time of injury
  » Mechanism (sharp, crush, avulsion, penetrating, or mixed)
  » Type of environment in which injury occurred — dirty/contaminated or clean
  » Treatment administered thus far — antibiotics, cleansing, local anesthetic use
  » Inconsistencies in history
    › Any inconsistencies on history should raise suspicion of nonaccidental injury (NAI) / child abuse (see Chapter 1.7, "Child Abuse").
- A general history should include:
  » Past medical history
  » Surgical history
  » Vaccination status
  » Current medications
  » Social history, including smoking, alcohol, and substance abuse
  » Previous hand injury or surgery, and any previously existing deficits
  » Hand dominance
  » Occupation, vocation (for adolescents)
  » Hobbies, sports
  » Tetanus status

Physical Exam

- Most anatomical structures of the upper limb can be examined clinically to rule out injury.
- Expose and inspect the entire upper extremity for:
  » Skin changes

  » Deformity
  » Lacerations
- In young and/or uncooperative toddlers, the examination is limited to observation; the patient may need to be sedated for a complete exam and management of the injury/wound.
- All anatomical structures lying deep and distal to the area of tissue damage need to be examined.
  » In sharp lacerations, the area of tissue damage is narrow and limited to the lacerated tissue.
  » In crush injuries, the area is wide and the damage extensive.

Laceration Exam

- All lacerations need to be **anesthetized** with local anesthetic and **explored**.
  » Topical local anesthetics can reduce the pain of injection.
  » Deep lacerations may appear superficial when skin flaps return to anatomical positions and are stuck down by dried blood.
  » Conversely, dried blood can make a superficial laceration appear more severe.
  » You **don't know** how deep a laceration is until you explore.
  » Failure to explore a laceration could miss deep injury or allow an infection to flourish.
- All wounds should be cleansed to remove debris and reduce microbial burden.
  » Use a 20-mL syringe with an 18-gauge angiocatheter, or an 18-gauge blunt tip needle to generate enough hydropressure to microdebride the wound.
  » Use a 1:1 mixture of povidone-iodine and normal saline.
  » Remember: "The washout is more important than the closure."
- Ensure appropriate tetanus prophylaxis (even for infections).

Vascular Exam

- Conduct a vascular exam, paying attention to:
  » Fingertip color
    › Dark pink or blue indicates venous congestion.
    › Pallor indicates arterial insufficiency.

» Capillary refill
› 1 to 3 seconds is normal.
» Warmth
› Cool digit suggests arterial insufficiency.
» Turgor
› Fingers with no blood flow become wrinkled as if soaked in water.
» Allen test
› This test is used for suspicions of radial or ulnar artery injury.
» Pencil Doppler
› When placed on pad of the fingertip, loud arterial pulsations should be produced.
› The absence of pulsation indicates arterial insufficiency.
» Pulse oximeter
› If the injured fingertip cannot obtain a good oximeter tracing or saturation compared to the noninjured fingers, this is an abnormal finding.

Note: If you are uncertain about what is normal for a patient, compare your findings to the noninjured hand/fingers for baseline.

Neurological Exam

- Test both the sensory and motor function of each terminal nerve — median, ulnar, and radial — to the hand.
- Moving two-point discrimination is the most sensitive test for sensory nerve injury.
  » It is unreliable in children < 8 years old.
  » Normal two-point discrimination is 3 to 5 mm in the fingertips.
  » If an abnormal two-point discrimination (i.e., > 5 mm) is found, repeat the test to determine consistency.
  » **Always test two-point discrimination before administering local anesthetic**.
  » If Tinel's sign is elicited over a laceration (i.e., electric shocks radiating distally), be highly suspicious for nerve laceration.
- If the patient is unable to cooperate with the sensory exam, submerge the hand in warm water.
  » The presence of skin wrinkling after several minutes implies intact innervation.
- The most reliable motor and sensory tests for each terminal nerve are:
  » Median nerve:
    › Motor test — "A-OK" sign
      · This tests the flexor pollicis longus (thumb interphalangeal [IP] joint flexion) and flexor digitorum profundus to index (index distal interphalangeal [DIP] joint flexion).
    › Sensory test — two-point discrimination on pad of index finger

» Ulnar nerve:
  › Motor test — "peace sign" (spread fingers)
    · This tests interossei muscles (abduction of index and middle finger).
  › Sensory test — two-point discrimination on pad of small digit
» Radial nerve:
  › Motor test — "thumbs up"
    · This tests the extensor pollicis longus (thumb extension).
  › Sensory test — light touch on the dorsum of first web space
- For injuries on the volar finger, test sensation on the radial and ulnar border of each fingertip.
  » Each finger has 2 volar digital nerves.

Tendon Exam

- The index through small fingers have 2 tendons each:
  1. Flexor digitorum superficialis (FDS)
    › The FDS flexes the proximal interphalangeal (PIP) joint.
  2. Flexor digitorum profundus (FDP)
    › The FDP flexes the PIP and DIP joints.
- The thumb has only 1 tendon that flexes the IP joint: the flexor pollicis longus.
- The hand has extrinsic extensor tendons with muscle bellies originating in the forearm, and intrinsic hand muscles — the lumbrical/interossei muscles — with muscle bellies originating in the hand.
  » Extrinsic extensor tendons extend the metacarpophalangeal (MCP) joints (extensor digitorum communis, extensor indices proprius, and extensor digiti minimi).
  » Lumbrical/interossei muscles flex the MCP joints and extend the PIP and DIP joints.
- Examine the cadence of the fingers (the resting posture) by having the patient relax their fingers.
  » Smooth cascade is normal; the small digit is most flexed, with increased extension moving to the radial digits.
  » Increased flexion or extension of 1 digit relative to the bordering digits should heighten suspicion for a flexor or extensor tendon laceration.
- When testing the FDS:
  » Test each finger individually
  » Extend the DIP joints of the digits not being tested and ask the patient to attempt bending their finger (pointing to the PIP joint helps)
    › This method eliminates FDP activation (common muscle belly), thus isolating the FDS.
    › Repeat maneuver for each digit.
- When testing the FDP:
  » Test each finger individually
  » Hold the PIP joint of the finger being tested in extension and ask the patient to flex the DIP joint

Note: Pain from a skin laceration can limit flexion, mimicking tendon laceration. Adequate local anesthesia is essential to your exam and eliminates confounding pain.

Caveat: Partial tendon laceration causes pain with flexion. An ultrasound of the digit can confirm partial flexor tendon lacerations.

- Damage to tendons of the wrist should be examined by active and resisted range-of-motion tests and palpation of the wrist joint.

Investigations

- All hand traumas, regardless of likelihood of fracture, require radiographs: 2 to 3 orthogonal views (3 is ideal) to rule out fracture or radio-opaque foreign body.
  - » For a single digit injury, request 3 views of that specific digit (anteroposterior [AP], lateral, oblique) and 1 AP view of the entire hand.
  - » For a metacarpal-phalangeal joint or palm injury, request 3 views of the hand.

NAILBED INJURIES

- Crushing mechanism is the most common cause of injury to nailbeds (e.g., in a door).
- *Nailbed* refers to the sterile and germinal matrix, while *nail plate* refers to the hard nail.
- Since the nailbed is very thin, minor nailbed injuries may easily expose the distal phalanx beneath.
- Order radiographs to rule out an underlying fracture.

Management

- Dislocation, fracture, or avulsion of the nail plate warrants complete removal.
- Failure to recognize exposed bone in a nailbed injury covered by an opacified nail plate could result in osteomyelitis.
- Employ basic wound management (cleanse, irrigate, debride devitalized tissue).
- Reapproximate the nailbed using absorbable sutures to cover exposed bone.
- Repair of the soft-tissue injury in the nailbed is often enough to reduce the fracture.
- Keep the injured nail plate — scrape and clean off the nail plate with a scalpel and soak it in povidone-iodine.
  - » After the repair of the nailbed, reinsert the nail plate beneath the eponychial fold to splint the nailbed. This acts as a splint and, if the fracture is not reduced already, is usually all that is required to reduce the distal phalanx fracture.
- Follow-up is required to ensure that healing is progressing well without infection.
- Beware of Seymour fracture (see "Seymour Fracture," below).

FINGER AMPUTATIONS

- Finger amputations may occur at any digit.
- Proper storage of an amputated piece minimizes warm ischemia time.
  - » Wrap the amputated piece in saline-soaked gauze, place it in a plastic bag, and then place the plastic bag in a bucket of ice.
  - » Never put the amputated piece in direct contact with ice.
- Order radiographs of the injured hand **with the injured piece** (multiple views).
- Surgical consultation is needed to determine the patient's replantation candidacy.
- If the digit is not replantable, the bone should be shortened and soft tissue closed over top.

FINGERTIP AMPUTATIONS

- If only the fingertip is involved and the amputated part is partially attached, suture back into place and insert the nail beneath the eponychial fold as per a nailbed injury.
- If only the fingertip is involved and the tip is completely amputated and:
  - » If no bone is exposed:
    - › Allow to heal by secondary intention (wound care)
  - » If bone exposed:
    - › Shorten bone and suture closed
  - » If amputated piece is available:
    - › For patients < 5 years of age, the entire piece (skin and fat with or without bone fragment) can be sutured back on as a graft
    - › For older children, only the removal fat and bone and the suturing of a graft of skin is required
- Surgical consultation is often warranted.

TENDON INJURIES

EXTENSOR TENDON LACERATION

- Extensor tendons are extremely close to the skin; dorsal lacerations with extensor lag are highly suspect for extensor tendon injury.
- In general, extensor tendons can be reapproximated using figure-of-eight stitches with a permanent, nonabsorbable suture (4–0 Mersilene or smaller in younger children).
- Division of the extensors into zones facilitates communication and guides management.
- Zones 1 through 8 are easily remembered; odd-numbered zones fall on top of joints:
  - » Zone 1 → DIP
  - » Zone 2 → middle phalanx
  - » Zone 3 → PIP

- » Zone 4 → proximal phalanx
- » Zone 5 → MCP
- » Zone 6 → metacarpals
- » Zone 7 → wrist
- » Zone 8 → forearm
- Postrepair, splint the hand in full extension. Splinting duration depends on zone:
  - » Zone 1 or 2 lacerations: 6 weeks of digit splinting in maximal extension
  - » Zones 3 through 5 lacerations: 4 weeks of hand splinting in a forearm-based splint (wrist in 40 degrees of extension, slight flexion at the MCP joints, full extension at the IP joints)

ZONE 1 (MALLET FINGER)

- Mallet finger manifests as an extensor lag at the DIP joint trauma.
- Order radiographs to determine the presence of a bony fragment.
- Salter-Harris III at the dorsal base of the distal phalanx is equivalent to an adult bony mallet.
- Non- or minimally-displaced fractures are treated with hyperextension splinting (4 to 6 weeks).
- Surgery is indicated with:
  - » A fragment that includes > 40% distal phalanx joint surface plus volar subluxation of distal phalanx
  - » > 1 to 2 mm of articular step-off

FLEXOR TENDON LACERATION

- Any laceration along the volar finger or palm should raise a high suspicion for flexor tendon injury and the flexor tendons need to be examined.

Note: Injury to digital arteries and nerves **frequently co-exist. Neurovascular examination** of the finger is critical. **Vascular compromise** of the fingertip requires emergency repair.

- Diagnosis of complete tendon laceration is made by simple clinical examination (see above).
- Painful flexion of PIP or DIP may indicate partial laceration.

Note: pain from the skin laceration can limit flexion and mimic flexor tendon injury. Ensure adequate local anesthesia of skin lacerations when examining tendons.

Management

- Lacerations are treated surgically, followed by strict rehabilitation.
  - » Consult a hand surgery team.
- Adherence to postsurgical rehabilitation is the biggest determinant of outcome.

SKIER'S THUMB

- Skier's thumb is the rupture of the ulnar collateral ligament (UCL) of the thumb MCP joint.
  - » The UCL is critical for thumb stabilization during pinch maneuvers.
- The mechanism of injury is thumb hyperextension in the dorsal or radial direction.
- Diagnosis is made clinically and/or radiologically (musculoskeletal ultrasound or MRI).
  - » A "tender mass" (avulsed ligament) is sometimes felt over the ulnar border on thumb MCP.
- Test the UCL by flexing the thumb MCP and applying a radial force to stress the UCL (may need local anesthesia — pain can induce spasm and confound the exam).
  - » In the case of complete UCL rupture, exam will demonstrate total laxity of the thumb MCP joint with no end point.
    - › Surgery is required.
  - » In the case of partial UCL rupture, exam will demonstrate laxity in a wider range compared to the noninjured contralateral thumb with a soft end point.
    - › Treatment is 6 weeks of thumb spica splinting.
  - » If uncertainty exists, obtain imaging.
- Always compare the injured thumb to the noninjured contralateral thumb.

HAND FRACTURES

- Males outnumber females in hand fractures 2:1.
- There is a bimodal age distribution for hand fractures (see Hastings, Simmons [1984]).
  - » The steepest increases are at age 5 (190 per 100 000 children per year) and age 10 (663 per 100 000 children per year), peaking at ages 14 to 15.
  - » Hand fractures in young children (ages 1 to 5) are usually caused by accidental crushing or lacerations while exploring the world around them.
  - » Hand fractures in older children (ages 10 to 15) are usually caused by sporting injuries, fights, or self-harm.
- Border digits are the most often injured (thumb and small finger).
- The majority of pediatric hand fractures are treated conservatively.
  - » 10% to 20% of patients require surgery.

Management

- The principle of management is to achieve closed or open reduction and maintain reduction until bone heals.
- Complete anesthesia is mandatory for phalangeal and metacarpal fracture reduction.
  - » Hematoma or digital nerve blocks work well.

- Closed reduction is achieved by longitudinal traction and reversal of the deforming force.
  - » Note the principle of ligamentotaxis: soft tissues (periosteum) provide support.
  - » High-energy injuries destroy periosteum, so closed reduction will likely be unsuccessful.
- A fracture is **unstable** and requires surgery if it fails to maintain adequate reduction after attempted closed reduction.
- High-risk fracture patterns requiring surgical consideration are:
  - » Articular fractures, including types III and IV Salter-Harris fractures
  - » Phalangeal neck fractures
  - » Open fractures
  - » Seymour fractures of the distal phalanx physis
  - » Multiple fractures
  - » Complete dislocation of the epiphysis (discussed below)
- Open fractures require a minimum of 1 dose of IV antibiotics.

FRACTURES OF THE PHYSIS

- Fractures of the physis are classified according to Salter-Harris classification, with the purpose of prognosticating growth plate (physis) fractures.
- Diaphyseal and metaphyseal fractures are not included in this classification.
- Prognosis according to Salter-Harris classification:
  - » Types I, II
    - › Prognosis is excellent; injury is treated with closed reduction, splinting, and follow-up.
  - » Types III, IV, and V
    - › Prognosis is poorer than Types I and II; there is a higher likelihood of growth arrest or deformity.
- The younger the child, the more years of growth remaining, and thus the more exaggerated a deformity will be from a disrupted growth plate.

Physical Exam

- Look for scissoring; this is a sign of a rotation or angulation deformity.
  - » Scissoring impairs function and rarely corrects itself.
  - » It is defined as abnormal over- or underlap of the affected digit.
  - » To assess, ask the patient to make a fist (easiest done after local anesthesia), and force the patient's finger into full flexion.
  - » If you are uncertain about scissoring, test the contralateral, uninjured hand.
  - » Be sure to retest for scissoring after reducing the fracture.
    - › Persistent scissoring signals an unstable fracture requiring surgery.

Note: Digits normally point toward the scaphoid, which may cause the small digit to underlap the ring and cause "pseudoscissoring." This is a normal finding and should correct itself in maximal fist flexion.

DISTAL PHALANX FRACTURES

- Distal phalanx fractures are classified into tuft, shaft, or physeal fractures.
- They are often accompanied by a nailbed injury; if nailbed injury is suspected or confirmed, treat as described in "Nailbed Injuries," above.
- Simple repair of the soft-tissue injuries is often enough to reduce the fracture.
- Displaced or intraarticular fractures warrant surgical consultation.
- Conservative, nonoperative treatment for distal phalanx fractures involves finger splinting for 4 weeks.

SEYMOUR FRACTURE

- In a Seymour fracture, the fracture line crosses the epiphyseal plate of the distal phalanx (i.e., Salter-Harris I).
  - » It is characterized by an unstable pattern in the distal phalanx: the terminal extensor tendon pulls the epiphysis dorsally, whereas FDP pulls the distal phalanx metaphysis volarly.

DISTAL PHALANX EPIPHYSEAL DISLOCATION

- Distal phalanx epiphyseal dislocation is the total avulsion and displacement of the epiphysis.
  - » It is characterized by "flake," "crescent," or poorly defined opacification dorsal to the DIP joint on lateral X-ray.
  - » Distal phalanx epiphyseal dislocation requires surgical repair.

MIDDLE AND PROXIMAL PHALANX FRACTURES

- The most unstable fracture patterns are:
  - » Intraarticular fractures (uni- or bicondylar fractures of the phalangeal head)
  - » Phalangeal neck fractures
  - » Pilon fractures at the phalangeal base

Management

- Generally, if the fracture is nondisplaced with no scissoring, it can be managed via closed reduction with splinting and **close follow-up** to ensure maintenance of the reduction is adequate.
- More than 5 to 10 degrees of angulation or 1 to 2 mm of articular step-off is an indication for surgery.
- Always splint the entire hand (thumb spica for thumb fractures, volar slab for index or ring finger fractures, and ulnar gutter for ring or small finger fractures).

- Unlike adults, children are more resistant to splinting-induced stiffness.
  » Even so, utilize a position of safety as much as possible.
- Splint for 4 weeks for conservative management.

METACARPAL FRACTURES

- The metacarpal bone is anatomically divided into the head, neck, shaft, and base.
- Neck fractures are most common (56% to 70%; see Vadivelu, Dias, Burke, and Stanton [2006]).
- Head fractures are likely intraarticular and warrant surgical consultation.
- Apex dorsal angulation occurs secondary to intrinsic muscular pull.
- Severely angulated metacarpal fractures cause:
  » Pseudo-claw deformity (inability to maximally extend MCP and PIP joints)
  » Discomfort with forceful grasp due to projection of the MC head into the palm

Management

- The Jahss maneuver is a maneuver for reducing metacarpal neck fractures.
  » Flex the MCP and PIP joint to 90 degrees and apply a dorsally directed force.
- The following indicate surgical management:
  » Failure of closed reduction
  » Scissoring of fingers
  » Incomplete extension (extensor lag) at the MCP joint
  » Excess angulation at the fracture site
  » Inadequate bone contact at the fracture site
  » Open fractures (require irrigation and debridement)
  » Multiple metacarpal fractures (unstable due to loss of intermetacarpal stability)
  » Unstable fractures (will displace even in splint immobilization)
  » Soft-tissue loss
  » Neurovascular damage
- Non- or minimally displaced fractures are treated with splint immobilization (3 to 4 weeks).

JOINT DISLOCATIONS OF THE DIGITS

- All dislocations need a **prereduction X-ray** to rule out a concomitant fracture and a **postreduction X-ray** to confirm alignment.
- Joints can only dislocate if one or more of the stabilizing ligaments are ruptured. Therefore, a dislocation is a ligament injury.
- The majority of isolated dislocations of the PIP, DIP, or MCP joints can be treated with closed reduction and buddy taping with active range of motion to prevent stiffness, if they are stable.
  » Stable dislocations are those which, after reduction, can move through the entire range of motion without redislocating or subluxing on postreduction X-rays.
- Complete analgesia of the affected joint with local anesthetic is a prerequisite to reduction.
- Dislocations that cannot be reduced by ligamentotaxis or reversing the mechanism of force likely have interposed soft tissue (ligament or joint capsule) blocking the reduction. Such dislocations require surgery.
- Dislocations that are unstable, nonreducible, or have a concomitant fracture require assessment by a specialist.

REFERENCES
Al-Qattan MM, Al-Qattan AM. A review of phalangeal neck fractures in children. *Injury.* 2015;46(6):935–944. https://doi.org/10.1016/j.injury.2015.02.018. Medline:25766097

Hastings H II, Simmons BP. Hand fractures in children: a statistical analysis. *Clin Orthop Relat Res.* 1984;(188):120–130. Medline:6467708

Lin CH, Aydyn N, Lin YT, Hsu CT, Lin CH, Yeh JT. Hand and finger replantation after protracted ischemia (more than 24 hours). *Ann Plast Surg.* 2010;64(3):286–290. https://doi.org/10.1097/SAP.0b013e3181b0bb37. Medline:20179474

Salter R, Harris R. Fractures involving the epiphyseal plate. *J Bone Joint Surg.* 1963;45(3):587–622. https://doi.org/10.2106/00004623-196345030-00019.

Vadivelu R, Dias JJ, Burke FD, Stanton J. Hand injuries in children: a prospective study. *J Pediatr Orthop.* 2006;26(1):29–35. https://doi.org/10.1097/01.bpo.0000189970.37037.59. Medline:16439897

6.5

Approach to a Child With a Limp

Eric Koelink

- Limp is characterized as a deviation from the usual walking pattern for a patient's age.
- It is a common complaint in the pediatric emergency department (ED).
- The ED physician must consider the location of the pain and contiguous joints (e.g., hip pain may be referred to the knee).
- Often a definitive diagnosis is not reached in the ED, and therefore follow-up with a primary care physician or subspecialist is very important.

History

- A good history will provide clues about the region on which to focus.
- Look for other areas of injury, and ask questions about symptoms around all areas of the lower limb.
- Specific information collected on history should include:
  » Site of injury or pain
  » Onset of symptoms
  » Character of the pain as well as any alleviating/exacerbating features
  » Nocturnal symptoms
  » Severity of pain
  » Impact on sports and school
  » History of fever or recent illness
  » Presence of rash
  » Radiating location

Red Flags

- Watch for these red flags on a patient's history:
  » Fever
  » Systemic illness
  » Waking from sleep
  » Progressively worsening limp
  » Night sweats
  » Weight loss

Physical Exam

- Assess the overall appearance of the child (e.g., well/unwell).
- Check vital signs (e.g., is the patient febrile or tachycardic?).
- Incorporate the look/feel/move approach.

- Examine the bony structures and contiguous muscles systematically:
  » Spine
    › Look for spine abnormalities including scoliosis (S-shape to the spine when erect; when bent forward at the waist one scapula appears elevated compared to the contralateral scapula [Adam's forward bend test]).
  » Pelvis
  » Hips
  » Femur
  » Knee
  » Tibia/fibula
  » Ankle joint
  » Foot
- Assess the characteristics of the pain.
  » On palpation, where does the patient localize the pain?
  » Is the pain diffuse or more focal?
- Feel for increased warmth over joints and palpate for an effusion.
- Assess stance and gait.
- Get the patient to walk in the ED pre- and postanalgesia.
- Perform neurological examination for tone, power, reflexes, and sensation.
- Special testing is dictated by clinical index of suspicion.
  » Consider Lachman and anterior drawer tests for knee injury (possible anterior cruciate ligament [ACL] tear).
  » Consider anterior drawer and talar tilt tests for ankle injuries (possible ligamentous laxity or instability due to injury to anterior talofibular ligament or calcaneofibular ligament).

Diagnosis

- Transient synovitis is a common cause of limp.
- Infections, especially septic arthritis and osteomyelitis, should be considered if the patient is febrile, has a warm joint, or is unable to bear weight.
- Rheumatic diseases such as juvenile idiopathic arthritis may also present with a limp.
- Disorders of the hip (which may cause a limp) include:
  » Developmental dysplasia

» Legg-Calvé-Perthes disease (see "Specific Hip Pathologies," below)

» Slipped capital femoral epiphysis

- Several potential life- or limb-threatening illnesses must be considered in the limping pediatric patient:
  » Septic arthritis
  » Osteomyelitis
  » Tumors (and X-ray findings):
    › Osteosarcoma
      · Osteosarcoma is usually in the metaphysis.
      · It is sclerotic and lytic in appearance.
      · It is characterized by the Codman triangle: a bone formation within the lesion.
    › Ewing sarcoma
      · These are lytic and destructive lesions that appear moth eaten.
      · They have an "onion skin" appearance (lamellated) from successive periosteal development.
    › Aneurysmal bone cyst
  » Epidural abscess
    › Although less common, epidural abscess has major consequences for a missed diagnosis and should always be considered.
  » Contiguous pathologies mimicking limp, such as:
    › Ruptured appendicitis
    › Psoas abscess

Investigations

- Investigations will vary depending on the clinical history and physical examination findings.

Imaging

- X-rays are a mainstay in the workup of a limping child.
  » Look for primary or secondary findings:
    › Fractures
    › Effusions
    › Lytic lesions
    › Periosteal reactions (osteomyelitis)
    › Avascular necrosis
  » A thorough history and physical examination usually direct the practitioner to a possible source of the limp.
    › This allows for targeted X-rays.
    › When there is no clear focus for the limp, the physician may begin the workup with X-rays of one or both lower limbs as an initial screen.
    › In older children, where the hip appears to be the source of the limp, anteroposterior (AP) and frog leg lateral views of the pelvis are recommended to rule out possible slipped capital femoral epiphysis.
- Consider advanced imaging.
  » Ultrasound may be useful for finding hip effusions (possible septic arthritis).
  » CT scan is useful for certain pathologies, such as intraarticular fractures, bony coalitions, or bone tumors.
  » MRI is the modality of choice for imaging the spinal cord, avascular necrosis, bone marrow disease, and osteomyelitis.

Bloodwork

- In cases with fever or systemic illness, consider:
  » Complete blood count (CBC), C-reactive protein (CRP), erythrocyte sedimentation rate (ESR)
  » Blood cultures (if febrile)
- Laboratory workups are also recommended in the absence of fever in a child with a limp for several days without evidence of trauma on plain films.
  » If laboratory findings are positive, consider further imaging or arthrocentesis for a definitive diagnosis.

Disposition

- Close follow-up of the limping child should be arranged prior to discharge from the ED once the initial workup, including X-rays and lab studies, is completely normal.

SPECIFIC HIP PATHOLOGIES

LEGG-CALVÉ-PERTHES DISEASE

- Legg-Calvé-Perthes disease is an idiopathic avascular necrosis of the femoral head.
- The disease is insidious in onset with a painless limp.
- It is typically seen in children 4 to 8 years of age.
  » The disease is more common in males than females (4:1).
  » It occurs bilaterally in 10% of cases.

Physical Exam

- Findings on physical examination include:
  » Hip stiffness with decreased internal rotation and abduction
  » Later finding of hip flexor contracture (positive Thomas test)
  » Antalgic or Trendelenburg gait (in severe cases)

Investigations

- X-ray findings are divided into 4 stages:
  1. Initial stage
     › The affected femoral head is smaller, the physeal plate is irregular, and the femoral head is radiolucent/sclerotic.
  2. Fragmentation stage
     › X-ray shows fragmentation of the epiphysis and increased density.
  3. Reossification from the subchondral stress fracture
     › Obvious changes to the femoral head and neck are visible.

MUSCULOSKELETAL EMERGENCIES

4. Healed stage
  › X-ray shows residual deformity of the femoral head.

Management

- Treatment is primarily nonoperative, with observation, activity restriction, and physiotherapy.
  » If conservative measures fail, referral to an orthopedic surgeon for consideration of operative management is appropriate.

TRANSIENT SYNOVITIS

- Transient synovitis is an aseptic inflammation of the synovium of the hip joint.
- The patient presents with hip pain, limp, decreased range of motion, and sometimes fever.
  » Fever is seen in < 10% of cases.
- Transient synovitis is more common in children 3 to 8 years of age.
  » Incidence is higher in males than females (2:1).
  » 95% of cases are unilateral.
  » There is equal incidence of left versus right hip.
- Transient synovitis is usually preceded by a viral illness.
  » This is typically an upper respiratory tract infection (URTI).
  » It is usually seen in the fall months.

Physical Exam

- Look for a decreased range of motion of the hip on internal and/or external rotation and abduction.

Investigations

- X-ray findings are often normal, but may show:
  » Widening of the joint space — a nonspecific finding
  » Loss of hip capsular shadow
- Ultrasound helps identify an effusion, if present.
  » 30% of cases show no evidence of an effusion.
- Laboratory findings include:
  » Mild leukocytosis
  » Elevated ESR
  » Normal or elevated CRP
- Patients with concerning clinical or laboratory findings should undergo a hip ultrasound and arthrocentesis to rule out septic arthritis.
  » Concerning findings include:
    › Inability to bear weight
    › Fever (temperature > 38.5°C)
    › CRP > 2 mg/dL
    › ESR > 20 mm/h

Diagnosis

- Due to its overlap in clinical presentation with septic arthritis, distinguishing transient synovitis from septic arthritis is difficult.

- Factors that suggest a diagnosis of septic arthritis include:
  » More severe pain to the point of resisting movement of the joint and refusing to bear weight
  » Unilateral presentation
    › 90% of septic hip joint cases are unilateral.
  » Febrile and unwell-looking patient
    › Fever seen in 60% to 70% of patients with septic arthritis.
  » Elevated inflammatory markers
  » Marked limited range of motion

Management

- Treatment includes activity modification and anti-inflammatory medications.
  » Recovery often occurs within 7 to 10 days.

SEPTIC ARTHRITIS

- Septic arthritis is an infection of the hip synovium and joint space, often seeded by hematogenous spread of bacteria.
  » The most common bacteria are *Staphylococcus aureus* and group A *Streptococcus* (*S. pyogenes*).
- Presenting features include hip pain, fever, and limp, which can make it difficult to differentiate septic arthritis from transient synovitis.
- Refer to Chapter 6.9 for more detailed information on septic arthritis.

SLIPPED CAPITAL FEMORAL EPIPHYSIS

- Slipped capital femoral epiphysis (SCFE) is the displacement of the proximal femoral epiphysis from the metaphysis of the femur due to abnormality of the physis.
- It has an estimated incidence of 1 per 10 000.
  » SCFE usually occurs in children 10 to 14 years of age.
  » 80% of cases occur during teen growth spurts.
  » It most commonly occurs on the left side.
  » Up to 25% of cases are bilateral.

Physical Exam

- Patients present with an antalgic limp, often holding the affected leg in external rotation.
  » Obligate external rotation as hip is flexed.

Risk Factors

- Risk factors for SCFE include:
  » Obesity
  » Polynesian and African ethnic groups
  » Male gender
  » Femoral retroversion
  » History of previous radiation to femoral head
  » Hypothyroidism
  » Renal osteodystrophy

Investigations

- X-rays should include AP and frog leg views.
- X-ray findings include:
  - » Classic "ice cream falling off the cone" with caudal displacement of femoral head
    - › This is confirmed by the lack of intersection of Klein's line drawn along the superior border of the femoral neck and the lateral aspect of the superior femoral epiphysis.
  - » Growth plate widening
  - » Blurring of proximal femoral metaphysis (sign of Steel)
  - » Angle of Southwick (the angle between the femoral head and shaft angle)
    - › A normal angle is 10° to 12°.
    - › The difference between the 2 angles gives the severity of SCFE:
      - · < 30° — mild
      - · 30° to 60° — moderate
      - · > 60° — severe

Management

- Treatment entails emergent orthopedic surgery with percutaneous in situ fixation.
  - » Often the surgeon will fix the contralateral side at the same time, especially in high-risk patients, due to the high rate of bilateral occurrence.

REFERENCES

Caird MS, Flynn JM, Leung YL, Millman JE, D'Italia JG, Dormans JP. Factors distinguishing septic arthritis from transient synovitis of the hip in children: a prospective study. *J Bone Joint Surg Am.* 2006;88(6):1251–1257. Medline:16757758

Chaudhry S, Phillips D, Feldman D. Legg-Calvé-Perthes disease: an overview with recent literature. *Bull Hosp Jt Dis (2013).* 2014;72(1):18–27. Medline:25150324

Dartnell J, Ramachandran M, Katchburian M. Haematogenous acute and subacute paediatric osteomyelitis: a systematic review of the literature. *J Bone Joint Surg Br.* 2012;94(5):584–595. https://doi.org/10.1302/0301-620X.94B5.28523. Medline:22529075

Del Beccaro MA, Champoux AN, Bockers T, Mendelman PM. Septic arthritis versus transient synovitis of the hip: the value of screening laboratory tests. *Ann Emerg Med.* 1992;21(12):1418–1422. https://doi.org/10.1016/S0196-0644(05)80052-6. Medline:1443834

Dodwell ER. Osteomyelitis and septic arthritis in children: current concepts. *Curr Opin Pediatr.* 2013;25(1):58–63. https://doi.org/10.1097/MOP.0b013e32835c2b42. Medline:23283291

Harris JC, Caesar DH, Davison C, Phibbs R, Than MP. How useful are laboratory investigations in the emergency department evaluation of possible osteomyelitis? *Emerg Med Australas.* 2011;23(3):317–330. https://doi.org/10.1111/j.1742-6723.2011.01413.x. Medline:21668719

Herman MJ, Martinek M. The limping child. *Pediatr Rev.* 2015;36(5):184–197, quiz 196–197. https://doi.org/10.1542/pir.36-5-184. Medline:25934907

Kienstra AJ, Macias C. Evaluation and management of slipped capital femoral epiphysis (SCFE). In: UpToDate, Wolters Kluwer. (Topic updated January 5, 2018.) Available from: https://www.uptodate.com/contents/evaluation-and-management-of-slipped-capital-femoral-epiphysis-scfe?source=search_result&search=scfe&selectedTitle=1~33

Kim MK, Karpas A. The limping child. *Clin Pediatr Emerg Med.* 2002;3(2):129–137. https://doi.org/10.1053/epem.2002.126756.

Kocher MS, Zurakowski D, Kasser JR. Differentiating between septic arthritis and transient synovitis of the hip in children: an evidence-based clinical prediction algorithm. *J Bone Joint Surg Am.* 1999;81(12):1662–1670. https://doi.org/10.2106/00004623-199912000-00002. Medline:10608376

Kost S. Limp. In: Fleisher GR, editor. *Textbook of pediatric emergency medicine.* 6th ed. Philadelphia, PA: Lippincott Williams and Wilkins; c2010. p. 372–377.

Nouri A, Walmsley D, Pruszczynski B, Synder M. Transient synovitis of the hip: a comprehensive review. *J Pediatr Orthop B.* 2014;23(1):32–36. https://doi.org/10.1097/BPB.0b013e328363b5a3. Medline:23812087

Pääkkönen M, Kallio MJ, Kallio PE, Peltola H. Sensitivity of erythrocyte sedimentation rate and C-reactive protein in childhood bone and joint infections. *Clin Orthop Relat Res.* 2010;468(3):861–866. https://doi.org/10.1007/s11999-009-0936-1. Medline:19533263

Perry DC, Bruce C. Evaluating the child who presents with an acute limp. *BMJ.* 2010;341(Aug 20):c4250. https://doi.org/10.1136/bmj.c4250. Medline:20729271

Plumb J, Mallin M, Bolte RG. The role of ultrasound in the emergency department evaluation of the acutely painful pediatric hip. *Pediatr Emerg Care.* 2015;31(1):54–58, quiz 59–61. https://doi.org/10.1097/PEC.0000000000000332. Medline:25560622

Souder C. Legg-Calvé-Perthes disease. Ortho Bullets. 2011. (Accessed on November 9, 2016.) Available from: http://www.orthobullets.com/pediatrics/4119/legg-calve-perthes-disease-coxa-plana

6.6

Joint Dislocations

Eric Koelink

SHOULDER DISLOCATIONS

- Shoulder dislocations are a common injury during sport activities.
- Approximately 20% of shoulder dislocations occur in patients < 20 years of age.
- The smaller size of the glenoid relative to the larger and more contoured humeral head leads to inherent instability.
  » As a result, the surrounding soft tissue structures and ligaments are required to provide additional stability
- The most common mechanism of injury occurs when the arm is forced into excessive abduction and external rotation, resulting in an anterior dislocation.
  » A Bankart lesion occurs when the attachment of the labrum to the glenoid is injured with an anterior dislocation.
    › A bony Bankart lesion occurs when there is also an associated fracture of the anterior glenoid rim.
  » A Hill-Sachs lesion occurs when there is a compression fracture of the humeral head posteriorly.
  » The dislocation may also disrupt the glenohumeral ligaments or cause a tear in the superior or posterior labrum.
- Posterior dislocations are from direct force to the anterior aspect of the shoulder.
  » Such dislocations are classically associated with electrocution / electrical injuries and seizures.
- True inferior dislocations (luxation erecta) are extremely rare.
- As ligaments are up to 7 times stronger than bone in young children, the skeletally immature patient is more susceptible to fractures.
  » Common types of fracture include Salter-Harris type II epiphyseal separations and metaphyseal fractures (see *Table 18.6.1* on page 330).

History

- A history should include the following:
  » Mechanism of injury
  » Pain/edema in neck or elbow
  » Paresthesias (suggestive of a "burner"/"stinger" or nerve injury)
  » Previous injury to the affected shoulder, including management
  » Patient having intrinsic ligamentous laxity (as suggested by dislocations of other joints)
- History often includes a traumatic injury associated with sudden onset of acute shoulder pain.
- A "popping out" sensation may be felt by the patient at the time of injury.

Physical Exam

- Swelling and deformity with loss of the usual rounding of the shoulder (called the sulcus sign) will be found on physical examination.
- On palpation, the humeral head will be felt anterior to the glenoid fossa in anterior dislocations.
- Signs of axillary nerve injury may be present in up to 42% of cases.
  » Always examine the axillary nerve pre- and postreduction.
    › A motor examination involves performing resisted shoulder abduction (deltoid) and external rotation of the shoulder with the shoulder adducted and elbow flexed to 90° (teres minor).
    › A sensory examination involves testing sensation over the deltoid patch (Sergeant's patch), which is innervated by the superior lateral cutaneous nerve.

Investigations

- Customary and axillary (Y-view) X-rays should be performed to best define the direction of dislocation.
- X-rays should be done to rule out a fracture prior to attempting reduction.
- This is especially important in younger children, as they are more prone to fractures.
- Postreduction films should be examined for the presence of:
  » Posterolateral humeral head impaction (Hill-Sachs lesion)
  » Osseous Bankart lesions
  » Other glenoid rim fractures
- A CT scan is rarely indicated.

- An MRI may be done in an outpatient setting to rule out associated soft tissue injuries, such as labral tears.
  » MR arthrograms are the modality of choice for labral tears.
    › One step more involved than plain MRI, MR arthrograms involve an intraarticular injection of contrast done just prior to the MRI.

Management

- Posterior dislocations are best reduced using:
  » Traction-countertraction method
  » Abduction of shoulder to 90° followed by external rotation
- Closed reduction of anterior dislocations can be accomplished by numerous techniques.

Anterior Dislocation Reduction Techniques

STIMSON TECHNIQUE

- This technique is done with significant analgesia on board.
- The patient lies prone on a table with the affected arm hanging over the side in a forward flexed position.
- A weight of approximately 4.5 kg is held in the patient's hand.
- The slow relaxation of muscles by the weight in the patient's hand allows spontaneous reduction.
- The Stimson technique has a 28% success rate.

KOCHER TECHNIQUE

- This is a slow, gradual technique that benefits from distraction techniques.
- The patient's elbow is flexed to 90°, arm adducted close to body.
- The physician slowly externally rotates the patient's shoulder to 70° to 85°, grasping wrist and elbow until resistance is felt.
- Once externally rotated, the shoulder is slowly abducted, then internally rotated while bringing the hand and elbow back down into an adducted position.
- The shoulder should now be relocated.
- The Kocher technique has a 97.5% success rate.

MATSEN TRACTION–COUNTERTRACTION TECHNIQUE

- With the shoulder brought into an abducted position, the physician applies firm traction to the affected arm.
- Countertraction is applied by a colleague to the chest of the patient using a folded sheet.
- The treating physician then alternates between both internal and external rotation to reposition the dislocated humeral head.

- The Matsen traction-countertraction technique has a 92.5% success rate.

CUNNINGHAM TECHNIQUE

- The patient is placed in a seated position with the elbow flexed to 90° and shoulder adducted to the body.
- The physician puts their hand in the patient's antecubital fossa and their forearm adjacent to the patient's forearm.
- A slow and steady, inferiorly-directed traction force is applied by the physician's hand at the patient's elbow.
- The physician's other hand applies a slow massage to the patient's shoulder, alternating between trapezius, deltoid, and biceps muscles until relaxation of the muscles occur.
- Once the muscles relax, the humeral head relocates into the glenoid fossa.
- With this technique, there may not be any clear indication that the shoulder has been reduced; in order to confirm relocation, the physician must observe and check regularly for the disappearance of the sulcus sign and a return to the normal contoured appearance of the shoulder.

Postreduction

- Postreduction, always repeat X-rays to:
  » Ensure that reduction was successful
  » Confirm the absence of fracture
  » Identify Hill-Sachs or bony Bankart lesions
- Always check neurovascular status after reduction, including axillary nerve.
- Postreduction, immobilize the shoulder in a sling for 1 to 3 weeks, as indicated.
- Management of a first-time dislocation of the shoulder is controversial; referral to an orthopedist/sports medicine physician is indicated.
- Chronic, recurrent subluxations/dislocations should also be referred to a subspecialist for further evaluation.

ELBOW DISLOCATIONS

- Posterior elbow dislocations account for approximately 5% of all elbow injuries in children.
- Elbow fractures happen more frequently because the elbow's ligaments and tendons are stronger than the surrounding bones.
  » 64% of dislocations have associated fractures.
- Radial artery transection and ulnar nerve injury comprise 2 of the major neurovascular injuries that can occur with elbow dislocation.
  » When the medial epicondyle is avulsed and then entrapped in the joint, it can injure the ulnar nerve.

» Median nerve entrapment can also occur but is much less common.

History

- The usual mechanism of injury involves a fall on an extended or partially flexed arm with the forearm in supination.
  » The radius and ulna are displaced posteriorly, tearing through the anterior capsule and rupturing the medial collateral ligament of the elbow.
- Associated fractures include:
  » Medial epicondyle
  » Coronoid process
  » Olecranon
  » Proximal radius
- On history, the physician must ask about:
  » Bleeding from injury site due to risk of possible open fracture
  » Paresthesias
  » Pain in joints above/below the affected elbow
  » Any previous injury to the elbow, and management of these injuries

Physical Exam

- Look for obvious deformity/swelling of the elbow with a foreshortened appearance.
- The ulnar notch can often be felt posteriorly and the humeral head can be felt anteriorly in the antecubital fossa.
- Thorough neurovascular examination must be performed, including:
  » Palpation of radial and ulnar artery pulses
  » Allen test for vascular compromise
  » Distal capillary refill
  » Motor and sensory examination of the radial, median, and ulnar nerves, focusing particularly on the area distal to the elbow

Investigations

- Immobilize the elbow to minimize the risk of further neurovascular injury prior to imaging.
- X-rays should be performed to confirm the dislocation and its direction, and to assess for any associated fractures.
- A CT or MRI is indicated in patients with unsuccessful reductions or significant instability, or to assess for occult injuries such as those resulting in entrapped intraarticular soft tissues.

Management

- Elbow dislocations are reduced via longitudinal traction of the arm, followed by flexion at the elbow.

Postreduction

- Obtain X-rays to look for associated fractures.
- Perform a neurovascular examination.
- Assess joint stability with passive elbow flexion and extension.
- Physician concerns about neurovascular compromise or discovery of a fracture associated with a dislocation constitutes an indication for prompt evaluation and treatment by an orthopedic surgeon.
- Simple, stable dislocations without associated neurovascular compromise or fracture should be placed in a posterior splint for 7 to 10 days, followed by active range of motion exercises or formal physiotherapy.
- The posterior splint should be applied with the elbow at 90° of flexion and the forearm in midpronation.

RADIAL HEAD SUBLUXATION (NURSEMAID ELBOW)

- Radial head subluxation most commonly occurs when a child's arm is pulled, often while being swung between 2 adults, with the child's arms in full extension.
- The radial head subluxes out of the annular ligament, leading to pain and decreased range of motion.

History

- Families will often report that the child simply and abruptly stopped using their arm.
- On history, the physician should ask about:
  » Mechanism of injury
  » Force applied
  » Any previous injury to the elbow and management
  » Previous incidences of this type of injury (making recurrence more likely)
  » Associated swelling (more likely indicative of a fracture)

Physical Exam

- The child often holds the affected elbow in a partially flexed, pronated position.
- The child is usually not markedly in pain as long as the elbow is not touched or moved.
- Tenderness is often mild at the radial head.
- Passive range of motion, if the patient can tolerate, is normal.
- As always, look at, feel, and move the other joints (and clavicle) on the affected side.

Investigations

- X-rays may be taken to rule out fracture or dislocation but are not suggestive of radiocapitellar subluxation.

Management

- Reduction techniques have varying efficacy. Supination/flexion and hyperpronation are 2 techniques for reduction of radial head subluxation. Both can be effective options.

Reduction Techniques

SUPINATION/FLEXION TECHNIQUE

- This is the most commonly used technique.
- With child's arm supported by the physician, pressure is applied to the radial head with a finger.
- With the opposite hand, the physician pulls on the child's arm with gentle traction, then supinates the forearm and flexes the elbow in a single movement.

HYPERPRONATION TECHNIQUE

- This technique is a potentially a less painful option and was found to be a more successful technique by a meta-analysis (RR 0.45, 95%; CI 0.28–0.73), but the quality of evidence was low.
- The physician supports the child's arm and applies pressure to the radial head with a finger.
- With the opposite hand, the physician hyperpronates the child's forearm.
- A subtle click may be felt by the physician at the point of the radial head when reduction is successful.

Postreduction

- Reduction is confirmed when the child begins to move the arm in a normal manner again.
- No further treatment or immobilization is needed for nursemaid elbow.
- Recurrence rates range from 27% to 39%, so anticipatory guidance must include recommendations to parents and caregivers to avoid pulling on the child's arm.
- No long-term consequences are associated with recurrent radial head subluxation. The annular ligament becomes thicker and stronger after age 5, making recurrence rare after this age.
- Multiple unsuccessful reduction attempts indicate referral.
  » If reduction is unsuccessful, obtain an X-ray to rule out associated fractures.
    › If X-rays are normal but the patient continues to refuse to use the arm, refer them to orthopedic surgery and place the affected arm in a sling for comfort.
- Nursemaid elbow may spontaneously reduce, and even if the subluxation goes unrecognized or untreated, no long-term consequences have been reported.

HIP DISLOCATIONS

- Dislocation of the hip in children and adolescents is uncommon.
- Most cases are posterior and are rarely associated with acetabular fractures.

History

- On history physician should ask about:
  » Mechanism of injury, including forces involved
  » Ability to weight bear
  » Paresthesias
  » Any previous injury to the hip and management
  » Any injuries or pain in other areas of the body/limb

Physical Exam

- The affected limb is often held in a foreshortened, externally rotated position.
- Inspect the limb for obvious hematoma, deformity, and bleeding.
- Range of motion testing will be painful in all directions.
- Ensure a thorough neurovascular examination is completed pre- and postreduction.

Investigations

- Plain X-rays should be performed to confirm the dislocation and assess for possible associated fractures (acetabular fractures are rare).
- A CT or MRI may be needed to confirm the adequacy of reduction or to assess for possible intraarticular entrapment of soft tissue.

Management

- Treatment delays of 6 hours or longer are associated with a 20-times increased risk of avascular necrosis (AVN) of the femoral head, necessitating prompt reduction in the emergency department (ED).
- Due to the risk of AVN, the ED physician should promptly perform closed reduction under sedation.
  » With the affected hip and knee flexed to 90°, apply a firm axial distraction force to the thigh.
- Confirmation of successful reduction is when the affected limb returns to a similar length as its contralateral counterpart and pain is significantly reduced.
- Detachment of the posterior labrum and capsule may occur with dislocation, which may result in entrapment of these tissues in the articular space.
  » This can lead to asymmetry of the joint space and unsuccessful reduction.
- Referral to orthopedic surgery is indicated if:
  » Reduction is unsuccessful
  » Tissue entrapment is suspected
  » There is a neurovascular injury

MUSCULOSKELETAL EMERGENCIES

PATELLAR DISLOCATIONS

- Patellar dislocations are relatively common compared to other dislocation injuries in children.
- Instability ranges from acute and traumatic to chronic and recurrent subluxation in patients with ligamentous laxity.
- The peak age for patellar dislocations is 15 to 19 years.
- Associated injuries include medial patellofemoral ligament tear, bone contusions, or fractures of the lateral femoral condyle and medial facet of the patella.
  » Fractures are present in approximately 39% of acute patellar dislocations.

History

- The mechanism of injury is often a flexion and rotation movement at the knee with the ipsilateral foot planted, combined with a strong contraction of the quadriceps muscle.
- Less commonly, there may be a direct blow to the medial aspect of the patella, but this occurs relatively rarely (in approximately 10% of cases).
- The patient will report acute knee pain, the sensation of the knee "popping out," swelling, and obvious deformity.
- There may be report of a second "pop" as the patella spontaneously reduces.
- On history, physicians should ask about:
  » Any previous episodes of subluxation/dislocation, including their management
  » Previous knee injuries, including fractures and management
  » Other acute joint pain/injuries above/below the knee
  » Paresthesias

Risk Factors

- Risk factors for this type of dislocation include:
  » Genu valgum (knock knee deformity; can be determined with the Q-angle)
  » Femoral anteversion
  » External tibial torsion
  » Ligamentous laxity (can be measured with the Beighton score)

Physical Exam

- The knee appears swollen with obvious deformity.
- On palpation, there is diffuse peripatellar tenderness and pain.
- The leg is usually held in partial flexion with the patella situated laterally.
- Points of maximal tenderness include the medial aspect of the patella, the medial epicondyle, and the lateral aspect of the lateral femoral condyle.
- There may be significant hemarthrosis if a fracture is present.
- Perform thorough neurovascular examination, especially the popliteal, dorsalis pedis, and tibialis posterior pulses.

Investigations

- Plain films, including anteroposterior (AP), lateral, and merchant views, should be obtained in the ED to diagnose any associated fractures.
- The physician may see an avulsion fracture representing the detachment of a small fragment of the medial patella at the medial patellofemoral ligament attachment site, best seen on merchant view.
- Subsequent outpatient MRI of the affected knee may be indicated (depending on clinical assessment), looking for any one of the constellation of injuries associated with patellar dislocations, including anterior cruciate ligament (ACL) and medial collateral ligament (MCL) tears.

Management

- Reduction of a patellar dislocation can be achieved by flexing the hip slightly and then gradually extending the knee with gentle, medially-directed pressure on the lateral aspect of the patella until it slips back into its normal position.
  » **Gentle force** must be used in order to avoid an associated iatrogenic fracture.
- Postreduction films must be performed to rule out an associated fracture.
- Place the affected leg in a knee immobilizer for 2 weeks with full weight bearing as tolerated.
- Subsequent outpatient assessment of all knee ligaments and cartilage should be performed as the mechanism of patellar dislocation (often plant and twist) may also cause associated injuries to, for example, the ACL, MCL, and menisci.
- After immobilization, a patellofemoral brace and physiotherapy are indicated.
- Anticipatory guidance should involve returning to sport approximately 6 to 12 weeks after the injury, depending on clinical assessment of recovery guided by the orthopedic surgeon, sports medicine physician, or physiotherapist.
- Chronic, recurrent subluxations are best managed with patellofemoral bracing, physiotherapy, and orthotics, if indicated.
- Indications for referral to orthopedic surgery include:
  » Complete avulsion of the vastus medialis oblique and/or medial patellofemoral ligament from the medial aspect of the patella
    › This may be diagnosed by appreciating a large gap of soft tissue on the medial side of the knee with a severely lateralized patella.
  » Fractures, including those with an intraarticular loose body or large fragment requiring fixation

» Recurrent instability
  › This may be considered if conservative treatment measures have been unsuccessful.

REFERENCES

Amar E, Maman E, Khashan M, Kauffman E, Rath E, Chechik O. Milch versus Stimson technique for nonsedated reduction of anterior shoulder dislocation: a prospective randomized trial and analysis of factors affecting success. *J Shoulder Elbow Surg.* 2012;21(11):1443–1449. https://doi.org/10.1016/j.jse.2012.01.004. Medline:22516569

Bishop JY, Flatow EL. Pediatric shoulder trauma. *Clin Orthop Relat Res.* 2005;(432):41–48. https://doi.org/10.1097/01.blo.0000156005.01503.43<. Medline:15738802

Cunningham NJ. Techniques for reduction of anteroinferior shoulder dislocation. *Emerg Med Australas.* 2005;17(5-6):463–471. https://doi.org/10.1111/j.1742-6723.2005.00778.x. Medline:16302939

Guler O, Ekinci S, Akyildiz F, et al. Comparison of four different reduction methods for anterior dislocation of the shoulder. *J Orthop Surg Res.* 2015;10(1):80. https://doi.org/10.1186/s13018-015-0226-4. Medline:26016671

Heyworth BE, Kocher MS. Shoulder instability in the young athlete. *Instr Course Lect.* 2013;62:435–444. Medline:23395048

Heyworth BE, Kocher MS. Intra-articular injuries of the knee. In: Flynn JM, Skaggs DL, Waters PM, editors. *Rockwood and Wilkins' fractures in children.* 8th ed. Philadelphia, PA: Wolters Kluwer; 2015.

Krul M, van der Wouden JC, van Suijlekom-Smit LW, Koes BW. Manipulative interventions for reducing pulled elbow in young children. *Cochrane Database Syst Rev.* 2012;1:CD007759. Medline:22258973

Li X, Ma R, Nielsen NM, Gulotta LV, Dines JS, Owens BD. Management of shoulder instability in the skeletally immature patient. *J Am Acad Orthop Surg.* 2013;21(9):529–537. Medline:23996984

Meyn MA Jr, Quigley TB. Reduction of posterior dislocation of the elbow by traction on the dangling arm. *Clin Orthop Relat Res.* 1974;103:106–108. https://doi.org/10.1097/00003086-197409000-00068. Medline:4415508

Moore BR, Bothner J. Radial head subluxation (nursemaid's elbow). In: UpToDate, Wolters Kluwer. (Accessed on December 16, 2016). Available from: https://www.uptodate.com/contents/radial-head-subluxation-nursemaids-elbow

Quick TJ, Eastwood DM. Pediatric fractures and dislocations of the hip and pelvis. *Clin Orthop Relat Res.* 2005;&NA;(432):87–96. https://doi.org/10.1097/01.blo.0000155372.65446.40. Medline:15738808

Stans AA, Lawrence JTR. Dislocations of the elbows, medial epicondylar humerus fractures. In: Flynn JM, Skaggs DL, Waters PM, editors. *Rockwood and Wilkins' fractures in children.* 8th ed. Philadelphia, PA: Wolters Kluwer; 2015.

6.7

Torticollis

Rahim Valani

- The incidence of torticollis is estimated to be between 1% and 16%.
- The condition is caused by unilateral shortening or fibrosis of the sternocleidomastoid muscle, resulting in an asymmetric posture of the head and neck.
  » Torticollis presents as a lateral flexion of the head toward the affected side with chin deviation to the opposite side.
- The sternocleidomastoid muscle originates from the sternum and clavicle, and inserts into the mastoid process and the occipital bone.
- The sternocleidomastoid muscle is innervated by cranial nerve XI and branches of C2 to C4.
- The sternocleidomastoid muscle can be divided into three areas, each of which has a different arterial supply:
  » Upper third — occipital artery
  » Middle third — superior thyroid artery
  » Lower third — superior thyroid, transverse scapular, and transverse cervical arteries

Etiology
- Torticollis can be classified as congenital or acquired.

CONGENITAL TORTICOLLIS
- Congenital torticollis is the third most common congenital musculoskeletal anomaly in infants (after congenital hip dysplasia and clubfoot).
- It is associated with craniofacial asymmetry in up to 80% of cases.
- Although the exact cause is unknown, it is thought to be a combination of:
  » Fetal malposition
  » Uterine compression
  » Birth trauma
  » Ischemic events involving the sternocleidomastoid muscle
- Sternocleidomastoid muscle tumor (fibrosis or hematoma) may be palpable.

ACQUIRED TORTICOLLIS
- Causes of acquired torticollis may be:
  » Traumatic — C1 fracture (see Chapter 18.2, "Cervical Spin Injury")
  » Infectious — Grisel syndrome (spontaneous subluxation of atlantoaxial joint following peripharyngeal inflammation)

› Specific infections include:
  · Pharyngitis (see Chapter 13.3)
  · Otitis media
  · Adenoiditis
  · Parotitis
  · Tonsillar or cervical abscess (See Chapter 10.10, "Cervical Lymphadenitis")
› Infection is also seen postsurgically in tonsillectomy/adenoidectomy.
» Ligamentous — lax ligaments seen with Down syndrome, mucopolysaccharidosis
» Inflammatory — thyroiditis, cervical adenitis
» Vascular — aneurysm, spinal epidural hematoma
» Muscular — cervical dystonia
» Drug reaction — neuroleptics, anti-emetics (Metoclopramide)
» Osseous — osteoblastoma, vertebral subluxation, Klippel-Feil syndrome due to osseous fusions
» Ocular — superior oblique palsy
» Psychiatric disorder — conversion disorder
» Neurologic disorder — posterior fossa tumor, acute disseminated encephalomyelitis (ADEM), increased intracranial pressure (ICP)
» Gastrointestinal (GI) — foreign body, Sandifer syndrome

BENIGN PAROXYSMAL TORTICOLLIS

- Benign paroxysmal torticollis occurs during infancy.
- Episodes recur from every few days to every few months, each episode lasting < 1 week.
- It resolves by age 3.
- It is associated with family history of migraines.

Management

- Management of torticollis depends on the cause and specific symptoms in each case.
- For trauma or neurologic symptoms:
  » Immobilize the neck
  » Obtain urgent imaging — CT or MRI
  » Consult with trauma or a spine surgeon
- For cervical mass:
  » Order bloodwork: complete blood count (CBC), erythrocyte sedimentation rate (ESR), C-reactive protein (CRP)
  » Consider blood culture
  » Obtain an ultrasound of the neck
- For cervical adenopathy:
  » If tender, consider treatment with antibiotics
  » If nontender or if suspicious for lymphoma, obtain bloodwork (lactate dehydrogenase [LDH] and uric acid) and a chest X-ray (CXR) to look for hilar nodes
- For abnormal neurologic or ophthalmologic exam:
  » Obtain a CT or MRI of the head
  » Lumbar puncture (LP) may be needed
- For dystonic reactions:
  » Give antibiotic therapy:
    › Diphenhydramine 1 mg/kg IV
    › Benztropine 0.02 mg/kg IV (to a maximum of 1 mg)
  » Consider alternative diagnosis if there is no improvement within 20 minutes
- Administer physiotherapy and nonsteroidal anti-inflammatory drugs (NSAIDs) if the cause of torticollis is muscular or benign.

REFERENCES

Hadjipanayis A, Efstathiou E, Neubauer D. Benign paroxysmal torticollis of infancy: an underdiagnosed condition. *J Paediatr Child Health.* 2015;51(7):674–678. https://doi.org/10.1111/jpc.12841. Medline:25644090

Kinon MD, Nasser R, Nakhla J, et al. Atlanotaxial rotatory subluxation: a review for the pediatric emergency physician. *Pediatr Emerg Care.* 2016;32(10):710–716. https://doi.org/10.1097/PEC.0000000000000817. Medline:27749670

Lepetsos P, Anastasopoulos PP, Leonidou A, et al. Surgical management of congenital torticollis in children older than 7 years with an average 10-year follow-up. *J Pediatr Orthop B.* 2017;26(6):580–584.

Per H, Canpolat M, Tümtürk A, et al. Different etiologies of acquired torticollis in childhood. *Childs Nerv Syst.* 2014;30(3):431–440. https://doi.org/10.1007/s00381-013-2302-6. Medline:24196698

Rosman NP, Douglass LM, Sharif UM, Paolini J. The neurology of benign paroxysmal torticollis of infancy: report of 10 new cases and review of the literature. *J Child Neurol.* 2009;24(2):155–160. https://doi.org/10.1177/0883073808322338. Medline:19182151

Salpietro V, Polizzi A, Granata F, Briuglia S, Mankad K, Ruggieri M. Upper respiratory tract infection and torticollis in children: differential diagnosis of Grisel's syndrome. *Clin Neuroradiol.* 2012;22(4):351–353. https://doi.org/10.1007/s00062-012-0145-2. Medline:22476653

Tomczak KK, Rosman NP. Torticollis. *J Child Neurol.* 2013;28(3):365–378. https://doi.org/10.1177/0883073812469294. Medline:23271760

6.8

Osteomyelitis

Rahim Valani

- Osteomyelitis affects the most vascularized regions of the growing skeleton due to the hematogenous spread of the infection.
  » The metaphysis is the primary site of infection.
- The rate of incidence is 8 to 10 per 100 000 in developed countries; in developing countries, the rate is 80 per 100 000.
  » Rates of osteomyelitis have been increasing in the past 2 decades; the rate of septic arthritis has remained stable.
- Most cases of osteomyelitis occur in children < 5 years of age.
  » It affects males more than females (2:1).
- There is a recent history of injury in about one-third of cases.
- 75% of osteomyelitis cases involve the lower limbs, which can present as difficulty ambulating.
  » The most common locations are:
    › Femur — 27%
    › Tibia — 26%
    › Humerus — 12%
    › Pelvis — 9%
    › Feet — 4% to 12%

Pathophysiology

- In children < 18 months of age, the epiphyseal and metaphyseal vessels are connected, which results in direct extension of the infection from the metaphysis to the epiphysis.
  » This results in destruction of:
    › Epiphyseal cartilage
    › Secondary ossification centers
    › Cells of the germinal zone of the physis
  » In this population, there is a higher incidence of adjacent septic arthritis (20% to 64%).
  » Infection extends into the subperiosteal space.
- A Brodie abscess is a limited area of subacute osteomyelitis.
  » It is characterized by a central area of necrosis with surrounding sclerotic rim and an outer halo of reactive tissue.
  » It is an avascular lesion, which helps distinguish it from other lesions.

Etiology

- Osteomyelitis is most commonly caused by a bacterial infection, such as:
  » *Staphylococcus aureus*
    › This is usually methicillin-sensitive *Staphlococcus aureus* (MSSA), but there is an increasing incidence of methicillin-resistant *Staphlococcus aureus* (MRSA).
    › MRSA osteomyelitis is more commonly associated with subperiosteal abscess, soft tissue involvement, multifocality, and deep vein thrombosis (DVT).
    › The following are risk factors for MRSA:
      · > 6 years of age
      · C-reactive protein (CRP) > 6
      · Location (spine / pelvis / lower extremity)
      · Sepsis
  » *Kingella kingae*
    › *Kingella kingae* is the most common cause of osteomyelitis in Europe and the Middle East.
    › It is usually seen in children 6 months to 4 years of age.
    › It is difficult to diagnose as routine blood cultures may not be positive.
    › Nucleic acid amplification or polymerase chain reaction (PCR) is required.
  » *Streptococcus pyogenes*
  » *Streptococcus pneumoniae*
- See *Table 6.8.1* for other specific causes are based on risk factors.

Table 6.8.1. ETIOLOGY OF OSTEOMYELITIS BASED ON RISK FACTORS

Risk factor	Organism
Neonate or young infant	• *Escherichia coli* • Group B *Streptococcus*
Puncture wound	• *Pseudomonas aeruginosa*
Sickle cell disease	• *Salmonella*
Immunocompromised patient	• *Candida* • *Mycobacteria* • *Bartonella henselae*
Tuberculosis-endemic area	• *Mycobacteria*
Chronic granulomatous disease	• *Serratia* • *Aspergillus*

History

- Clues on history include:
  - » Recent trauma
  - » Fever
  - » Erythema
  - » Refusal to ambulate

Physical Exam

- Patient may present with:
  - » Fever
  - » Focal tenderness
  - » Decreased range of motion for joints with effusion / septic arthritis
  - » Erythema
  - » Lymphadenopathy

Investigations

Bloodwork

- Initiate bloodwork:
  - » Complete blood count (CBC)
    - › Only 36% of patients will have elevated white cell count.
  - » Erythrocyte sedimentation rate (ESR) and CRP
    - › Sensitivity of 98% if both are elevated

Cultures

- Blood cultures are positive in up to 40% of cases.
- Pharyngeal cultures are useful for identifying *K. kingae*.
- Bone/joint cultures can increase sensitivity to 70%.

Imaging Studies

- Plain X-rays are diagnostic in < 20% of cases.
  - » Findings on plain films include:
    - › Local bony changes
    - › Periosteal reaction — usually seen 1 to 2 weeks after onset of osteomyelitis
    - › Soft tissue involvement
    - › Concerning features such as neoplasm or fracture
    - › Lytic lesions — need 50% to 75% depletion of bone mineral density to be visible on plain films
- MRI is the imaging of choice.
  - » MRI has low signal intensity on T1 image with high signal intensity on STIR or T2 images.
  - » It has reduced marrow enhancement.
- Consider ultrasound.
  - » Ultrasounds is useful for imaging deep soft tissue swelling.
  - » Use Doppler ultrasound to look for DVT.
- Consider CT scan.
  - » Radiation dose is an issue.
  - » CT scan has a sensitivity of 66% and a specificity of 97%.
  - » It easily identifies sequestration and larger abscesses.
- Consider triple-phase bone scan.

Management

- Prompt and targeted therapy leads to better outcomes.

Antibiotic Therapy

- Give patients 30 days of IV antibiotics.
- New studies suggest giving 2 to 4 days of IV antibiotics followed by 20 days of oral therapy.
  - » Patients must be stable, with no pyrexia and significant reduction in CRP.
  - » This method decreases complication rates of having a central line.

SPECIFIC ANTIBIOTIC THERAPIES

- Give empiric treatment until specific cultures are obtained, or for particular risks.
  - » For patients > 3 months old, give:
    - › Cefazolin 100 mg/kg per day divided and given every 8 hours (to a maximum of 6 g/day)
  - » For neonates give:
    - › Cefotaxime 150 to 200 mg/kg per day divided and given every 8 hours (to a maximum of 10 g/day)
    — and —
    - › Vancomycin 40 mg/kg per day divided and given every 6 to 12 hours (to a maximum of 2 g/day)
  - » For sickle cell patients, give:
    - › Ceftriaxone 75 to 100 mg/kg per day every 24 hours (to a maximum of 2 g/day)
  - » For MRSA, give:
    - › Clindamycin 25 to 40 mg/kg per day divided and given every 6 to 8 hours (to a maximum of 2.7 g/day)
    — or —
    - › Vancomycin 40 mg/kg per day divided and given every 6 to 12 hours (to a maximum of 2 g/day)
  - » For *Kingella*, give:
    - › Ampicillin 200 mg/kg per day divided and given every 6 hours (to a maximum of 12 g/day)

Surgical Management

- Consider surgical management for moderate to large abscesses.
- Surgical management is indicated when patients fail to improve after 48 to 72 hours of IV antibiotics.

Complications

- Osteomyelitis has a complication rate of 6%.
- Other infections associated with osteomyelitis are:
  - » Multiple bony abscesses
  - » Myositis/pyomyositis
  - » Necrotizing fasciitis (see Chapter 6.2)
- Other complications of osteomyelitis include:
  - » Avascular necrosis

» Physeal damage (1.8%)
» Pathological fractures (1.7%)
» Chronic osteomyelitis (1.7%)
  › Chronic osteomyelitis is defined as infection last-ing < 6 months.
  › It is characterized by:
    · Necrotic bone (sequestrum) surrounded by pus and reactive bone sclerosis (involucrum)
    · A linear defect on the bone that penetrates the cortex (cloaca)
  › It may also develop a sinus tract that allows direct drainage to the skin surface.
» Sepsis
» DVT (0.4% to 6%)
  › There is a higher incidence of DVT with MRSA osteomyelitis.
  › Risk factors for DVT include:
    · MRSA infection
    · CRP > 6
    · Spine / pelvis / lower limb infection

REFERENCES

Arnold JC, Bradley JS. Osteoarticular infections in children. *Infect Dis Clin North Am.* 2015;29(3):557–574. https://doi.org/10.1016/j.idc.2015.05.012. Medline:26311358

Branson J, Vallejo JG, Flores AR, et al. The contemporary microbiology and rates of concomitant osteomyelitis in acute septic arthritis. *Pediatr Infect Dis J.* 2017;36(3):267–273. https://doi.org/10.1097/INF.0000000000001417. Medline:27870814

Castellazzi L, Mantero M, Esposito S. Update on the management of pediatric acute osteomyelitis and septic arthritis. *Int J Mol Sci.* 2016;17(6):855. https://doi.org/10.3390/ijms17060855. Medline:27258258

Chiappini E, Camposampiero C, Lazzeri S, Indolfi G, De Martino M, Galli L. Epidemiology and management of hematogenous osteomyelitis in a tertiary pediatric centre. *Int J Environ Res Public Health.* 2017;14(5):477. https://doi.org/10.3390/ijerph14050477.

Funk SS, Copley LAB. Acute hematogenous osteomyelitis in children: pathogenesis, diagnosis, and treatment. *Orthop Clin North Am.* 2017;48(2):199–208. https://doi.org/10.1016/j.ocl.2016.12.007. Medline:28336042

Jaramillo D, Dormans JP, Delgado J, Laor T, St Geme JW III. Hematogenous osteomyelitis in infants and children: imaging of a changing disease. *Radiology.* 2017;283(3):629–643. https://doi.org/10.1148/radiol.2017151929. Medline:28514223

Johnston JJ, Murray-Krezan C, Dehority W. Suppurative complications of acute hematogenous osteomyelitis in children. *J Pediatr Orthop B.* 2017;26(6):491–496. https://doi.org/10.1097/BPB.0000000000000437. Medline:28181919

Okubo Y, Nochioka K, Testa M. Nationwide survey of pediatric acute osteomyelitis in the USA. *J Pediatr Orthop B*; 2017;26(6):501–506.

Spruiell MD, Searns JB, Heare TC, et al. Clinical care guideline for improving pediatric acute musculoskeletal infection outcomes. *J Pediatric Infect Dis Soc.* 2017;6(3): e86–e93. https://doi.org/10.1093/jpids/pix014

6.9

Septic (Bacterial) Arthritis

Ahmed Mater

- Children are affected by septic arthritis more commonly than adults.
- The peak incidence of septic arthritis is in children 2 to 6 years of age.
- Septic arthritis is more common in males than females (male to female ratio of 1.2–2:1).
- The incidence in children for septic arthritis is estimated at 5 to 37 per 100 000.
- In most cases, the site of infection is in a single joint (knee, hip, or ankle in 80% of cases).
  » Bilateral hip arthritis may occur.
  » ≤ 10% of cases are polyarticular.
    › When polyarticular cases are seen, it is usually in neonates.
- More than 80% of infections occur in the lower limbs:
  » Ankles — 23%
  » Knees — up to 40%
  » Hips — up to 30%

Risk Factors

- Risk factors for septic arthritis in neonates are:
  » Umbilical vessel catheterization
  » Central lines
  » Femoral vein access
  » Osteomyelitis
- Risk factors for septic arthritis in older children are:
  » Immunodeficiency
  » Joint surgery
  » Sickle cell disease (SCD)

» Juvenile idiopathic arthritis
» Insulin-dependent diabetes mellitus (IDDM)

Pathophysiology

- Bacteria reach the joint space through 1 of 3 possible mechanisms:
  1. Hematogenous spread
     › This is the most common mechanism in pediatric patients.
     › Hematogenous spread may occur because of:
       · Bacteremia (from pneumonia, tonsillitis, cellulitis, etc.)
       · Joint manipulation (aspiration or surgery)
  2. Direct inoculation
     › Direct inoculation may be polymicrobial.
     › It may occur after a skin wound has healed.
     › Direct inoculation may be the result of joint surgery or trauma.
  3. Extension from osteomyelitis
     › Septic arthritis may complicate osteomyelitis in up to 64% of cases.
- The most common causative organisms are similar to the culprits that cause bacteremia:
  » *Staphylococcus aureus* — methicillin-sensitive *Staphlococcus aureus* (MSSA) and methicillin-resistant *Staphlococcus aureus* (MRSA)
    › These are the most common causative organisms across all age groups.
  » *Haemophilus influenzae* type B
    › This was the second most common until the introduction of the vaccine.
  » *Kingella kingae*
    › *Kingella kingae* is a gram-negative bacterium.
    › It is more common in children aged 1 to 2 years of age.
  » *Streptococcus pneumoniae*
  » Beta-hemolytic *Streptococcus*

History

- On history, the physician should ask about:
  » Usual history items for fever (e.g., onset, duration, height, etc.)
  » Contact with sick individuals
  » Joint pain, including:
    › Level of pain (could range from mild to severe)
    › Inability to use limb or weight bear
    › Joint trauma (animal bite, needle puncture, laceration, etc.)
  » Skin lesions
    › Skin lesions may provide a clue to organism (impetigo and cellulitis with *S. aureus*, *Streptococcus pyogenes*; rash with *Neisseria meningitidis*, *Neisseria gonorrhoeae*).
  » Recent antibiotic use
    › This may mask the clinical picture.

- Additional factors to include:
  » Recent illness
    › Recent illness may indicate alternate diagnosis (upper respiratory tract infection [URTI] with transient synovitis; postinfectious arthritis).
  » Family history
    › Rheumatologic disease or inflammatory bowel disease (IBD) may suggest alternate diagnosis.
  » Travel history
    › Specifically, ask about travel to Lyme disease — or tuberculosis (TB) — endemic areas.
  » Animal exposure, particularly to:
    › Cats — risk of *Bartonella* and *Pasteurella*
    › Livestock — risk of Q fever
    › Reptiles — risk of *Salmonella*
  » Unpasteurized dairy intake
    › Patients are at higher risk of brucellosis.
  » Immunization status
  » Recent or concurrent strep throat
  » Recent or intercurrent diarrhea
    › This may indicate *Salmonella* infection.

Physical Exam

- Assess the joint involved and signs of injury.
- Infants and young children may appear sick, holding the joint in a position of comfort and refusing to move.
  » Patients often hold the affected hip in a position of partial flexion, abduction, and external rotation.
- Examine skin for specific lesions (e.g., *N. gonorrhoeae*, *N. meningitidis*, Lyme disease).
- An eye exam may help identify an alternative diagnosis (e.g., nonpurulent conjunctivitis in Kawasaki disease, uveitis in idiopathic arthritis).
- Conduct an abdominal exam; hepatomegaly indicates brucella arthritis.
- Examine all joints.
  » Look for injury, swelling, and redness.
  » Palpate, looking for hot, swollen, tender joints.
  » Test passive and active range of motion.
    › Pain with range of motion suggests bacterial arthritis.
  » Assess joints for pain with maneuvers that increase intracapsular pressure (compression of femoral head into acetabular joint).

Neonates and Infants

- Signs of septic arthritis in neonates and infants are:
  » Subtle or nonspecific signs (e.g., fussiness, poor feeding)
  » Septicemia (irritability, lethargy, poor feeding)
  » Cellulitis
  » Fever or hypothermia
  » Lack of use of extremity or crying with handling of a limb or joint

» Swelling of joint or limb
» Polyarticular
» Adjacent osteomyelitis
  › This is found in up to 60% to 100% of infants < 3 months of age with septic arthritis.

Older Children and Adolescents

- Signs of septic arthritis in older children and adolescents are:
  » Swelling, pain, and limited joint movement
  » Acute fever and malaise, irritability, poor appetite, tachycardia
  » Pain with active or passive movement
- Consider septic arthritis in any child with fever and joint pain, limping, or decreased movement of a limb or joint.
- Look for associated infection in children 6 months to 2 years of age.
- Meningitis may be present in up to 20% if *Haemophilus influenzae* is isolated in culture.

Investigations

Bloodwork

- Initiate bloodwork:
  » Complete blood count (CBC) and differential
    › Usually white blood cell (WBC) count is elevated.
  » C-reactive protein (CRP) and/or erythrocyte sedimentation rate (ESR)
    › CRP is elevated in most patients.
      · A normal CRP could be a good indicator that bacterial arthritis is less likely.
      · A normal CRP has a negative predictive value (NPV) of 87% for positive synovial fluid culture.
      · CRP is used to monitor disease response to therapy.
      · Levels peak within 1 to 2 days of onset of infection.
      · Levels fall to normal within 1 week of successful treatment.
    › ESR may remain elevated up to 30 days.
  » Blood culture
    › An aerobic blood culture must be done in all patients.
      · This culture is positive in 40% of patients.
    › An anaerobic culture should be collected if an anaerobic organism is suspected (central vein access, direct inoculation).

Synovial Fluid

- Synovial fluid analysis (cell count, Gram stain, and culture) should be performed as soon as possible to confirm the diagnosis and isolate the pathogen:
  » Cell count
    › WBC > 50 ×10^9/L with > 90% neutrophils suggests bacterial arthritis.

    › This is neither specific nor sensitive.
    › Lower counts may be present with bacterial arthritis.
  » Gram stain
    › This is not diagnostic, but it is important even if culture is negative because synovial fluid has bacteriostatic properties.
  » Aerobic and anaerobic culture
    › Cultures are positive in 50% to 60% of cases.
    › The physician may use blood culture bottles to enhance growth, especially in children < 36 months of age.

Kocher Criteria

- The Kocher criteria can help differentiate between septic arthritis and transient synovitis.
- The Kocher criteria are:
  » Temperature > 38.5°C
  » WBC > 12 × 10^9/L
  » ESR > 40 mm/h
  » Inability to bear weight

Table 6.9.1. KOCHER CRITERIA FOR SEPTIC ARTHRITIS OF THE HIP

Number of criteria met	Predicted probability of septic arthritis (%)
1	3.0
2	40.0
3	93.1
4	99.6

- Caird et al. (2006) added CRP to the Kocher criteria.
  » If CRP > 23.81 mol/L, this is another predictor of septic arthritis.
    › The best predictor of septic arthritis is fever > 38.5°C, followed by CRP > 19 mol/L.

Specific Tests

- The physician should also conduct the following investigations based on history and physical examination:
  » Lyme disease serology
  » Fungal culture (immune compromised)
  » TB testing (if TB exposure)
  » Polymerase chain reaction (PCR) of synovial fluid for *K. kingae*
  » Culture oropharynx, rectum, cervix for *N. gonorrhoeae*
  » Antistreptolysin O titer (ASOT) — if streptococcal arthritis is suspected

Imaging

- Imaging can confirm effusion of joints that are difficult to examine (hip, shoulder, sacroiliac [SI] joints).
- Plain X-ray findings may include:
  » Possible signs of trauma
  » Soft tissue swelling

- » Widened joint space
- » Increased opacity in a joint
- » Subluxation
- » Findings of osteomyelitis: erosion of epiphysis or metaphysis or subchondral bone 2 to 4 weeks after onset
- X-ray may help to exclude other possible diagnoses.
- Ultrasound and MRI are sensitive for joint effusion.
  - » Ultrasound:
    - › Is easily available
    - › Does not require sedation
    - › Has a high negative predictive value (NPV)
    - › Can guide joint aspiration
    - › Gives a false negative if performed < 24 hours from onset or with inadequate imaging

Note: When looking for infection, remember that:

- Neither presence of an effusion nor sonographic fluid appearance (echolucent vs echogenic) correlate with presence of infection
- Increased blood flow suggests infection, but normal flow does not exclude infection

- » MRI:
  - › Is highly sensitive for early joint effusion
  - › Is not readily available and more costly
  - › May show findings of osteomyelitis or another diagnosis
- Bone scan is generally not used to diagnose septic joints.
  - » It may be used if concomitant osteomyelitis is suspected.

Diagnosis

- A definitive diagnosis is made via:
  - » A positive synovial fluid culture
  - » A positive blood culture in the presence of clinical manifestations and elevated synovial fluid WBC count (usually > 50 $\times 10^9$/L).
- A probable diagnosis is indicated by:
  - » Negative blood and synovial fluid cultures
  - » Clinical manifestations consistent with septic arthritis
  - » Supporting laboratory workups (WBC > 50 $\times 10^9$/L in synovial fluid)
  - » Radiologic features
  - » Excluding other diagnoses
- A probable diagnosis should be managed as a confirmed case.

Management

- Permanent articular changes may occur if prompt surgical drainage is not done.
- Seek an emergent orthopedic consultation.
  - » The goal of orthopedic consultation is:
    - › Sterilization and decompression of the joint space
    - › Removal of inflammatory debris to relieve pain and prevent deformity
      - · Arthrotomy is immediately indicated if joint aspiration reveals pus, regardless of Gram stain result.
  - » Definitive drainage by orthopedics is indicated if:
    - › Hip or shoulder joints are affected
    - › Patient fails to improve after 48 hours of antibiotic therapy
    - › Synovial fluid culture is persistently positive
- Consider infectious disease consultation in cases of:
  - » Postoperative infection
  - » Chronic joint infection
  - » Penetrating injury (unusual organisms)
  - » Unusual pathogens on cultures (e.g., *Pasteurella multocida*, *Propionibacterium acnes*, fungi)
  - » Antibiotic allergies

Antibiotic Therapy

- Coverage for *S. aureus* (most common organism) is indicated for all ages.
  - » Give cefazolin 100 mg/kg per day divided in 3 doses (to a maximum of 6 g per day).
- If MRSA is suspected, then give:
  - » Vancomycin
    - › For patients 1 month to 11 years of age: 10 to 15 mg/kg per dose IV every 6 to 8 hours
    - › For patients 12 to 16 years of age: 1 g every 12 hours IV

  — or —

  - » Clindamycin
    - › For infants/children: 25 to 40 mg/kg per day IV divided and given every 6 to 8 hours
- Other coverage is based on age, clinical picture, and Gram stain.

Complications

- Complications of septic arthritis include:
  - » Sepsis
  - » Osteonecrosis of femoral head and neck
  - » Premature arthritis
  - » Physeal closure and growth disturbances

REFERENCES

Agarwal A, Aggarwal AN. Bone and joint infections in children: septic arthritis. *Indian J Pediatr.* 2016;83(8):825–833. https://doi.org/10.1007/s12098-015-1816-1. Medline:26189923

Arnold JC, Bradley JS. Osteoarticular infections in children. *Infect Dis Clin North Am.* 2015;29(3):557–574. https://doi.org/10.1016/j.idc.2015.05.012. Medline:26311358

Caird MS, Flynn JM, Leung YL, Millman JE, D'Italia JG, Dormans JP. Factors distinguishing septic arthritis from transient synovitis of the hip in children: a prospective study. *J Bone Joint Surg Am.* 2006;88(6):1251–1257. Medline:16757758

Castellazi L, Mantero M, Esposito S. Update on management of pediatric acute osteomyelitis and septic arthririst. *Int J Mol Sci.* 2016;17(6):855. https://doi.org/10.3390/ijms17060855.

Joffe MD, Loiselle JM. Septic arthritis: infectious disease emergencies. In: Fleisher G, Ludwig S, Henretig F, editors. *Textbook of pediatric emergency medicine.* 5th ed. Philadelphia: Lippincott Williams & Wilkins; 2006.

Krogstad P. Bacterial arthritis: treatment and outcome in infants and children. In: Up to Date, Wolters Kluwer. (Topic last updated Aug 3, 2017.) Available from: https://www.uptodate.com/contents/bacterial-arthritis-treatment-and-outcome-in-infants-and-children?source=search_result&search=septic%20arthritis&selectedTitle=2~150

Krogstad P. Bacterial arthritis: clinical features and diagnosis in infants and children. In: Up to Date, Wolters Kluwer. (Topic last updated Aug 4, 2017.) Available from: https://www.uptodate.com/contents/bacterial-arthritis-clinical-features-and-diagnosis-in-infants-and-children?source=search_result&search=septic%20arthritis&selectedTitle=1~150#H17

Krogstad P. Bacterial arthritis: epidemiology, pathogenesis, and microbiology in infants and children. In: Up to Date, Wolters Kluwer. (Topic last updated Mar 7, 2017.) Available from: https://www.uptodate.com/contents/bacterial-arthritis-epidemiology-pathogenesis-and-microbiology-in-infants-and-children?source=search_result&search=septic%20arthritis&selectedTitle=3~150

Wheeless CR, editor. Wheeless' textbook of orthopaedics. Duke University Medical Center's Division of Orthopaedic Surgery. Available from: http://www.wheelessonline.com

MUSCULOSKELETAL EMERGENCIES

7.1

Diabetic Ketoacidosis

Sarah Reid

The publication of the PECARN DKA FLUID trial in June 2018 will lead to new recommendations regarding fluid therapy in pediatric DKA.

Recommendations from the Canadian Diabetes Association and International Society of Pediatric and Adolescent Diabetes will be updated accordingly. If there are any further changes to the therapy outlined in this chapter, updates will be made as required and posted as an online adendum at www.brusheducation.ca/pediatrics.

- Type 1 diabetes mellitus (DM) is primarily a result of pancreatic beta cell destruction.
- Individuals with type 1 DM are prone to diabetic keto-acidosis (DKA).
- Insulin insufficiency leads to the increased lipolysis, ketogenesis, glycogenolysis, hyperglycemia and dehydration that results in ketoacidosis.
- DKA is a common complication of type 1 DM (and increasingly type 2 diabetes).
  - » It is usually seen in new onset diabetes that has not yet been recognized, or by a failure to take insulin or poor management of diabetes with an intercurrent illness.
- Ketoacidosis is the leading cause of morbidity and mortality in children with type 1 DM.

Diagnosis

- DKA is diagnosed with all of the following 3 criteria:
  1. Acidosis (defined as pH < 7.3 and/or bicarbonate level < 15 mmol/L on venous or capillary blood gas)
  2. Moderate to large ketones on urine dipstick or routine urinalysis
  3. New onset (random plasma glucose > 11.1 mmol/L and symptoms of diabetes) or existing diabetes

Table 7.1.1. SEVERITY OF DKA

Severity	Mild	Moderate	Severe
pH	7.2 to 7.29	7.1 to 7.19	< 7.1
Bicarbonate level	10 to 14 mmol/L	5 to 9 mmol/L	< 5 mmol/L

Physical Exam

- Clinical features of DKA are:
  - » Dehydration (usually moderate, 5% to 9% loss of total body water)
  - » Tachycardia
  - » Tachypnea, Kussmaul respirations
  - » Ketotic breath
  - » Nausea, vomiting (may mimic early gastroenteritis)
  - » Abdominal pain (may mimic appendicitis)
  - » Confusion, drowsiness, decreased level of consciousness

Investigations

- Initiate initial investigations:
  - » Plasma glucose, pH, pCO_2, bicarbonate, sodium, potassium, chloride, urea, creatinine, serum osmolality
  - » Urinalysis for ketones, glucose
- Consider hemoglobin A1c (HbA1c), thyroid stimulating hormone (TSH), thyroid antibodies.
- Recall that corrected Na = measured Na + 2 [(plasma glucose − 5.6)/5.6] mmol/L.

Management

- Use an up to date, published, pediatric-specific protocol.
- Initiate early communication with a pediatric diabetes specialist at the referral site.
- The goals of therapy are:

» Correcting dehydration
» Correcting acidosis and reversing ketosis
» Restoring blood glucose to near normal
» Monitoring patient for complications of DKA and providing treatment
» Identifying and treating any precipitating event

Administering Fluids

- The PECARN DKA FLUID trial did **not** find a difference in incidence of cerebral edema between DKA patients treated with a slow or fast rehydration protocol using either hypotonic or isotonic fluid.
- All patients **except for those exhibiting signs of cerebral edema / brain injury** (see "Cerebral Edema and DKA," below) should receive a bolus of normal saline 0.9% (10 mL/kg) over 30 minutes and their perfusion should be reassessed.
- Patients who are persistently hypotensive or poorly perfused should receive a second bolus of normal saline 0.9% (20 mL/kg to a maximum of 1000 mL); discuss further management with pediatric referral site.
- After the initial fluid bolus has been given, calculate the patient's fluid deficit at 10% of body weight and subtract the bolus already given. Divide the remaining deficit: half will be replaced over the first 12 hours (plus maintenance) and half over the next 24 hours (plus maintenance). This replicates the fast protocol in the PECARN DKA FLUID trial.
- IV composition and rate are then adjusted as per specific patient needs as metabolic derangements are repaired.
- Give nothing by mouth if acidosis is severe.

Other Management

POTASSIUM

- Patients will have a total body deficit of potassium from depletion of the intracellular pool caused by:
  » Transcellular shifts from increased plasma osmolality, insulin deficiency, and acidosis
  » Loss from body through vomiting and osmotic diuresis
- Add 40 mmol/L potassium chloride if plasma potassium < 5 mmol/L and patient is not anuric.
- Some patients may require potassium phosphate or potassium acetate to avoid a persistent hyperchloremic metabolic acidosis as rehydration proceeds.
- Consider an electrocardiogram (ECG) to look for abnormal T waves.

INSULIN

- Delay start of IV insulin infusion until 1 hour after intravenous fluid is started (not longer than 2 hours).
- Give 0.1 U/kg per hour (regular insulin).

- Boluses of IV insulin are contraindicated as they increase the risk of cerebral edema.

BICARBONATE

- The use of sodium bicarbonate is contraindicated as it increases the risk of cerebral edema.
- Some references state that sodium bicarbonate can be **considered** in patients with cardiovascular collapse/arrest or life-threatening hyperkalemia.

Monitoring

- Initiate monitoring via:
  » Cardiorespiratory monitor
  » Hourly blood glucose
  » Electrolytes and blood gas every 2 to 4 hours after IV therapy has started
  » Hourly intravenous fluid intake and urine output
  » Close neurological observation

Disposition

- DKA patients should be admitted to hospital.
- Only a small, select population can be discharged home.
  » Older children with very mild DKA may be treated in the emergency department (ED) with subcutaneous insulin and monitoring in consultation with a pediatric diabetes specialist.
  » These patients may be discharged following resolution of acidosis and arrangement of close follow-up.
- Considerations for transfer to PICU are:
  » Severe DKA (see *Table 7.1.1*, above) with or without signs of cerebral edema / brain injury
  » Children < 5 years of age
    › These patients are at high risk of cerebral edema / brain injury and are often admitted to PICU for close observation.

CEREBRAL EDEMA AND DKA

- Cerebral edema / brain injury may complicate any episode of DKA.
- Imaging studies reveal that subclinical cerebral edema may be quite common in patients with DKA.
- Up to 1% of episodes of DKA are complicated by symptomatic cerebral edema / brain injury.
  » 95% of episodes occur in individuals < 20 years of age.
  » One-third of episodes occur in children < 5 years of age.
  » Two-thirds occur in children with new-onset DM who are in DKA.
  » Episodes are rarely reported in adults.
- Cerebral edema / brain injury is the most feared complication as it has high morbidity and mortality.

Physical Exam

- Clinical features of cerebral edema / brain injury are:
  » Headache
  » Vomiting
  » Confusion
  » Glasgow Coma Scale (GCS) < 15 (see *Table 18.1.1* on page 316).
  » Irritability in young children (not consolable by caregiver)

Risk Factors

- Risk factors related to the patient are:
  » Age < 5 years
  » New-onset diabetes
  » Sick appearance
  » Longer duration of symptoms
  » More dehydrated (high urea, higher hematocrit)
  » Greater acidosis (lower pCO_2, lower pH)
- Risk factors related to management are:
  » IV bolus of insulin
  » Early IV insulin infusion (within first hour of IV fluids)
  » Failure of serum sodium to rise during treatment
  » Administration of sodium bicarbonate

Pathophysiology

- The pathophysiology of cerebral edema / brain injury is likely multifactorial.
- Historically, cerebral edema in pediatric DKA was felt to be due to hyperosmolarity, with the creation of intra-cellular idiogenic osmoles that cause brain cells to swell with rehydration.
  » Treatment was implicated.
  » This mechanism likely only plays a minor role in cerebral edema in pediatric DKA.
- More recent studies suggest that dehydration and hypo-perfusion are a more important cause of brain injury and cerebral edema is likely a consequence of this injury, thus the move to liberalize fluid therapy.

Management

- Monitor vital signs, airway, breathing, circulation, pupils, and GCS closely.
- Severe headache, change in sensorium, dilated pupils, bradycardia, hypertension, irregular breath-ing, posturing, and incontinence are all signs of acute deterioration.
- If a patient is demonstrating signs of cerebral edema / brain injury, adjust the fluid administration rate as needed to maintain normal blood pressure and avoid excessive fluid administration that might increase cere-bral edema formation.
  » Avoid hypotension that might compromise cerebral perfusion pressure.

  » In a normotensive patient who is well perfused, a conservative approach would be to decreased the fluid rate to maintenance.
- Elevate the head of the bed to 30°.
- Call for help (from provincial transport service, PICU, anesthesia).
  » These patients need to be in an intensive care setting.
- Administer 3% normal saline at a dose of 5 mL/kg IV over 15 minutes (may be given more rapidly in the case of acute herniation) **and/or** mannitol at a dose of 0.5 to 1 g/kg IV over 20 minutes.
- Obtain head CT scan when patient is stable at pediatric referral site.

Intubation

- Intubation should only be performed in consultation with provincial transport service/PICU/anesthesia support.
- Patients with cerebral edema / brain injury are at high risk for deterioration/arrest, especially during intubation.
  » A sudden increase of pCO_2 during or following intubation may cause cerebrospinal fluid (CSF) pH to decrease and contribute to worsening cerebral edema.
- In the case of acute cerebral herniation (blown pupil, hemiparesis, decreased level of consciousness, Cush-ing's reflex) intubation and brief mild hyperventila-tion (keep pCO_2 30–35 mmHg) may be used as a temporizing measure prior to emergent neurosurgical intervention.

Prevention

- The best ways to prevent DKA and its complications are:
  » Better management and recognition of new-onset DM
  » Better compliance and management of known DM
  » Early recognition of DKA
  » Following a pediatric-specific DKA protocol and avoid medical interventions that may increase the risk of cerebral edema / brain injury

REFERENCES

Chua HR, Schneider A, Bellomo R. Bicarbonate in diabetic ketoacidosis – a systematic review. *Ann Intensive Care.* 2011;1(1):23. https://doi.org/10.1186/2110-5820-1-23. Medline:21906367

Diabetes Canada Clinical Practice Guidelines Expert Committee. Diabetes Canada 2018 clinical practice guidelines for the prevention and management of diabetes in Canada. *Can J Diabetes.* 2018:42(Suppl 1):S1–S325.

Edge JA, Jakes RW, Roy Y, et al. The UK case-control study of cerebral oedema complicating diabetic ketoacidosis in children. *Diabetologia.* 2006;49(9):2002–2009. https://doi.org/10.1007/s00125-006-0363-8. Medline:16847700

Glaser NS, Wootton-Gorges SL, Buonocore MH, et al. Subclinical cerebral edema in children with diabetic ketoacidosis randomized to 2 different rehydration protocols. *Pediatrics*. 2013;131(1):e73–e80. https://doi.org/10.1542/peds.2012-1049. Medline:23230065

Kuppermann NS, Ghetti S, Schunk JE, et al. *Pediatric Emergency Carae Applied Research Network (PECARN) DKA FLUID Study Group*. Clinical trial of fluid infusion rates for pediatric diabetic ketoacidosis. *N Engl J Med*. 2013;378(24):2275–2287. https://doi.org/10.1056/NEJMoa1716816.

Reid S; Translating Emergency Knowledge for Kids. Bottom line recommendations: diabetic ketoacidosis (DKA). Winnipeg, MB; Children's Hospital Research Institute of Manitoba John Buhler Research Centre; 2016 (for review 2018). Available from: https://kte01.med.umanitoba.ca/assets/trekk/assets/attachments/159/original/dka-blr-reformatted-aug-2017.pdf?1505224804

Ugale J, Mata A, Meert KL, Sarnaik AP. Measured degree of dehydration in children and adolescents with type 1 diabetic ketoacidosis. *Pediatr*

Crit Care Med. 2012;13(2):e103–e107. https://doi.org/10.1097/PCC.0b013e3182231493. Medline:21666534

Watts W, Edge JA. How can cerebral edema during treatment of diabetic ketoacidosis be avoided? *Pediatr Diabetes*. 2014;15(4):271–276. https://doi.org/10.1111/pedi.12155. Medline:24866063

Wherrett D, Huot C, Mitchell B, Pacaud D; Canadian Diabetes Association Clinical Practice Guidelines Expert Committee. Type 1 diabetes in children and adolescents. *Can J Diabetes*. 2013;37(Suppl 1):S153–S162. https://doi.org/10.1016/j.jcjd.2013.01.042. Medline:24070940

Wolfsdorf JI, Allgrove J, Craig ME, et al; International Society for Pediatric and Adolescent Diabetes. ISPAD clinical practice consensus guidelines 2014 compendium. Diabetic ketoacidosis and hyperglycemic hyperosmolar state. *Pediatr Diabetes*. 2014;15(Suppl 20):154–179. https://doi.org/10.1111/pedi.12165. Medline:25041509

7.2

Hypoglycemia

Ahmed Ali Nahari, Karen McAssey

- Hypoglycemia is defined as a plasma glucose level of < 2.77 mmol/L at any age except during the first 72 hours of life.
- A low glucometer (capillary) blood glucose level must always be confirmed by a more accurate laboratory determination of blood glucose.
- Prolonged or repeated hypoglycemia in childhood may cause irreversible brain damage and permanently impair neurologic development.
- Obtain "critical" laboratory blood specimens before treatment is begun to confirm the diagnosis and to evaluate the etiology of the hypoglycemia.
- During therapy for hypoglycemia, a blood glucose level > 3.89 mmol/L should be achieved.
- Most hypoglycemia in childhood occurs during fasting, when adaptive mechanisms (glycogenolysis, gluconeogenesis, and/or fatty acid oxidation and ketogenesis) fail to maintain normal glucose homeostasis.

History

- Children with hypoglycemia may be asymptomatic or may present with severe central nervous system (CNS) and cardiorespiratory dysfunction.
- In infants, the signs of hypoglycemia are nonspecific (e.g., irritability, lethargy, jitteriness, tachypnea, cyanosis, hypothermia, or unresponsiveness).
- Autonomic nervous system activation (neurogenic symptoms) is the early manifestation of hypoglycemia:
  » Sweating
  » Tachycardia
  » Palpitations
  » Tremor, jitteriness
  » Anxiety
  » Pallor
  » Hunger, nausea, vomiting
  » Perspiration
  » Weakness
- Neuroglycopenia develops with prolonged or severe hypoglycemia:
  » Lethargy
  » Headache
  » Dizziness
  » Incoordination, ataxia
  » Seizure, hemiparesis
  » Confusion, irritability
  » Coma

Etiology

- Hypoglycemia may be the result of:
  » Infection
  » Acute brain injury — seizure, encephalitis, trauma, hemorrhage, hypoxia
  » Hypoxemia, hypotension, septic shock
  » Hepatic dysfunction
  » Alcohol intoxication, salicylate intoxication, beta-blockers, exogenous insulin, sulfonylurea
  » Hyperinsulinism
  » Inborn errors of metabolism — e.g., galactosemia,

ENDOCRINE EMERGENCIES

fructose intolerance, glycogen storage disease, amino or organic acid metabolism
» Growth hormone or cortisol deficiency
» Inadequate stores — small for gestational age (SGA) and preterm newborns, malnutrition, anorexia
• In childhood, idiopathic ketotic (substrate deficient) hypoglycemia and easily depleted glycogen stores, in combination with inadequate production of glucose through gluconeogenesis, contribute to hypoglycemia.

Investigations

• Obtain a critical (archival) blood sample immediately before therapeutic intervention.
• Collect the first urine void during or following hypoglycemia for urine ketones, organic acids, reducing substance, and toxicology screen as indicated.
• Order bloodwork.
» Basic bloodwork should include complete blood count (CBC), electrolytes, liver function tests, serum glucose, venous blood gases, ammonia, and lactate.
» Additional bloodwork should include insulin, cortisol, growth hormone, free fatty acids, beta-hydroxybutyrate, C peptide, total and free carnitine, and acylcarnitine.

Management

• Initial treatment focuses on management of ABCs and good supportive care.
• If the patient is conscious and able to tolerate oral fluids, then give rapidly absorbed carbohydrate (90–120 ml of formula or juice); repeat if they are still hypoglycemic in 10 to 15 minutes.
» If hypoglycemia does not improve in 15 to 30 minutes, then parental glucose is required.
• If the patient presents with an altered state of consciousness:
» Infuse an IV bolus of dextrose for moderate to severe hypoglycemia to provide 0.20 to 0.5 g/kg of dextrose (maximum single dose: 25 g)
› Give:
· A 10% dextrose bolus of 2 to 5 mL/kg IV/IO
— or —
· A 25% dextrose bolus of 1 to 2 mL/kg IV/IO
— or —
· A 50% dextrose bolus of 0.5 to 1.0 mL/kg IV/IO
› Administer IV bolus slowly to avoid rebound hypoglycemia.
» Following IV bolus, provide a continuous infusion of a dextrose-containing solution to provide glucose at 6 to 9 mg/kg per minute (usually a minimum of 10% dextrose)
› The rate of glucose infusion (mg/kg per minute) can be calculated as:

$$\frac{\text{dextrose in solution} \times 10 \times \text{rate of infusion}\,(\text{mL}/\text{hr})}{\text{weight}\,(\text{kg}) \times 60\,(\text{min/hr})}$$

» Monitor the patient's blood glucose every 15 to 30 minutes
» If the hypoglycemia does not resolve, increase the dextrose infusion to provide 10 to 15 mg/kg per minute
• A dextrose requirement above 10 mg/kg per minute is very suspicious for hyperinsulinism.
• Additional treatment options for persistent hypoglycemia (and particularly for hyperinsulinism) are:
» Glucagon — 0.5 to 1.0 mg subcutaneous or intramuscular, 1 to 2 mg IV over 24 hours
» Diazoxide — 5 to 20 mg/kg per day PO divided and given every 8 hours
» Octreotide — 2 to 20 mcg/kg per day SC divided and given every 6 to 8 hours
• Consider admission to hospital if the patient presents with any of the following:
» Difficulty maintaining normal glucose level by oral intake
» Ingestion of hypoglycemic agents
» Overdose with long-acting insulin
» Recurrent hypoglycemia
» Unknown cause of hypoglycemia requiring further investigation

REFERENCES

Aynsley-Green A, Hussain K, Hall J, et al. Practical management of hyperinsulinism in infancy. *Arch Dis Child Fetal Neonatal Ed.* 2000;82(2):F98–F107. https://doi.org/10.1136/fn.82.2.F98. Medline:10685981

Flykanaka-Gantenbein C. Hypoglycemia in childhood: long-term effects. *Pediatr Endocrinol Rev.* 2004;1(Suppl 3):530–536. Medline:16444188

Fournet JC, Junien C. The genetics of neonatal hyperinsulinism. *Horm Res.* 2003;59(Suppl 1):30–34. Medline:12566718

Haymond MW, Sunehag A. Controlling the sugar bowl. Regulation of glucose homeostasis in children. *Endocrinol Metab Clin North Am.* 1999;28(4):663–694. https://doi.org/10.1016/S0889-8529(05)70096-7. Medline:10609114

Laron Z. Hypoglycemia due to hormone deficiencies. *J Pediatr Endocrinol Metab.* 1998;11(Suppl 1):117–120. https://doi.org/10.1515/JPEM.1998.11.S1.117. Medline:9642649

Losek JD. Hypoglycemia and the ABC'S (sugar) of pediatric resuscitation. *Ann Emerg Med.* 2000;35(1):43–46. https://doi.org/10.1016/S0196-0644(00)70103-X. Medline:10613939

Lteif AN, Schwenk WF. Hypoglycemia in infants and children. *Endocrinol Metab Clin North Am.* 1999;28(3):619–646, vii. https://doi.org/10.1016/S0889-8529(05)70091-8. Medline:10500934

Stanley CA, Rozance PJ, Thornton PS, et al. Re-evaluating "transitional neonatal hypoglycemia": mechanism and implications for management. *J Pediatr.* 2015;166(6):1520–1525.e1. https://doi.org/10.1016/j.jpeds.2015.02.045. Medline:25819173

Thornton PS, Finegold DN, Stanley CA, Sperling MA. Hypoglycemia in the infant and child. In: Sperling MA, editor. *Pediatric endocrinology.* 2nd ed. Pennsylvania: Saunders; 2002. p. 367.

van den Berghe G. Disorders of gluconeogenesis. *J Inherit Metab Dis.* 1996;19(4):470–477. https://doi.org/10.1007/BF01799108. Medline:8884571

7.3

Water Balance

Ahmed Ali Nahari, Karen McAssey

- 75% to 80% of the body weight of term neonates and young infants is water.
- The adult distribution of intracellular (40%), extracellular (20%), and total body water (60%) is achieved during childhood.
- Water losses occur through the respiratory tract and skin (insensible losses), the gastrointestinal (GI) tract, and urine.
  » Normal net water loss is approximately 1500 mL/m^2 per day.
- Osmolar homeostasis is achieved by thirst / arginine vasopressin, whereas volume homeostasis is regulated primarily by the renin-angiotensin-aldosterone system.

DIABETES INSIPIDUS

- Patients with diabetes insipidus (DI) present with:
  » Polyuria with inappropriately dilute urine
  » Hypernatremia
  » Increased serum osmolality
  » Dehydration
- DI can be due to:
  » Arginine vasopressin (AVP) deficiency — central DI
  » AVP resistance — nephrogenic DI

History

- On history, ask about:
  » Polyuria (urine output of > 4 mL/kg per hour in children and 6 mL/kg per hour in neonates)
  » Thirst
  » Irritability
  » Fever
  » Weakness
  » Dehydration
  » Vomiting
  » Constipation
  » Failure to thrive

CENTRAL DIABETES INSIPIDUS

Etiology

- Central DI may be caused by:
  » A central nervous system (CNS) tumor
  » A congenital midbrain abnormality (e.g., pituitary agenesis, septo-optic dysplasia, holoprosencephalic syndrome)
  » Trauma or surgery to the base of the brain
  » Infiltrative lesions (e.g., Langerhans cell histiocytosis, lymphocytic neurohypophysitis)
  » Infections involving the base of the brain
  » Genetics
  » Drugs (e.g., ethanol, phenytoin, opiate antagonists, halothane, and α-adrenergic agents)
- The etiology of central DI may also be idiopathic.

Diagnosis

- The diagnosis of central DI is established if the serum osmolality is > 300 mmol/kg and urine osmolality is < 300 mmol/kg.
- This diagnosis is unlikely if the patient's serum osmolality is < 270 mmol/kg or the urine osmolality is > 600 mmol/kg.
- If the patient's serum osmolality is < 300 mmol/kg but > 270 mmol/kg, and pathologic polyuria and polydipsia are present, a water deprivation test is indicated to establish the diagnosis of DI and to differentiate central from nephrogenic causes.

Management

Fluid Therapy

- With an intact thirst and free access to oral fluids, a person with DI can maintain normal plasma osmolality and high normal serum sodium with high fluid intake.
- Neonates and young infants are often best treated solely with fluid therapy, given their requirement for large volumes of nutritive fluid (3 L/m^2 per 24 hours).

Vasopressin Analogs

- The use of vasopressin analogs in patients with obligate high fluid intake is contraindicated given the risk of life-threatening hyponatremia.
- Treatment of central DI in children is best accomplished with the use of the long-acting vasopressin analog desmopressin (DDAVP).
- Under most circumstances, total fluid intake **must be** limited to 1 L/m^2 per 24 hours during antidiuresis.

- DDAVP is available:
  - » PO: 25 to 100 mcg/dose
  - » IV/SC: 0.25 to 1 mcg/dose (to a maximum of 4 mcg/dose)
  - » IN: 2.5 to 10 mcg/dose
    - › This can be administered by rhinal tube (allowing dose titration) or by nasal spray.
- Treatment should begin with the lowest amount that gives the desired antidiuretic effect.
- These are initial doses; the dose and frequency of administration must be determined based on patient response and are usually given every 12 to 24 hours.
- To prevent water intoxication, patients should have at least 1 hour of urinary breakthrough between doses each day.

Hydrochlorothiazide

- Hydrochlorothiazide is an alternative therapy to DDAVP in infants.
- In neonates (< 6 months of age), give 1 to 2 mg/kg per day, divided and given orally 2 to 3 times daily (to a maximum of 37.5 mg/day).
- Chlorothiazide 5 to 10 mg/kg per day may be used instead.

NEPHROGENIC DIABETES INSIPIDUS

- Nephrogenic DI usually presents in the first few weeks of life.
- Additional renal disorders may include:
  - » Nonobstructive hydronephrosis
  - » Hydroureter
  - » Megabladder

Etiology

- Nephrogenic DI may be caused by:
  - » Genetic etiologies
  - » Acquired electrolyte disturbance (e.g., hypercalcemia, hypokalemia, protein malnutrition)
  - » Medications (e.g., lithium, demeclocycline, foscarnet, clozapine, amphotericin, methicillin, and rifampin)
  - » Kidney disease (e.g., ureteral obstruction, ischemic injury, polycystic kidney disease)

Diagnosis

- The diagnostic criteria for nephrogenic DI are the same as central DI; see "Diagnosis" under "Central Diabetes Insipidus," above.

Management

- If possible, eliminate the underlying disorder or medication.

- Ensure the intake of adequate calories for growth and avoid severe dehydration.
- Pharmacologic approaches to the treatment of nephrogenic DI include the use of thiazide diuretics, which are intended to decrease the patient's overall urine output.
- Indomethacin and amiloride may be used in combination with thiazides to further reduce polyuria.

SYNDROME OF INAPPROPRIATE ANTIDIURETIC HORMONE (SIADH)

- Syndrome of inappropriate antidiuretic hormone (SIADH) is characterized by oliguria with urine hyperosmolity, hyponatremia, serum hyposmolality, and euvolemia or mild hypervolemia resulting from the inappropriate release or excess activity AVP.
- SIADH can result in severe hyponatremia.
- Patients with SIADH fail to suppress AVP secretion even when plasma osmolality falls below the normal osmotic threshold for stimulated AVP release.
  - » This results in impaired renal free water clearance, total body free water excess, and hyponatremia.

History

- On history, ask about:
  - » Decreased urine output
  - » Volume status is normal to increased
  - » Generalized muscle weakness
  - » Seizure
  - » Coma

Etiology

- SIADH may be caused by:
  - » CNS surgery or traumatic injury
  - » Neuroendocrine tumor
  - » Hydrocephalus
  - » CNS infection (e.g., meningitis, encephalitis, tuberculous meningitis, brain abscess)
  - » Pulmonary disorders (e.g., acute respiratory failure, severe asthma, respiratory syncytial virus [RSV] bronchiolitis, cystic fibrosis [CF] exacerbation, and pneumonia)
  - » Drugs (e.g., lisinopril, carbamazepine, oxcarbazepine, valproic acid, cisplatinum, cyclophosphamide, vinblastine, vincristine, amantadine, trihexyphenidyl, haloperidol, thioridazine, acetaminophen, clofibrate, chlorpropamide, tolbutamide, fluoxetine, sertraline, imipramine, amitriptyline, and ecstasy)
  - » Emesis, pain, physiologic stress, hypoxia
  - » Cancer

Diagnosis

- The following are diagnostic criteria for SIADH:
  - » Hyponatremia

» Decreased plasma osmolality (plasma osmolality < 275 mmol/kg)
» Inappropriately concentrated urine > 100 mmol/kg
» Normal renal function
» Normal-to-high urine sodium
» Low serum uric acid
» Normal acid-base and potassium balance
- Exclude:
  » Hypothyroidism and adrenal insufficiency
    › Both can cause an SIADH-like syndrome due to impairment of free water excretion.
  » Heart failure
  » Cirrhosis of the liver
  » Nephrotic syndrome

Management

- Restrict the patient's fluid intake to less than insensible losses plus urine output.
- If IV fluid is required, use normal saline.
- If serum sodium is < 120 mmol/L, consider using hypertonic saline.
- Treat any underlying cause, if possible.
- Frequent monitoring of fluid input, serum sodium, and urine output and osmolality is required.
- Aim for the cautious correction of hyponatremia. The rate of serum sodium correction should not exceed 8 to 12 mmol/L per 24 hours.
- For symptomatic hyponatremia:
  » Fluid restriction should be instituted and hypertonic saline infusion used to raise serum sodium level more rapidly until symptoms remit
    › Give a 3% sodium chloride IV bolus of 1 to 2 mL/kg (usual maximum: 150 mL/dose) over 10 minutes (3% sodium chloride = 514 mmol/L sodium concentration); repeat if necessary.
- For chronic hyponatremia:
  » Rapid correction has been associated with central pontine myelinolysis

REFERENCES

Brook CGD, Brown RS. *Handbook of clinical pediatric endocrinology.* Wiley; 2008.

Di Iorgi N, Napoli F, Allegri AE, et al. Diabetes insipidus—diagnosis and management. *Horm Res Paediatr.* 2012;77(2):69–84. https://doi.org/10.1159/000336333. Medline:22433947

Duffett M, editor. *Pediatric critical care medication handbook.* Hamilton, Ontario: McMaster Children's Hospital; 2014. Available from: https://fhs.mcmaster.ca/pediatrics/documents/PICUDrugHandbook201416-Jun-14.pdf

Gross P. Clinical management of SIADH. *Ther Adv Endocrinol Metab.* 2012;3(2):61–73. https://doi.org/10.1177/2042018812437561. Medline:23148195

Hamilton Health Sciences. Pediatric critical care medication handbook. 2014.

Haycock G. Hypernatraemia: diagnosis and management. *Arch Dis Child Educ Pract Ed.* 2006;91(1):ep8. https://doi.org/10.1136/adc.2004.066928.

Haycock G. Hypernatraemia: diagnosis and management. *Arch Dis Child Educ Pract Ed.* 2006;91(2):ep37–ep41. https://doi.org/10.1136/adc.2005.086132.

Muhsin SA, Mount DB. Diagnosis and treatment of hypernatremia. *Best Pract Res Clin Endocrinol Metab.* 2016;30(2):189–203. https://doi.org/10.1016/j.beem.2016.02.014. Medline:27156758

Sperling MA. *Pediatric endocrinology.* 4th ed. Milton, ON: Elsevier; 2014.

7.4

Congenital Adrenal Hyperplasia

Kenneth Van Dewark

- Congenital adrenal hyperplasia (CAH) is a result of cortisol and occasionally aldosterone deficiency.
- It is a form of adrenal insufficiency.
- CAH has a high morbidity and mortality rate if not clinically recognized and treated.
- It is an autosomal recessive congenital disorder and is the result of the mutation or deletion of the gene coding for an enzyme involved in the conversion of precursor substrates into hormones produced by the adrenal medulla.
- In CAH, the endocrinological disruption can manifest as abnormalities in phenotypic sexual differentiation.
  » This is secondary to the disruption of the synthesis of androgen precursors used to synthesize aldosterone and cortisol.
- The prevalence of CAH in the United States is estimated at 1 per 15 000 live births.
- The most common cause of CAH is a deficiency in 21-hydroxylase (95%) followed by a deficiency in 11β-hydroxylase (4%).

» CAH is most commonly seen among those of Hispanic, Balkan, and Ashkenazi descent.

Normal Physiology

- The adrenal gland is a crucial endocrine organ, producing:
  » Aldosterone (adrenal cortex)
  » Cortisol (adrenal cortex)
  » Androstenedione/androstenediol (adrenal cortex) — testosterone precursors
  » Epinephrine/norepinephrine (adrenal medulla)
- The hypothalamic-pituitary axis regulates cortisol secretion.
  » Stress input to the hypothalamus releases corticotrophin-releasing hormone (CRH) → triggering the release of adrenocorticotrophic hormone (ACTH) from the anterior pituitary → triggering the release of cortisol from the adrenal medulla → leading to metabolic stress responses.
- Aldosterone secretion is regulated by the renin-angiotensin-aldosterone system and is a key mediator in renal electrolyte and blood pressure regulation.
- The production of all hormones within the adrenal cortex share a common pathway of precursor substrates.
  » Pregnenolone is the precursor of aldosterone, cortisol, and androstenedione.
  » Aldosterone is created through a series of intermediate steps mediated by 3β-hydroxysteroid dehydrogenase, 21-hydroxylase, 18-hydroxylase, 11β-hydroxylase and aldosterone synthetase.
  » Cortisol and testosterone precursors are produced by the conversion of pregnenolone by 17α-hydroxylase.

Pathophysiology

- CAH is caused by a mutation or deletion in the various CYP P450 enzymes involved in synthesizing aldosterone and cortisol.
  » These congenital disorders are autosomal recessive in inheritance.
- The majority of cases of CAH are caused by a congenital deficiency in 21-hydroxylase, with a mutation or deletion in the gene CYP21A.
- The acute symptoms of CAH are caused by a deficiency in cortisol and or aldosterone production.
- Disruption of aldosterone or cortisol synthesis can result in excess or deficiencies in the precursor substrate involved in the synthesis of androgens by the adrenal medulla.
  » Disruption in testosterone synthesis during fetal development can result in ambiguous genitalia or genitalia opposite from karyotypic sex.
  » The disruption of testosterone can also manifest during childhood and puberty.

- Deficiencies in 17α-hydroxylase and 11β-hydroxylase can result in pseudohyperaldosteronism.
  » This results in an accumulation of deoxycorticosterone, which can act as a mild mineralocorticoid.

Diagnosis

- The presentation of CAH can vary from severe to mild depending on the mutation affecting the enzyme involved in steroidogenesis.
- Clinical features are a consequence of the loss of cortisol and androstenedione production, with variable preservation of aldosterone production.
- Symptoms and clinical signs of cortisol deficit are:
  » Malaise
  » Weakness
  » Fatigue
  » Weight loss
  » Vomiting
  » Hypoglycemia
  » Hyperpigmentation
- Symptoms and clinical signs of aldosterone deficiency are:
  » Hypovolemic shock / hypotension / orthostasis
  » Hyperkalemia
  » Hyponatremia
  » Contraction alkalosis
  » Hyperchloremic acidosis
  » Physiologic stress — exacerbates symptoms of adrenal insufficiency
- Children with 11β-hydroxylase deficiency can present in the first month of life with a salt-wasting crisis with profound hypovolemic shock and electrolyte disturbance.
- Deficiencies in 17α-hydroxylase and 11β-hydroxylase can demonstrate findings of hypermineralocorticoidism after the first month of life secondary to an accumulation of deoxycorticosterone, which acts as a mineralocorticoid.
- Fluid resuscitation refractory hypotension is an important clinical sign for recognizing CAH.
- Symptoms can be dependent on sex:
  » Females
    › If there is a dysfunction in 3β-hydroxysteroid dehydrogenase, 21-hydroxylase, or 11β-hydroxylase, virilization of the genitalia or ambiguous genitalia can be seen at birth.
    › In milder cases of 21-hydroxylase deficiency, delayed symptoms can be seen in adolescence (hirsutism, accelerated growth, precocious pubic hair, oligomenorrhea).
    › If there is a dysfunction in 17α-hydroxylase, genitalia appear normal at birth, but absence of breast development and amenorrhea can be seen during puberty.

» Males
› Deficiency in 21-hydroxylase results in normal-appearing genitalia at birth, but during adolescence or childhood, accelerated growth, early bone maturation, and precocious puberty can result.
› Deficiency in 3β-hydroxysteroid dehydrogenase or 17α-hydroxylase can result in ambiguous or female genitalia at birth; these children are often diagnosed secondary to delayed onset of puberty.

Investigations

- Recommended investigations, as appropriate, are:
  » Electrolytes and extend electrolytes
  » Creatinine and blood urea nitrogen
  » Venous blood gas and lactate
  » Capillary glucose
  » Septic and metabolic workup in undifferentiated presentations
  » Plasma renin activity
  » Androstenedione and testosterone level
  » Progesterone level
  » ACTH stimulation test
- Subacutely, the evaluation of inappropriate levels of precursor substrate can assist in determining diagnosis.
  » Elevated 17-hydroxyprogesterone (> 1200 ng/dL) suggests 21-hydroxylase deficiency.
  » Elevated 11-deoxycortisol and deoxycorticosterone suggests 11β-hydroxylase deficiency.
- The role of imaging is limited outside a septic workup.
  » Consider an abdominal CT scan if bilateral adrenal hemorrhage is on the differential diagnosis.
  » Consider pelvic ultrasound for evaluation of ambiguous genitalia.
- Karyotyping may be done to determine genetic sex.

Management

- Assess the hemodynamic stability of the patient and manage hypotension initially with fluid resuscitation while other investigations are being completed.
- Within the emergency department (ED), the main goals of treatment are:
  » Glucocorticoid replacement
  › This will assist in correcting acidosis, hypotension, hyperkalemia.
  › Correct these conditions with hydrocortisone 1 to 2 mg/kg IV loading dose.
  › Do not delay administration if CAH is suspected and patient is unstable.
  » Fluid resuscitation
  › Give a normal saline bolus of 20 mL/kg IV.
  · Repeat as needed if the patient is hypotensive.
  » Correct hypoglycemia and electrolyte abnormalities
  › Correct glucose with 5mL/kg 10% dextrose solution IV followed by a 5% dextrose infusion.

» Mineralocorticoid replacement
› Do not give acutely if patient is hypotensive.
› Aggressive fluid resuscitation and glucocorticoids are initial therapy.
› Replace if patient is stable and has known aldosterone deficiency.
· Correct this deficiency with fludrocortisone 0.05 to 0.2 mg PO.

- Depending on the etiology of the CAH, long-term replacement of glucocorticoid and possibly mineralocorticoid should be initiated by a pediatric specialist.
- Stress dosing of hydrocortisone is required for children with known CAH.
  » Parental stress dosing:
  › 25 mg (< 1 year of age)
  › 50 mg (1 to 4 years of age)
  › 100 mg (> 4 years of age)
- Exogenous gonadotropin-releasing hormone and androgen inhibitors can be initiated later by a pediatric specialist if growth abnormalities or precocious puberty occur.

Disposition

- Children with suspected CAH should be evaluated by a pediatric endocrinologist and geneticist.
- Patients with acute presentations of CAH should be admitted to hospital for continued management by a pediatric specialist.
- Long-term management requires a multidisciplinary approach to determine a definitive diagnosis, pharmaceutical management, dietary management, genetic counseling, and overall goals of care during childhood and puberty.

REFERENCES

Auchus RJ. The classic and nonclassic concenital adrenal hyperplasias. *Endocr Pract.* 2015;21(4):383–389. https://doi.org/10.4158/EP14474. RA. Medline:25536973

Hannah-Shmouni F, Chen W, Merke DP. Genetics of congenital adrenal hyperplasia. *Endocrinol Metab Clin North Am.* 2017;46(2):435–458. https://doi.org/10.1016/j.ecl.2017.01.008. Medline:28476231

Raff H, Sharma ST, Nieman LK. Physiological basis for the etiology, diagnosis, and treatment of adrenal disorders: Cushing's syndrome, adrenal insufficiency, and congenital adrenal hyperplasia. *Compr Physiol.* 2014;4(2):739–769. https://doi.org/10.1002/cphy.c130035. Medline:24715566

Torre JJ, Bloomgarden ZT, Dickey RA, et al; AACE Hypertension Task Force. American Association of Clinical Endocrinologists medical guidelines for clinical practice for the diagnosis and treatment of hypertension. *Endocr Pract.* 2006;12(2):193–222. Medline:16718944

Witchel SF. Congenital adrenal hyperplasia. *J Pediatr Adolesc Gynecol.* 2017;30(5):520–534. https://doi.org/10.1016/j.jpag.2017.04.001. Medline:28450075

ENDOCRINE EMERGENCIES

7.5

Disorders of the Thyroid Gland

Ahmed Ali Nahari, Karen McAssey

HYPOTHYROIDISM

- Hypothyroidism results from the deficient production of thyroid hormone or a defect in thyroid hormone receptor activity.
- Thyroid hormone production by the thyroid gland is regulated by the hypothalamus and the pituitary gland.
- Hypothyroidism may be manifest from birth or acquired.

CONGENITAL HYPOTHYROIDISM

- Congenital hypothyroidism is one of the most common preventable and treatable causes of intellectual disability.
- The prevalence of congenital hypothyroidism is approximately 1:2000 to 1:4000 newborns.
- Most babies with congenital hypothyroidism are asymptomatic, even if there is complete agenesis of the thyroid gland.
- Retardation of physical and mental development will progress with any delay in the initiation of treatment.

Etiology

- Congenital hypothyroidism may be caused by:
  » Primary hypothyroidism due to:
    › Thyroid dysgenesis (most common cause)
    › Dyshormonogenesis (defective synthesis and secretion of thyroxine)
    › Resistance to thyroid stimulating hormone (TSH)
  » Defects in thyroid hormone transport or action
  » Central hypothyroidism
  » Transient congenital hypothyroidism

Diagnosis

- Primary hypothyroidism is characterized by:
  » Elevated serum TSH
  » Low free thyroxine (T_4)
- Central hypothyroidism is characterized by:
  » Low or normal serum TSH
  » Low free T_4
- Other investigations to be considered:
  » Serum thyroglobulin assay
  » Tests for thyroid autoantibodies
  » Ultrasonography
  » Thyroid radionuclide uptake

Clinical Presentation (Neonates)

- Neonates with congenital hypothyroidism may present with:
  » Prolongation of physiologic jaundice
  » Feeding difficulties
  » Puffy (myxedematous) facies
  » Macroglossia
  » Large fontanelle
  » Hypotonia
  » Dry skin
  » Umbilical hernia
  » Goiter — in some types of dyshormonogenesis
  » Associated congenital anomalies (e.g., cardiac, central nervous system [CNS], or eye)
  » Low-voltage P and T waves with diminished amplitude of QRS complexes demonstrated in electrocardiogram
  » Poor left ventricular function and pericardial effusion — in severe cases

Management

- Levothyroxine (T_4) is the treatment of choice.
  » The recommended starting dose in neonates is 10 to 15 mcg/kg per day (typically to a maximum of 25 to 50 mcg/day).
  » For neonates, the levothyroxine (T_4) pill should be crushed and mixed with a small amount of breast milk or cow's milk formula.
    › It should not be administered with iron or soy protein formula, which can bind T_4 and inhibit its absorption.
- Serum TSH and free T_4 should be maintained in the normal range according to age.
- Overtreatment may risk craniosynostosis.

ACQUIRED HYPOTHYROIDISM

- Autoimmune thyroid disease is the most common cause of acquired hypothyroidism, affecting 6% of children aged 12 to 19 years.

- Although typically seen in adolescence, autoimmune thyroid disease occurs as early as the first year of life.
- It occurs more often in females versus males (2:1).
- Autoimmune thyroid disease may be part of a polyglandular syndrome.
  » Children with Down, Klinefelter, or Turner syndromes, as well as those with celiac disease or type 1 diabetes, are at higher risk for associated autoimmune thyroid disease.

Etiology

- Autoimmune etiologies include:
  » Chronic lymphocytic thyroiditis (Hashimoto thyroiditis) — the most common autoimmune etiology
  » Polyglandular autoimmune syndrome, types 1 and 2
- Iatrogenic etiologies include:
  » Radioiodine
  » Thyroidectomy
  » Irradiation
  » Medications:
    › Methimazole
    › Propylthiouracil
    › Iodine
    › Lithium
    › Amiodarone
    › Phenytoin
    › Phenobarbital
    › Valproate
- Other etiologies of acquired hypothyroidism are:
  » Hypothalamic-pituitary dysfunction
  » Histiocytic infiltration of the thyroid (Langerhans cell histiocytosis)
  » Thyroid hormone resistance

Diagnosis

- Primary hypothyroidism is characterized by:
  » Elevated serum TSH
  » Low free T_4
- Subclinical hypothyroidism is characterized by:
  » Elevated serum TSH
  » Normal free T_4
- Central hypothyroidism is characterized by:
  » Normal or low serum TSH
  » Low serum free T_4
- The measurement of antithyroglobulin and antithyroperoxidase antibodies may indicate autoimmune hypothyroidism.
- Generally, there is no indication for thyroid imaging unless a nodule is detected clinically.

Clinical Presentation

- Patients with acquired thyroid disease may present with:
  » Bradycardia

  » Goiter
  » Myxedematous changes of the skin
  » Constipation
  » Cold intolerance
  » Decreased energy
  » Weight gain
  » Deceleration of growth
  » Delayed osseous maturation
  » Delayed puberty
  » Galactorrhea or pseudoprecocious puberty — in young children

Management

- Levothyroxine (T_4) is the treatment of choice.
- Serum TSH and free T_4 should be maintained in the normal range according to age.

Table 7.5.1. ORAL THYROXINE DOSE IN CHILDREN ACCORDING TO AGE

Age	Dose (per day)
1 to 5 years	5 to 6 mcg/kg
6 to 12 years	4 to 5 mcg/kg
Older than 12 years; growth and puberty incomplete	2 to 3 mcg/kg
Older than 12 years; growth and puberty complete	1.6 mcg/kg

MYXEDEMA COMA

- Myxedema coma (myxedema crisis) is a rare condition caused by severe hypothyroidism.
- The condition may be precipitated by an acute illness in a child who has preexisting hypothyroidism or long-standing untreated hypothyroidism.
- Myxedema coma is characterized by organ decompensation and is associated with a high mortality rate.

Diagnosis

- Diagnosis of myxedema coma is made via:
  » Clinical signs, symptoms, and corresponding abnormal thyroid function tests
  » Low free T_4 and T_3
  » Elevated TSH
    › This is a usual finding, but TSH may be low or even normal.
  » Other laboratory findings:
    › Hyponatremia
    › Hypoglycemia
    › Elevated creatine kinase
    › Anemia

Clinical Presentation

- Patients in a myxedema crisis may present with:
  » Altered mental status
  » Hypothermia
  » Generalized edema

ENDOCRINE EMERGENCIES

» Hypotension
» Bradycardia
» Cardiogenic shock
» Coma

Management

- Manage ABCs and give appropriate supportive care and monitoring.
  » Give IV fluids.
  » Use warming blankets to counter hypothermia.
- Treat the underling or precipitating illness.
- Correct hypoglycemia.

Specific Therapies

THYROID HORMONE REPLACEMENT

- IV is preferred if available.
- Levothyroxine (T_4) and T_3 are most commonly used:
  » Give levothyroxine (T_4) 3 mcg/kg IV.
    › Levothyroxine (T_4) is converted to T_3 in extrathyroidal tissue.
    › It has a half-life of 7 days.
- Give T_3, 5 to 25 mcg PO, daily (can be divided and administered every 8 hours)
  » 100 mcg of levothyroxine (T_4) is equivalent to 25 mcg of T_3 (for PO formulation).
    › Advantages of using T_3 include a more rapid onset of action and clinical improvement within 24 hours.

STRESS DOSE GLUCOCORTICOIDS

- Adrenal impairment is seen with severe hypothyroidism.
- Give hydrocortisone 100 mg/m^2 IV.
  » Dosing is age-based:
    › 0 to 3 years of age: hydrocortisone 25 mg
    › 3 to 12 years of age: hydrocortisone 50 mg
    › > 12 years of age: hydrocortisone 100 mg

HYPERTHYROIDISM

Etiology

- Graves disease is the most common cause of hyperthyroidism in the pediatric age group.
  » Graves disease is characterized by diffuse goiter, hyperthyroidism, and occasionally ophthalmopathy.
  » It occurs as a result of the stimulation of the thyroid gland by immunoglobulins.
  » 80% of pediatric Graves disease is found in children ≥ 10 years of age, predominantly in females.
- Other etiologies of thyrotoxicosis include:
  » Autonomously functioning thyroid nodule
  » Thyroiditis

» McCune-Albright syndrome
» Thyroid hormone ingestion
» Neonatal thyrotoxicosis
» TSH-producing pituitary adenomas

Diagnosis

- Graves disease is diagnosed via:
  » Clinical signs, symptoms, and corresponding abnormal thyroid function tests
  » Elevated serum free T_4
  » Suppressed TSH
  » Presence of TSH receptor antibodies

Clinical Presentation

- Patients with hyperthyroidism may present with:
  » Weight loss
  » Tremor
  » Tachycardia
  » Heat intolerance
  » Hyperactivity
  » Increased appetite
  » Palpitation
  » Exophthalmos

Management

- Treat Graves disease with antithyroid medication (e.g., methimazole).
  » Avoid using propylthiouracil (PTU) because of PTU-related hepatotoxicity.
  » The typical starting dose of methimazole is 0.2 to 0.5 mg/kg per day.
    › Possible side effects are agranulocytosis and hepatotoxicity.
- Before initiating therapy, obtain a complete blood count (CBC) and differential, serum aspartate transaminase (AST), alanine transaminase (ALT), and gamma-glutamyl transferase (GGT).
- If the patient develops a fever, jaundice, or pharyngitis, the medication should be stopped and a physician contacted.
- Consider radioactive iodine (^{131}I) therapy.
  » The goal of ^{131}I therapy for Graves disease is to induce hypothyroidism.
- Consider thyroidectomy.
  » Surgery is preferred in young children (< 5 years of age) when definitive therapy is needed and can be performed by an experienced thyroid surgeon.

THYROID STORM

- Thyroid storm (thyrotoxic crisis) is the most severe state of thyrotoxicosis.
- It is most commonly seen in children with underlying Graves disease.

- Thyroid storm may be precipitated by an acute illness, trauma, surgery, or medication.
- It is a rare condition associated with a high mortality rate.

Diagnosis

- Thyroid storm is diagnosed via:
  » Clinical signs and symptoms with corresponding abnormal thyroid function tests
  » Elevated free T_4 and T_3
  » Suppressed TSH

Clinical Presentation

- Patients with thyroid storm may present with:
  » Fever
  » Irritability
  » Tachycardia
  » Cardiac arrhythmia
  » Congestive heart failure
  » Diarrhea, nausea, vomiting, abdominal pain
  » Jaundice, abnormal liver function
  » Agitation, delirium, seizures

Management

- Put the patient under intensive care monitoring.
- Give supportive management (fluids, cooling, and electrolyte replacement).
- Treat the underlying or precipitating illness.

Specific Therapies

METHIMAZOLE

- Methimazole is used to inhibit hormone synthesis.
  » Use methimazole rather than PTU because of PTU-related hepatotoxicity.
- The typical dose of methimazole is 1 to 1.5 mg/kg PO daily, divided and administered every 6 hours.

POTASSIUM IODIDE OR LUGOL'S SOLUTION

- Use potassium iodide or Lugol's solution to inhibit hormone release.
  » Start one hour **after** giving methimazole.
  » Give 2 to 10 drops (based on body weight) every 6 hours.

BETA-BLOCKERS

- Use beta-blockers (propranolol) to inhibit peripheral effects of excess thyroid hormone.
  » Propranolol is contraindicated in bronchial asthma or peripheral vascular disease.
  » Propranolol dosing:
    › 0.015 mg/kg IV over 10 minutes
      · This can be repeated 3 times to a maximum cumulative dose of 5 mg.

HYDROCORTISONE

- Hydrocortisone reduces peripheral conversion of T_4 to T_3.
- Give 100 mg/m² IV.
  » Dosing is age based:
    › 0 to 3 years of age: hydrocortisone 25 mg
    › 3 to 12 years of age: hydrocortisone 50 mg
    › > 12 years of age: hydrocortisone 100 mg

OTHER THERAPIES

- Consider thyroidectomy (in difficult cases).
- Consider radioactive iodine treatment (dependent on patient's age).

REFERENCES

Alm J, Hagenfeldt L, Larsson A, Lundberg K. Incidence of congenital hypothyroidism: retrospective study of neonatal laboratory screening versus clinical symptoms as indicators leading to diagnosis. *Br Med J (Clin Res Ed)*. 1984;289(6453):1171–1175. https://doi.org/10.1136/bmj.289.6453.1171. Medline:6437473

Bakker B, Bikker H, Vulsma T, de Randamie JS, Wiedijk BM, de Vijlder JJ. Two decades of screening for congenital hypothyroidism in the Netherlands: TPO gene mutations in total iodide organification defects (an update). *J Clin Endocrinol Metab*. 2000;85(10):3708–3712. https://doi.org/10.1210/jcem.85.10.6878. Medline:11061528

Barker JM, Bajaj L. Hypo and hyper: common pediatric endocrine and metabolic emergencies. *Adv Pediatr*. 2015;62(1):257–282. https://doi.org/10.1016/j.yapd.2015.04.008. Medline:26205117

Buckingham BA, Costin G, Roe TF, Weitzman JJ, Kogut MD. Hyperthyroidism in children. A reevaluation of treatment. *Am J Dis Child*. 1981;135(2):112–117. https://doi.org/10.1001/archpedi.1981.02130260004003. Medline:7468542

Carroll R, Matfin G. Review: endocrine and metabolic emergencies: thyroid storm. *Ther Adv Endocrinol Metab*. 2010;1(3):139-145.

Collu R, Tang J, Castagné J, et al. A novel mechanism for isolated central hypothyroidism: inactivating mutations in the thyrotropin-releasing hormone receptor gene. *J Clin Endocrinol Metab*. 1997;82(5):1561–1565. Medline:9141550

Dorreh F, Chaijan PY, Javaheri J, Zeinalzadeh AH. Epidemiology of congenital hypothyroidism in Markazi Province, Iran. *J Clin Res Pediatr Endocrinol*. 2014;6(2):105–110. https://doi.org/10.4274/jcrpe.1287. Medline:24932604

Fadeyev V, Karseladse E. Hyperthyroidism and other causes of thyrotoxicosis: management guidelines of the American Thyroid Association and American Association of Clinical Endocrinologists. *Clin Exp Thyroidol*. 2011;7(4):8–18. https://doi.org/10.14341/ket2011748-18.

Jaruratanasirikul S, Leethanaporn K, Sriplung H. Thyrotoxicosis in children: treatment and outcome. *J Med Assoc Thai*. 2006;89(7):967–973. Medline:16881428

Léger J, Olivieri A, Donaldson M, et al; ESPE-PES-SLEP-JSPE-APEG-APPES-ISPAE; Congenital Hypothyroidism Consensus Conference Group. European Society for Paediatric Endocrinology consensus guidelines on screening, diagnosis, and management of congenital hypothyroidism. *J Clin Endocrinol Metab*. 2014;99(2):363–384. https://doi.org/10.1210/jc.2013-1891. Medline:24446653

Rivkees SA, Sklar C, Freemark M. Clinical review 99: The management of Graves' disease in children, with special emphasis on radioiodine treatment. *J Clin Endocrinol Metab*. 1998;83(11):3767–3776. Medline:9814445

ENDOCRINE EMERGENCIES

Hematology/Oncology Emergencies

8.1

Febrile Neutropenia

Kenneth Van Dewark

- Febrile neutropenia in a pediatric patient carries a high risk of morbidity and mortality.
- The incidence of febrile neutropenia in pediatric patients receiving chemotherapy and presenting with fever ranges from 10% to 40%.
- The condition is defined as having both fever and neutropenia.
  » Fever presents with oral temperatures of 38.0°C or greater.
    › Avoid taking temperatures rectally in any patient known or suspected to be neutropenic to reduce the risk of bleeding or infection.
  » Diagnosis of neutropenia is based on the absolute neutrophil count (ANC).
    › ANC varies by age.
      · The lower limit of normal in the first 24 hours of life is 0.6 cells/L.
      · Consensus guidelines most often suggest an ANC cutoff for febrile neutropenia of < 0.5 cells/L.
    › Neutropenia can be categorized as:
      · Mild — ANC 1 to 1.5 cells/L
      · Moderate — ANC 0.5 to 1 cells/L
      · Severe — ANC < 0.5 cells/L
- The emergency physician plays a critical role in identifying and initiating treatment. Delays in diagnosis and empiric treatment negatively impacts morbidity and mortality.

Etiology

- The cause of the febrile neutropenia can be due to:
  » Underlying malignancy or treatment:
    › Chemotherapeutic agents
    › Hematopoietic stem cell transplantation
  » Nonmalignant hematologic etiologies:
    › Medications — analgesics, anti-inflammatories, anticonvulsants, antidepressants, antipsychotics

    › Viral infections
    › Autoimmune conditions
    › Bone marrow failure syndromes — aplastic anemia and Fanconi anemia
    › Alloimmune neutropenia — between birth and 3 months of age
    › Congenital conditions — Kostmann syndrome, cyclic neutropenia

History

- History should focus on identifying potential sites of infection.
- Symptoms and features to consider on history:
  » Last chemotherapy session and agents used
  » Presence of central venous access (port, PICC, or central line)
  » History of bone marrow or stem cell transplantation
  » Prior infections
  » Use of medications
  » Onset of fever
  » Symptoms suggestive of source — upper respiratory tract infection (URTI) symptoms, erythematous skin, urinary symptoms, vomiting/diarrhea, etc.

Physical Exam

- The physical exam, like the history, should focus on identifying potential sites of infection.
- Look for the source of infection:
  » Upper and lower respiratory tract
  » Site of indwelling catheters
  » Abdominal examination
  » Genitourinary and rectal area
- Neutropenia is a relative contraindication for a rectal exam.
- Signs of infectious foci may be reduced due to immunosuppression.

Complications

- Relative immunosuppression caused by neutropenia increases the risk for opportunistic infections leading to fever.
- Bacteremia is the most common serious infection.
  - » Approximately 15% to 25% of patients with febrile neutropenia have bacteremia.
  - » The most commonly isolated organisms are:
    - › Gram-positive:
      - · Coagulase-negative staphylococci
      - · Viridans streptococci
      - · *Staphylococcus aureus* — including methicillin-resistant *S. aureus* (MRSA)
    - » Gram-negative:
      - · *Escherichia coli*
      - · *Klebsiella*
      - · *Pseudomonas*
      - · *Enterobacter*
- In approximately 80% of children with fever and neutropenia, no infectious etiology is identified.
  - » Nevertheless, all children presenting with neutropenia and fever should undergo a comprehensive workup for infectious foci.
- Common sites of infection include:
  - » Blood
  - » Upper and lower respiratory tract
  - » Urinary tract
  - » Gastrointestinal tract
  - » Skin
  - » Indwelling catheter sites

Investigations

- All patients with suspicion of febrile neutropenia should be investigated urgently.
  - » Initiate immediate cell count to determine if the patient is neutropenic.
  - » Determine possible foci of infection or an occult infection; all children presenting with neutropenia and fever should undergo comprehensive investigations for infectious foci.
- Order the following tests:
  - » Complete blood count (CBC) with differential
  - » Electrolytes and liver transaminases
  - » Creatinine and urea nitrogen
  - » Cultures from the following sites:
    - › Blood
    - › Catheters
    - › Urine
    - › Stool, sputum, and skin — consider based on clinical presentation
  - » Urinalysis
    - › Diagnostic yield can be reduced due to neutropenia causing decreased pyuria.
- Consider a chest X-ray (CXR) if respiratory symptoms are present.
- Consider virology and a lumbar puncture based on clinical presentation.
- Evidence for additional biomarkers is undefined in the current literature.

Management

- Ensure that the patient is hemodynamically stable.
  - » Provide adequate resuscitation with IV fluids and vasopressors as needed.

Antibiotic Therapy

- All patients with a suspicion of febrile neutropenia should receive empiric antibiotics.
- Empiric monotherapy is preferred as it is not inferior to combination therapy and carries fewer side effects.
- Investigations should not delay administration of antibiotics.
- Current guidelines recommend antibiotics be given within 60 minutes of presentation to the ED.
  - » All patients with a suspect diagnosis should receive empiric gram-negative coverage:
    - › Ceftriaxone 75 to 100 mg/kg given every 24 hours (to a maximum of 2 g/day).
  - » If high-risk features are present (see "High-risk Features," below), then empiric coverage for *Streptococcus viridians* and *Pseudomonas* should be administered:
    - › Piperacillin-tazobactam 300 mg/kg per day (based on piperacillin component) divided and given every 8 hours

      — **or** —
    - › Imipenem 100 mg/kg per day divided and given every 6 hours (to a maximum of 1 g/day)

HIGH-RISK FEATURES

- Suggested high-risk features indicating the use of Piperacillin-tazobactam empirically:
  - » ANC < 500 cells/µL
  - » Comorbidities
  - » Hepatic or renal dysfunction
  - » Neurologic symptoms
  - » Hemodynamic instability
  - » Recent central line
  - » Recent stem cell transplant
  - » Infants
  - » Vancomycin should not be used routinely, but should be added if:
    - › Catheter infection is suspected
    - › Soft tissue infection is present
    - › Pneumonia is suspected
    - › Patient is hemodynamically unstable
    - › History of colonization with MRSA

> › History of recent antibiotic use
> › There are high local rates of MRSA

Antifungal Therapy

- Empiric use of antifungals is reserved for patients with a history or physical exam suggestive of a fungal etiology.
  - » If fever persists for > 96 hours, neutropenia persists > 7 days postantibiotics, or cultures or imaging suggest a fungal infection, then antifungal therapy should be promptly initiated.

Antiviral Therapy

- Reserve empiric antivirals for:
  - » Patients with a history of exposure to influenza or presenting with influenza-like symptoms
  - » Patients for whom there is high suspicion of herpes simplex or varicella zoster infection or exposure
  - » Patients who are considered high risk or have hemodynamic instability

Other Management

COLONY-STIMULATING FACTORS

- There is no evidence to suggest that colony-stimulating factors have any benefit in mortality rates; however, these agents decrease admission duration, improve neutrophil recovery rate, and decrease duration of antibiotics administered.

INFECTIOUS FOCISOURCE REMOVAL

- Any catheter or indwelling line suspected of being a focus of infection must be promptly removed and replaced if still needed.

Disposition

- Patients with febrile neutropenia should be admitted, and empiric antibiotics continued and tailored to culture sensitivities when available.
- Some studies suggest low-risk patients can be stepped down to oral antibiotics with possible outpatient follow up. There is currently no validated method for risk stratifying such low-risk patients, so admission of these patients is currently the recommended standard of care.

REFERENCES

Barton CD, Waugh LK, Nielsen MJ, Paulus S. Febrile neutropenia in children treated for malignancy. *J Infect.* 2015;71(Suppl 1):S27–S35. https://doi.org/10.1016/j.jinf.2015.04.026. Medline:25917801

Dubos F, Delebarre M, Martinot A. Predicting the risk of severe infection in children with chemotherapy-induced febrile neutropenia. *Curr Opin Hematol.* 2012;19(1):39–43. https://doi.org/10.1097/MOH.0b013e32834da951. Medline:22123661

Haeusler GM, Sung L, Ammann RA, Phillips B. Management of fever and neutropenia in paediatric cancer patients: room for improvement? *Curr Opin Infect Dis.* 2015;28(6):532–538. https://doi.org/10.1097/QCO.0000000000000208. Medline:26381997

Ku BC, Bailey C, Balamuth F. Neutropenia in the febrile child. *Pediatr Emerg Care.* 2016;32(5):329–334. https://doi.org/10.1097/PEC.0000000000000809. Medline:27139294

Loeffen EA, Te Poele EM, Tissing WJ, Boezen HM, de Bont ES. Very early discharge versus early discharge versus non-early discharge in children with cancer and febrile neutropenia. *Cochrane Database Syst Rev.* 2016;2:CD008382. Medline:26899263

Mhaskar R, Clark OA, Lyman G, Engel Ayer Botrel T, Morganti Paladini L, Djulbegovic B. Colony-stimulating factors for chemotherapy-induced febrile neutropenia. *Cochrane Database Syst Rev.* 2014;(10):CD003039. Medline:25356786

8.2

Sickle Cell Disease

Andrea Estey, Sarah McKillop

- Sickle cell disease (SCD) is a chronic autosomal-recessive genetic disorder of hemoglobin molecules characterized by hemolysis; unpredictable, life-threatening, acute complications; and chronic organ damage (see *Table 8.2.1*).

Table 8.2.1. IMPORTANT CLINICAL MANIFESTATIONS OF SICKLE CELL DISEASE

Acute manifestations	Chronic manifestations
• Bacterial sepsis or meningitis	• Anemia
• Recurrent VOC	• Jaundice
• Splenic sequestration	• Splenomegaly
• Aplastic crisis	• Functional asplenia
• Acute chest syndrome	• Cardiomegaly, functional murmurs
• Stroke	• Hyposthenuria and enuresis
• Priapism	• Proteinuria
• Ocular complications	• CKD
	• Cholelithiasis
	• Delayed growth and maturation
	• Restrictive lung disease
	• Pulmonary hypertension
	• Avascular necrosis
	• Proliferative retinopathy
	• Leg ulcers
	• Transfusional hemosiderosis

CKD chronic kidney disease. **VOC** vasoocclusive crisis.

- Approximately 5% of the world's population are carriers of SCD or thalassemia.
- The majority affected are of African ancestry.
  - » A minority are of Hispanic, Southern European, Middle Eastern, Asian, or Indian descent.
- Approximately 5000 Canadians live with SCD; this number is increasing due to immigration from countries with a high prevalence of the condition and improved patient survival.
  - » 95 to 100 babies with SCD are born in Canada every year.
  - » Patients with SCD represent 1% of emergency department (ED) visits.
- SCD is detectable via universal newborn screening in the majority of Canadian provinces.
- >90% of children with SCD survive into adulthood, but their lives are shortened by 2 to 3 decades.
- In a retrospective cohort of SCD patients, 71% had at least 1 ED visit in a single year, whereas 16.9% had 3 or more.

Pathophysiology

- Normal adult hemoglobin (HbA) contains 2 alpha-globin and 2 beta-globin chains and is the predominant hemoglobin (Hb) after 6 months of age.
  - » Hemoglobin F (HbF) predominates in the fetal and infant periods and contains 2 alpha-globin and 2 gamma-globin chains.
- Hemoglobin S (HbS) is the result of a point mutation that alters beta globin chains (beta^s).
- HbS polymers change shape when oxygen is off-loaded, causing the normally crescent-shaped red blood cells (RBCs) to become sickle-shaped. This results in:
  - » Less deformability
  - » Shortened half-life
  - » Increased adhesivity
- Homozygous hemoglobin S (HbSS) and HbS-beta^0 thalassemia result in the most common and most severe forms of SCD.
  - » Other forms include HbS-beta$^+$ thalassemia and HbSC.
- Disease severity varies widely depending on the relative concentrations of HbF, HbS, and other hemoglobins, as well as genetic and environmental factors.
- Sickling can be exacerbated by:
  - » Dehydration
    - › Dehydration causes hyperviscosity due to a reduction in plasma volume, promoting and sustaining sickling and predisposing the patient to stroke.
  - » Intercurrent illness
  - » Fever
  - » Surgery
  - » Cold exposure
  - » Changes in weather
  - » Overexertion
  - » Psychological stress
- Sickled cells are detrimental in 2 main ways:
  1. Vasoocclusion
     › Vasoocclusion occurs primarily in the postcapillary venule, where hemoglobin oxygen concentration is low and blood vessels are at their narrowest.

› Sickled cells can block circulation in any organ, causing ischemia, pain, and damage.

2. Hemolysis
  › Damaged red cell membranes shorten the cells' lifespans.
  › Increased cell breakdown results in anemia.

- Heterozygous individuals have sickle cell trait; this is generally benign and asymptomatic.
- Diagnosis of SCD is made by:
  » Hemoglobin electrophoresis
  » Microscopy
    › Microscopy demonstrates sickled cells.
  » Sickle "prep" test
    › This test is helpful in ruling out sickle cell disease.
    › A positive test requires definitive testing with electrophoreses to differentiate whether the patient has SCD or trait.

Physical Exam

- Children with SCD may present with a variety of signs and symptoms, termed *crises*.
- Due to potential severity and rapid deterioration, as well as disease complexity, SCD patients should be assessed with priority in the ED.
  » Local pediatric hematology service should be consulted as appropriate.
- The exam should focus on areas of pain and include a careful examination for signs of infection, especially pneumonia, osteomyelitis, and sepsis.
- Evaluate males for priapism.
  » Note that they may be reluctant to report this symptom (see "Priapism," below).
- Examination of the spleen is critical.
  » Normal spleens usually cannot be palpated.
  » With enlargement, the anterior pole of the spleen descends below the rib cage, across the abdomen, and toward the right iliac fossa.

History

- SCD results in chronic anemia, and the baseline hemoglobin varies widely per patient.
  » Knowing an individual patient's baseline hemoglobin value or "steady state" is important.
  » Acute anemia is a decrease in hemoglobin by ≥ 20 g/L from baseline.
- History should focus on:
  » Precipitating factors
  » Location
  » Intensity
  » How the current presentation compares to usual episodes
- Changes in usual characteristics, especially of pain, should prompt a broader differential diagnosis.

- Further items to consider on history are:
  » Medications
    › Twice-daily antibiotic prophylaxis with penicillin-VK or amoxicillin is recommended for all children with SCD from age 2 months to at least 5 years, and often longer.
      · Strict patient compliance helps greatly reduce bacterial infection.
    › Most patients are on folic acid supplementation due to increased folate utilization with increased RBC turnover.
    › Hydroxyurea is used to reduce related complications by increasing the concentration of HbF in red blood cells, which leads to less sickling of RBCs.
      · This has the potential side effect of bone marrow suppression.
  » Transfusions
    › Required frequency of and previous need for exchange transfusions will help inform the physician of disease severity and past crises.
  » History of ICU admission
    › This is a red flag for disease severity.
  » Immunization
    › In addition to the routine immunization schedule and annual influenza vaccine, immunization against the following is recommended:
      · *Streptococcus pneumoniae* with pneumococcal conjugate vaccine (PCV13) and pneumococcal polysaccharide vaccine (PPV23)
      · *Neisseria meningitidis* with meningococcal conjugate ACYW-135 vaccine (MCV4) and meningococcal conjugate B vaccine
      · Hepatitis A and B — immunization during infancy
      · *Salmonella typhi* — for travelers

Management

- Management of specific crises is described in further sections.
- For all cases:
  » Thoroughly address the ABCs
  » Do not delay pain management
  » Supplement oxygen if saturation is ≤ 95%
  » Reassess the patient frequently as the condition may evolve rapidly
  » Consult the local pediatric hematology service
- Depending on the presenting symptoms, consider the following investigations:
  » Complete blood count (CBC) with differential and reticulocyte count
  » Cultures as required — blood, urine, throat
  » Bilirubin (total and direct) and liver enzymes
  » Blood urea nitrogen (BUN) and creatinine
  » Venous blood gas, lactate

- » Blood type and screen (cross match as needed)
- » Quantitative %HbS and %HbF
- » Parvovirus B19 serology
- » Chest X-ray (CXR) or other imaging studies

Fluid Management

- A careful assessment of hydration status is prudent
- SCD patients are more susceptible to dehydration due to hyposthenuria — an inability to concentrate urine maximally due to the loss of deep juxtamedullary nephrons — as well as increased insensible losses and reduced fluid intake.
- No randomized controlled trials have assessed the safety and efficacy of extra fluids in SCD.
- Fluid boluses should be given to restore euvolemia in suspected sepsis and other fluid loss states but should be avoided in acute chest syndrome and stroke.

Transfusion

- Transfusion is indicated to treat severe exacerbations of anemia and to treat and/or reduce the complications of SCD.
- Complications of transfusion include:
  - » Transfusion reactions — acute and delayed
  - » Hyperhemolysis — posttransfusion RBC destruction resulting in hemoglobin below pretransfusion levels
  - » Hyperviscosity — hypertension with congestive heart failure, altered mental status, seizures, signs of stroke
  - » Iron overload
- Transfuse with phenotypically-matched sickle-negative RBCs, if available, to reduce risk of alloimmunization and hemolytic transfusion reactions.
- Use caution to avoid volume overload; consider a pre-transfusion diuretic.
- Indications for transfusion include:
  - » Hemoglobin decrease to < 50 to 60 g/L
  - » Symptoms of heart failure, dyspnea, hypotension, or marked fatigue regardless of hemoglobin level
  - » Trauma
  - » Aplastic crisis
  - » Splenic or hepatic sequestration crisis
  - » Acute chest syndrome
  - » Acute ischemic stroke
  - » Retinal occlusion
  - » Priapism lasting > 4 hours that is unresponsive to other measures, and when surgical intervention is ineffective or not immediately available
- Hemoglobin concentration should not be increased over the patient's baseline or 100 to 110 g/L.
- Exchange transfusion may be required to achieve the traditional HbS% goal of < 30% without exceeding the desired hemoglobin concentration.

VASOOCCLUSIVE CRISIS (VOC)

- VOCs are acute, painful episodes that occur without warning and are caused by the stasis of sickled cells in capillaries and small veins.
  - » They often last 3 to 9 days.
- VOC is the most common complication of SCD and the most common reason for admission to hospital.
- Young children (< 5 years of age) commonly present with dactylitis (painful swelling of the fingers or toes) due to multiple phalangeal, metacarpal, and metatarsal infarcts.
  - » They may present with irritability, refusal to walk, and crying when touched or held.
- Patients often present with swelling, mild erythema, warmth, localized tenderness, and low-grade fever.
  - » Fever associated with pain should not be considered a VOC until infection has been ruled out.
- Common VOC locations include the long bones, ribs, sternum, spine, and pelvis.
  - » Infarcts can occur in any bone.
- Other causes of pain occur frequently in SCD and should be considered:
  - » Osteomyelitis
  - » Avascular necrosis (AVN)
  - » Pneumonia
  - » Cholelithiasis
  - » Constipation
  - » Acute chest syndrome
  - » Stroke
- Bone pain in SCD is 50 times more likely to be due to VOC than to osteomyelitis.
  - » Imaging studies are only needed to rule out other diagnoses if the physician is concerned.
  - » Do not delay pain relief while considering alternate diagnoses.
  - » MRI is the imaging of choice to help distinguish between osteomyelitis and bone crisis.

Management

- The primary management of VOC consists of fluid management, oxygen, and pain management.
- Empiric antibiotic therapy is not indicated in a simple pain event without the presence of fever or other signs of infection.
- Red blood cell transfusion is not indicated.
- Inhaled nitric oxide, corticosteroids, or magnesium sulfate have not been proven effective during pain crises.

FLUID MANAGEMENT

- Initiating hydration with oral fluids is preferable if tolerated.
- If IV fluids are required, a hypotonic solution is preferred (unless there are concerns of hyponatremia).

OXYGEN

- Oxygen should be provided if saturation is < 95% or if respiratory symptoms are present.
- Encourage the use of incentive spirometry and ambulation as soon as possible to help avoid acute chest syndrome.

PAIN MANAGEMENT

- Canadian guidelines suggest initiation of appropriate pain control within 30 minutes of ED arrival.
- Consider multimodal analgesia (acetaminophen, nonsteroidal anti-inflammatory drugs [NSAIDs]) as an adjunct to opioids.
  » Most patients will have treated themselves with acetaminophen, NSAIDs, or oral morphine prior to ED presentation; do not delay aggressive, appropriate analgesia (i.e., IV opioids).
- For moderate to severe pain:
  » Start with morphine bolus of 0.1 mg/kg IV
  » Give continuous infusion of 10 to 40 mcg/kg per hour IV
  » Consider a patient-controlled analgesia pump in older patients
- Response to treatment and medication titration should be assessed frequently.
- Respiratory status and excessive sedation must be monitored closely in patients receiving high-dose opiates.
  » High-dose opiates result in increased risk of acute chest syndrome.
- Use adjunctive nonpharmacologic approaches to treat pain (i.e., heat or ice packs, distraction, consultation with a child life specialist, relaxation, acupuncture, self-hypnosis).

FEVER/SEPSIS

- Children with SCD are at increased risk for severe infections from encapsulated bacteria (*Streptococcus pneumoniae*, *Neisseria meningitidis*, *Haemophilus influenzae* B, and nontyphi *Salmonella*) due to reduced or absent splenic function.
- Splenic impairment begins by 2 to 3 months of age.
- Functional asplenia occurs in 94% of patients by age 5.

Investigations

- Initiate investigations as indicated by presentation; consider:
  » Throat culture, stool culture, lumbar puncture, evaluation for osteomyelitis, screening for malaria
  » Urine culture in children < 3 years of age
  » CXR for all patients with cough, chest pain, fever, and/or oxygen saturation < 96%

High-risk Factors

- Signs and symptoms of high-risk patients include:
  » Unwell appearance or hemodynamic instability
  » Fever ≥ 40°C
  » Age < 6 months
  » Any of:
    › Leukopenia — white blood cells (WBC) < 5 × 10⁹/L
    › Leukocytosis — WBC > 30 × 10⁹/L
    › Thrombocytopenia — platelet count < 100 × 10⁹/L
    › Hb < 50 g/L
    › A decline in Hb ≥ 20 g/L from baseline
  » Respiratory distress or hypoxia
  » Concern of meningitis, osteomyelitis, ACS, or splenic sequestration
  » Pulmonary infiltrate on CXR
  » History of pneumococcal sepsis and/or meningitis
  » Severe pain
  » Severe dehydration
  » ≥ 2 visits to the ED for the same episode

Management

- High-risk patients should be admitted to hospital and treated parenterally until afebrile and cultures are negative.
  » Patients should also be admitted if unsafe for discharge or if close follow-up cannot be assured.
- IV fluid boluses should be administered as required to restore euvolemia.
- Low-risk patients (those with no high-risk factors; see "High-risk Factors," above) can be discharged home after receiving a 24-hour dose of ceftriaxone in the ED.
  » Patients should be observed for a minimum of 2 hours for ceftriaxone-induced hemolysis.
  » Ensure proper follow-up plans are in place if discharging the patient home (i.e., repeat antibiotic dose, follow-up with clinic).

Antibiotics

- Canadian guidelines suggest appropriate parenteral antibiotics be administered within 30 minutes of ED arrival, immediately after blood culture.
- Antibiotics should not be delayed if a blood culture is unattainable.
- Second- or third-generation cephalosporins are the antibiotic of choice:
  » Ceftriaxone 100 mg/kg IV/IM every 24 hours (to a maximum of 2 g/dose)
- If the patient has an allergy to cephalosporins, give:
  » Levofloxacin IV/PO every 12 hours
    › 10 mg/kg per dose for patients aged 6 months to 5 years
    › 5 mg/kg per dose for patients aged ≥ 5 years
- In areas with intermediate or high levels of

penicillin-resistant pneumococcal infection and in patients who are unwell, hemodynamically unstable, or suspected of having meningitis, vancomycin is recommended:

» Vancomycin 15 mg/kg IV every 6 hours (to a maximum of 1 g/dose)

- Patients > 5 years of age with respiratory symptoms should also receive a macrolide (consider in younger children if clinical suspicion is high):

» Clarithromycin 15 mg/kg per day divided and given twice daily

- Consider antivirals if influenza is suspected.

ACUTE CHEST SYNDROME

- Acute chest syndrome (ACS) is defined as a new infiltrate on CXR associated with one or more of:
  » Fever, cough, sputum production, tachypnea, dyspnea, chest pain, or new onset hypoxia
  » Other symptoms, including wheezing, chills, abdominal pain, rib pain, and extremity pain
- What would be considered pneumonia in a patient without SCD usually meets the criteria for ACS.
- Overall incidence of ACS is estimated at 10.5 per 100 patient years.
- ACS is most common in patients 2 to 4 years of age.
- ACS is potentially fatal and requires a high index of suspicion.
  » It is the most common cause of death in SCD.
  » It can develop acutely or insidiously.
  » It is often complicated by neurologic events.
  » It rapidly progresses to respiratory failure.
- ACS should be managed in a tertiary care center with ICU availability.
- Recurrent ACS is associated with an increased risk of stroke.

Etiology

- Etiology is unknown and possibly multifactorial:
  » Infection (often atypical organisms)
    › *Chlamydophila* and *Mycoplasma* are the most common isolated organisms.
  » Pulmonary infarction
  » Fat embolism
  » Pulmonary embolism
    › Consider this in at-risk patients due to similar presentations.

Risk Factors

- Risk factors include:
  » Overhydration
  » Immobility
  » Hypoventilation or splinting
  » Surgery
  » Comorbid asthma
  » Younger age
  » Lower HbF level
  » Degree of anemia (higher steady-state hemoglobin level)
  » Higher steady-state WBC count

Management

- Consult PICU immediately in any patient suspected of ACS.
- For fluid management:
  » Avoid fluid bolus
  » Carefully monitor fluid balance
    › Overhydration is associated with pulmonary edema and worsening clinical status.
  » Ensure that IV plus PO equals 75% to 100% of maintenance rate
- Treat the condition empirically with bronchodilators and incentive spirometry.
- Administer oxygen to maintain saturations ≥ 95%.
- Treat pain appropriately.
  » Beware of hypoventilation as it is a risk factor for precipitating ACS.
- If the patient is febrile, obtain cultures and start broad-spectrum antibiotics (including a macrolide).
- RBC transfusion results in improved oxygenation and should be pursued after a discussion with hematology.
  » Avoid relative polycythemia (Hb > 100 to 110).
- Exchange transfusion should be considered in severe or rapidly progressing cases.
- Use of corticosteroids is not routinely recommended.

APLASTIC CRISIS

- Aplastic crisis is profound reticulocytopenia (typically < 1%) following a viral illness.
- It is most commonly caused by parvovirus B19, which destroys erythrocyte precursors in bone marrow (usually without characteristic rash).
- It resolves after 1 week with the introduction of protective antibodies.
- A significant fall in hemoglobin occurs prior to reticulocyte recovery due to decreased sickled RBC lifespan.
- Patients present with gradual onset fatigue, shortness of breath, and occasionally syncope; fever is common.
- Physical exam shows lethargy, tachycardia, and occasionally heart failure.
- Hemoglobin is often 30 to 60 g/L and far below the patient's baseline. Reticulocyte count is reduced or even zero.
- RBC transfusion may be required if the patient is symptomatic or has Hb < 50 g/L.

» This results in a compensatory increase in plasma volume.
» Transfuse cautiously to avoid volume overload.
- Consider other causes of acute anemia in the differential diagnosis:
  » Splenic, hepatic, or pulmonary sequestration
  » Accelerated hemolysis due to delayed hemolytic transfusion reaction
  » Septicemia or other serious infections
  » ACS
  » VOC

SPLENIC SEQUESTRATION CRISIS

- Splenic sequestration crisis is an acute and life-threatening complication of SCD.
- Most episodes occur in patients 6 months to 5 years of age but can occur in all ages.
- Trapping of sickled cells in splenic sinusoids can result in massive, painful splenic enlargement over a period of hours.
- The condition is characterized by an enlarging spleen and a sudden drop in hemoglobin.
- Presentation includes sudden weakness, pallor, tachycardia, tachypnea, abdominal fullness, left upper quadrant pain, and palpable splenomegaly.
  » Back pain, left flank pain, chest pain, and obtundation are less common presentations.
- Laboratory studies reveal reticulocytosis, increased nucleated RBCs, and less commonly thrombocytopenia and leukopenia.
  » The mean decline in hemoglobin is usually ≥ 30 g/L from baseline.
- Recurrent crises occur in 50% of patients, with risk of mortality increasing with each episode.

Management

- If not urgently treated, splenic sequestration crises cause death from hypovolemic shock and anemia.
- Immediate transfusion is required.
  » While waiting for blood, give normal saline 10 to 20 mL/kg IV to manage hypovolemia.
  » To avoid accidental polycythemia and hyperviscosity, consider packed red blood cells (PRBCs) in smaller volumes (i.e., 3 to 5 mL/kg IV).
  » Reassess hemoglobin level before any additional transfusions.
    › Avoid excessive transfusion (Hb > 80 g/L).
  » Do not raise hemoglobin excessively or rapidly as the spleen will involute, causing autotransfusion, markedly increasing hemoglobin and hyperviscosity.
  » Emergency splenectomy should be performed if patient does not respond to PRBC transfusion, as signaled by:
    › Inability to maintain hemoglobin level
    › Increasing splenic size
    › Persistent hypovolemia

HEPATIC SEQUESTRATION CRISIS

- Less commonly, hepatic sequestration crisis may occur, resulting in rapid liver enlargement.
  » Laboratory studies reveal reticulocytosis and a conjugated hyperbilirubinemia.
  » Alkaline phosphatase and transaminases may also be increased.
- Two-thirds of SCD patients have mild baseline hepatomegaly; change in size should be monitored.
- Treatment is cautiously administered PRBC transfusions.

STROKE AND NEUROLOGIC COMPLICATIONS

- SCD patients are at risk for ischemic and hemorrhagic stroke, transient ischemic attack, silent cerebral infarction, cerebral vasculopathy, and moyamoya disease.
- Any acute neurologic symptom, even if transient, requires urgent evaluation.
- SCD is the most common cause of pediatric stroke.
  » Annual screening of SCD patients with transcranial Doppler (TCD) ultrasound should be started at age 2.
- Patients with HbSS disease have an 11% chance of having a stroke by age 20.
- The first and second highest incidences of first stroke occur, respectively, at 2 to 5 years of age and at 6 to 9 years of age.

Management

- Management depends on the type of stroke (see Chapter 4.2).
  » Most strokes in patients with SCD are ischemic.
- Presenting signs of acute ischemic stroke include focal weakness (hemiparesis); seizure; altered level of consciousness and mentation; confusion; and visual, speech, and sensory disturbances.
  » Symptoms may be transient.
- Presenting signs of acute hemorrhagic stroke include severe headache, nausea or vomiting, nuchal rigidity, seizures, focal neurological deficits, and altered level of consciousness.

ACUTE ISCHEMIC STROKE

- Administer oxygen to keep saturations ≥ 95%.
- Hydrate at maintenance rates.
- Maintain normothermia, normal blood pressure, and normoglycemia.
- Control seizures.

- Consider MRI and MR angiography if CT and CT angiography are negative.
- Pursue exchange RBC transfusion to target HbS < 30%.
- Thrombolytic therapy is not routinely recommended.

ACUTE HEMORRHAGIC STROKE
- Give supportive care as for ischemic stroke.
- There is no clear evidence for exchange blood transfusion.
- Obtain urgent neurosurgical consultation.

PRIAPISM
- Priapism is a common complication affecting 35% of males with SCD.
- Refer to Chapter 16.2 for further details.

REFERENCES
Baskin MN, Goh XL, Heeney MM, Harper MB. Bacteremia risk and outpatient management of febrile patients with sickle cell disease. *Pediatrics*. 2013;131(6):1035–1041. https://doi.org/10.1542/peds.2012-2139. Medline:23669523

Brousseau DC, Owens PL, Mosso AL, Panepinto JA, Steiner CA. Acute care utilization and rehospitalizations for sickle cell disease. *JAMA*. 2010;303(13):1288–1294. https://doi.org/10.1001/jama.2010.378. Medline:20371788

Canadian Haemoglobinopathy Association (CanHaem). Consensus statement on the care of patients with sickle cell disease in Canada (Version 2.0) [Internet]. Ottawa, ON: Canadian Haemoglobinopathy Association; 2015. Available from: http://sicklecellanemia.ca/pdf_2016/CANHAEM.pdf

Canadian Organization for Rare Disorders. Newborn screening in Canada status report [Internet]. Toronto, ON: Canadian Organization for Rare Disorders; 2012 [cited 2017 Feb 12]. Available from: https://www.raredisorders.ca/content/uploads/Canada-NBS-status-updated-Sept.-3-2015.pdf.

McGrath PJ, Walco GA, Turk DC, et al; PedIMMPACT. Core outcome domains and measures for pediatric acute and chronic/recurrent pain clinical trials: PedIMMPACT recommendations. *J Pain*. 2008;9(9):771–783. https://doi.org/10.1016/j.jpain.2008.04.007. Medline:18562251

National Heart, Lung and Blood Institute. Evidence-based management of sickle cell disease: expert panel report 2014 [Internet]. Bethesda, MD: U.S. Department of Health and Human Services, National Institutes of Health; 2014. Available from: https://www.nhlbi.nih.gov/sites/www.nhlbi.nih.gov/files/sickle-cell-disease-report.pdf

Okomo U, Meremikwu MM. Fluid replacement therapy for acute episodes of pain in people with sickle cell disease. *Cochrane Database Syst Rev*. 2015;(3):CD005406. Medline:25764071

Rogovik AL, Friedman JN, Persaud J, Goldman RD. Bacterial blood cultures in children with sickle cell disease. *Am J Emerg Med*. 2010;28(4):511–514. https://doi.org/10.1016/j.ajem.2009.04.002. Medline:20466235

Section on Hematology/Oncology Committee on Genetics, American Academy of Pediatrics. Health supervision for children with sickle cell disease. *Pediatrics*. 2002;109(3):526–535. https://doi.org/10.1542/peds.109.3.526. Medline:11875155

Shihabuddin BS, Scarfi CA. Fever in children with sickle cell disease: are all fevers equal? *J Emerg Med*. 2014;47(4):395–400. https://doi.org/10.1016/j.jemermed.2014.06.025. Medline:25161094

Zempsky WT. Evaluation and treatment of sickle cell pain in the emergency department: paths to a better future. *Clin Pediatr Emerg Med*. 2010;11(4):265–273. https://doi.org/10.1016/j.cpem.2010.09.002. Medline:21499553

8.3

Hereditary Bleeding Disorders

Rahim Valani

HEMOPHILIA
- Hemophilia is an X-linked factor deficiency that causes a delay in the formation of a clot.
- Hemophilia A and B are the most common inherited blood disorders.
  - » Hemophilia A (80%) is caused by factor VIII deficiency.
    - › It occurs in 1 in 5000 to 10 000 male births.
  - » Hemophilia B (20%) is caused by factor IX deficiency.
    - › It occurs in 1 in 30 000 to 50 000 male births.
  - » Hemophilia C (autosomal recessive) is caused by factor XI deficiency.
    - › It is most frequently encountered in individuals of Ashkenazi descent.
  - » Deficiencies of factors VIII, IX, XI, and XII have prolonged partial thromboplastin time (PTT) with a normal prothrombin time (PT).
- Severity is classified based on factor levels (see *Table 8.3.1*).

Table 8.3.1. SEVERITY CLASSIFICATION FOR HEMOPHILIA

Factor level	Severity	Symptoms
> 5%	Mild	• Bleeding with severe injury or surgery • Hemarthrosis is rare
1% to 5%	Moderate	• Bleeding with minor injury
< 1%	Severe	• Spontaneous bleeding unrelated to injury • Hemarthrosis is characteristic

Physical Exam

- Patients present with an unknown bleeding disorder.
  » 30% of males with hemophilia will have prolonged bleeding from the circumcision site.
- Patient may or may not have a history of trauma.
- The most frequent presentations in patients with a known bleeding disorder are:
  » Intracranial hemorrhage
    › This is the most common cause of death.
  » Hemarthrosis
    › This is the most common complication.
    › Knees, ankles, and elbows are the most frequent sites.
  » Hematuria
    › Hematuria is usually atraumatic and painless.
    › It may lead to anemia.
  » Oral bleeding
    › Oral bleeding is common in young patients.
    › It is often due to falls.

Investigations

- Bloodwork will help identify the type of bleeding disorder.
  » Initiate coagulation studies:
    › Platelet count
    › PT
    › PTT
    › Bleeding
    › Fibrinogen
  » Test von Willebrand factor (vWF) (see "Von Willebrand Disease," below).
  » If PTT is prolonged, obtain specific factor VIII and IX levels.
  » Screening tests can help identify the cause of the bleeding disorder (see *Table 8.3.2*).

Table 8.3.2. EXPECTED TEST RESULTS FOR THE DIFFERING BLEEDING DYSCRASIAS

Pathology	PT	PTT	Bleeding time	vWF testing	Platelet count
Hemophilia	Normal	Prolonged	Normal	Normal	Normal
von Willebrand disease	Normal	Prolonged	Normal or prolonged	Abnormal	Normal or reduced
Platelet	Normal	Normal	Prolonged	Normal	Reduced

PT prothrombin time. **PTT** partial thromboplastin time. **vWF** von Willebrand factor.

Management

- Replacement therapy is the mainstay of management.
- Treat hemophilia early and aggressively.
  » For suspected intracranial bleeds, treat on suspicion; do not wait for a CT scan.
    › Patients with normal neurologic exam and a significant mechanism of injury need treatment and a CT scan.
  » For hemarthrosis:
    › Treat based on the patient's perception of joint bleeding as signs (bruising, swelling) may be absent early
    › Immobilize the affected joint
  » For hematuria:
    › Treat with factor and bedrest if painless
    › Treat and investigate further if traumatic (ultrasound or CT scan as needed)
    › Avoid aminocaproic acid (Amicar)
  » For oral bleeding:
    › Administer Amicar 100 mg/kg every 6 hours (to a maximum of 24 g/day) for 5 days
  » Enquire whether patients have antibodies to certain products and treat accordingly.
  » Avoid agents that cause platelet dysfunction (e.g., ASA, clopidogrel).
  » Target the correction of factor level based on specific injuries (see *Table 8.3.3*).

Table 8.3.3. TARGET FACTOR LEVEL AND DURATION OF THERAPY FOR HEMOPHILIA PATIENTS

Injury	Factor target level	Duration of treatment
Joint hemorrhage	40 to 50% • Target joint bleeding protocol corrects to 100% on day 1 and 40% to 50% on days 1 to 3.	1 to 3 days
Muscle hemorrhage	40% to 50%	2 to 3 days
Iliopsoas (retroperitoneal) hemorrhage	80% to 90%	7 to 14 days
Head injury / intracranial bleed	80% to 100%	14 days
Throat/neck hemorrhage, severe tonsillitis	80% to 100%	
Acute GI bleed	80% to 100%	7 to 10 days
Epistaxis	Local control	
Laceration	Local wound care if minor • If the wound is deep, consider replacement to 50%.	5 to 7 days (depending on depth and location)

GI gastrointestinal.

HEMOPHILIA A

- Management of hemophilia A involves:
  » Factor VIII / recombinant factor replacement
    › 1 U/kg raises plasma factor VIII levels by 2%.
    › Half-life is 8 to 12 hours.

» Desmopressin
  › Desmopressin is useful only for mild hemophilia with ≥ 5% factor VIII levels.
» Antifibrinolytic therapy
  › Give tranexamic acid:
    · 10 mg/kg IV
    — or —
    · 15 to 20 mg/kg PO given 3 times a day
• Cryoprecipitate should be avoided (it has not undergone viral attenuation).

HEMOPHILIA B

• Management of hemophilia B involves:
  » Factor IX / recombinant factor replacement:
    › 1 U/kg raises plasma factor VIII levels by 1%.
  » Fresh frozen plasma (FFP)
    › FFP should not be used unless factor IX is not available and the situation is a life-threatening emergency.
    › Administer FFP 15 mL/kg.
  » Antifibrinolytic therapy
    › Tranexamic acid:
      · 10 mg/kg IV
      — or —
      · 15 to 20 mg/kg PO given three times daily
  » Prothrombin complex
    › Three-factor (F-II, IX, X) or 4-factor (F-II, VII, IX, X) concentrates may be used.
    › These are not used often given the availability of recombinant F-IX.

Disposition

• Ensure that the hematology service is involved in the care of patients with hemophilia.
• Ideally, patients with known bleeding disorders will have a care plan with them or filed at their local emergency department (ED).
  » Some patients may be placed on prophylactic therapy.
• Patients may need repeat dosing and clinical reassessment after 24 hours.
• Unique complications for hemophilia patients include:
  » Synovitis
  » Chronic arthropathy
  » Pseudotumors
  » Inhibitors to F-VIII or F-IX
    › Risk factors for developing inhibitors include:
      · Severity of hemophilia (past exposure to factors, intensity of exposure, age of first use)
      · Family history of inhibitors
      · Use of prophylaxis factor replacement
      · Use of plasma-derived factor replacement

VON WILLEBRAND DISEASE (vWD)

• Von Willebrand disease is caused by an abnormality in the von Willebrand factor (vWF).
  » vWF is a protein produced in megakaryocytes and endothelial cells.
    › It binds to platelet GP Ib/IX receptors that help it adhere to damaged endothelium.
    › It interacts with GP IIb/IIIa receptor on platelets to help with platelet aggregation.
    › It also acts as a carrier for F-VIII.
• The transmission of von Willebrand disease is autosomal dominant and occurs equally in males and females.
• It is a common cause of heavy menstrual bleeding postmenarche.

Pathophysiology

• Six subtypes are related to the function or level of vWF (see *Table 8.3.4*):
  » Type 1
    › The prevalence is 1% in the general population.
    › It is the most common variant of the disease (70% to 80%).
    › Deficiency of vWF is heterozygous.
    › vWF is structurally normal but in reduced concentration.
  » Type 2A
    › vWF undergoes accelerated proteolysis and has abnormal size (smaller).
  » Type 2B
    › vWF binds spontaneously to platelets and is cleared from circulation.
    › Patients have low platelet count as a result.
  » Type 2N
    › vWF is abnormal and cannot bind to F-VIII.
  » Type 2M
    › Abnormal binding site for platelet GP Ib receptor results in reduced ristocetin cofactor activity.
  » Type 3
    › Levels of vWF are extremely low.

Table 8.3.4. CLASSIFICATION OF VON WILLEBRAND FACTOR (VWF) DISEASE

vWD type	Abnormality	vWF:RCo	vWF:Ag	F-VIII level
1	Reduced concentration	< 30	< 30	Low or normal
2A	Smaller size and early proteolysis	< 30	< 30 to 200	Low or normal
2B	Increased affinity for GP Ib	< 30	< 30 to 200	Low or normal
2M	Abnormal GP Ib binding site	< 30	< 30 to 200	Low or normal
2N	Inability to bind to factor VIII	30–200	30 to 200	Low
3	Deficient vWF	< 3	30 to 50	Low

Ag antigen. **GP** glycoprotein. **RCo** ristocetin cofactor. **vWD** von Willebrand disease. **vWF** von Willebrand factor.

History

- Family members may have a bleeding problem.
  - » vWD is the most common inherited bleeding disorder.
- Adolescent patients may also have a history of prior hemostatic challenges such as excessive bleeding during surgery or delivery (postpartum hemorrhage), and after dental extractions.
- Patients may also have epistaxis, gingival bleeding, and bleeding that lasts for more than 15 minutes after trivial wounds.
- There may also be bleeding into joints or muscles.

Physical Exam

- Patients usually have mucocutaneous and surgical bleeding (from oral injury or dental extractions).
- Patients frequently present with epistaxis.
- Bruising is often present.
- Menorrhagia is a common symptom.

Investigations

- Initiate bloodwork and studies:
  - » Complete blood count (CBC) with platelet count
  - » PT and PTT
- If bleeding history is strong, consider performing a vWD assay — vWF:Ag, vWF:RCo, and factor VIII.

Management

- Avoid NSAIDs or other platelet-inhibiting medications.
- Prophylaxis is not recommended.
- There are 3 broad categories of management:
  - » Category 1 — promote the endogenous release of vWF
  - » Category 2 — enhance alternative prothrombotic pathways
  - » Category 3 — replace with exogenous vWF

Category 1 — Promote the Endogenous Release of von Willebrand Factor

DESMOPRESSIN

- Desmopressin (DDAVP) is a synthetic derivative of vasopressin.
- DDAVP is used to promote the release of vWF from endothelial cells.
- It is not recommended for patients < 2 years of age.
- It is mainly useful for types 1, 2A, and 2M.
- Dosing:
  - » IV:
    - › 0.3 mcg/kg in 50 mL normal saline over 30 minutes
  - » IN:
    - › 150 mcg for patients < 50 kg
    - › 300 mcg for patients ≥ 50 kg
  - » SC:
    - › 0.3 mcg /kg
- Most type 1 patients will respond to DDAVP.
- In type 2B, DDAVP can result in transient thrombocytopenia — use with caution.
- Side effects of DDAVP include:
  - » Facial flushing
  - » Headache
  - » Hypertension or hypotension
  - » Hyponatremia with repeat doses

COMBINED ORAL CONTRACEPTIVES

- Higher doses of estrogen increase endogenous production of vWF.
- Combined oral contraceptive (COC) therapy is excellent for management of menorrhagia.
- It is also helpful for type 3 patients.

Category 2 — Enhance Alternate Prothrombotic Pathways

CRYOPRECIPITATE

- Cryoprecipitate contains vWF and F-VIII.
- There is a risk of infection with the use of cryoprecipitate.

ANTIFIBRINOLYTIC AGENTS — TRANEXAMIC ACID

- Tranexamic acid prevents the conversion of plasminogen to plasmin and stabilizes the clot.
- Dose at 15 mg/kg every 8 hours for 5 days.

Category 3: Replace With Exogenous vWF

- Category 3 management is indicated if:
  - » DDAVP is ineffective or contraindicated
  - » Risk of bleeding is high
  - » Hemostatic support is needed for > 2 days
- Products approved by Health Canada are:
  - » Humate-P
  - » Wilate
    - › Both have a half-life of approximately 12 hours.

REFERENCES

American Society of Hematology. Quick reference: 2012 clinical practice guideline on the evaluation and management of von Willebrand disease. Washington, DC: American Society of Hematology; 2012.

Curnow J, Pasalic L, Favaloro EJ. Treatment of von Willebrand disease. *Semin Thromb Hemost.* 2016;42(2):133–146. https://doi.org/10.1055/s-0035-1569070. Medline:26838696

National Heart Lung and Blood Institute. The diagnosis, evaluation, and management of von Willebrands disease. National Institute of Health. Publication No: 08-5832. 2007.

Neff AT, Sidonio RF. Management of VWD. *Hematology.* 2014;2014(*1*):536–541. https://doi.org/10.1182/asheducation-2014.1.536.

Ng C, Motto DG, Di Paola J. Diagnostic approach to von Willebrand disease. *Blood.* 2015;125(*13*):2029–2037. https://doi.org/10.1182/blood-2014-08-528398. Medline:25712990

Peyvandi F, Garagiola I, Young G. The past and future of haemophilia: diagnosis, treatments, and its complications. *Lancet.* 2016;388(*10040*):187–197. https://doi.org/10.1016/S0140-6736(15)01123-X. Medline:26897598

Schwartz KR, Rubinstein M. Hemophilia and von Willebrand disease in children: emergency department evaluation and management. *Pediatr Emerg Med Pract.* 2015;12(*9*):1–20, quiz 20–21. Medline:26284379

Tengborn L. *Fibrinolytic inhibitors on the management of bleeding disorders.* Revised ed. Montreal: World Federation of Hemophilia; 2012.

World Federation of Hemophilia. Protocols for the treatment of hemophilia and von Willebrand disease. 3rd ed. Montreal: World Federation of Hemophilia; 2008.

8.4

Tumor Lysis Syndrome

Rahim Valani

- Tumor lysis syndrome (TLS) is the most common disease-related emergency for hematological cancers.
- It occurs when the destruction of large numbers of cancer cells results in the release of intracellular contents.
- It can be related to:
  » Rapidly accumulating tumor cells that undergo apoptosis
  » Destruction of sensitive tumor cells by cytotoxic drugs
- The highest incidence is seen with B-cell acute lymphoblastic leukemia (ALL) (approximately 25% of cases).
- The initiation of chemotherapy, radiotherapy, or steroid therapy can trigger TLS.
  » TLS can also occur spontaneously.
- Complications include:
  » Acute kidney injury
  » Seizures
  » Arrhythmias

Pathophysiology

- Cell lysis results in metabolic and electrolyte disturbances that cause the toxic effects:
  » Release of nucleic acids
    › Nucleic acids are broken down into xanthine and then uric acid by xanthine oxidase.
    › Uric acid deposits in the kidneys (deposition and crystallization are worse in an acidic urine environment).
  » Hyperkalemia
    › Hyperkalemia results from high intracellular potassium release.
    › In the presence of acute kidney injury, symptoms of hyperkalemia worsen and can lead to cardiac dysrhythmias.
  » Hyperphosphatemia
    › Hyperphosphatemia is due to high intracellular concentration of phosphate.
    › It is further exacerbated by renal insufficiency.
    › It causes secondary hypocalcemia due to calcium-phosphate precipitation.
      · Crystals can deposit in the renal tubules as well, further exacerbating renal injury.

Risk Factors

- Tumor-related risk factors include:
  » Malignancy type — ALL, acute myelogenous leukemia (AML), Burkitt lymphoma
  » High tumor burden — bulky lymphatic disease, elevated lactate dehydrogenase (LDH), elevated white blood cells (WBC)
  » High sensitivity of the tumor to chemotherapy
- Risk factors related to patient characteristics are:
  » Small child with large tumor
  » Volume depleted
  » Renal function — having an elevated baseline creatinine, administration of nephrotoxic drugs, or preexisting renal condition
  » Elevated baseline uric acid level

Diagnosis

- Diagnosis involves both laboratory and clinical criteria (see *Table 8.4.1*).
- TLS is usually seen 3 to 7 days after chemotherapy starts, but patients should be screened at presentation for all new suspected leukemias or lymphomas.

HEMATOLOGY/ONCOLOGY EMERGENCIES

Table 8.4.1. CAIRO-BISHOP CLASSIFICATION OF TUMOR LYSIS SYNDROME (TLS)

Adapted from Cairo and Bishop (2004)

Laboratory criteria	Clinical criteria
Uric acid > 476 μmol/L	Creatinine 1.5 times upper limit
Potassium > 6.0 mmol/L	Cardiac arrhythmia
Phosphorous > 2.1 mmol/L	Seizure, tetany, or other symptoms of hypocalcemia
Calcium 1.75 mmol/L	

Management

- TLS is best managed with preventative measures; however, acute management is sometimes necessary.

Fluid Resuscitation

- Fluid resuscitation is used for both acute management and prevention.
  » Fluid resuscitation aids in the clearance of uric acid and hyperkalemia.
  » Administer 2 times maintenance to achieve urine output of 2 to 3 mL/kg per hour.

Management of Electrolyte Imbalances

HYPERKALEMIA

- Obtain an urgent electrocardiogram (ECG) to see if any ECG abnormalities are present:
  » Peaked T-waves, shortened QT interval, prolonged PR interval, ST segment changes, and widening of the QRS complex
- If ECG abnormalities are present, then consider:
  » IV Calcium gluconate at 60 mg/kg
    › If using a 10% gluconate solution, this would be equivalent to 0.6 mL/kg.
  » Salbutamol (nebulized) starting with 2.5 mg and repeating as needed while other medications are being drawn and started
  » Insulin/glucose combination
    › Give insulin at 0.1 U/kg with 400 mg/kg of glucose, both given IV.
  » Kayexalate at 1 g/kg PO
- Consider hemodialysis in severe refractory cases.

HYPERPHOSPHATEMIA

- Hydrate the patient.
- Administer oral phosphate binders:
  » Aluminum hydroxide 100 mg/kg per day divided and administered every 6 hours
- Initiate dialysis (see "Dialysis," below).

HYPOCALCEMIA

- Initiate IV calcium (only if symptomatic). Administer:
  » 20 mg/kg of calcium chloride (or 0.2 mL/kg 10% chloride solution)

— or —
  » 60 mg/kg of calcium gluconate (or 0.6 mL/kg 10% gluconate solution)

Xanthine Oxidase Inhibitors (Allopurinol)

- Allopurinol is a purine analogue functions that functions as a xanthine oxidase inhibitor.
- The purpose is to decrease the conversion of xanthine to uric acid.
- Toxic effects include:
  » Stevens-Johnson syndrome
  » Hepatitis
  » Marrow suppression
  » Allopurinol hypersensitivity syndrome
- Allopurinol is more often used for prophylaxis to prevent TLS.

Recombinant Urate Oxidase (Rasburicase)

- Rasburicase metabolizes uric acid to allantoin, carbon dioxide, and hydrogen peroxide.
- Allantoin is readily excreted by the kidneys.
- Dose at 0.15 to 2 mg/kg in 50 mL of normal saline over 30 minutes.
- Rasburicase reduces uric acid levels within 4 hours.
- Avoid giving rasburicase to patients with G6PD deficiency as it may cause hemolysis.

Dialysis

- Dialysis is useful for:
  » Augmenting the clearance of potassium, uric acid, and phosphate
  » Acid-base balance
  » Calcium disorders
  » Therapy for acute renal injury
  » Volume overload

Other Considerations

- Diuretics are only useful in the setting of volume overload.
- Urinary alkalinization is no longer recommended.
  » No studies have shown any benefit.
  » It can exacerbate renal injury due to the precipitation of calcium phosphate crystals.
- Consider admitting the patient to a telemetry bed or the ICU.

REFERENCES

Cairo MS, Bishop M. Tumor lysis syndrome: new therapeutic strategies and classification. *Br J Haematol.* 2004;127(1):3–11. https://doi.org/10.1111/j.1365-2141.2004.05094.x.

Criscuolo M, Fianchi L, Dragonetti G, Pagano L. Tumor lysis syndrome: review of pathogenesis, risk factors and management of a medical emergency. *Expert Rev Hematol.* 2016;9(2):197–208. https://doi.org/10.1586/17474086.2016.1127156. Medline:26629730

McCurdy MT, Shanholtz CB. Oncologic emergencies. *Crit Care Med.* 2012;40(7):2212–2222. https://doi.org/10.1097/CCM.0b013e31824e1865. Medline:22584756

Mirrakhimov AE, Voore P, Khan M, Ali AM. Tumor lysis syndrome: a clinical review. *World J Crit Care Med.* 2015;4(2):130–138. https://doi.org/10.5492/wjccm.v4.i2.130. Medline:25938028

Wagner J, Arora S. Oncologic metabolic emergencies. *Emerg Med Clin North Am.* 2014;32(3):509–525. https://doi.org/10.1016/j.emc.2014.04.003. Medline:25060247

Wilson FP, Berns JS. Onco-nephrology: tumor lysis syndrome. *Clin J Am Soc Nephrol.* 2012;7(10):1730–1739. https://doi.org/10.2215/CJN.03150312. Medline:22879434

8.5

Superior Vena Cava Syndrome

Rahim Valani

- Superior vena cava (SVC) syndrome is an oncologic emergency in which the SVC cannot drain the blood supply from the head and upper limbs into the right atrium.
- Superior mediastinal syndrome is an SVC obstruction that occurs together with tracheal compression.

Etiology

- 80% to 90% of cases of SVC are associated with malignancies.
  » They are most commonly seen with anterior mediastinal masses.
  » There is an incidence of 2% to 5% in the following malignancies:
    › Non-Hodgkin and Hodgkin lymphoma
    › T-lymphoblastic lymphoma
    › T-cell acute lymphoblastic leukemia
- Other causes include:
  » Central venous catheters / port line–related complications
  » Total parenteral nutrition lines
  » Pacemakers

Pathophysiology

- The SVC carries about one-third of the venous return to the heart.
- The vessel can be easily compressed by adjacent structures or tumors.
  » Extrinsic obstruction is usually malignancy-related.
  » Intrinsic obstruction is usually from a thrombus.
- Obstruction of the SVC causes impaired venous drainage from the head, neck, and upper extremities.
- Collateral vessels develop and become engorged over time to help drain the upper limbs and head.
- The symptoms and severity of the clinical findings depend on how quickly the obstruction occurs.

- Symptoms will also be more severe if the level of obstruction is below where the azygos vein drains.
  » If the blockage is above where the azygos vein drains, then blood can flow through collateral vessels, enter the azygos vein, and drain farther down the SVC.
- Symptoms occur from compression caused by venous drainage into the mediastinum, and include:
  » Facial and neck edema
  » Dilation of proximal veins
  » Collateral vessels
  » Plethora
  » Cyanosis
  » Dyspnea
  » Persistent cough
  » Stridor
  » Chest pain
  » Headache

Investigations

Imaging Studies

CHEST X-RAY

- 84% of SVC obstruction patients will have an abnormal chest X-ray (CXR).
- 64% will show a widened mediastinum.

CT SCAN

- CT scan is a better imaging choice that CXR but having the patient recumbent can worsen symptoms.

ELECTROCARDIOGRAM

- Electrocardiogram (ECG) is used to rule out pericardial effusion.

DOPPLER ULTRASOUND

- This can demonstrate flow reversal of the internal thoracic vein.

HEMATOLOGY/ONCOLOGY EMERGENCIES

Tissue Studies

- Tissue samples may help identify underlying malignancies for which SVC syndrome is the initial presentation; this can guide treatment.
- Consider the following tissue studies:
  » Biopsy of peripheral nodes
  » Pericardiocentesis
  » Bone marrow aspiration

Management

- If there is evidence of respiratory compromise:
  » Keep the patient upright
  » Provide supplemental oxygen
  » Start parenteral steroids immediately
- If there is evidence of impending airway obstruction, prepare for difficult intubation and call anesthesia for assistance.
- Consider:
  » Radiation therapy
  » Treating the underlying malignancy/thrombus/ infection
  » Interventional vascular procedures (stenting)
- For stable patients, it is important to know the cause of the SVC obstruction.
  » If the cause is thrombotic in nature (due to central line or catheter):
    › Remove the offending central line / catheter, if possible
    › Administer thrombolytics
      · Patients respond best when this is started within a few days of the onset of symptoms.
    › Begin anticoagulation therapy

- If SVC is associated with malignancy:
  › Provide oxygen to maintain saturation levels and to prevent anxiety
  › Elevate head of bed
    · Symptoms worsen when patients are recumbent.
  › Administer parenteral steroids
  › Consider diuretics
  › Consult the oncology team

REFERENCES

Haut C. Oncological emergencies in the pediatric intensive care unit. *AACN Clin Issues.* 2005;16(2):232–245. https://doi.org/10.1097/00044067-200504000-00013. Medline:15876890

Henry M, Sung L. Supportive care in pediatric oncology: oncologic emergencies and management of fever and neutropenia. *Pediatr Clin North Am.* 2015;62(1):27–46. https://doi.org/10.1016/j.pcl.2014.09.016. Medline:25435110

McCurdy MT, Shanholtz CB. Oncologic emergencies. *Crit Care Med.* 2012;40(7):2212–2222. https://doi.org/10.1097/CCM.0b013e31824e1865. Medline:22584756

Rachapalli V, Boucher L-M. Superior vena cava syndrome: role of the interventionalist. *Can Assoc Radiol J.* 2014;65(2):168–176. https://doi.org/10.1016/j.carj.2012.09.003. Medline:23415716

Sonavane SK, Milner DM, Singh SP, Abdel Aal AK, Shahir KS, Chaturvedi A. Comprehensive imaging review of the superior vena cava. *Radiographics.* 2015;35(7):1873–1892. https://doi.org/10.1148/rg.2015150056. Medline:26452112

Straka C, Ying J, Kong F-M, Willey CD, Kaminski J, Kim DW. Review of evolving etiologies, implications and treatment strategies for the superior vena cava syndrome. *Springerplus.* 2016;5(1):229. https://doi.org/10.1186/s40064-016-1900-7. Medline:27026923

Talapatra K, Panda S, Goyle S, Bhadra K, Mistry R. Superior vena cava syndrome: a radiation oncologist's perspective. *J Cancer Res Ther.* 2016;12(2):515–519. https://doi.org/10.4103/0973-1482.177503. Medline:27461602

Warner P, Uberoi R. Superior vena cava stenting in the 21st century. *Postgrad Med J.* 2013;89(1050):224–230. https://doi.org/10.1136/postgradmedj-2012-131186. Medline:23322744

8.6

Hemolytic Anemia

Louise Guolla, Kevin Chan

- Typical nonnucleated red blood cells (RBCs) have a lifespan of between 100 and 120 days.
- To maintain homeostasis and a stable hemoglobin level, the expected destruction of about 1% of circulating RBCs each day is balanced by the production of RBCs in the bone marrow as reticulocytes.
- When excessive destruction (hemolysis) occurs and RBC lifespan is shortened, the marrow responds by increasing RBC production, which presents as reticulocytosis.
- If the body cannot respond adequately or rapidly enough, anemia results.

Pathophysiology

- Many inherited conditions that predispose an individual to chronic hemolysis (i.e., hemoglobinopathies)

achieve homeostasis by having hyperactive bone marrow with evidence of reticulocytosis.
- » Reticulocytes are elevated by 2% to 3%.
- » Anemia may be mild or not apparent if full compensation is achieved.
- Acute insults to the body such as infection or exposure to toxins may precipitate a rapid worsening of chronic hemolysis for which the body is unable to compensate, and a hemolytic crisis may occur.

EXTRAVASCULAR HEMOLYSIS
- Extravascular hemolysis is characterized by the removal of RBCs from circulation via phagocytosis of abnormal RBCs by macrophages in the spleen or Kupffer cells in the liver.
- Phagocytosed RBCs are eventually broken down into biliverdin, leading to an increased bilirubin level in the body.
- Most hemolytic anemias have an extravascular component, especially autoimmune hemolytic anemia, sickle cell disease (SCD), and other inherited disorders of RBC structure.

INTRAVASCULAR HEMOLYSIS
- Intravascular hemolysis is characterized by the damage and destruction of RBCs within the vasculature itself.
- It may be secondary to mechanical factors such as shear stress, complement-mediated hemolysis, or toxins, as in hemolytic uremic syndrome (HUS), which is associated with the Shiga toxin.
- Lysis of RBCs results in free-floating extracellular hemoglobin.
- Hemoglobin is bound by haptoglobin, resulting in lowered serum haptoglobin levels.
- If hemolysis is excessive and haptoglobin–binding capacity is exceeded, hemoglobin is excreted by the kidneys, resulting in hemoglobinuria (dark urine).

Diagnosis
- Features of anemia are:
  - » Fatigue
  - » Pallor
  - » Shortness of breath
  - » Exercise intolerance
  - » Dizziness or lightheadedness
- Features of hemolysis are:
  - » Jaundice or scleral icterus
  - » Dark urine (hemoglobinuria)
  - » Abdominal pain
  - » Hepato- and/or splenomegaly
- The features of an underlying cause (such as infection or malignancy) may be present.

- Chronic hemolysis predisposes an individual to cholelithiasis with pigmented gallstones secondary to elevated bilirubin. This must be considered if features of gallbladder disease are present.

SEVERE CASES OF HEMOLYSIS (HEMOLYTIC CRISIS)
- In cases of hemolytic crisis, hemolysis is rapid and extensive, having a similar effect to a significant hemorrhage.
  - » This is most often seen in chronic hemolytic conditions with acute decompensation (e.g., glucose-6-phosphate dehydrogenase [G6PD] deficiency with oxidative exposure).
- Features of congestive heart failure or hypovolemia may be present.
- Cerebral injury with features of stroke may occur.

APLASTIC CRISIS
- Aplastic crises occur with acute myelosuppression and are often secondary to parvovirus B19 in patients who have chronic hemolysis (such as SCD).
- Aplastic crisis is indicated in patients who present with evidence of bone marrow failure.
  - » These patients may be unable to compensate for their underlying hemolysis.

Investigations
- If hemolysis is suspected, it is important to consider all the investigations that must be done to determine a diagnosis **before** transfusion is provided.
- Consultation with a pediatric hematologist is recommended.
- Initial investigations should include:
  - » Complete blood count (CBC) and differential
    - › These tests will show evidence of normocytic anemia; some macrocytosis is possible due to reticulocytes.
  - » Peripheral blood smear
  - » Reticulocyte count
    - › This should be elevated unless myelosuppression or reticulocyte destruction is present.
  - » Markers of hemolysis (some or all may be present):
    - › Elevated total and direct bilirubin
    - › Elevated lactate dehydrogenase (LDH)
    - › Low levels of haptoglobin (in children > 18 months of age)
- Further diagnostic tests include:
  - » Direct antiglobulin test (DAT), both for IgG and complement (C3)
  - » Hemoglobin electrophoresis
  - » Enzyme assays (i.e., G6PD)
  - » Osmotic fragility test

Figure 8.6.1. HEMOLYTIC ANEMIAS

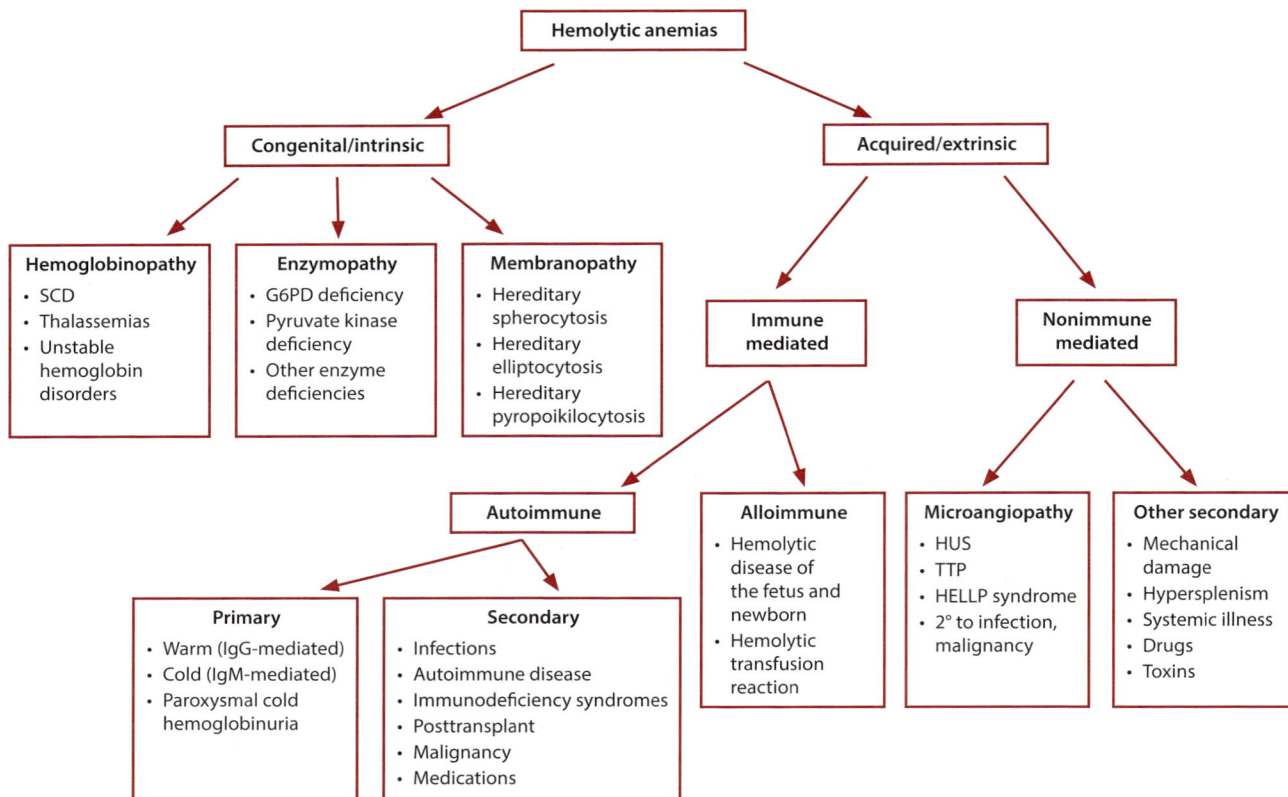

G6PD glucose-6-phosphate dehydrogenase. **HELLP** hemolysis, elevated liver enzymes, and low platelet count. **HUS** hemolytic uremic syndrome. **SCD** sickle cell disease. **TTP** thrombotic thrombocytopenic purpura.

Management

- Provide supportive care (ABCs).
- Treat the underlying cause if hemolysis is secondary to infection or other disease.

Transfusion Guidelines

- Consider transfusion in any patient with hemodynamic compromise, independent of hemoglobin level.
- In hemodynamically stable children and neonates, several randomized control trials have demonstrated that a restrictive hemoglobin transfusion threshold of 70 g/L is safe and effective.
  - » In children who are actively hemolyzing and hemoglobin is expected to continue to fall, a higher threshold may be appropriate.

Special Cases

MANAGEMENT CONSIDERATIONS FOR SICKLE CELL DISEASE

- Two special cases associated with SCD must be considered:
  1. Hyperhemolysis

› Hyperhemolysis is typically treated with transfusion and supportive strategies.
› Immunosuppression may play a role, with IV Ig, steroids, and rituximab all having been used.
› Erythropoietin may also be effective.
2. Splenic sequestration and aplastic crisis
› Both conditions may cause life-threatening anemia.
› Treat with transfusion and supportive strategies.
› Aplastic crisis secondary to parvovirus B19 typically self-resolves in 10 to 14 days.

MANAGEMENT CONSIDERATIONS FOR AUTOIMMUNE HEMOLYTIC ANEMIA

- Despite the likelihood of significant cross-reactivity between donor and recipient on initial testing, it has been shown that hemolytic transfusion reactions are unlikely when cross-reactivity is due solely to the presence of RBC autoantibodies, provided alloantibodies are not also present.
  - » Specialized tests exist to indicate which antibodies are present.
- Indications for transfusion in autoimmune hemolytic anemia are similar to those for non–autoimmune hemolytic anemia conditions.

CHRONIC HEMOLYSIS AND LONG-TERM STRATEGY

- Management of chronic hemolysis includes folic acid supplementation and splenectomy in certain conditions.

INTRINSIC HEMOLYSIS / CONGENITAL HEMOLYTIC DISORDERS

HEMOGLOBINOPATHIES

SICKLE CELL DISEASE (SCD)

- Refer to Chapter 8.2 for further information on SCD.
- SCD is a broad category of diagnoses characterized by inherited variants in hemoglobin that are predisposed to agglutination, resulting in the sickling of RBCs in response to stressors.
  » The most common and most severe form is HbSS disease.
- SCD presents with chronic hemolytic anemia with a variable baseline hemoglobin level that may wax and wane in response to illness and other stressors.
- Clinical manifestations of SCD include:
  » A variety of crises secondary to vasoocclusion (e.g., pain crises, acute chest syndrome)
  » Splenic sequestration events resulting in a sudden drop in hemoglobin
  » Sepsis secondary to splenic dysfunction
  » Stroke
  » Aplastic crisis secondary to myelosuppression
- In all cases, rapid drops in hemoglobin may occur and can worsen symptoms and outcomes.
  » Transfusion is often necessary to restore baseline hemoglobin levels.
- Treatment of SCD is aimed at preventing these events with hydroxyurea and, in some individuals, chronic transfusion (see "Management Considerations for Sickle Cell Disease," above).

THALASSEMIAS AND UNSTABLE HEMOGLOBIN DISORDERS

- Thalassemias and unstable hemoglobin disorders are a spectrum of disorders with mutation in α- or β-globin, resulting in absent or decreased production of the globin chain.
  » This leads to precipitation of remaining hemoglobin particles, causing oxidative damage to RBCs and hemolysis.
- Thalassemias and unstable hemoglobin disorders are characterized by microcytic anemia.
- They manifest as chronic hemolysis.
- They are managed with transfusion.

ENZYME DEFICIENCIES

- There are several enzymopathies that result in impaired production of adenosine triphosphate (ATP).
  » RBCs cannot meet metabolic requirements and are destroyed.
- Most enzymopathies are autosomal recessive and result in mild disease or are asymptomatic (e.g., pyruvate kinase deficiency).
  » An exception is G6PD deficiency.

G6PD DEFICIENCY

- G6PD deficiency is a common X-linked recessive condition that primarily affects males.
  » There is a high prevalence in malaria-endemic areas (as G6PD is protective against severe malarial infection).
- G6PD deficiency severity depends on enzyme activity.
  » < 10% of cases are considered severe.
- Severe G6PD deficiency may manifest as chronic hemolytic anemia or intermittent episodes of hemolysis.
- Milder forms present with hemolytic events triggered by oxidant exposure.
- Common stressors include:
  » Drugs (especially sulfa medications, antimalarials, nitrofurantoin, isoniazid, dapsone, rasburicase)
  » Henna
  » Illnesses
    › Bacterial or viral infections
  » Toxins
  » Naphthalene
  » Other oxidizing agents such as fava beans
- Patients must be diagnosed when well as the enzyme level may be falsely elevated during episodes of acute hemolysis.

CELL MEMBRANE DEFECTS

HEREDITARY SPHEROCYTOSIS

- Hereditary spherocytosis is the most common membranopathy, affecting about 1 in 2000 people in North America.
- Affected RBCs are spherical, less deformable, and sensitive to osmotic changes.
  » Diagnostic workup should include osmotic fragility test or flow cytometry.
- Spherocytes are retained and cleared by the spleen, often leading to splenomegaly.
- Disease severity has a wide range, from mild/asymptomatic to severe with transfusion dependence.
  » Acutely, it may present with worsened hemolysis in the context of illness.

HEREDITARY LYMPHOCYTOSIS

- Hereditary lymphocytosis is the second most common membranopathy.
  - » A rare variant is hereditary pyropoikilocytosis.
- There is a range of disease severity, though most cases are mild and asymptomatic.
  - » In the neonatal period, patients may have severe hyperbilirubinemia and anemia.

EXTRINSIC HEMOLYSIS

ALLOIMMUNE HEMOLYTIC ANEMIA

HEMOLYTIC DISEASE OF THE FETUS AND NEWBORN

- Hemolytic disease results in the destruction of neonatal RBCs after maternal IgG antibodies cross the placenta and attach to antigens present on neonatal RBCs.
- It may occur both before and after birth.
- Maternal antibodies may be directed against incompatible Rhesus factor (Rh D antigen), ABO blood type, or minor blood groups (i.e., Kell, Duffy, etc.).
- The majority of cases are mild to moderate in severity, presenting as hyperbilirubinemia and anemia in the neonatal period.
  - » Transfusion is only occasionally required.
  - » DAT is usually positive.

HEMOLYTIC TRANSFUSION REACTIONS

- Hemolytic transfusion reactions result from the destruction of recipient RBCs due to the presence of donor antibodies in transfused plasma or packed red blood cells (PRBCs).
- Reactions occur rapidly after the initiation of transfusion, presenting with fever, chills, and abdominal pain.

AUTOIMMUNE HEMOLYTIC ANEMIA — PRIMARY

- See "Management Considerations for Autoimmune Hemolytic Anemia," above.

WARM AUTOIMMUNE HEMOLYTIC ANEMIA (IGG-MEDIATED)

- Warm autoimmune hemolytic anemia is an autoimmune-mediated condition caused by IgG antibodies.
  - » DAT (IgG) is positive in most cases.
- First-line treatment:
  - » Corticosteroids
- Second-line treatment:
  - » Rituximab
  - » Splenectomy
- Transfusion may be required if hemolysis is severe.

COLD AUTOIMMUNE HEMOLYTIC ANEMIA (IGM-MEDIATED)

- Cold autoimmune hemolytic anemia is a cold agglutinin disease mediated by IgM antibodies that bind only at temperatures below 37°C and are most reactive at even colder temperatures.
- Hemolysis is mediated by complement.
  - » DAT is positive for C3, not for IgG.
- Treatment is focused on avoiding cold and ensuring warming of any IV solutions.

PAROXYSMAL COLD HEMOGLOBINURIA

- Paroxysmal cold hemoglobinuria is a rare, self-limited form of autoimmune hemolytic anemia caused by Donath-Landsteiner (DL) antibody (cold-reactive IgG) and usually preceded by a viral upper respiratory tract infection (URTI).
- It is diagnosed with a DL test, which is not universally available, and may be negative beyond the first few days of illness.

AUTOIMMUNE HEMOLYTIC ANEMIA — SECONDARY

- Autoimmune hemolytic anemia is triggered by underlying disease or illness about 60% of the time.
- Infections are a common trigger (e.g., Epstein-Barr virus (EBV), cytomegalovirus (CMV), mycoplasma, pneumococcus, etc.).
  - » These are often mediated by cold agglutinins (IgM).
- Other triggers include:
  - » Underlying autoimmune disease
  - » Immunodeficiency syndromes
  - » Posttransplant of stem cells or organs
  - » Malignancy (e.g., leukemia, lymphoma)
  - » Medications

MICROANGIOPATHIC HEMOLYTIC ANEMIA

HEMOLYTIC UREMIC SYNDROME (HUS)

- Refer to Chapter 17.1 for more information on HUS.
- HUS is mediated by Shiga-toxin (produced by *E. coli*), which causes massive release of von Willebrand factor (vWF) multimers that accumulate in small vessels, causing organ damage (e.g., renal dysfunction leading to electrolyte disturbance).
- Hemolysis also occurs due to shear stress on RBCs filtering through affected glomeruli.
- It requires supportive treatment.

THROMBOTIC THROMBOCYTOPENIC PURPURA (TTP)

- Thrombotic thrombocytopenic purpura (TTP) is caused by an excess of large protein precipitate (secondary to cleaving enzyme–deficiency), causing thrombosis.

» The condition can be acquired (due to autoantibodies) or inherited.

OTHER CAUSES OF MICROANGIOPATHIC HEMOLYTIC ANEMIA

- Microangiopathic hemolytic anemia may also be secondary to infection or malignancy.
- It has been associated with pregnancy (i.e., HELLP syndrome) and disseminated intravascular coagulation (DIC).

OTHER NONIMMUNE CAUSES OF HEMOLYSIS

- Rarely, mechanical damage may cause hemolysis of RBCs. This can be seen in the setting of mechanical heart valves or Kasabach-Merritt syndrome.
- An enlarged spleen may also cause anemia, both through sequestration of RBCs and increased destruction of RBCs because of increased baseline activation.
- Systemic disease (e.g., liver or renal dysfunction) can independently contribute to RBC destruction, as can systemic infection.
- Certain drugs and toxins may induce hemolysis, usually through oxidative mechanisms.
  » Common drugs: rifampin, nitrites, antiviral/antimalarials, ceftriaxone
  » Toxins: lead, copper, snake/insect bites

REFERENCES

Bain BJ. Diagnosis from the blood smear. *N Engl J Med.* 2005;353(5):498–507. https://doi.org/10.1056/NEJMra043442. Medline:16079373

Beris P, Picard V. Non-immune hemolysis: diagnostic considerations. *Semin Hematol.* 2015;52(4):287–303. https://doi.org/10.1053/j.seminhematol.2015.07.005. Medline:26404441

Gehrs BC, Friedberg RC. Autoimmune hemolytic anemia. *Am J Hematol.* 2002;69(4):258–271. https://doi.org/10.1002/ajh.10062. Medline:11921020

Haley K. Congenital hemolytic anemia. *Med Clin North Am.* 2017;101(2):361–374. https://doi.org/10.1016/j.mcna.2016.09.008. Medline:28189176

Ibrahim M, Ho SK, Yeo CL. Restrictive versus liberal red blood cell transfusion thresholds in very low birth weight infants: a systematic review and meta-analysis. *J Paediatr Child Health.* 2014;50(2):122–130. https://doi.org/10.1111/jpc.12409. Medline:24118127

Lacroix J, Hébert PC, Hutchison JS, et al; TRIPICU Investigators; Canadian Critical Care Trials Group; Pediatric Acute Lung Injury and Sepsis Investigators Network. Transfusion strategies for patients in pediatric intensive care units. *N Engl J Med.* 2007;356(16):1609–1619. https://doi.org/10.1056/NEJMoa066240. Medline:17442904

Nahar A, Ravindranath Y. Approach to severe anemia in children in the emergency room. *Therapy.* 2008;5(4):475–484. https://doi.org/10.2217/14750708.5.4.475

New HV, Berryman J, Bolton-Maggs PHB, et al; British Committee for Standards in Haematology. Guidelines on transfusion for fetuses, neonates and older children. *Br J Haematol.* 2016;175(5):784–828. https://doi.org/10.1111/bjh.14233. Medline:27861734

Noronha SA. Acquired and congenital hemolytic anemia. *Pediatr Rev.* 2016;37(6):235–246. https://doi.org/10.1542/pir.2015-0053. Medline:27252179

Novelli EM, Gladwin MT. Crises in sickle cell disease. *Chest.* 2016;149(4):1082–1093. https://doi.org/10.1016/j.chest.2015.12.016. Medline:26836899

Petz LD. Emergency transfusion guidelines for autoimmune hemolytic anemia. *Lab Med.* 2005;36(1):45–48. https://doi.org/10.1309/NE3BH8U3K6N1149V

8.7

Immune Thrombocytopenia Purpura

Krista Helleman

- Immune thrombocytopenia purpura (ITP) was previously known as idiopathic thrombocytopenic purpura.
- It is an acute and generally self-limiting thrombocytopenia in children.
- ITP is one of the most common forms of autoimmune disease in children and one of the more common acquired bleeding disorders in childhood.
- It is seen in children from 1 to 9 years of age, with a peak incidence between 2 and 5 years of age.
  » It occurs with the same frequency in both males and females.

Pathophysiology

- ITP is generally seasonal in nature, which suggests that an infectious or environmental agent is responsible for this condition.
- The unknown agent may trigger an immune response, which results in the production of platelet-reactive autoantibodies 4 to 8 weeks following the infection.

Physical Exam

- The patient often presents with diffuse, nonpalpable bruising and petechiae.

- Epistaxis is another common presentation.
  - » Occasionally, patients may present with other mucous membrane bleeds such as menorrhagia, gastrointestinal bleeding, or oral blood blisters.
- Symptoms are rapid in onset.
- Patients are usually systemically well at the time of presentation (no fever, respiratory, or gastrointestinal symptoms).
  - » The patient does, however, usually have a history of a previous illness, allergies, immunizations, or a viral illness in a family member.
- There is no other explanation for the bruising, bleeding, or petechiae, such as systemic lupus erythematosus or HIV infection.
- The patient does not have jaundice, pallor, or hepatosplenomegaly.
- The typical course in an untreated child is a resolution of bleeding symptoms 3 to 10 days after diagnosis, regardless of platelet count, and an increase in platelet count in 1 to 3 weeks.

Complications

- Most children have minimal bleeding, but severe complications can arise such as:
  - » Intracranial hemorrhage (incidence of 0.1% to 0.5%)
  - » Epistaxis requiring surgical intervention
  - » Gross hematuria
  - » Other life-threatening hemorrhage

Investigations

- Complete blood count (CBC) and peripheral blood smear findings include:
  - » Presence of an isolated thrombocytopenia (platelets $< 100 \times 10^9/L$)
  - » Large platelets — seen on the smear
  - » Normal morphology of all other cell lines
  - » Mild anemia — may be present if severe bleeding has occurred
- While only the CBC and peripheral smear are needed for diagnosis, a few other tests may be ordered for confirmation; findings in a patient with ITP are the following:
  - » Bleeding time — prolonged
  - » International normalized ratio (INR) — normal
  - » Partial thromboplastin time (PTT) — normal
- Bone marrow aspiration is **not** necessary when clinical and laboratory features are classic; likewise, bone marrow examination is not recommended for children who fail therapy with intravenous immunoglobulin (IVIG).

Diagnosis

- ITP is a diagnosis of exclusion.
- The patient's history should be consistent with the above-noted clinical presentation of a sudden onset of bruising, petechiae, or bleeding in a previously healthy child, with no other explanation for the symptoms.
- Physical examination reveals only nonpalpable bruises and petechiae, with no evidence of hepatosplenomegaly, lymphadenopathy, or the stigmata of congenital conditions.
- Laboratory study results should be consistent with those listed above.

Differential Diagnosis

- The following should be considered in the differential diagnosis:
  - » Congenital thrombocytopenia
  - » HIV infection
  - » Systemic lupus erythematosus
  - » Evans syndrome (an autoimmune destruction of blood cells)
  - » Leukemia or lymphoma

Management

- The goal of all treatment strategies is to achieve a platelet count that is associated with adequate hemostasis; a normal platelet count is **not** the goal.
- Treatment should involve:
  - » Watchful waiting
    - › Patients with no bleeding or mild bleeding, and with skin manifestations only, such as petechiae and bruising, are eligible for watchful waiting.
    - › The majority of patients should be treated with observation alone, regardless of the platelet count because:
      - · There is little risk of life-threatening hemorrhage in children with ITP
      - · Therapy has not been definitively proven to prevent severe hemorrhage
      - · ITP is usually self-resolving
  - » Corticosteroids
    - › A short course of corticosteroids may be given, if necessary, for management.
    - › Steroids lead to a more rapid rise in platelet count than observation alone.
    - › Long courses of steroids are not recommended due to their side effects.
  - » IVIG 0.8 to 1.0 g/kg
    - › IVIG causes a more rapid and sustained rise in platelet count than steroids.
    - › Use IVIG when a rapid rise in platelets is desired.
    - › IVIG treatment is expensive.
  - » Anti-D immunoglobulin
    - › Anti-D immunoglobulin may produce severe hemolysis.
    - › It should not be used in patients with bleeding causing a decline in hemoglobin, or in those with evidence of autoimmune hemolysis.
    - › Anti-D immunoglobulin may be considered

for first-line therapy in Rh+, unsplenectomized children.

Treatment of Life-threatening Hemorrhage in Children with ITP

- Apply measures such as direct pressure for local control of bleeding.
- IVIG and/or intravenous methylprednisolone should be given to increase the platelet count.
- Platelet transfusion can be considered with severe bleeds, though this is a temporizing measure.
- An emergency splenectomy may be necessary if the above methods fail to achieve hemostasis.

Disposition

- The majority of ITP patients can be managed on an outpatient basis.
- Hospitalization is necessary only for life-threatening bleeding.

Prognosis

- The thrombocytopenia resolves spontaneously in ≤ 6 months in 85% of cases.
- 15% of children will develop chronic ITP, with platelet counts remaining below normal levels beyond 6 months from the onset of the disorder.

REFERENCES

Medeiros D, Buchanan GR. Idiopathic thrombocytopenic purpura: beyond consensus. *Curr Opin Pediatr.* 2000;12(1):4–9. https://doi.org/10.1097/00008480-200002000-00002. Medline:10676767

Neunert C, Lim W, Crowther M, Cohen A, Solberg L Jr, Crowther MA; American Society of Hematology. The American Society of Hematology 2011 evidence-based practice guideline for immune thrombocytopenia. *Blood.* 2011;117(16):4190–4207. https://doi.org/10.1182/blood-2010-08-302984. Medline:21325604

Nugent DJ. Childhood immune thrombocytopenic purpura. *Blood Rev.* 2002;16(1):27–29. https://doi.org/10.1054/blre.2001.0177. Medline:11913990

Tarantino MD. Acute immune (idiopathic) thrombocytopenic purpura in childhood. *Blood Rev.* 2002;16(1):19–21. https://doi.org/10.1054/blre.2001.0175. Medline:11913988

HEMATOLOGY/ONCOLOGY EMERGENCIES

Rheumatological Emergencies

9.1

Kawasaki Disease

Krista Helleman

- Kawasaki disease is a systemic vasculitis that mainly affects medium-sized arteries, particularly the coronary arteries.
- It is the second most common cause of vasculitis in children, after Henoch-Schönlein purpura.
- Kawasaki disease is the leading cause of acquired heart disease for children in most developed countries.
- It predominantly affects children < 5 years of age, with a peak in incidence between 18 and 24 months.

Risk Factors
- Risk factors for Kawasaki disease are:
  » Male gender
  » Asian descent, especially East Asian

Pathophysiology
- Kawasaki disease is a systemic vasculitis of unknown etiology.
- The disease may be triggered by an infectious agent in genetically susceptible individuals.
- Three distinct vascular processes are involved:
  » Necrotizing arteritis
  » Subacute or chronic vasculitis
  » Luminal myofibroblastic proliferation

Diagnosis
- Kawasaki disease is a clinical diagnosis. The diagnostic criteria are as follows:
  » Fever for ≥ 5 days
  — and —
  » 4 of the 5 findings listed below:
    › Conjunctivitis — nonpurulent, bulbar, bilateral
    › Lymphadenopathy — usually cervical, > 1.5 cm
    › Rash — polymorphous, no vesicles or crusting
    › Changes in lips or oral mucosa — red, dry, cracked lips; "strawberry" tongue or diffuse erythema of the oropharynx; nonpurulent pharyngitis

› Changes in extremities
  · Initial stage: erythema and edema of palms and soles
  · Convalescent stage: peeling of skin from the fingertips and toes

Note: Kawasaki disease may be diagnosed with < 4 of these features if coronary artery abnormalities are detected (see "Incomplete Kawasaki Disease" and "Atypical Kawasaki," below).

- Infants < 6 months of age may present with a prolonged fever and few other clinical criteria. As a result, the diagnosis should be considered for any infant with a fever lasting ≥ 7 days for which no other etiology has been found.
  » Laboratory tests and an echocardiogram can help to confirm the diagnosis in this age group.
- Other common clinical findings include:
  » Irritability (almost always present)
  » Erythema and induration at the site of previous bacillus Calmette-Guérin (BCG) immunization
  » Congestive heart failure
  » Myocarditis
  » Pericarditis
  » Valvular regurgitation
  » Arthritis
  » Aseptic meningitis
  » Pneumonitis
  » Uveitis
  » Gastroenteritis
  » Hepatic enlargement and jaundice
  » Meatitis and dysuria
  » Otitis media
  » Transient unilateral peripheral facial nerve palsy
  » Gallbladder hydrops

Differential Diagnosis

- Infections often resemble Kawasaki disease; the most common of these are:
  » Scarlet Fever (Group A streptococcal [GAS] infection)
  » Adenovirus
  » Measles
  » Dengue Fever
  » Epstein-Barr Virus
  » Toxic Shock Syndrome
- Other conditions that can mimic Kawasaki disease include:
  » Drug hypersensitivity reactions
  » Stevens-Johnson syndrome
  » Juvenile rheumatoid arthritis
  » Mercury hypersensitivity reactions
  » Hemophagocytic lymphohistiocytosis

INCOMPLETE KAWASAKI DISEASE

- Incomplete Kawasaki disease occurs when a fever has been present for ≥ 5 days but only 2 or 3 of the other diagnostic criteria are present.
- A diagnosis of incomplete Kawasaki disease can be made if the following criteria are met, along with the above clinical criteria:
  » C-reactive protein (CRP) ≥ 30 mg/L and/or erythrocyte sedimentation rate (ESR) ≥ 40 mm/hr
  » ≥ 3 supplemental laboratory criteria (see "Investigations," below)
  » Positive findings on echocardiogram (only required if < 3 supplemental laboratory criteria are present)

ATYPICAL KAWASAKI

- Atypical Kawasaki may be diagnosed in patients who present with findings not usually seen with Kawasaki disease, which include:
  » Unilateral facial palsies
  » High-frequency sensorineural hearing loss
  » Hepatomegaly with jaundice
  » Acalculous gallbladder distention
  » Testicular swelling
  » Pulmonary nodules
  » Pleural effusion

Investigations

- While not diagnostic, these laboratory values indicating inflammation can support the diagnosis:
  » Elevated ESR — ≥ 40 mm/hr
  » Elevated CRP — ≥ 30 mg/L
  » Elevated white blood cell (WBC) count — ≥ 15×10^9/L
  » Thrombocytosis — ≥ 450×10^9/L
    › Thrombocytosis may not be present initially but is often present after 7 days of illness.

- Other possible laboratory abnormalities include:
  » Thrombocytopenia early in the illness
  » Anemia
  » Hyperbilirubinemia
  » Elevated transaminases, especially an elevated alanine transferase (ALT)
  » Hypoalbuminemia (≤ 30 g/L)
  » Sterile pyuria (≥ 10 WBCs / high-power field)

Management

- Consider an urgent electrocardiogram (ECG) to evaluate possible coronary artery involvement.

Acetylsalicylic Acid

- Acute phase of illness
  » Give 80 to 90 mg/kg ASA per day, in 4 divided doses, along with IVIG.
  » Continue this dose until the child has been afebrile for 48 to 72 hours.
- Convalescent phase of illness
  » Give 3 to 5 mg/kg ASA per day.
  » Continue until the patient shows no evidence of coronary changes (by 6 to 8 weeks after the onset of illness) or indefinitely (if coronary abnormalities persist).

Intravenous Immunoglobulin (IVIG)

- A single infusion of 2 g/kg is given over 12 to 24 hours, along with ASA.
- If possible, therapy should be initiated within the first 10 days of illness, and preferably within the first 7 days of the start of symptoms.
- Treatment of Kawasaki disease before day 5 of illness has not been shown to prevent the cardiac complications of this disease and may be associated with the need for further IVIG therapy.
- IVIG reduces the incidence of coronary artery abnormalities from 18% to 4%.
- The failure rate of this therapy is approximately 13% (defined as fever present after 36 hours posttreatment).
  » When patients fail to respond, retreatment with IVIG at 2 g/kg is recommended.

Steroids

- The benefit of steroid therapy is uncertain in acute Kawasaki disease, and steroid use is currently not recommended as a first-line therapy.
- Consider using steroids in IVIG-resistant patients.
  » Steroids may be used when ≥ 2 infusions of IVIG have been ineffective.
    › Methylprednisolone 30 mg/kg IV is administered over 2 to 3 hours, once daily, for 1 to 3 days.

Other Treatments

- Other treatments that may be used when IVIG therapy fails (i.e., when ≥ 2 infusions of IVIG have been ineffective) are:
  » Plasma exchange
  » Infliximab
  » Cyclosporin A

Complications

- It is important to recognize that the most important complications relate to the coronary vessels.
  » In the short term, Kawasaki disease can cause coronary artery aneurysms (either fusiform or saccular).
  » Other coronary complications include coronary artery fistula formation and coronary artery dilation.
- Coronary artery aneurysms occur in 15% to 25% of untreated cases.
- The aneurysms can lead to myocardial infarction, ischemic heart disease, or sudden death.
- In the long term, coronary artery stenosis or obstruction may occur.

Prognosis

- The long-term prognosis is good for children who have no coronary artery involvement or only minimal dilatation 6 weeks after the onset of symptoms.
- Patients with persistent coronary dilatation and aneurysms are at risk of coronary artery thrombosis or stenosis.

- 50% to 70% of coronary artery aneurysms resolve in 1 to 2 years after the onset of the illness.
- Giant aneurysms never resolve completely.
- Children with persistent aneurysms require long-term ASA therapy unless the aneurysms resolve.

REFERENCES

Eleftheriou D, Levin M, Shingadia D, Tulloh R, Klein NJ, Brogan PA. Management of Kawasaki disease. *Arch Dis Child.* 2014;99(1):74–83. https://doi.org/10.1136/archdischild-2012-302841. Medline:24162006

Ho CL, Fu YC, Lin MC, Jan SL. Early immunoglobulin therapy and outcomes in Kawasaki disease: a nationwide cohort study. *Medicine (Baltimore).* 2015;94(39):e1544. https://doi.org/10.1097/MD.0000000000001544. Medline:26426619

Kawasaki T. Kawasaki disease. *Int J Rheum Dis.* 2014;17(5):597–600. https://doi.org/10.1111/1756-185X.12408. Medline:25042617

Newburger JW, Takahashi M, Gerber MA, et al. Diagnosis, treatment, and long-term management of Kawasaki disease: a statement for health professionals from the Committee on Rheumatic Fever, Endocarditis, and Kawasaki Disease, Council on Cardiovascular Disease in the Young, American Heart Association. *Pediatrics.* 2004;114(6):1708–1733. https://doi.org/10.1542/peds.2004-2182. Medline:15574639

Singh S, Newburger JW, Kuijpers T, Burgner D. Management of Kawasaki disease in resource-limited settings. *Pediatr Infect Dis J.* 2015;34(1):94–96. https://doi.org/10.1097/INF.0000000000000600. Medline:25741801

Yim D, Curtis N, Cheung M, Burgner D. An update on Kawasaki disease II: clinical features, diagnosis, treatment and outcomes. *J Paediatr Child Health.* 2013;49(8):614–623. https://doi.org/10.1111/jpc.12221. Medline:23647873

Zhu FH, Ang JY. The clinical diagnosis and management of Kawasaki disease: a review and update. *Curr Infect Dis Rep.* 2016;18(10):32. https://doi.org/10.1007/s11908-016-0538-5. Medline:27681743

9.2

Henoch-Schönlein Purpura

Melissa Chan

- Henoch-Schönlein purpura (HSP) is the most common systemic vasculitis in the pediatric population.
- It is an immunoglobulin A (IgA)–mediated small vessel vasculitis that typically affects the skin, joints, and renal and gastrointestinal (GI) systems.
- The onset is typically preceded by a viral illness.
- HSP shows seasonal variation.
  » It is more common in winter, spring, and fall.
- Occurrence peaks around 3 to 8 years of age.
  » HSP is more common in males than in females.
  » HSP is rarely seen in individuals of African ancestry.

Pathophysiology

- HSP is caused by IgA deposition into different organ systems, including the skin, kidneys, intestines, and joints.
- It triggers a complex inflammatory process that includes:
  » Complement pathway
  » Clotting cascade
  » Prostaglandins, cytokines, and chemotactic factors

Diagnosis

- Palpable purpura occurs with 1 or more of:
  - » Arthritis or arthralgia
  - » Renal involvement (proteinuria, hematuria, increased creatinine)
  - » Abdominal pain
  - » Positive histopathology showing deposition of IgA

Physical Exam

- On physical exam, look for:
  - » Dermatologic symptoms
    - › Palpable purpura is most typically found on lower limbs and buttocks or other dependent areas of affected children.
  - » Musculoskeletal symptoms — joint pain
    - › Arthritis is the most common manifestation, seen in 65% to 80% of cases.
    - › It typically affects knees and ankles.
  - » GI symptoms
    - › GI symptoms originate from IgA deposition in the bowel wall and resulting submucosal and subserosal edema and hemorrhage.
    - › Look for intussusception from a pathogenic lead point, which is ileoileal in 70% of cases.
    - › 50% to 75% of patients present with abdominal pain.
  - » Renal symptoms
    - › Patients may exhibit hypertension or edema (e.g., scrotum, periorbital edema).

Investigations

- Suggested laboratory studies are:
  - » Complete blood count (CBC)
  - » Serum IgA
  - » Coagulation studies
    - › Prothrombin time (PT) and partial thromboplastin time (PTT)
    - › International normalized ratio (INR)
  - » Electrolytes and renal function
    - › Urea and creatinine
  - » Urinalysis
  - » 24-hour urine for protein
- In a patient with HSP, the physician should expect these findings:
  - » Normal INR/PTT and platelet count
  - » Urea/creatinine may be normal or elevated
  - » CBC may show increased white blood cells (WBCs) and/or mild normocytic anemia
  - » Urine analysis may show hematuria, casts, or proteinuria
  - » 24-hour urine protein collection may be high

Management

- Treatment is mainly supportive as HSP tends to self-resolve after 6 to 8 weeks.
  - » If no renal or GI symptoms or complications are present, use nonsteroidal anti-inflammatory drugs (NSAIDs) for joint pain and painful purpura.
  - » Close outpatient monitoring of renal function (with urine dipsticks) and blood pressure is required as many renal complications do not occur until later in life.
- GI complications occur in approximately 50% to 75% of cases.
  - » If the patient has abdominal pain alone, some evidence suggests that a short course of steroids may decrease pain.
  - » If there are concerns of intussusception, refer the patient to radiology or a surgical consult.
    - › The most commonly found intussusceptions are ileoileal; thus, ultrasound is the first-line investigation rather than a contrast enema.
  - » Patients with GI bleeding should be stabilized, and general surgery consulted.
- Renal complications occur in about one-third of cases, usually within the first 4 weeks.
  - » Early short-term steroid use has not been shown to prevent or alter the course of mild renal disease.
  - » If there are concerns regarding renal complications (e.g., signs of nephritis), then a pediatric nephrologist should be consulted for further management.
- HSP recurs in one-third of cases.
  - » Recurrence usually happens in the first 4 months after the original presentation.

REFERENCES

Barut K, Sahin S, Kasapcopur O. Pediatric vasculitis. *Curr Opin Rheumatol.* 2016;28(1):29–38. https://doi.org/10.1097/BOR.0000000000000236. Medline:26555448

Bluman J, Goldman RD. Henoch-Schönlein purpura in children: limited benefit of corticosteroids. *Can Fam Physician.* 2014;60(11):1007–1010. Medline:25551129

Hahn D, Hodson EM, Willis NS, Craig JC. Interventions for preventing and treating kidney disease in Henoch-Schönlein Purpura (HSP). *Cochrane Database Syst Rev.* 2015;8(8):CD005128. Medline:26258874

Hernstadt HM, Bartlett M, Kausman JY, Macgregor D, Akikusa JD. Complicated Henoch-Schönlein purpura. *J Paediatr Child Health.* 2015;51(6):639–642. https://doi.org/10.1111/jpc.12786. Medline:25510813

Ozen S, Pistorio A, Lusan SM, et al. EULAR/PRINTO/PRES criteria for Henoch-Schönlein purpura, childhood polyarteritis nodosa, childhood Wegener granulomatosis and childhood Takayasu arteritis: Ankara 2008. Part II: Final classification criteria. *Ann Rheum Dis.* 2010;69(9):798–806.

Infectious Disease Emergencies

10.1

Fever in the Returning Traveler

Sowmith Rangu, Kevin Chan

- Every year, millions of children travel internationally with their families, many to developing countries, to visit friends and relatives.
- Approximately 22% to 64% of travelers report illness after visiting a developing country.
  - » 8% of all travelers will seek healthcare upon their return, and of those, 28% will have associated fever.
- The 2011 report from the 54 GeoSentinel sites highlighted that there are 5 major categories in which travelers present:

  1. Systemic febrile illness without localizing findings
  2. Acute diarrhea
  3. Dermatologic disorders
  4. Chronic diarrhea
  5. Nondiarrheal gastrointestinal disorders

- The study also noted that the 2 most common specific diagnoses were malaria (21%) and dengue fever (6%).
- Excellent resources for travel information include the Centers for Disease Control and Prevention's *Yellow Book* and the World Health Organization's *International Travel and Health*.

History

- When assessing a patient who has returned from international travel, obtain:
  - » A detailed travel history, including:
    - › Geographic region of travel
    - › Season of visit
    - › Duration of stay
    - › Activities and exposures (e.g., swimming, camping)
    - › Preparation for travel and any prophylactic medications or vaccinations taken
    - › Travel routes
    - › Areas where meals were eaten (e.g., hotels, campsites, rural areas)
  - » A history of travel to high-risk locations (e.g., areas where Ebola is present)
    - › If patient has recently traveled to such regions, containment measures should be put in place.
  - » The exact pattern of fever
    - › To determine incubation periods, see *Table 10.1.1* below.
    - › Identify any pattern to the fever (e.g., cyclical, prolonged [> 5 days]).

Note:

- The longer the symptoms persist, the less likely they are to be associated with travel, although some conditions such as vivax malaria may present months after the patient's return.
- Almost all life-threatening conditions after travel present with fever.
  - » Although malaria is the most important of these to rapidly exclude, other potential serious tropical infections that cause fever include dengue, typhoid, rickettsioses, and leptospirosis
  - » Rarely, serious infections other than these are encountered.
- The incubation period gives critical clues to the etiology of fever in travelers.

Physical Exam

- Remember to isolate the patient appropriately and protect yourself with the appropriate equipment.
- Conduct a complete physical examination, looking specifically for:
  - » Altered mental status
    - › Altered mental status indicates possible central nervous system (CNS) involvement.
  - » Presence of rash and type of rash
    - › Maculopapular rash indicates dengue fever.
    - › Petechiae or purpura indicates hemorrhagic fevers.

Table 10.1.1. MOST COMMON INFECTIOUS DIAGNOSES RELATED TO RETURNING TRAVELER

Infection	Incubation period	Diagnostic test	Management
Malaria	• Usually < 14 days, but may be 30 days for vivax and ovale	• Thick and thin smear	• (See Chapter 10.2)
Diarrheal illness (more commonly bacterial cause)		• Stool culture for culture and sensitivity • Ova and parasites	• Antibiotics, depending on cause
Respiratory tract infections		• CXR • Nasopharyngeal swab • Sputum culture	• Depends on cause
Dengue fever		• Acute and convalescent serology	• Supportive treatment
Typhoid fever	• Average 14 days	• Blood and stool culture	• Supportive treatment • Amoxicillin or trimethoprim/sulfamethoxazole can be used for susceptible strains
Rickettsioses	• < 14 days	• Clinical diagnosis (if eschar present) • Acute and convalescent serology	• Doxycycline

CXR chest X-ray.

› Jaundice indicates malaria.
» Conjunctival or retinal changes
» Hepatomegaly or splenomegaly
  › These indicate malaria or typhoid.
» Lymphadenopathy
» Genital lesions
• Concerning findings include:
  » Signs of hemorrhage
  » Respiratory distress
  » Persistent cough
  » Persistent diarrhea
  » Persistent vomiting
  » Jaundice
  » Evidence of shock
  » Neurological findings — confusion, lethargy, meningismus or a bulging fontanelle, paralysis, or focal neurological signs

Investigations

• The combination of history, location of exposure, and estimation of incubation periods help narrow the differential diagnosis.
• If warranted, and if there is concern about an infectious disease, consider:
  » Complete blood count (CBC)
  » Liver function tests
  » Electrolytes and creatinine
  » Urinalysis and urine culture
  » Blood culture
  » Peripheral blood smears and rapid diagnostic tests for malaria
• Additional testing may include:
  » Stool culture
  » Ova and parasites
  » Chest X-ray (CXR)

» Specific serologic assays, such as those for dengue fever

COMMON CAUSES OF FEVER IN THE RETURNING TRAVELER

• Consider common childhood diseases first, such as an upper respiratory tract infection (URTI), otitis media, pneumonia, gastroenteritis, and urinary tract infections.

MALARIA

• See Chapter 10.2 for further information on malaria.

DENGUE

• Dengue is the most common diagnosis in febrile travelers who have returned from any tropical region except Africa.

Diagnosis

• A "breakbone" fever that develops within 7 days of entering an endemic area is unlikely to be caused by malaria, whereas a fever that develops more than 2 weeks after leaving an endemic area should not be caused by dengue.
• The dengue virus has a short incubation period.
• Common laboratory findings include leukopenia and thrombocytopenia.

Physical Exam

• Dengue is generally a self-limited illness.
• The patient should have 2 of the following:
  » Nausea and vomiting
  » Rash
  » Aches and pains

» Warning signs:
  › Severe abdominal pain
  › Persistent vomiting
  › Mucosal bleeding
  › Liver enlargement
  › Clinical fluid accumulation
  › Lethargy or restlessness
  › Increase in hematocrit with a decrease in platelet count
• Although severe dengue (hemorrhagic and shock syndrome) may occur in some travelers, particularly those who have had the disease before, it is rare in first-time travelers.

Management
• Nonsevere dengue is self-limited and requires supportive care.
• Severe dengue requires hospitalization and intensive management focused on early recognition and treatment of shock.

MEASLES
• Measles is common in areas with poor vaccination rates (e.g., Africa, South Asia).
• Diagnosis is clinical.
• Signs and symptoms of measles are:
  » Head-to-toe maculopapular rash
  » Fever
  » Cough
  » Coryza
  » Conjunctivitis
  » Possible Koplik spots — white papular rash inside the buccal mucosa

Management
• Give vitamin A.
• Administer supportive treatment, depending on other symptoms.

OTHER CAUSES OF FEVER

TYPHOID AND PARATYPHOID FEVER
• Fever and fatigue are the hallmarks of typhoid and paratyphoid fever.
  » The fever usually has a "stepladder" pattern, with febrile temperature progressively increasing over the day (lowest in the morning and highest in the early evening).
• Typhoid fever ("rickettsia"):
  » Occurs in areas with poor hygiene
  » Is sometimes known as "jail fever"
  » Is a severe but nonspecific febrile illness with abdominal pain

» Presents with a cough, arthritis, nausea and vomiting, and headache
» Causes a dull, red, spreading rash in about 50% of patients
• Other signs, include:
  » Relative bradycardia — normal heart rate despite fever
  » Headache
  » Malaise
  » Anorexia
  » Abdominal pain
  » Vomiting and diarrhea
  » Maculopapular rash ("rose spots")

TRAVELER'S DIARRHEA
• Traveler's diarrhea is a common complaint.
• It is most commonly caused by viral infections, but bacterial and/or parasitic causes are also common.
• The key component to remember is to rehydrate the patient promptly with supportive electrolytes, if needed.
  » Consider antibiotics if bloody diarrhea is present.

MENINGOCOCCUS
• About 50% of patients with meningococcus present with meningitis.
• Meningococcemia with fever and petechiae or a purpuric rash occurs in 20% of patients and progresses to shock, adrenal hemorrhage, and multiorgan failure.

CHIKUNGUNYA
• Many cases of chikungunya are asymptomatic, but the disease causes a febrile arthralgia syndrome.
• Severe disease is rare, particularly in children.
• It is usually self-limited, but substantial joint pain may persist.

YELLOW FEVER
• About 15% of infected patients have fever, jaundice, renal failure, shock, and disseminated intravascular coagulation (DIC).

DIPHTHERIA
• Patients present with mild fever 2 to 5 days after contact with the bacteria.
• Patients can develop a sore throat, drooling, and painful swallowing.
• Rarely, patients develop pseudomembranes about 2 to 3 days after the onset of the illness.
  » Pseudomembranes affect the tonsils, pharynx, and larynx, but can sometimes invade the trachea, leading to upper airway obstruction.

PLAGUE

- Patients present after 2 to 7 days with chills, fever, malaise, headache, muscle pain, and seizures.
- There are 3 major types of plague:
  1. Bubonic
     › Bubonic plague is characterized by small, painful lymph nodes.
  2. Pneumonic
  3. Septicemic

LEPTOSPIROSIS

- Patients present 2 days to 3 weeks postexposure.
- Patients in the early phase (< 7 days) present with fever, headache, epistaxis, diarrhea, abdominal pain, and myalgia.
- A characteristic symptom is retro-orbital pain with conjunctival inflammation and photophobia.
- The disease may progress to jaundice, renal failure, hemorrhage, and even death.

VIRAL HEMORRHAGIC FEVERS

- Viral hemorrhagic fevers include Ebola, Lassa, dengue, and yellow fevers.
- All present with bleeding.
- Symptoms may include flushing of the face and chest, petechiae, shock, malaise, myalgia, headache, vomiting, and diarrhea.

TRYPANOSOMIASIS

- Trypanosomiasis is also known as "sleeping sickness."
- It is endemic in sub-Saharan Africa.
- Trypanosomiasis presents with fever, headache, malaise, myalgia, facial edema, pruritus, lymphadenopathy, and weight loss.
- There is also CNS involvement, including headache, mood disorders, behavioral change, and focal deficits with somnolence.

ARBOVIRAL DISEASES

- Arboviral diseases have high fatality rates.
- They are rare in travelers because of availability of effective vaccines.
- Most patients present with subclinical infection.

SYSTEMATIC LEISHMANIASIS

- Systematic leishmaniasis can take weeks to months to present.
- Patients present with fever, weight loss, hepatosplenomegaly, and pancytopenia.

FILARIASIS ("ELEPHANTIASIS")

- There are 2 types of filariasis:
  1. Acute adenolymphangitis — lymphadenopathy with associated fever and a significantly swollen limb
  2. Filiarial fever — fever without lymphadenitis

CHAGAS DISEASE

- Chagas disease presents a week after exposure and lasts for 60 days.
- Most patients are asymptomatic.
- The disease may develop years after exposure.
- Patients may present with fever, swelling, and malaise.
- Patients may also have heart arrhythmia, heart failure, constipation and abdominal pain, hepatosplenomegaly, lymphadenopathy, and swallowing difficulties.

SCHISTOSOMIASIS ("KATAYAMA FEVER")

- Patients may present with fever, chills, lymphadenopathy, and/or hepatosplenomegaly.
- They may also have bloody diarrhea, abdominal pain, dysuria, and hematuria.

REFERENCES

Cavagnaro CS, Brady K, Siegel C. Fever after international travel. *Clin Pediatr Emerg Med.* 2008;9(4):250–257. https://doi.org/10.1016/j.cpem.2008.09.002.

Centers for Disease Control and Prevention. CDC Yellow Book 2018 [Internet]. New York: Oxford University Press; 2017 May [updated 2017 July 31]. Available from: https://wwwnc.cdc.gov/travel/page/yellowbook-home

Hagmann S, Neugebauer R, Schwartz E, et al; GeoSentinel Surveillance Network. Illness in children after international travel: analysis from the GeoSentinel Surveillance Network. *Pediatrics.* 2010;125(5):e1072–e1080. https://doi.org/10.1542/peds.2009-1951. Medline:20368323

Halbert J, Shingadia D, Zuckerman JN. Fever in the returning child traveller: approach to diagnosis and management. *Arch Dis Child.* 2014;99(10):938–943. https://doi.org/10.1136/archdischild-2012-303196. Medline:24667950

Harvey K, Esposito DH, Han P, et al. Surveillance for travel-related disease—GeoSentinel Surveillance System, United States, 1997–2011. *Morbidity and Mortality Weekly Report: Surveillance Summaries.* 2013;62(3):1–15.

Hill DR. Health problems in a large cohort of Americans traveling to developing countries. *J Travel Med.* 2000;7(5):259–266. https://doi.org/10.2310/7060.2000.00075. Medline:11231210

Nield LS, Stauffer W, Kamat D. Evaluation and management of illness in a child after international travel. *Pediatr Emerg Care.* 2005;21(3):184–195, quiz 196–198. Medline:15744199

Steffen R, deBernardis C, Baños A. Travel epidemiology: a global perspective. *Int J Antimicrob Agents.* 2003;21(2):89–95. https://doi.org/10.1016/S0924-8579(02)00293-5. Medline:12615369

Summer A, Stauffer WM. Evaluation of the sick child following travel to the tropics. *Pediatr Ann.* 2008;37(12):821–826. https://doi.org/10.3928/00904481-20081201-12. Medline:19143333

Tolle MA. Evaluating a sick child after travel to developing countries. *J Am Board Fam Med.* 2010;23(6):704–713. https://doi.org/10.3122/jabfm.2010.06.090271. Medline:21057065

West NS, Riordan FA. Fever in returned travellers: a prospective review of hospital admissions for a 2(1/2) year period. *Arch Dis Child.* 2003;88(5):432–434. https://doi.org/10.1136/adc.88.5.432. Medline:12716718

Wilson ME, Weld LH, Boggild A, et al; GeoSentinel Surveillance Network. Fever in returned travelers: results from the GeoSentinel Surveillance Network. *Clin Infect Dis.* 2007;44(12):1560–1568. https://doi.org/10.1086/518173. Medline:17516399

World Health Organization. International travel and health [Internet]. Update 2018. Available from: http://www.who.int/ith/en/.

INFECTIOUS DISEASE EMERGENCIES

10.2

Malaria

Rahim Valani

- Malaria is caused by an intraerythrocyte parasite of the *Plasmodium* genus.
  » There are 5 main species of malaria:
    1. *P. falciparum*
    2. *P. vivax*
    3. *P. ovale*
    4. *P. malariae*
    5. *P. knowlesi*
  » *P. falciparum* and *P. vivax* are the most common species worldwide and pose the greatest public health challenge.
- Malaria is a disease of the tropics, transmitted by the female *Anopheles* mosquito.
- There are an estimated 214 million cases globally, with 438 000 deaths annually.
  » 89% of cases occur in sub-Saharan Africa.

Pathophysiology

- The female mosquito injects sporozoites into the bloodstream of a human.
  » The sporozoites travel to the liver and infect hepatocytes.
  » They proliferate in hepatocytes over the next 1 to 2 weeks, maturing into schizonts.
  » The mature schizonts in the liver rupture and release thousands of merozoites, which then infect erythrocytes.
- This results in:
  » Lysis of erythrocytes, which in turn causes:
    › Anemia
      · As anemia worsens, it can result in hemodynamic compromise.
    › Severe intravascular hemolysis
      · This results in hemoglobinuria, which can precipitate acute renal failure.
  » Inflammatory response — proinflammatory state
  » Sequestration of erythrocytes and adherence to vascular endothelium
    › Patients may present with poor perfusion and hypoxic state due to poor or obstructed flow.
    › The effects may be responsible for cerebral malaria and renal failure.

Physical Exam

- Patients can present with varying symptoms, depending on the species of mosquito and severity of the infection.
- Malaria presents as paroxysms of fever, chills, rigor, and headache.
  » These classically occur in a cyclical pattern every 3 days.
- Pallor and jaundice may be evident with hemolysis.
- Hepatomegaly or splenomegaly may be present.
- Other symptoms can range from nonspecific, viral-like symptoms to altered mental status; they may include:
  » GI symptoms — nausea, vomiting, diarrhea, abdominal pain
  » Respiratory symptoms — tachypnea, cough
  » Musculoskeletal symptoms — arthralgias, myalgias
  » Neurologic symptoms — confusion, seizures

Investigations

- Order bloodwork, including:
  » Complete blood count (CBC), electrolytes, blood urea nitrogen (BUN), creatinine
  » Venous blood gas and lactate
  » Glucose
  » Thick and thin smears for malaria
  » Blood cultures

Diagnosis

- Look for the presence of the parasite on a blood smear.
- Obtain both thick and thin smears.
  » Use thick smear to identify the presence of the parasite.
  » Use thin smear to determine the species and parasite load.
- If the initial smear is negative, repeat smears every 24 hours for 3 days.
- Severe malaria is defined as any of:
  » > 5% parasitemia load
  » Central nervous system (CNS) symptoms
  » Any evidence of end-organ damage
  » Shock
  » Metabolic acidosis — lactate > 5 mmol/L or bicarbonate < 15 mmol/L
  » Hypoglycemia — glucose < 2.2 mmol/L
  » Severe anemia — hemoglobin < 50 g/L
  » Hemoglobinuria secondary to kidney injury

Management

- Ensure adequate resuscitation of the patient, based on clinical symptoms and vital signs.
- Give IV fluids if the patient shows signs of dehydration; use caution in cases of severe malaria.
- Give antipyretics for fever.
- Give IV dextrose solution for hypoglycemia.
  » If blood sugar is < 3 mmol/L, treat with 5 mL/kg of 10% dextrose solution.
- In patients with cerebral findings, consider other causes of altered levels of consciousness (see Chapter 2.2).
- Manage seizures with benzodiazepines.
  » If seizures do not stop, consider phenytoin or phenobarbital.
  » Seizures are seen in 30% of severe malaria cases in children.
- Patients with severe malaria (see "Diagnosis," above) should be managed aggressively.
- Patients with a hematocrit of < 12% or a hemoglobin ≤ 40 g/L should be transfused.

Main Considerations for Therapy

PARASITE LOAD

- A parasite load > 5% is categorized as severe malaria.
- Ensure adequate resuscitation by treating shock and preventing or minimizing end organ damage.
- Administer IV artesunate at 2.4 mg/kg per dose until the parasite load is < 1%.
  » Consider IV quinine as second-line treatment with a loading dose of 5.8 mg/kg of base in 100 mL of 5% dextrose solution over 30 minutes, followed by 8.3 mg/kg of base in 500 mL of 5% dextrose solution every 8 hours.
    › All subsequent infusions after the bolus dose are run over 2 to 4 hours.
- Check for hypoglycemia and treat appropriately.
- Avoid rapid fluid boluses unless the patient is in shock state.
  » Fluid therapy is guided by urine output with a goal of > 1 mL/kg per hour.
- Consult ICU for admission.

SPECIES

- P. falciparum is the main cause of severe malaria, but it can also be seen with P. vivax and P. knowlesi.

DRUG RESISTANCE

- There is high chloroquine resistance worldwide.
- Options for treatment depend on where the patient has traveled to, resistance patterns, and availability of medications; consider:
  » Atovaquone or proguanil

  » Quinine
    › IV quinine can be used for patients with non-severe malaria who are unable to tolerate PO medications.
  » Doxycycline
  » Primaquine
    › Avoid primaquine in pregnant patients or in patients with G6PD deficiency.
  » Clindamycin
  » Mefloquine

Advice for Travelers to Endemic Areas

- Individuals traveling to areas where malaria is endemic should consult with a travel medicine clinic to ensure appropriate prophylaxis, travel advice, and immunizations.
- The risk to travelers varies depending on:
  » Region of travel and accommodations
  » Duration of travel
  » Use of preventative measures (below)
- The 3 pillars of malaria prevention are:
  1. Vector control
    › Chemical barriers:
      · Mosquito nets treated with insecticide (permethrin)
      · Topical repellents (20% to 30% DEET or 20% icaridin)
    › Indoor residual spraying
    › Physical barriers
      · Wearing long-sleeved tops and long pants
  2. Chemoprophylaxis (see Table 10.2.1)
  3. Prompt diagnosis and treatment in a returning traveler (see "Management," above)

Table 10.2.1. MALARIA CHEMOPROPHYLAXIS

Agent	When to start	When to stop
Atovaquone/Proguanil	1 to 2 days prior to travel	1 week after return
Doxycycline	1 to 2 days prior to travel	4 weeks after return
Primaquine	1 to 2 days prior to travel	3 days after return
Mefloquine	2 weeks prior to travel	4 weeks after return

REFERENCES

Committee on Infectious Diseases, American Academy of Pediatrics. *Red book 2015.* 30th ed. Illinois: AAP; 2015.

Olivero RM, Barnett ED. Malaria. In: Cherry JD, Demmler-Harrison GJ, Kaplan SL, Steinbach WJ, Hotez P, editors. *Feigin and Cherry's textbook of pediatric infectious diseases.* 7th ed. Philadelphia, PA: Saunders; 2014.

Public Health Agency of Canada. Canadian recommendations for the prevention and treatment of malaria [Internet]. Ottawa, ON: Public Health Agency of Canada; 2014. Available from: http://publications.gc.ca/collections/collection_2014/aspc-phac/HP40-102-2014-eng.pdf

World Health Organization. *Management of severe malaria: a practical handbook.* 3rd ed. Geneva: WHO; 2012.

World Health Organization. *World malaria report 2015.* Geneva: WHO; 2015.

INFECTIOUS DISEASE EMERGENCIES

10.3

Pediatric Tuberculosis

Amita Misir, Ian Kitai

- Tuberculosis (TB) infection and disease is caused by *Mycobacterium tuberculosis*, a fastidious, aerobic, acid-fast bacillus that can affect nearly any body system.
- Tuberculosis (TB) is currently the leading infectious cause of death worldwide.
  - » The World Health Organization estimates there were 9.6 million new cases of TB infections and 1.2 million deaths in 2014.
  - » The Canadian rate of TB is 4.6 per 100 000, and the global rate is 133 per 100 000.
- Childhood TB is paucibacillary (i.e., requires only few bacilli) and difficult to diagnose.
  - » Best estimates suggest that children < 15 years of age account for 11% of the burden of disease globally.
- In Canada, pediatric TB is relatively uncommon but demonstrates significant regional variation.
  - » In 2010, overall (child and adult) incidence rates ranged from a low of 0.7 per 100 000 on Prince Edward Island to a high of 106.1 per 100 000 in the northern territories combined.
- In Canada, pediatric TB is largely a disease affecting:
  - » Foreign-born children
  - » Children of foreign-born parents
  - » Indigenous children

Risk Factors

- Risk factors for TB disease include:
  - » Close contact with a confirmed or suspected case of infectious TB
    - › This is the most important risk factor.
  - » Being of Indigenous ancestry
  - » Being foreign-born
  - » Children with foreign-born parents
  - » Travel to endemic areas (i.e., Asia, Africa, Latin America, countries of the former Soviet Union), especially with prolonged stay or contact (> 1 week) with the local population
- There is an increased risk of progression from TB infection to TB disease in the following populations and contexts:
  - » Infants and adolescents
  - » Those having been recently infected (within the past 2 years)
  - » Immunodeficient patients (including prolonged steroid use or chemotherapy) or HIV-positive patients
  - » IV drug users
  - » Those with certain diseases or other medical conditions, including lymphoma, diabetes mellitus, chronic renal failure, and malnutrition

Pathophysiology

TB Incubation and Infection

- Children < 4 years of age may rapidly develop serious forms of TB, including miliary disease and TB meningitis, often within 2 to 3 months.
- The primary local infection is usually accompanied by an occult, subclinical bacteremia that seeds distant sites, including the apices of the lungs, lymph nodes, and central nervous system.
- More rarely, patients may display hypersensitivity reactions (e.g., fever, erythema nodosum, phlyctenular keratoconjunctivitis) during this time.
- Patients will generally display immune-conversion as manifested by the tuberculin skin test (TST) and/or interferon-gamma release assay (IGRA) 3 to 8 weeks after exposure, provided the above infectious process is initiated.

0 TO 6 WEEKS: EXPOSURE AND INCUBATION

- Individuals are exposed via inhalation from an individual with pulmonary or laryngeal TB.
- An asymptomatic incubation period ensues after exposure.

1 TO 3 MONTHS: PRIMARY DISEASE

- Inhaled bacteria are taken up by alveolar macrophages and, if not immediately destroyed, primary local infection of the lung ensues.
- Small parenchymal lesions develop in the periphery, middle, and lower lung zones (the most ventilated areas).
- Lesions are accompanied by regional lymphadenopathy (often perihilar or mediastinal).
- Patient may recover spontaneously from primary local infection with minimal, self-limiting symptoms (i.e., mild, viral-like) and transient chest X-ray (CXR) changes.
  - » Changes may not be detected if CXR is not done when changes are present.

Latent TB Infection

- Pulmonary TB and extrapulmonary sites of infection may result in latent TB infection.
- Approximately 10% of untreated adults with latent TB infection will develop the reactivated disease over their lifetime.
  - » Up to 40% of children < 12 months of age will reactivate and present with TB, much of which will be extrapulmonary or disseminated.
- There is no confirmatory test for latent TB infection.
- A child with latent TB infection is considered to have no symptoms related to the infection.
  - » Diagnosis is typically made by fulfillment of all the following criteria:
    - › Positive TST or IGRA
    - › No clinical evidence of disease
    - › CXR that is either normal or demonstrates evidence of remote infection (calcified parenchymal nodule and/or a calcified intrathoracic lymph node)
    - › No history of receiving adequate treatment for latent TB infection

TB Disease

- Bacilli spread throughout the lungs and pleura, resulting in symptomatic intrathoracic TB disease.

- Bacilli may also travel to other sites in the body (most commonly the lymphatic system, meninges, bones and/or joints, and abdomen), causing extrathoracic TB disease.
- The risk of progression to TB disease is inversely related to age.
  - » Infants have the highest risk at 50%.
  - » Children > 10 years old have the lowest risk at 10% to 20%.
- In the vast majority of cases (> 90%), TB disease occurs within 1 year after the primary infection and most commonly manifests as intrathoracic disease.
  - » Rarely, disseminated disease develops within 3 to 6 months from the time of primary infection, especially in children < 4 years of age.
- The classical distinction between TB infection and TB disease is not always easy; this distinction can be somewhat artificial and may be better conceptualized as a series of clinical syndromes (see *Figure 10.3.1*).

Clinical Presentation

- TB disease generally presents in 2 ways in North America:
  1. It is detected via contact, immigration, or other screening; or
  2. It presents as symptomatic TB disease

Figure 10.3.1. CLINICAL SYNDROMES ASSOCIATED WITH PEDIATRIC TB INFECTION AND DISEASE

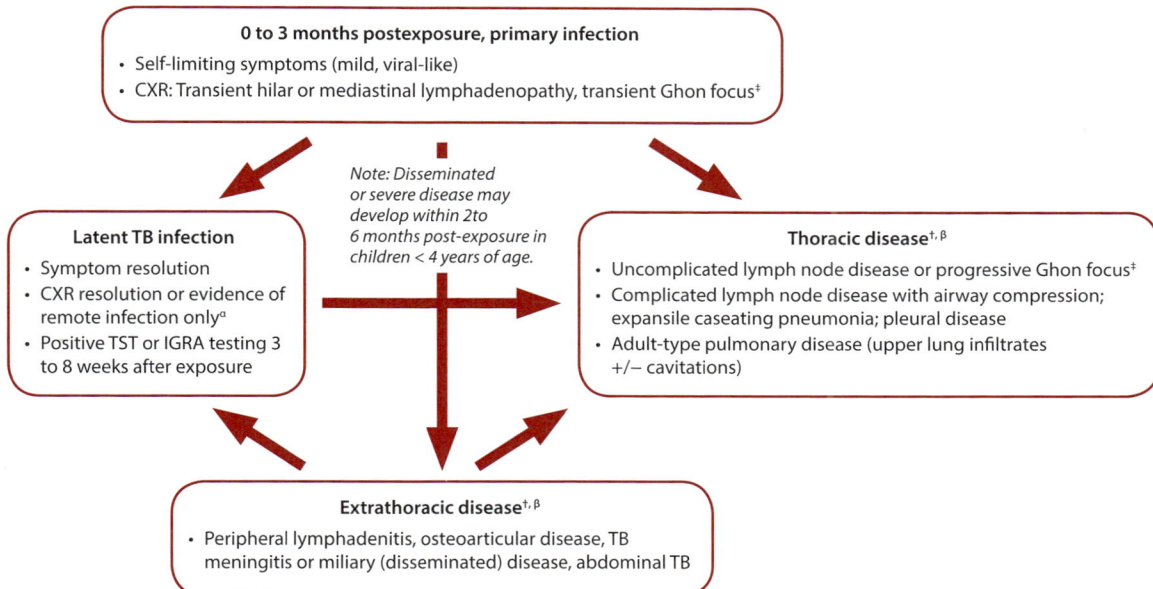

0 to 3 months postexposure, primary infection
- Self-limiting symptoms (mild, viral-like)
- CXR: Transient hilar or mediastinal lymphadenopathy, transient Ghon focus[‡]

Note: Disseminated or severe disease may develop within 2 to 6 months post-exposure in children < 4 years of age.

Latent TB infection
- Symptom resolution
- CXR resolution or evidence of remote infection only[a]
- Positive TST or IGRA testing 3 to 8 weeks after exposure

Thoracic disease[†, β]
- Uncomplicated lymph node disease or progressive Ghon focus[‡]
- Complicated lymph node disease with airway compression; expansile caseating pneumonia; pleural disease
- Adult-type pulmonary disease (upper lung infiltrates +/− cavitations)

Extrathoracic disease[†, β]
- Peripheral lymphadenitis, osteoarticular disease, TB meningitis or miliary (disseminated) disease, abdominal TB

[†]At least 90% of disease manifestations occur within 12 months of infection.

[‡]A Ghon focus (also known as a Ghon lesion) represents a calcified tuberculous caseating granuloma (tuberculoma) and represents the sequelae of primary pulmonary tuberculosis infection.

[a]Evidence of remote infection is defined as a calcified parenchymal nodule and/or calcified intrathoracic lymph node.

[β]Because test results may be negative in certain clinical situations where disease exists, a negative TST or IGRA cannot be used to rule out disease.

Contact and Screening

- Screening by TST or CXR is **not** part of routine screening for children immigrating to Canada.
- Contact with a TB case should be evaluated by history, physical examination, and CXR.
  » This can help rule out worrisome symptoms (e.g., cough lasting > 2 weeks, weight loss, fever, pain, vomiting, altered mental status) that would require more urgent further evaluation and/or hospital admission.
- Disposition of a TB-exposed patient who does not demonstrate signs or symptoms suggestive of TB disease is further discussed in "Management" and "Disposition," below.

Symptomatic TB Disease

- Clinical manifestations of TB disease will most often appear 1 to 6 months after exposure or infection, with at least 90% of disease manifestations occurring within 12 months after infection (up to 18 months for osteoarticular disease).
- Presentation may be protean and can involve almost any system in the body.
  » Nonspecific symptoms present a diagnostic challenge.
- Most common symptoms include fever, cough, weight loss or poor weight gain, and growth delay.
- The most common presentation of symptomatic TB disease is pulmonary:
  » Cough lasting > 2 weeks
  » Fever
  » Hemoptysis and night sweats (uncommon in children)
  » Possible normal physical exam
- Extrapulmonary TB accounts for 20% to 35% of adolescent TB in low-burden settings.

MENINGITIS AND CENTRAL NERVOUS SYSTEM TB SYMPTOMS

- Subacute presentation over days or weeks includes fever, behavioral changes, and headache.
- Patients may also develop hydrocephalus, basilar meningitis, basal ganglia infarct, and tuberculomas (space-occupying lesions) with increased intracranial pressure.

PLEURAL DISEASE

- Patients may present with pleuritic chest pain.

BONE AND JOINT TB SYMPTOMS

- TB may affect any bone in the body and mimic subacute or chronic bacterial osteomyelitis, with spine involvement in nearly 50% of pediatric skeletal TB cases.

LYMPHATIC SYSTEM TB SYMPTOMS

- Lymphadenitis (most commonly cervical) is the most common form of extrapulmonary TB.
- Lymphadenitis usually presents with painless and progressive swelling, sometimes with constitutional symptoms.
- Skin discoloration is also seen in nontuberculous mycobacterial lymphadenitis, which can occur with *Mycobacterium bovis*.

ABDOMINAL TB SYMPTOMS

- The most common abdominal symptoms are abdominal pain, fever, and weight loss.
- Acute presentations represented 55% of all abdominal cases in one review.
- Gastrointestinal TB symptoms include:
  » Acute-onset colicky abdominal pain, nausea and vomiting, diarrhea with weight loss (mimics inflammatory bowel disease), right lower-quadrant abdominal pain, anorexia, and fever
- Peritoneal TB is more common in children.
  » "Wet type" peritoneal TB is characterized by significant ascites.
  » "Dry type" peritoneal TB has adhesions or obstruction; fibrotic type has omental thickening and loculated ascites.
  » Patients may have palpable abdominal mass.
  » Peritoneal TB can be asymptomatic.

CONSTITUTIONAL SYMPTOMS

- Constitutional TB is characterized by failure to thrive, reduced playfulness, and low-grade or intermittent fevers.

Diagnosis

Latent TB Infection

- There is no confirmatory test for latent TB infection.
- A child with latent TB infection is considered to have no symptoms related to the infection.
  » Diagnosis is typically made by fulfillment of all the following criteria:
    › Positive TST or IGRA
    › No clinical evidence of disease
    › CXR that is either normal or demonstrates evidence of remote infection (calcified parenchymal nodule and/or a calcified intrathoracic lymph node)
    › No history of receiving adequate treatment for latent TB infection

TB Disease

- A positive culture from sputum or other sample(s) from affected sites confirms the disease and remains the gold standard for diagnosis.

» With drug-resistant TB, it is best to make every attempt to obtain specimens before starting therapy.
• Because childhood TB is often paucibacillary, it is often culture-negative (50% to 75% of cases).
  » Diagnosis often rests on the basis of:
    › Positive TST or IGRA
    › Abnormal CXR
    › History of contact with a case of infectious TB, in addition to compatible clinical signs or symptoms
• Criteria for the diagnosis of confirmed, probable, and possible childhood intrathoracic TB have been proposed by an international expert panel in the context of clinical research; however, these criteria are not yet used or validated for clinical application.

Investigations

• A CXR should be ordered for all patients with suspected TB or who have had contact with a known or suspected case of TB.
  » Hilar lymphadenopathy is the hallmark of TB in children < 10 years old and may be accompanied by parenchymal focus.
  » In older children and adolescents, TB is more likely to present with upper-lobe airspace disease with possible cavitating lesions.
  » A CXR that "looks worse than the patient" is more suggestive of TB than other more common bacterial etiologies.

• For symptomatic patients presenting to the emergency department (ED):
  » Perform TST and/or IGRA
  » Obtain other imaging as clinically indicated, which may include:
    › MRI or CT head with contrast
      · Detection of basilar meningitis and hydrocephalus
    › Abdominal ultrasound demonstrating hypoechogenic lymphadenopathy — may be a clue to gastrointestinal TB
  » Efforts should be made to obtain samples for bacterial stain and culture from all appropriate site(s)
  » Obtain and send for TB culture ≥ 1 sputum specimen(s) from any child able to expectorate.
    › Specimens should preferably be obtained by sputum induction.
    › Specimens can be obtained as little as 1 hour apart and should preferably be obtained by sputum induction procedures (i.e., administration of 200 mcg of bronchodilator, nebulization of 5 mL of hypertonic saline, followed by chest percussion if necessary).
    › 3 serial early morning gastric aspirates after at least 6 hours of sleep has traditionally been the diagnostic procedure of choice in young children who are unable to produce sputum.
    › Sputum induction followed by collection of nasopharyngeal aspirates has been used in infants as young as 1 month of age.

Table 10.3.1. APPROACHES TO DIAGNOSIS OF TB DISEASE

Diagnosis of TB disease is based on:		
• Positive culture of Mycobacteria tuberculosis from sputum or other fluid/tissue sample (gold standard) — and/or —		
• Clinical diagnosis based on combination of the following:		
Criteria	**Assessment**	**Comments**
Immunological evidence of tuberculosis exposure	Either TST and/or IGRA may be used. TST must be administered and interpreted according to clinical context (see Menzies D [2014] chapter 4; Morris SK et al. [2015] for details). Where available, IGRA is the preferred test for those under 5 years of age who have been BCG vaccinated, however TST is a good test for close contacts.	In cases of significant clinical suspicion, both tests may be applied. A negative test result for TST and/or IGRA does not rule-out disease; up to 10-20% of immunocompetent children with culture-proven TB disease will initially be TST/IGRA negative.
Chest radiography abnormalities	Anterior-Posterior and Lateral views of the chest should be obtained looking for: • Uncomplicated lymph node disease • Progressive Ghon focus • Lymph node disease with airway compression • Lymph node disease with bronchopneumonia or expansile lobar pneumonia • Disseminated (miliary) disease • Pleural or pericardial effusion • Adult-type pulmonary disease with cavitating lesions in upper lung zones	Chest radiograph should be interpreted by an experienced paediatric radiologist. Rarely CT or MRI of thorax may be helpful in making diagnosis of intra-thoracic TB.
History of contact with an infectious case of TB	History of contact with a known or suspected case of TB especially within the last 2 years	Risk increases with increasing proximity and duration of exposure.
Compatible clinical signs or symptoms	As noted in "Clinical Presentation," above	Any organ system may be involved.

BCG bacillus Calmette–Guérin. **IGRA** interferon gamma release assay. **TST** tuberculin skin test.

» Conduct arthrocentesis of any joint effusions
» Send biologic samples for both staining (fluorescent staining is preferred over acid-fast) and culture in both solid and liquid media
» Consider nucleic acid amplification technologies (NAATs) or polymerase chain reaction (PCR) as they give faster results than cultures
  › Complementary bacterial cultures on cerebrospinal fluid (CSF) collected for suspected TB meningitis are especially important to send if NAAT/PCR is done.
  › These tests generally appear to be specific but are not very sensitive.

Management

Infection Control

- TB is one of the few infections (including measles and varicella) that is transmitted by an airborne route via small-droplet nuclei that remain suspended in the air for long periods of time.
- Ensure that airborne precautions are followed for everyone who comes into contact with the patient.
  » The patient should be isolated in an airborne infectious isolation room.
    › An airborne infectious isolation room is a negative-pressure room with a minimum of 9 air exchanges per hour and high-efficiency particulate air (HEPA) filtration to minimize transmission.
    › Both the patient and caregivers should wear surgical masks, and all attendant healthcare personnel should wear an N95 mask or the equivalent.
- If an active respiratory TB case is suspected or confirmed, the patient should remain in hospital until and unless home isolation conditions are met.

Initial Management of Suspected or Confirmed TB Disease

- Ensure appropriate isolation of the patient.
- Notify the local public health unit.
- Involve a multidisciplinary TB team and experts whenever possible (telephone consultation at minimum).
- Draw the following baseline laboratory studies:
  » Liver tests — alanine aminotransferase, aspartate transaminase, bilirubin
  » HIV serology
- Once the decision is made to initiate therapy for TB disease and after specimens are obtained, the principles of therapy will involve directly observed therapy (DOT), typically with a 4-drug regimen (isoniazid, rifampin/rifampicin, pyrazinamide, and ethambutol).
- Ensure prompt treatment of TB meningitis to minimize complications.

Complications

- Patients on TB therapy may present with deterioration after weeks to months of the initiation of therapy.
- Emergent complications include:
  » Airway obstruction — enlarging intrathoracic lymphadenopathy often leads to severe airway compromise
  » Focal neurologic signs or deficits — formation of tuberculomas in TB meningitis despite effective therapy
  » Peripheral neuropathy or intractable seizures
    › Pyridoxine (B_6) deficiency cause by isoniazid therapy, especially in young children, exclusively breastfed infants, or children on meat- or milk-deficient diets.
  » Hepatotoxicity
    › Isoniazid (INH) is the most common cause of hepatotoxicity during TB treatment.
    › Note that hepatotoxicity is rare in children (approximately 1 in 1000 patients).
    › Hepatotoxicity presents with anorexia, abdominal pain, and vomiting; jaundice is a late finding.
    › Maintain a high index of suspicion and a low threshold for checking liver enzymes and bilirubin even with early, nonspecific symptoms.
- Deterioration after the initiation of therapy may be due to what is termed the "paradoxical reaction" or immune response inflammatory syndrome (IRIS), which reflects the immunopathologic basis of many of these episodes but is difficult to differentiate from acquired drug resistance or treatment failure.
  » In these cases, treatment with steroids may be initiated after expert consultation.

Disposition

- If a TB-exposed patient does not exhibit signs or symptoms suggestive of TB disease, the patient may be discharged with an outpatient referral to a public health and/or a pediatric infectious disease specialist; this follow-up is needed to complete the evaluation of latent TB infection for the patient and to ensure adequate control of any infectious TB cases in the community.
- An asymptomatic patient should be urgently referred (i.e., with follow-up assured within 1 to 7 days) if the patient:
  » Is a TB-exposed child < 4 years of age
    › Such patients are at high risk of developing severe or disseminated disease and the "window period" for medical prophylaxis may be indicated for up to 8 weeks postexposure until a reliable TST or IGRA may be obtained.
  » Has an abnormal CXR

REFERENCES

Alvarez GG, Clark M, Altpeter E, Douglas P, Jones J, Paty MC, Posey DL, Chemtob D. Pediatric tuberculosis immigration screening in high-immigration, low-incidence countries. *Int J Tuberc Lung Dis.* 2010;14*(12)*:1530–1537. Medline:21144237

Birnbaum B, Marquez L, Hwang KM, Cruz AT. Neurologic deterioration in a child undergoing treatment for tuberculosis meningitis. *Pediatr Emerg Care.* 2014;30*(8)*:566–567. https://doi.org/10.1097/PEC.0000000000000190. Medline:25098802

Clark M, Hui C. Children from Baffin Island have a disproportionate burden of tuberculosis in Canada: data from the Children's Hospital of Eastern Ontario (1998-2008). *BMC Pediatr.* 2010;10*(1)*:102. https://doi.org/10.1186/1471-2431-10-102. Medline:21192806

Cruz AT, Ong LT, Starke JR. Emergency department presentation of children with tuberculosis. *Acad Emerg Med.* 2011;18*(7)*:726–732. https://doi.org/10.1111/j.1553-2712.2011.01112.x. Medline:21762235

Delisle M, Seguin J, Zeilinski D, Moore DL. Paediatric abdominal tuberculosis in developed countries: case series and literature review. *Arch Dis Child.* 2016;101*(3)*:253–258. https://doi.org/10.1136/archdischild-2015-308720. Medline:26699532

Kimberlin D, ed. *RedBook: 2015 report of the Committee on Infectious Diseases.* 30th ed. Elk Grove Village, IL: American Academy of Pediatrics; 2015.

Matlow A, Robb M, Goldman C. Infection control and paediatric tuberculosis: A practical guide for the practicing paediatrician. *Paediatr Child Health.* 2003;8*(10)*:624–626. https://doi.org/10.1093/pch/8.10.624. Medline:20019856

Menzies D, ed. *Canadian tuberculosis standards.* 7th ed. Ottawa, ON: Public Health Agency of Canada; 2014.

Morris SK, Demers AM, Lam R, Pell LG, Giroux RJ, Kitai I. Epidemiology and clinical management of tuberculosis in children in Canada. *Paediatr Child Health.* 2015;20*(2)*:83–88. https://doi.org/10.1093/pch/20.2.83. Medline:25838781

Perez-Velez CM, Marais BJ. Tuberculosis in children. *N Engl J Med.* 2012;367*(4)*:348–361. https://doi.org/10.1056/NEJMra1008049. Medline:22830465

Thampi N, Stephens D, Rea E, Kitai I. Unexplained deterioration during antituberculous therapy in children and adolescents: clinical presentation and risk factors. *Pediatr Infect Dis J.* 2012;31*(2)*:129–133. https://doi.org/10.1097/INF.0b013e318239134c. Medline:22016079

World Health Organization, Global Tuberculosis Programme. Global tuberculosis report WHO [Internet]. Geneva: Global Tuberculosis Programme, World Health Organization; 2015 [cited 2016 Oct 10]. Available from: http://www.who.int/tb/publications/global_report/en/

Zar HJ, Hanslo D, Apolles P, Swingler G, Hussey G. Induced sputum versus gastric lavage for microbiological confirmation of pulmonary tuberculosis in infants and young children: a prospective study. *Lancet.* 2005;365*(9454)*:130–134. https://doi.org/10.1016/S0140-6736(05)17702-2. Medline:15639294

10.4

Tetanus

E. Vicky Fera

- Tetanus is caused by a neurotoxin produced by *Clostridium tetani* bacteria. It is characterized by tonic muscle contractions.
- Tetanus spores are found ubiquitously in the environment, particularly in soil and dust.
  » Transmission requires only a breach in the skin.
- The disease occurs primarily in unvaccinated individuals or in those with lapsed immunity.

Pathophysiology

- *C. tetani* is harmless until spores find their way into a warm, oxygen-deprived environment such as devitalized tissue from a crush injury, penetrating wound, laceration, or foreign body.
  » In this environment, the spores germinate and release toxins, including the neurotoxin tetanospasmin.
  » The toxin enters the nervous system through presynaptic terminals and reaches the central nervous system through retrograde axonal transport.
- The neurotoxin prevents inhibition of the motor neurons, resulting in spasms and rigidity.
  » Binding at the junctions is irreversible.

- Muscles with the shortest neuronal pathways are the first affected.
- The incubation period varies but typically ranges from 3 to 21 days.
- Mortality is due to autonomic dysfunction.

Physical Exam

- There are 4 clinical patterns:
  1. Generalized
     › The generalized pattern is the most common form.
     › It presents with trismus (lockjaw), risus sardonicus (facial muscle spasm causing a "sarcastic smile"), and rigid abdominal muscles.
     › It can progress to the paraspinal muscles, causing extreme back arching (opisthotonos), which is painful and can compromise respiratory status.
     › Spasms are intermittent and painful; they are brought on by sensory stimuli.
     › Autonomic symptoms begin a few days later and are the main cause of mortality.
  2. Localized
     › The localized pattern is less common.
     › Muscle at the site of inoculation becomes painful

and weak, then rigid within 2 to 3 days after the injury.
› This can last weeks to months.
› Localized tetanus rarely progresses to generalized tetanus.

3. Cephalic
› This is a rare form of localized tetanus that occurs from a head wound.
› It typically affects the lower motor facial nerve.
› It results in facial palsy, dysphasia, and extraocular muscle paresis.

4. Neonatal
› This is the neonatal version of generalized tetanus.
› It typically presents on days 7 to 14 of life.
› It occurs in infants born to mothers with inadequate immunity.
› Inoculation occurs at the umbilical stump and is due to poor obstetrical care (nonsterile procedures) or traditional practices such as placing cow dung or a coin on the umbilicus.
› Patients present with a weak suck and general weakness.
› Symptoms quickly progress to general rigidity and opisthotonoid back arching.

Diagnosis

- Diagnosis is primarily based on clinical presentation.
- There is no test that will diagnose tetanus with certainty.
  » The organism is very difficult to isolate and is not significant in an immunized individual as it is ubiquitous in soil.
  » Antibody detection is not useful as patients can have antibody levels above the protective concentration and still be affected.

Differential Diagnosis

- Consider the following conditions that mimic tetanus:
  » Strychnine intoxication (glycine antagonizer)
    › Strychnine is found in street drugs, homeopathic medications, and animal pesticides.
    › It is the only true mimic of tetanus; toxicology testing on serum and urine will distinguish the conditions.
  » Dystonic reaction
    › This may be from antipsychotic medication or dopamine antagonists such as antiemetics.
    › It causes neck stiffness similar to tetanus, but the patient's head will be turned laterally (a position that is rare in tetanus).
    › Treat patients with an anticholinergic agent (benztropine or diphenhydramine) to distinguish the condition from tetanus.
  » Dental infection
    › Dental infection can cause trismus (lockjaw) similar to tetanus, but other clinical findings of tetanus are not present.

Management

- There is no specific treatment for tetanus.
- The aim of management is to:
  » Stabilize the patient from a cardiorespiratory standpoint
  » Prevent autonomic instability (tachycardia and hypertension)
  » Prevent muscle fatigue by inhibiting muscle spasms
  » Neutralize circulating neurotoxin
  » Stop further neurotoxin production

Medications Used for Supportive Care

BENZODIAZEPINES

- Benzodiazepines are the mainstay of supportive care for tetanus.
- They control muscle spasms as well as provide sedative and anxiolytic effects.

NEUROMUSCULAR BLOCKADES

- Neuromuscular blockades are used when sedation from benzodiazepines does not achieve adequate effect.
- Longer-acting agents such as pancuronium can worsen autonomic instability, so continuous infusion of short-acting vecuronium is preferred.

MAGNESIUM SULFATE

- Magnesium sulfate is a calcium blocker that causes vasodilatation and acts as an anticonvulsant by causing presynaptic neuromuscular blockade.
- It may help control muscle spasms and autonomic dysfunction, but does not reduce the need for ventilatory support or reduce overall mortality and requires frequent monitoring for toxicity.

Other Medications

BACLOFEN

- Baclofen has been used in small trials.
- It does not cross the blood-brain barrier well, so it is administered intrathecally, which is costly and can lead to secondary infection.

BETA-BLOCKERS

- Labetalol has shown moderate effects on autonomic instability, but in some cases has had to be combined with clonidine for a more complete effect.

MORPHINE

- The analgesic effect of morphine can decrease anxiety and stabilize autonomic dysfunction, but only small trials have been conducted.
- All survivors should receive a tetanus vaccination series.

Table 10.4.1. TETANUS MANAGEMENT PROTOCOL

Adapted from Mandel (2010)

	Action	Laboratory workups	Medications
Initial management: 1st hour of presentation	1) Monitor ventilation closely, protect airway. • A single spasms can cause respiratory arrest. • Intubate if necessary. 2) Rule out dystonic reaction to dopamine antagonist. 3) Minimize muscle spasm and decrease rigidity. 4) Minimize stimulation to minimize spasms — transfer to dark, quiet ICU room.	• Tetanus antibody level • Electrolytes • Renal function • Urine myoglobin • Blood for strychnine and dopamine antagonist assay	• If intubating — sedate with benzodiazepine and paralyze with short-acting neuromuscular blockade (vecuronium) • Benztropine or diphenhydramine IV to rule out dystonic reaction. • Benzodiazepine IV at sedating dose (intubate if airway becomes compromised)
Management: following 24 hours	1) Neutralize circulating neurotoxin. 2) Stop further toxin production — debride wound thoroughly, remove foreign body (umbilical stump **should not** be excised).* 3) Continue sedation.		• Human tetanus immunoglobin (TIg) IM in doses of 3000 to 6000 IU (4)† • Tetanus vaccine (even if patient has a history of vaccination) IM at different site than TIg • Metronidazole IV every 6 hours (penicillin is an acceptable alternative; cephalosporins are not reliable) • Benzodiazapine

*There is no benefit to infiltrating the wound with immunoglobulin or antibiotics.

† Contact the local Medical Officer of Health to obtain TIg.

Prevention

- Primary tetanus prevention involves primary vaccinations followed by a booster every 10 years.
- Secondary tetanus prevention involves giving vaccine and immunoglobulin at the time of a high-risk injury, if warranted (see *Table 10.4.2*, below).

Table 10.4.2. MANAGEMENT OF ACUTE WOUND INJURY

Adapted from Public Health of Canada (2014)

	Clean, minor wounds		All other wounds	
Tetanus immunization history	Tetanus vaccine	TIg*	Tetanus vaccine	TIg*
Unknown, < 3 doses	Yes	No	Yes	Yes
≥ 3 doses, < 5 years since booster	No	No	No	No
≥ 3 doses, > 5 but < 10 years since booster	No	No	Yes	No
≥ 3 doses, > 10 years since booster	Yes	No	Yes	No

*The recommended dose of tetanus immunoglobulin for adults and children ≥ 7 years of age is 250 units IM (deltoid or lateral thigh); for children > 7 years old, use 4 units/kg.

- Tertiary tetanus prevention involves giving vaccine and immunoglobulin after the symptoms of tetanus have developed.
  - » Patients that have recovered from tetanus should receive the full vaccine series as having the illness does not result in immunity.

Prognosis

- A shorter time interval from the time of injury to the onset of symptoms results in a worse prognosis.

GENERALIZED TETANUS

- The patient's condition worsens over the first 2 weeks, then slowly resolves over 3 to 5 weeks following the regeneration of new neuromuscular junctions.

LOCALIZED TETANUS

- The prognosis for localized tetanus is good; patients recover spontaneously after 3 to 5 weeks.

CEPHALIC TETANUS

- The prognosis for cephalic tetanus is poor.
- The condition has been described even in vaccinated individuals.

NEONATAL TETANUS

- The prognosis for neonatal tetanus is poor.
- Mortality is > 90% within 1 to 2 weeks; survivors suffer from developmental delays.

REFERENCES

American Academy of Pediatrics. Section 3: summaries of infectious diseases. In: Pickering LK, Baker CJ, Long SS, McMillan JA, editors. *Red book: 2012 report of the Committee on Infectious Diseases*. 29th ed. Elk Grove Village, IL: American Academy of Pediatrics;–777.

Bleck TP, Reddy P. Clostridium botulinum (botulism). In: Mandel GL, Bennett JE, Dolin R, editors. *Principles and practice of infectious diseases*. 7th ed. Philadelphia, PA: Churchill Livingstone;–3095.

Public Health Agency, Manitoba Health. Communicable disease management protocol: tetanus. Winnipeg, MB; 2001 [cited 2016 Mar 7]. Available from: https://www.gov.mb.ca/health/publichealth/cdc/protocol/tetanus.pdf

Public Health Agency of Canada. Canadian immunization guide: part 4 – active vaccines, tetanus toxoid. Public Health Agency of Canada; 2014 [cited 2016 Mar 9]. Available from: https://www.canada.ca/en/public-health/services/publications/healthy-living/canadian-immunization-guide-part-4-active-vaccines/page-22-tetanus-toxoid.html

Rodrigo C, Fernando D, Rajapakse S. Pharmacological management of tetanus: an evidence-based review. *Crit Care*. 2014;*(2)*:217. https://doi.org/10.1186/cc13797. Medline:25029486

10.5

HIV

Sarah Khan

- Pediatric HIV can present in neonates, children, or adolescents.
- The prevention of vertical transmission (from mother to child) has significantly reduced the number of incident cases in high-income (developed) countries.
- Risk factors for HIV in pregnancy include:
  » IV drug use
  » High-risk sexual behaviors
  » Immigration from a country where HIV is endemic
- The risk of vertical transmission with no preventive interventions is 25%.
  » This can be reduced to < 2% with maternal combination antiretroviral treatment during pregnancy, intrapartum IV zidovudine, and avoidance of breastfeeding.
- Pediatric HIV continues to be an issue in children from lower- and middle-income countries and should be considered in children coming from areas where HIV is endemic.
- Sexual transmission should be considered when risk factors are present in children or adolescents.

Pathophysiology

- HIV transmission through sexual, blood-borne, or vertical transmission leads to infection into T lymphocytes using the CD4 receptor to enter the cell.
- As an RNA virus, HIV reverse-transcribes itself into DNA using a reverse transcriptase enzyme, integrating itself into the host cell genome.
- Once activated, the viral genome replicates, and viral proteins are produced using host cell machinery.
- The cell ruptures and dies as the mature virions are released, going on to infect other cells (lymphocytes, monocytes, macrophages) with CD4 receptors.

Primary Infection

- Upon initial infection, the HIV virus typically rapidly replicates, and a peak viral load is reached after a few weeks to months.
- This peak can be accompanied by an acute retroviral illness consisting of fever and flu-like symptoms.
- The rapid replication of the virus typically declines,

and the viral load drops to a set-point level, where it plateaus.
  » Once it has plateaued, clinical latency occurs, which is typically asymptomatic or mildly symptomatic.

Viral Progression

- HIV DNA remains in infected cell host genomes, acting as a reservoir of infection, even if the peripheral plasma (HIV RNA) viral load is controlled or undetectable with medications.
  » This HIV reservoir is thought to play a role in the inability to remove or cure HIV infection despite rapid initiation of combination antiretroviral medication in newly infected infants.
  » HIV may be present in genital secretions and breast milk despite undetectable plasma viral loads.
- The incubation period from time of infection to presentation with symptoms varies from weeks to years.
- Often years after primary infection, the virus is stimulated to replicate again and a rapid rise in viral load occurs, concomitant with a decline in CD4 T lymphocytes, which will progress to AIDS without intervention.
- Clinical latency usually lasts 8 to 10 years after infection; without treatment, immune function begins to decline and constitutional symptoms begin to appear, followed by opportunistic diseases.
- Depending on immune factors, the rapidity of this progression can be categorized as:
  » Rapid — patient dies within 5 years
  » Average — clinical latency lasting 8 to 10 years
  » Slow — clinical latency lasting more than 10 years
  » Nonprogressor — patient remains healthy with a normal CD4 count for > 15 years without treatment
  » Viremic or elite controller — a rare exception in which patient maintains a low or undetectable viral load without treatment

HIV-1 and HIV-2

- There are 2 strains of HIV: HIV-1 and HIV-2.
- HIV-2 infection is endemic in Angola, Mozambique, West African countries (Cape Verde, Ivory Coast, Gambia, Guinea-Bissau, Mali, Mauritania, Nigeria, Sierra Leone, Benin, Burkina Faso, Ghana, Guinea, Liberia,

Niger, Nigeria, Sao Tome, Senegal, and Togo), and parts of India.

» It also occurs in countries such as France and Portugal, which have large numbers of immigrants from these regions.

- HIV-1 and HIV-2 coinfections may also occur but are rare outside areas where HIV-2 is endemic.

- HIV-2 is rare in North America.

- Accurate diagnosis of HIV-2 can be problematic but is clinically important because HIV-2 strains are naturally resistant to several antiretroviral drugs developed to suppress HIV-1.

Diagnosis

- The preferred method of diagnosis is with antigen/antibody combination immunoassay (serology).

  » The p24 antigen is a viral core protein and is the antigen component in the antigen/antibody serologic blood test.

  » In addition, an HIV virologic blood test (viral load) should also be done as a confirmation using a reverse transcriptase polymerase chain reaction (RT-PCR) assay. The viral load can quantify the amount of virus circulating in the plasma.

    › All HIV tests have a "window period" where a false negative may occur very early in HIV infection. For serology the window period is 2 to 4 weeks, whereas virologic testing has a shorter window period of 1 to 2 weeks.

  » In certain remote settings without laboratory access, rapid point-of-care combination antigen/antibody tests are available but are less sensitive.

- Generally, 2 tests are needed to confirm HIV status (2 serologic immunoassays, followed by virologic testing if a discrepancy is found).

- Once HIV infection is confirmed, drug-resistance testing should be performed (genotypic testing is preferred over phenotypic testing).

  » 15% to 20% of newly infected patients have at least one drug-resistance mutation.

  » Nonnucleoside reverse transcriptase inhibitor resistance is more common compared to protease inhibitor resistance mutations.

- The HIV-exposed infant requires virologic testing prior to 18 months of age, as serologic testing may merely reflect the transplacental passage of maternal antibodies.

  » HIV-1 p24/antibody combination immunoassays are not sensitive or specific in the first months of life compared to HIV virologic tests.

  » HIV DNA polymerase chain reaction (PCR) detects HIV viral DNA in peripheral blood mononuclear cells and is highly sensitive, with 99.8% specificity at birth and 100% specificity at ages 1, 3, and 6 months.

- Certain conditions have been defined by the Centers for Disease Control (CDC) to be considered AIDS-defining illnesses.

  » For more information, see "Appendix A: AIDS-Defining Conditions" in *Morbidity and Mortality Weekly* Volume 57 RR-10, accessible via www.cdc.gov.

Clinical Presentation

- Lymphadenopathy and hepatosplenomegaly are non-specific manifestations.

- During the first year of life, oral candidiasis, failure to thrive, and developmental delay are other common presenting features of HIV infection.

- The most common AIDS-defining conditions observed among children with vertically acquired HIV infection include:

  » *Pneumocystis jirovecii* pneumonia (PJP)

  » Recurrent bacterial infections

  » Wasting syndrome

  » Esophageal candidiasis

  » HIV encephalopathy

  » Cytomegalovirus pneumonia, colitis, encephalitis, or retinitis

- See below for further information on these AIDS-defining conditions.

Management

- All children with HIV should be treated with antiretroviral therapy, but the strength of the recommendation varies by age and pretreatment CD4 cell count due to fewer data being available regarding the benefits and risks of immediate therapy in asymptomatic HIV-infected children compared to adults.

- Several factors need to be considered in making decisions about the urgency of initiating and changing antiretroviral therapy (ART) in children, including:

  » Severity of HIV disease and risk of disease progression, based on:

    › Age

    › Presence or history of HIV-related illnesses (as described above)

    › Degree of CD4 immunosuppression

    › Level of HIV plasma viremia

  » Availability of appropriate (and palatable) drug formulations

  » History of antiretroviral treatment use

  » Drug resistance

  » Presence of comorbidity

  » Potential antiretroviral drug interactions with other medications

  » Compliance

- The treatment of choice for HIV-infected children is a regimen containing at least 3 drugs from at least 2 classes of antiretroviral drugs.

» The regimen typically involves 2 nucleoside reverse transcriptase inhibitor (NRTI) drugs and a third drug from another class.

Drug Classes

- There are 6 main classes of medications that work on different components of the viral life cycle:
  1. Nucleoside reverse transcriptase inhibitors (NRTIs)
  2. Nonnucleoside reverse transcriptase inhibitors (NNRTIs)
  3. Protease inhibitors
  4. Integrase inhibitors (INSTIs)
  5. Fusion inhibitors
  6. Chemokine receptor antagonists (CCR5 antagonists)

Infant Feeding

- In Canada, exclusive formula feeding is currently recommended for infants born to mothers living with HIV irrespective of maternal clinical, immunologic, and virologic status or antiretroviral therapy received.
- Healthcare providers should assist patients in accessing formula, some provinces have funded formula programs for infants born to mothers living with HIV.

PNEUMOCYSTIS JIROVECII PNEUMONIA

- 50% of all AIDS-defining conditions are diagnosed in the first year of life.
- The disease typically develops at CD4 < 200 cells/μL or CD4 < 15%.
- Symptoms include low-grade fever, tachypnea, non-productive cough, and progressive shortness of breath.
- Physical examination shows normal to severe rales and rhonchi.
- Chest X-ray (CXR) shows bilateral interstitial infiltrations.
- CT scan demonstrates ground-glass opacities and patchy distributions affecting the central lung.
- PJP is diagnosed using stains for PJP in pulmonary fluid or tissue (bronchial alveolar lavage [BAL], lung biopsy, sputum induction, endotracheal tube [ETT] aspirate).

Management

- The mortality rate is 5% to 40% if treated, 100% if untreated.
- Initiate empiric therapy while awaiting test results if clinical suspicion is high.
- First-line treatment is trimethoprim-sulfamethoxazole (TMP-SMX).
  » An adjunctive steroid is suggested if disease is moderate to severe (observational data only).

» Chemoprophylaxis is TMP-SMX 2.5 to 5 mg/kg per dose given twice daily (dose based on the TMP component); do not exceed 320 mg TMP given 3 days per week.

» Chemoprophylaxis is recommended for:
  › All children aged 4 to 6 weeks to 12 months of age with confirmed HIV infection regardless of CD4 count or percentage (due to high risk in this age group)
  › HIV-infected children aged 1 to < 6 years with CD4 count < 500 cells/μL or CD4 < 15%
  › HIV infected children aged 6 to 12 years with CD4 < 200 cells/μL or < 15%

RECURRENT BACTERIAL INFECTIONS

- Pneumonia and bacteremia are the most frequently seen infections.
- Pathogens include *Streptococcus pneumonia*, *Salmonella* species, *Staphylococcus aureus*, *Hemophilus influenza* B (Hib), and *Pseudomonas*.
- Prevention includes administration of pneumococcal, meningococcal, and Hib vaccines.
- If patient presents with hypogammaglobulinemia (IgG < 400 mg/dL), consider administering intravenous immunoglobulin (IVIG) at 400 mg/kg every 2 to 4 weeks.

FAILURE TO THRIVE (WASTING SYNDROME)

- The condition is diagnosed with one of the following 3 criteria:
  1. Persistent weight loss > 10% from baseline
  2. Downward crossing of 2 or more major percentile lines on the weight-for-age chart
  3. < 5th percentile on weight-for-height chart on 2 consecutive measurements 30 or more days apart, plus chronic diarrhea or documented fever
- Failure to thrive can severely impact growth and development.
- Patients are at high risk for HIV disease progression and short-term mortality.

ESOPHAGEAL CANDIDIASIS

- Risk factors for esophageal candidiasis include prior oral candidiasis, low CD4, and antibiotic use.
- The disease presents with the following:
  » Odynophagia
  » Retrosternal pain
  » Fever
  » Nausea/vomiting

» Drooling/dehydration
» Hoarseness
» Gastrointestinal bleeding

- Diagnosis is made via upper endoscopy with biopsy and culture.
- Treat with IV fluconazole.
  » Administer an initial dose of 6 mg/kg PO, then 3 to 12 mg/kg daily to a maximum of 400 mg/day.
  » Continue treatment for > 3 weeks total, and for > 2 weeks after symptom resolution.
- No prophylaxis is recommended due to the potential for azole resistance to develop.

MYCOBACTERIUM AVIUM COMPLEX

- *Mycobacterium avium* is an environmental organism that can be ingested, inhaled, or inoculated and can disseminate in immunocompromised hosts.
- The organism causes fever, weight loss, persistent GI symptoms, adenitis, bone marrow suppression, hepatosplenomegaly, and lymphadenopathy.
- It is isolated in the blood by mycobacterial culture or from the biopsy of normally sterile sites (bone marrow, lymph nodes).
- Prophylaxis is:
  » Clarithromycin 7.5 mg/kg (to a maximum of 500 mg) PO given twice daily
  — or —
  » Azithromycin 20 mg/kg (to a maximum of 1200 mg) PO once weekly
- Prophylaxis is indicated in patents based on age and CD4 cutoff:
  » < 1 year of age with CD4 count < 750 cells/μL
  » 1 to < 2 years of age with CD4 count < 500 cells/μL
  » 2 to < 6 years of age with CD4 count < 75 cells/μL
  » > 6 years of age with CD4 count < 50 cells/μL

HIV ENCEPHALOPATHY

- HIV encephalopathy can present with any of the following:
  » Failure to attain developmental milestones, loss of milestones, or loss of cognitive ability
  » Impaired brain growth or acquired microcephaly as determined by head circumference measurements, or brain atrophy as demonstrated by CT scan or MRI:
    › Focal changes, typically including cerebral atrophy and basal ganglia calcifications
  » Acquired symmetric motor deficits manifested by 2 or more of the following:
    › Paresis
    › Pathologic reflexes
    › Ataxia
    › Gait disturbances
- HIV encephalopathy can be static or progressive.
  » Static HIV encephalopathy is more common and involves global cognitive and motor deficits with a normal rate of learning.
  » Progressive HIV encephalopathy, the most severe form of HIV encephalopathy, occurs almost exclusively in patients with untreated HIV and involves severe developmental delay or regression of developmental milestones.
- > 50% of children who develop HIV encephalopathy are symptomatic by 1 year of age, indicating the importance of early antiretroviral therapy.
- HIV encephalopathy increases mortality risk.

CYTOMEGALOVIRUS (CMV) DISEASE

- In HIV-positive children, cytomegalovirus (CMV) disease can range from asymptomatic, prolonged fever to pneumonitis, colitis, encephalitis, and/or retinitis.
- CMV may act as an immunomodulator and accelerate the progression of HIV.
- Treatment includes IV ganciclovir or PO valganciclovir, depending on the severity of the disease.

OTHER CLINICAL MANIFESTATIONS OF HIV

- Other clinical manifestations of HIV include:
  » Cryptosporidiosis
  » Chronic HSV
  » Kaposi sarcoma
  » Lymphoid interstitial pneumonia
  » Cytopenias
  » Skin infections — fungal, bacterial, viral
  » Parotitis
  » HIV-associated nephropathy, nephrotic syndrome
  » Cardiomyopathy, pericardial effusion, myocarditis
- Early diagnosis and treatment of HIV-infected infants dramatically decreases morbidity and mortality.
- Long-term comorbidities include:
  » Mental health concerns
  » Dyslipidemia
  » Cardiovascular complications — accelerated atherosclerosis, cardiomyopathy
  » Insulin resistance, diabetes mellitus
  » Decrease bone mineral density
  » Renal disease

REFERENCES

Bitnun SA, et al. Guidelines for the prevention of mother-to-child HIV transmission, information and practice guidance for health practitioners in Ontario: working with HIV-infected women with inadequate control of HIV, and women with unknown HIV status who present in labor, Version date: January 6, 2017. Available from: http://www.ohtn.on.ca/wp-content/uploads/2017/02/MTCT-prevention-guidelines-January-20-2017.doc

Burchett SK, Pizzo PA. HIV infection in infants, children, and adolescents. *Pediatr Rev.* 2003;24(6):186–194. https://doi.org/10.1542/pir.24-6-186. Medline:12777610

CDC. Revised classification system for human immunodeficiency virus infection in children less than 13 years of age. *Morb Mortal Wkly Rep.* 1994;43(RR-12):1–10. https://www.cdc.gov/MMWR/preview/mmwrhtml/00032890.htm

CDC. Appendix A: AIDS-defining conditions. [No. RR-10] *Morb Mortal Wkly Rep.* 2008;57(RR-10):9. https://www.cdc.gov/mmwr/preview/mmwrhtml/rr5710a2.htm.

De Clercq E. The design of drugs for HIV and HCV. *Nat Rev Drug Discov.* 2007;6(12):1001–1018. https://doi.org/10.1038/nrd2424. Medline:18049474

Fauci AS, Pantaleo G, Stanley S, Weissman D. Immunopathogenic mechanisms of HIV infection. *Ann Intern Med.* 1996;124(7):654–663. https://doi.org/10.7326/0003-4819-124-7-199604010-00006. Medline:8607594

10.6

Bites

Sarah Khan

- Bites account for 1% of all emergency department (ED) visits.
- The majority of bites are inflicted by:
  » Dogs — 60% to 90%
  » Cats — 5% to 20%
  » Rodents — 2% to 3%
  » Humans — 2% to 3%
- Only 10% of individuals with bite wounds seek medical attention, and the delay increases the risk of infection.
  » 10% of patients require suturing and follow-up care.
  » 1% to 2% of patients require admission to hospital.
- Posttraumatic stress disorder can occur in some patients from the bite.
- Pathogens in animal bite wounds are polymicrobial and include:
  » Pathogens from the oral flora of the biting animal
  » Human skin flora
- The most common pathogens are:
  » *Pasteurella* species
    › These tend to be more severe presentations with fever and lymphadenopathy.
  » *Staphylococcus* species
  » *Streptococcus* species
  » Anaerobic bacteria
  » Other relevant but less common pathogens, which include:
    › *Capnocytophaga canimorsus* — a fastidious gram-negative rod that can cause fatal sepsis after animal bites in asplenic patients, individuals who abuse alcohol, or those with hepatic disease
    › *Bartonella henselae* — the catscratch disease organism, which can be transmitted by cat bites
    › *Eikenella corrodens* — a gram-negative anaerobe that can be transmitted by human bites.

DOG BITES

- Dog bites are likely to be caused by animals known to the victim.
- Bites to the head and neck are common in children because of their proximity to the level of the animal's mouth.
- Children often have uninhibited behavior around dogs, making them more vulnerable to bites.
- Bites can vary from minor wounds to deep, open lacerations, tissue avulsions, and crush injuries caused by animals with large jaws capable of exerting strong force.

CAT BITES

- Cats usually cause wounds with their teeth or claws; bites are more likely than not the result of provocation.
- Bites are typically to the upper extremities and face.
- Injuries range from scratches to deep puncture wounds caused by long, slender, sharp teeth, resulting in direct inoculation into bone.
- Small wounds may appear insignificant and result in delay in seeking medical care.

HUMAN BITES

- A semicircular or oval area of erythema or bruising is characteristic of human bites.
  » A wound with an intercanine distance of 3 cm is an adult bite.

- Human bites are at higher risk for infection if they penetrate the dermis.
- Small wounds over the metacarpophalangeal joints typically arise from fistfights.
  - » Potential exists for infection into the deep compartments and tendon spaces of the hand.
- Patients with human bites tend to delay seeking medical attention.

OTHER BITES
- Small animals (e.g., squirrels, rodents, rabbits) often cause injuries similar to cat bites, with deep penetration.
- Reptile bites can be associated with *Salmonella* infections.
- Shark bites are associated with *Vibrio* infections.

History
- The following information should be gathered on the patient's history:
  - » Type of animal, whether the bite was provoked or not, the location of the animal, and its owner
  - » Time since injury
  - » Symptoms or complaints since the bite (e.g., neurovascular, pain, bleeding, fever, wound concerns)
  - » Patient's medical condition (e.g., immunosuppressed, asplenic, diabetes, vascular insufficiency)
  - » Patient's allergies
  - » Patient's tetanus status

Physical Exam
- A physical examination should evaluate the following:
  - » Skin site for depth of penetration and crush injury
  - » Nerve and tendon function
  - » Vascular supply and lymph nodes
  - » Underlying joints for penetration
- Photograph or draw a diagram of the wounds.

Investigations
- Obtain radiological imaging.
  - » X-rays may show evidence of fracture, presence of tooth fragment, or joint disruption.
  - » Ultrasound may reveal underlying abscess or foreign body.
- Initiate bloodwork as needed.
  - » Request a complete blood count (CBC).
    - › C-reactive protein (CRP) may be elevated if patient has cellulitis, septic arthritis, osteomyelitis, or bacteremia.
  - » Aerobic and anaerobic blood cultures should be considered.

- Send wound cultures only if the bite appears infected prior to initiating antibiotics.
  - » A CT scan may be required for dog bites to the head due to the potential for depressed skull fractures.
    - › Evaluate the patient for signs of fracture, puncture through the outer plate of the skull, and pneumocephalus.

Management

Initial Management
- Initial management of bite wounds involves:
  - » Stabilization
    - › Apply pressure to actively bleeding wounds.
    - › Perform neurovascular assessment distal to the wound.
  - » Wound preparation
    - › Local anesthesia facilitates wound cleansing with 1% povidone iodine or benzalkonium chloride.
    - › Irrigate the wound with saline and debride any devitalized tissue.
  - » Wound exploration
    - › Identify any injury to underlying structure.
    - › Remove any foreign bodies.
    - › Puncture wounds are challenging to debride.
      - · Use high pressure.
      - · Soak the wound for 15 minutes in an antiseptic solution to help cleanse.

Wound Closure
- Maintain concern over the closure of wounds given the high risk of infection.
  - » Primary closure of dog bite lacerations may be considered.
  - » Never close the following wounds primarily (usually allowed to heal by secondary intention):
    - › Infected wounds
    - › Crush injuries
    - › Puncture injuries
    - › Bites to hands and feet
    - › Wounds more than 12 hours old (> 24 hours on face)
    - › Cat or human bites (except those to the face)
    - › Bite wounds in immunocompromised patients (asplenic, venous stasis, diabetic adults, cancer patients)
- Obtain a surgical consultation for:
  - » Deep wounds that penetrate bones, tendons, joints, or major structures
  - » Complex facial lacerations
  - » Neurovascular compromise
  - » Complex infections (abscess, osteomyelitis, joint involvement)

Table 10.6.1. ANTIBIOTIC DOSES

Medications	IV Dosing	PO Dosing
Piperacillin-tazobactam	• 200 to 300 mg/kg per day (based on piperacillin component) divided and given every 8 hours (to a maximum of 16 g/day or 4.5 g [4 g of piperacillin + 0.5 g tazobactam every 8 hours])	• N/A
Ceftriaxone	• 50 to 75 mg/kg every 24 hours (to a maximum of 2 g/day) • Consider CNS dosing if bite is to the head	• N/A
Clindamycin	• 30 to 40 mg/kg per day divided and given every 8 hours (to a maximum of 900 mg/dose)	• 10 to 20 mg/kg per day divided and given every 8 hours (to a maximum of 450 mg/dose)
Metronidazole	• 20 to 30 mg/kg per day divided and given every 12 hours (to a maximum of 1 g/day)	• 20 to 30 mg/kg per day divided and given every 12 hours (to a maximum of 1 g/day)
Amoxicillin-clavulanic acid	• N/A	• 25 to 40 mg/kg per day (based on amoxicillin component) divided and given every 8 hours (to a maximum of 500 mg/dose)
Doxycycline	• 2 to 4 mg/kg per day divided and given every 12 hours	• 2 to 4 mg/kg per day divided and given every 12 hours
Trimethoprim-sulfamethoxazole	• 8 mg/kg per day (based on trimethoprim component) divided and given every 12 hours	• 8 mg/kg per day (of trimethoprim component) divided and given every 12 hours
Moxifloxacin	• 10 mg/kg IV every 24 hours (to a maximum dose of 400 mg)	• 10 mg/kg every 24 hours (to a maximum dose of 400 mg)

CNS central nervous system.

Prophylaxis

ANTIBIOTIC PROPHYLAXIS

• Antibiotic prophylaxis should be considered for the following:
  » Deep puncture wounds (e.g., cat bites)
  » Moderate to severe crush injuries
  » Wounds in areas of underlying venous and/or lymphatic compromise
  » Wounds on hands, genitalia, face, or in close proximity to bone or joint
  » Wounds requiring closure
  » Bite wounds in immunocompromised patients
  » Human bites through the dermis
• Prophylaxis should include staphylococcal, streptococcal, and anaerobic coverage.
  » Common IV antibiotics include:
    › IV piperacillin-tazobactam
    › IV ceftriaxone and clindamycin or metronidazole
  » Common PO antibiotic options include:
    › Amoxicillin-clavulanic acid
    › Doxycycline
    › Trimethoprim-sulfamethoxazole
    › Moxifloxacin and clindamycin or metronidazole
  » Avoid cephalexin, cloxacillin, and macrolides as they do not cover *Pasteurella* or *Eikenella*.

TETANUS PROPHYLAXIS

• Tetanus prophylaxis should be considered if the bite has penetrated the skin (see Chapter 10.4).
  » Prophylaxis should be determined based on the patient's immunization status.
  » Whether or not tetanus toxoid (vaccine) or tetanus immunoglobulin (TIg) is given should be assessed based on the patient's vaccination history (number of doses and date of last dose).

Table 10.6.2. TETANUS POSTEXPOSURE PROPHYLAXIS (TOXOID/VACCINE AND IMMUNOGLOBULIN)

Previous number of doses	Clean, minor wounds		All other wounds	
	Tetanus toxoid	TIg	Tetanus toxoid	TIg
< 3 doses or unknown	Yes	No	Yes	Yes
> 3 doses	Only if last dose was > 10 years ago	No	Only if last dose was > 5 years ago	No

• For further information on tetanus, see Chapter 10.4.

RABIES PROPHYLAXIS

• Rabies prophylaxis is a concern if an animal is ill, wild, or stray (nonvaccinated) or if the attack was unprovoked.
• See Chapter 10.7 for more detailed information on rabies.

VIRAL PROPHYLAXIS

• Viral prophylaxis should be considered after human bites.
• Hepatitis B can be transmitted from an HBsAg-positive host in unvaccinated victims.
  » If the biter is not known or is unable to be tested, hepatitis B vaccine should be administered.
• Hepatitis C and HIV transmission via saliva is extremely unlikely.
  » HIV postexposure prophylaxis is generally not indicated; discuss with a local infectious disease or HIV expert.

INFECTED BITES

- Remove any suture material if the bite has been previously repaired.
- Obtain a Gram stain and aerobic and anaerobic cultures from the depth of the infected puncture or laceration prior to initiating antibiotics, noting on the lab requisition that the culture is from a bite wound.
- Draw blood cultures as well if there are signs of systemic infection.
- Consult surgery for operative exploration, debridement, abscess drainage, or infected bone; send intraoperative cultures from pus and tissue.
- Administer empiric antibiotics PO or IV depending on the severity of the bite for a total of 10 to 14 days or until resolution of the injury.

REFERENCES

Dendle C, Looke D. Review article: animal bites: an update for management with a focus on infections. *Emerg Med Australas*. 2008;20(*6*):458–467. doi: 10.1111/j.1742-6723.2008.01130.x.

Endom E, et al. Initial management of animal and human bites. [cited 2016]. Available from: http://www.uptodate.com/contents/clinical-manifestations-and-initial-management-of-animal-and-human-bites

Griego RD, Rosen T, Orengo IF, Wolf JE. Dog, cat, and human bites: a review. *J Am Acad Dermatol*. 1995;33(*6*):1019–1029. https://doi.org/10.1016/0190-9622(95)90296-1. Medline:7490347

10.7

Rabies

E. Vicky Fera

- Rabies is a zoonotic infection caused primarily by the rabies virus (genus *Lyssavirus*), leading to fatal encephalitis.
- There are 70 000 reported deaths per year.
  - » 60% of cases are from India.
  - » 40% of cases are pediatric.
- In developing countries, the rabies virus is usually contracted from unvaccinated dogs and is most common in children < 15 years of age, as they are more likely to be bitten.
- In North America, bats are the most common reservoir of the virus.

Pathophysiology

- Transmission can occur by:
  - » A bite from an infected animal
  - » Exposure of human mucous membrane to the virus
  - » Aerosol transmission of the virus
    - › This is a rare form of transmission.
- Saliva infected with the virus enters the body via a bite wound, scratch, or contact with mucosal tissue, where it replicates in neighboring muscle cells for weeks or months.
- The virus then penetrates the neuronal system, traveling in retrograde fashion along peripheral nerves to the central nervous system (CNS).
- Finally, the virus spreads to the rest of the body via peripheral nerves to the highly innervated salivary glands, where the virus replicates.
- Rabies causes characteristic inflammatory changes of the neurons and eosinophilic inclusion bodies (Negri bodies).

Physical Exam

- Incubation usually lasts 3 months, though periods of a few days to 19 years have been reported.
- The disease progresses faster from bites that are closer to the CNS.
  - » Facial bites progress more rapidly than those to lower limbs.
- Prodrome lasts 4 to 10 days, with typical symptoms of viral illness such as fever, headache, and upper respiratory tract infection (URTI) symptoms.
- There are two forms of rabies: furious and paralytic.

FURIOUS (ENCEPHALITIC) RABIES

- Furious rabies accounts for 80% of cases.
- It primarily affects the brain.
- It is characterized by periods of hyperexcitabilty are interspersed with lucid phases; patients may present with:
  - » Aggressive behavior (biting, hitting, and agitation)
  - » Anxiety
  - » Hallucinations
  - » Bizarre behavior
- Other symptoms include:
  - » Hydrophobia

- » Aerophobia
- » Hyperventilation.
- » Autonomic instability:
  - › Hypersalivation
  - › Diaphoresis
  - › Pupillary dilatation
- » Cardiac arrhythmias, including premature atrial and ventricular beats
- » Symptom of inappropriate antidiuretic hormone (SIADH) / diabetes insipidus (DI)
- Furious rabies is fatal within 7 of 14 days of presentation of initial symptoms.

PARALYTIC RABIES

- Paralytic rabies is characterized by ascending flaccid paralysis.
- It accounts for 20% of cases.
- There is a high burden on the spinal cord, nerve roots, and peripheral nerves.
- Paralytic rabies progresses to quadriparesis, facial weakness, and hydrophobia.
  - » It can be confused with Guillain-Barré syndrome.
- Paralytic rabies is fatal within 21 days of onset of symptoms.

History

- Patients will have had contact with a rabid animal either by bite or by contact with mucous membranes.
- Domestic animals (dogs, cats, ferrets) can be infected with rabies.
- Individuals that touch, are sprayed by, or come into contact with rabid animal feces, urine, or blood are not at risk of infection.
  - » Spelunkers that have extensive respiratory exposure to bat habitats are considered an exception.

Risk Factors

- Risk assessment can be based on the following 4 factors:
  1. Category of exposure — World Health Organization classification
     - › Category 1 — Touch or mucous contact (e.g., licking) with intact skin
     - › Category 2 — Nibbling on uncovered skin, minor scratches or abrasions
     - › Category 3 — Break in skin and contact or contamination with saliva or mucosa of an infected animal
  2. Animal exposure
     - › Determine what the offending animal was.
     - › Animal risk factors in Canada are:
       - · Bats — constitute the highest risk as they carry the highest burden of infection

- · Raccoons, coyotes, foxes, and skunks — depending on geographic location, these are considered an increased risk for exposure to the virus
- · Dogs, cats, ferrets — constitute a very low risk of exposure if domesticated and vaccine status is up to date; stray animals constitute an only slightly higher risk.
- · Rodents such as squirrels, chipmunks, rats, and mice — constitute very low risk as these animals will likely be eaten by the larger rabid animal that infected them
  3. Local rabies epidemiology
     - › Check local rabies epidemiology with local public health agencies.
       - · The incidence of rabid raccoons is higher near the Ontario–United States border compared to northern Ontario, for example.
  4. Offending animal behavior and circumstances surrounding the event.
     - › For example, if a person (particularly a child) is found in a room with a bat and exposure by bite, scratch, or mucosal membrane cannot be reliably ruled out, then the individual is considered at risk (see "Postexposure Prophylaxis," below).

Diagnosis

- To help with patient diagnosis:
  - » If the offending animal is a domesticated animal such as a dog or a cat, then, when possible, the animal should be observed for 10 days regardless of vaccine status (either at the owner's home or at a veterinary clinic).
    - › If rabid behavior develops, the animal should be humanely euthanized and the brain tissue preserved for viral testing.
  - » If the offending animal is a wild animal, animal control should, if possible, capture and euthanize the offending animal to test it for rabies.
    - › Wild animals are difficult to observe for rabid behavior.

Investigations

- Direct fluorescent antibody staining (DFA) of the brain tissue of a human or rabid animal is the gold standard for determining the presence of the rabies virus.
- Antirabies antibodies or the presence of rabies virus RNA may be found via RT-PCR testing in any of:
  - » Serum
  - » Tissue (nuchal skin biopsy)
  - » Cerebrospinal fluid (CSF)
    - › CSF may be normal or show a viral meningoencephalitic profile.
    - › CSF may show pleocytosis with a predominance of mononuclear cells.

- Brain imaging is usually normal until late in the course of the disease.
  - » MRI findings are nonspecific but can show moderate T2 enhancement of the brain stem, thalamus, hippocampus, and gray matter of the cord as the virus is tropic to these areas.
  - » The 2 subtypes of rabies show no difference in lesions on MRI.
  - » The brachial plexus can show enhancement in the prodromal phase of the disease.

Management

- There is no definitive treatment once the rabies virus has penetrated the neurologic system and encephalitis has developed.
- Treatment is mainly supportive in an intensive care setting.
- Rabies vaccine and immunoglobulin are not recommended.
- Benzodiazepines or morphine is used to minimize spasms and agitations in ferocious rabies.
- The Milwaukee protocol is no longer recommended.
- Antiviral medications such as ribavirin and amantadine have been used, but there is no evidence in case reports that they are effective.

Prophylaxis

- In some areas of Ontario, all cats and dogs are required by law to obtain rabies vaccine every 3 years.
  - » This is recommended in other parts of Canada.

Preexposure Prophylaxis

- Preexposure prophylaxis is recommended for veterinarians and travelers to areas with a high prevalence of rabies and minimal accessibility to medical services.
  - » The vaccination is given as a 3-dose course on days 0, 7, and 21 or 28 IM / intradermal (ID).
    - › A booster is given every 2 to 3 years.

Postexposure Prophylaxis

- All cases of suspected rabies exposure are managed in consultation with local public health agencies.
- Refer to provincial/state guidelines to determine who qualifies for postexposure prophylaxis (PEP).
- As the virus must replicate locally at the site of inoculation prior to penetrating the CNS, thorough cleaning and prompt local administration of neutralizing antibodies is critical to prevent spread.
- Cleaning the wound thoroughly can reduce the risk of infection by 90%.
  - » Wash the wound with a 20% soap solution and irrigate with a virucidal agent (e.g., povidone-iodine) or 70% ethanol.

- » Avoid suturing the wound closed.
- » Ensure that the patient's tetanus vaccination is up to date.
- » Consider antibiotics if indicated.
- Administer human rabies immunoglobulin (HRIG).
  - » Dosage of HRIG is weight-based: 20 IU/kg.
  - » Infiltrate as much volume into the wound as possible.
    - › The remainder is given IM away from the vaccination site.
  - » If HRIG is not given concurrently with immunization, it can be given up to 7 days after first administration of vaccine.
  - » Equine rabies immunoglobulin (ERIG) is cheaper, just as effective, and well tolerated, but is usually only used outside North America.
    - › Dose is weight-based: 40 IU/kg.
- Administer rabies vaccine (postexposure protocol).
  - » Give a 4-dose vaccination course (if there has been no previous preexposure prophylaxis) on days 0, 3, 7, 14.
  - » A 5-dose vaccination course is recommended for patients taking chloroquine and immunocompromised patients on days 0, 3, 7, 14, and 28.
  - » If previously vaccinated, patients only receive the vaccine on days 0 and 3 without rabies immunoglobulin.

REFERENCES

American Academy of Pediatrics. Section 3: summaries of infectious diseases. In: Pickering LK, Baker CJ, Long SS, McMillan JA, editors. *Red book: 2015 report of the Committee on Infectious Diseases.* 30th ed. Elk Grove Village, IL: American Academy of Pediatrics;–665.

Bassin SL, Rupprecht CE, Bleck TP. Rhabdoviruses. In: Mandel GL, Bennett JE, Dolin R, editors. *Principles and practice of infectious diseases.* 7th ed. Philadelphia: Churchill Livingstone;–2258.

Canadian Food Inspection Agency. Rabies in Canada – 2015 (archived). Available from: http://www.inspection.gc.ca/animals/terrestrialanimals/diseases/reportable/rabies/rabies-in-canada-2015/eng/1455315254510/1455315255675

Hankins DG, Rosekrans JA. Overview, prevention, and treatment of rabies. *Mayo Clin Proc.* 2004;79(5):671–676. https://doi.org/10.4065/79.5.671. Medline:15132411

Jackson AC. Human rabies: a 2016 update. *Curr Infect Dis Rep.* 2016;18(38). https://doi.org/10.1007/s11908-016-0540-y. Medline:27730539

Mahadevan A, Suja MS, Mani RS, Shankar SK. Perspectives in diagnosis and treatment of rabies viral encephalitis: insights from pathogenesis. *Neurotherapeutics.* 2016;13(3):477–492. https://doi.org/10.1007/s13311-016-0452-4. Medline:27324391

Ontario Ministry of Health and Long-Term Care. Guidance document for the management of suspected rabies exposures; 2013 (accessed 2016 March 7). Available from: http://www.health.gov.on.ca/en/pro/programs/publichealth/oph_standards/docs/guidance/gd_mng_suspected_rabies_exposures.pdf

Zhu S, Guo C. Rabies control and treatment: from prophylaxis to strategies with curative potential. *Viruses.* 2016;8(11): 279. https://doi.org/10.3390/v8110279. Medline:27801824

10.8

Botulism

E. Vicky Fera

- Botulism is a rare, life-threatening neuroparalytic illness.
- It is caused by *Clostridium botulinum,* a spore-forming, anaerobic, gram-positive bacillus found ubiquitously in soil and animal intestines.
- The organism releases a neurotoxin that is known to be one of the most poisonous substances by weight.
- There are 8 distinct organism subtypes: A, B, C_α, C_β, D, E, F, G.
  » Subtypes A, B, E, and F cause human disease.
  » The neurotoxicity and mechanism of action of all subtypes are similar.
- The spores are dormant, but when placed in a favorable environment, they germinate, releasing neurotoxin.
  » Favorable conditions for germination are:
    › pH > 4.5
    › Sodium chloride concentration < 3.5%
    › Low nitrite level
    › Anaerobic environment
    › Minimum temperature of 10°C, although subtype E can produce toxins at temperatures as low as 5°C
- Although the spores are heat resistant, the toxins are heat labile.
  » A temperature of 80°C for 30 minutes will destroy the toxin.
- The most common cause of botulism is home-canned foods.
  » To prevent spore germination, phosphoric acid or citric acid is used in canned or bottled foods.
- Injectable modified forms of the toxin are used therapeutically; indications include:
  » Blepharospasm
  » Strabismus
  » Cervical dystonia
  » Achalasia
  » Sialorrhea
  » Upper or lower limb spasticity
  » Anal fissure
  » Bladder dysfunction
  » Tardive dyskinesia
  » Chronic migraine
  » Primary axillary hyperhidrosis
  » Cosmetic procedures

Pathophysiology

- Botulism toxicity presents as acute, afebrile, symmetric, descending paralysis.
- The neurotoxin enters the preganglionic nerve terminal and binds irreversibly to the cell membrane.
- The toxin inhibits calcium-dependent exocytosis, which prevents the release of acetylcholine.
  » The toxin acts as a zinc-dependent protease that cleaves polypeptides essential for acetylcholine release.
- The effects are mainly in the peripheral nervous system, with no effects centrally or on axonal conduction.
  » This makes anticholinergic medications of limited use in treatment.
- *Table 10.8.1,* below, summarizes the 4 most common forms of botulism, with details of each.
- Two less common forms of botulism are:
  » Inhalational botulism
    › Inhalation botulism results from the inhalation of preformed toxin.
    › It could be used in bioterrorism, though pulmonary delivery is inefficient.
  » Iatrogenic botulism
    › Iatrogenic botulism result from an overdose of injectable toxin and is extremely rare.

Investigations

- Initiate routine laboratory tests.
- Cerebral spinal fluid (CSF) and CT or MRI scan of brain are normal.
- Clinical suspicion of botulism should lead to prompt treatment as waiting for culture results can delay treatment.

Diagnosis

- Diagnosis is based on the presence of descending paralysis along with any 1 of the following:
  » Typical electromyography findings — brief, small, abundant motor unit action potentials with normal nerve conduction velocity
  » *C. botulinum* in stool or wound
  » Botulinum toxin in serum, stool, wound, or food samples
  » Epidemiological link to a confirmed case

Table 10.8.1. THE 4 MOST COMMON FORMS OF BOTULISM

Type	Notes	Mechanism	Neurotoxin source	Risk factors	Incubation	Symptoms
Foodborne	• Foodborne botulism is the most common type of botulism in Canada.	• Oral ingestion of neurotoxin	• Preformed toxin in food products contaminated with spores that germinated in anaerobic conditions	• Poorly preserved foods (e.g., smoked meats, preserved fish, home-canned goods)	• 12 to 72 hours	• Initially: nausea, vomiting, diarrhea (as the toxin is absorbed through the gut) • Followed by: » Cranial nerve palsies: diplopia, dysarthria, dysphonia, dysphagia, and xerostomia » Descending symmetrical flaccid paralysis leading to asphyxia and death • Condition is usually afebrile
Infant	• Infant botulism is the second most common type of botulism in Canada.	• Oral ingestion of spores	• Neurotoxin is produced in intestines	• Soil- or dust-contaminated foods (e.g., honey, formula powder, peanut butter)	• Unknown; condition has slow onset as spores need to germinate in the intestines to form the neurotoxin	• Initially: acute onset of poor feeding (most common symptom), constipation (often but not always associated) • Followed by: weak cry, poor suck, facial weakness, decreased tears despite normal urine output, flushed skin despite septic appearance, progressive hypotonia with pronounced head lag due to decreased muscle tone ("floppy baby syndrome) • Condition is usually afebrile
Wound	• Wound botulism is uncommon in Canada, though there is increasing incidence among IV drug users.	• Soil-contaminated, improperly cleaned or debrided wound • Severe trauma	• Neurotoxin is produced in devitalized tissue or abscess	• Illicit drug injection	• 4 to 18 days	• Cranial nerve palsies and weakness • Fever can be present due to associated tissue infection
Adult	• This is the least common cause of botulism in Canada	• Oral ingestion of spores	• Neurotoxin is produced in intestines	• Anatomical or functional intestinal irregularities • Disruption to intestinal function or immunocompromised state » Normal gut is protected from colonization by *C. botulinum* • Recent antibiotic treatment	• Unknown; like infant botulism, the condition has a slow onset as spores need to germinate in the intestines to form the neurotoxin.	• Initially: nausea and vomiting • Followed by: descending symmetrical flaccid paralysis starting with cranial nerves • Condition is usually afebrile

- The differential diagnosis for botulism includes:
  » Guillain-Barré syndrome
  » Stroke
  » Myasthenia gravis
  » Tick paralysis
  » Lambert-Eaton myasthenic syndrome
- See *Table 4.7.2* (page 95) to differentiate between myasthenia gravis, GBS, and botulism.

FOODBORNE BOTULISM

- Neurotoxin may be found in serum, gastric aspirate, stool, and contaminated food products.

- *C. botulinum* may also be cultured from gastric aspirate, stool, and contaminated food products.
  » Isolation of *C. botulinum* in food product cultures is a helpful sign but is not diagnostic as spores are ubiquitous in food products.

INFANT BOTULISM

- Diagnosis is confirmed by identification of the neurotoxin or *C. botulinum* in the stool.
  » As constipation is a common presentation, Public Health Canada also accepts analyte taken from rectal swab or a soiled diaper.
  » Serum is usually negative for neurotoxin in infants but is included in testing.

WOUND BOTULISM

- Neurotoxin can be identified in serum or *C. botulinum* can be cultured from the wound.
  » Ensure that anaerobic cultures are obtained.

Management

- Mortality from untreated botulism results from respiratory failure.
- With prompt treatment and supportive care, mortality is < 8%.
- Recovery depends on the type of toxin; subtype A tends to last longer than subtypes B and E.

Supportive Care

- For foodborne botulism, gastric lavage and cathartic agent can be beneficial within 1 hour of ingestion.
  » Consider a high enema if patient has no symptoms of ileus.
- For wound botulism, significantly debride devitalized tissue or wound.
- Close monitoring in ICU of respiratory function is imperative.
  » Check for gag reflex, pulse oximetry, negative inspiratory force, and forced vital capacity (FVC).
  » Intubate at 30% FVC.
    › Approximately half of patients require mechanical ventilation.
  » If the patient is not intubated, position them with head tilted up.
- Provide nasogastric tube / parenteral feeding unless patient presents with severe ileus.

Antitoxin (For Patients > 1 Year of Age)

- Antitoxin binds only to unbound neurotoxin.
  » It is effective against botulism subtypes A, B, and E.
- In cases of foodborne, wound, or adult botulism, equine-derived botulism antitoxin is given to patients who have developed symptoms of botulism within 24 hours.
  » Several forms of equine-derived botulism antitoxin exist and are available only through the Special Access Program.
  » Severe reaction may occur, including anaphylaxis and serum sickness.

Immunoglobulin (For Patients < 1 Year of Age)

- Antitoxin is not given to patients < 1 year of age due to concerns of anaphylaxis.
- For cases of infant botulism, give human-derived botulism immune globulin (BIG-IV or BabyBIG) as a single infusion IV.
  » This therapy is only approved for infants < 1 year of age.
  » BIG-IV is only available in Canada through Special Access Program.
- **Do not** treat with antibiotics as bacterial lysis may increase toxin release.

Antibiotics

- Antibiotic treatment is only recommended for treatment of wound botulism.
- Penicillin G is the antibiotic of choice.
  » Prescribe metronidazole for penicillin-allergic patients.

Prognosis

- Recovery occurs over several months when nerve endings regrow.

Prevention

- Ensure that safe food handling and canning practices are followed.
- Avoid giving honey to infants < 1 year of age.
- The toxin is destroyed in air within 12 hours, by exposure to the sun within 3 hours, or by boiling heat-canned or jarred food for 10 minutes.
- The spores are extremely resilient and are only destroyed with autoclaving at 160°C or by irradiation.

Contact Information

- If botulism is suspected, contact Health Canada's Botulism Reference Service in Ottawa: (613) 957–0902 or after hours (613) 296–1139.

REFERENCES

American Academy of Pediatrics. Section 3: summaries of infectious diseases. In: Pickering LK, Baker CJ, Long SS, McMillan JA, eds. *Red book: 2012 report of the Committee on Infectious Diseases.* 29th ed. Elk Grove Village, IL: American Academy of Pediatrics; 2012. 257–260

Bleck TP, Reddy P. Clostridium botulinum (botulism). In: Mandel GL, Bennett JE, Dolin R, eds. *Principles and practice of infectious diseases.* 7th ed. Philadelphia: Churchill Livingstone; 2010. 3097–3101

Chalk CH, Benstead TJ, Keezer M. Medical treatment for botulism. [review]. *Cochrane Database Syst Rev.* 2014;2(2):CD008123. Medline:24558013

Leclair D, Fung J, Isaac-Renton JL, et al. Foodborne botulism in Canada, 1985-2005. *Emerg Infect Dis.* 2013;19(6):961–968. https://doi.org/10.3201/eid1906.120873. Medline:23735780

Ontario Ministry of Health and Long-Term Care. *Infectious diseases protocol, appendix A: botulism, revised 2014.* Toronto, ON: Queen's Printer for Ontario; 2014.

Public Health Agency of Canada. Botulism: guide for healthcare professionals. Ottawa (ON): Health Canada; 2014 [cited 2016 March 7]. Available from: http://www.hc-sc.gc.ca/fn-an/legislation/guide-ld/botulism-botulisme-prof-eng.php

Rossetto O, Pirazzini M, Montecucco C. Botulinum neurotoxins: genetic, structural and mechanistic insights. *Nat Rev Microbiol.* 2014;12(8):535–549. https://doi.org/10.1038/nrmicro3295. Medline:24975322

10.9

General Approach to Sexually Transmitted Infections

Samantha Woodrow Mullett, Kevin Chan

- Sexually transmitted infections (STIs) are a growing public health concern in Canada, particularly for young adults.
- Emergency departments (EDs) have been identified as areas where screening should take place because of the infrequent use of healthcare services by adolescents.
- When an STI is identified in a child, sexual abuse needs to be considered; conversely, if child abuse is suspected, consider screening the patient for STIs (see Chapter 1.7, "Child Abuse").
- Adolescents who are pregnant should be screened for STIs.

Epidemiology

- Although the incidence of STIs was declining, there have been increases in the rates of reported cases of chlamydia, gonorrhea, and syphilis in Canada since the year 2000.

- The most common STIs in young people are:
  » Chlamydia
  » Gonorrhea
  » Human papillomavirus (HPV)
  » Genital herpes
- Females are usually affected at a younger age.
- More males are affected by gonorrhea, whereas more females are affected by genital herpes.
- Although overall rates of HIV are low, and males who have sex with males still represent the largest number and proportion of those affected, females represent an increasing proportion of positive HIV reports, with the largest rise in females aged 15 to 19.
  » For more information on HIV infection, see Chapter 10.5.
- Special consideration should be given to infants born to mothers who are hepatitis B–positive as they are at increased risk of contracting the infection.

Table 10.9.1. EPIDEMIOLOGY OF STIS IN CANADA

Infection	Frequency in clinical practice	Trends in incidence	Most affected population(s)
Chlamydia	• Most commonly diagnosed and reported bacterial STI • Cases reported in Canada in 2014: 109 263	• Rate of incidence has been steadily increasing in Canada since 1997.	• Females aged 15 to 24 years • Males aged 20 to 29 years

Gonorrhea	• Second most commonly diagnosed and reported bacterial STI
	• Cases reported in Canada in 2014: 16 285
		• Rate of incidence has been steadily increasing in Canada since 1997; from 2005 to 2014, the rate of incidence increased by 61.3%.
		• Antimicrobial resistance has been steadily increasing:
		  » Quinolone resistance has increased from < 1% in the early 1990s to 15.7% in 2005 (national rate in Canada).
		  » Shifts in minimal inhibitory concentrations for third-generation and oral cephalosporins have been increasing in Canada and globally
			• Males
			  » Males account for two-thirds of reported cases but infection rates are increasing more rapidly among females than males.
			  » Most affected are males aged 20 to 24 years and females aged 15 to 19 years.
			• Increase in cases in males who have sex with males
			• Males aged 20 to 29
			• Females aged 15 to 24

Infectious syphilis	• Previously rare in Canada • Cases reported in Canada in 2014: 2357 • Cases reported in Canada 2006: 1493	• Dramatic national increases have been noted since 1997 related to regional outbreaks across Canada.	• Males who have sex with males (HIV positive and negative) aged 30 to 39 • Sex workers and their clients • Acquisition in endemic regions
Chancroid	• Exceedingly rare in Canada	• Stable	• Acquisition in endemic regions
Granuloma inguinale	• Exceedingly rare in Canada	• Stable	• Acquisition in endemic regions

Table 10.9.1 continues on next page.

Infection	Frequency in clinical practice	Trends in incidence	Most affected population(s)
Lymphogranuloma venereum	• Previously rare in Canada	• Unknown • Recent outbreaks in Canada have resulted in the development and implementation of an enhanced surveillance system.	• Males who have sex with males • Acquisition in endemic regions
Human papilloma virus (HPV)	• Very common » 70% of the adult population will have had at least 1 genital HPV infection over their lifetime.	• The true rate of incidence is not known, as HPV is not a reportable disease.	• Adolescent and young adult females and males (but affects females and males of all ages)
Genital herpes (HSV-1 and -2)	• Common	• The true rate of incidence is not known, as HSV is not a reportable disease. • Seroprevalence studies indicate rates of at least 20%.	• Very common in both adolescent and adult males and females » Females are more affected than males
HIV	• Rare in general practice • In 2014 there were an estimated 2570 new cases in Canada and estimated 75 500 Canadians living with HIV (20% of whom are undiagnosed).	• There has been a 20% rise in number of HIV+ test reports in Canada (2000 to 2004). • Since 2005 the estimated number of new HIV infections is declining.	• Males who have sex with males • Acquisition in endemic regions • Injection drug users • Females aged 15 to 19
Hepatitis B	• Low to moderate in general practice and varies in different populations • Approximately 700 acute cases per year in Canada	• Incidence of acute hepatitis B is twice as high for males as for females. • Peak incidence rates are found in the 30 to 39 age group.	• Infants born to HBsAg+ mothers • Injection drug users who share equipment • Persons with multiple sexual partners • Acquisition in endemic regions • Sexual and household contacts with an acute or chronic carrier

HBsAg hepatitis B surface antigen. **HPV** human papilloma virus. **HSV** herpes simplex virus. **STI** sexually transmitted infection.

Prevention

- Primary prevention strategies include:
  » Vaccination:
    › Hepatitis B
    › HPV
    › Hepatitis A — if patient will be traveling to endemic areas
  » Condom use
  » Behavioral change such as increasing the age of sexual initiation, decreasing number of partners, and/or decreasing other high-risk activities such as substance abuse that can increase the risk of unsafe sex
- Secondary prevention strategies include:
  » Partner notification
  » Treatment and screening for STIs in asymptomatic young adults

Screening

- Pediatric EDs should screen patients for STIs.
  » Although many adolescents have primary care providers, they often rely heavily on EDs for care.
  » In the U.S., adolescents and young adults 15 to 24 years of age represent 25% of the sexually active population but 50% of all new STI cases.
  » In a recent study, 10% of asymptomatic youth presenting to an ED were found to have chlamydia and/or gonorrhea.
  » STIs can cause problems such as pelvic inflammatory disease, ectopic pregnancy, infertility, genitorectal cancers, facilitation of HIV infection, and increased transmission of disease, leading to overall increases in healthcare costs.

ASYMPTOMATIC PATIENTS

- Screening should be carried out in all sexually active adolescents. As well, if a patient's history includes one or more of the features listed below they are at an increased risk for acquiring an STI:
  » Being a victim of sexual assault or abuse
  » History suggestive of sexual contact with a person with a known STI
  » History of previous STI
  » Previously having been a patient of an STI clinic
  » Having a new sexual partner or > 2 sexual partners in the last year
  » Injection drug use and/or other substance use, especially if associated with sexual activity
  » Unsafe sexual practices (e.g., unprotected sex) or sexual activities with risk of blood exchange (e.g., sadomasochism or sharing of sex toys)
  » Anonymous sexual partnering (e.g., meeting online, in a bathhouse, at a rave)
  » Engaging in sex work / hiring sex workers
  » "Survival sex" (sex in exchange for money, shelter, clothing, food)
  » History of street involvement or homelessness
  » Having spent time in a detention facility
  » Being a victim of sexual assault or abuse

SYMPTOMATIC PATIENTS

- All patients with a presenting complaint suggestive of

an STI should be tested, regardless of their history of sexual activity.

- Symptoms include:
  » Penile or vaginal discharge
  » Dysuria
  » Abdominal pain
  » Testicular pain
  » Genital rashes
  » Genital lesions
  » Systemic symptoms — fever, weight loss, lymphadenopathy
- Particular attention should be paid to adolescent females presenting with lower abdominal pain or genitourinary (GU) symptoms.

Screening Tests

CHLAMYDIA

- Nucleic acid amplification testing (NAAT) can be performed on urine, urethral swabs, and vaginal or cervical swabs.
- Culture of cervical or urethral specimen is the test of choice for medico-legal cases (e.g., child abuse).

GONORRHEA

- Use NAAT.

SYPHILIS

- Use serologic testing.
  » Treponema-specific enzyme immunoassay (EIA) (e.g., FTA-ABS and TP-PA) is more sensitive than nontreponemal tests (e.g. RPR, VDRL), but testing algorithms vary across jurisdictions.
  » A second test is required to confirm an initial positive result.

HIV

- Conduct a serum EIA initial screening test followed by western blot or other confirmatory test.

Diagnosis

- Identify the presenting complaint.
- Obtain a brief history and STI risk assessment (see the screening guidelines above for asymptomatic and symptomatic patients to guide questioning).
  » It is important to attempt to speak with adolescents without a parent or caregiver present.
  » Be sure to discuss the limits of confidentiality.
- Perform a focused physical exam based on the findings from the patient's history.

Physical Exam

- Parent/caregiver may be present for the exam if patient desires.

- Asymptomatic adolescent patients do not require a genital exam.
- General assessment of adolescents involves:
  » Assessing patient for systemic signs of STIs:
    › Weight loss, fever, enlarged lymph nodes
  » Examining:
    › Mucocutaneous regions, including pharynx
    › External genitalia for cutaneous lesions, inflammation, genital discharge, and anatomical irregularities
    › Perianal area
  » Considering anoscopy or digital rectal exam if anal symptoms are present

Males

- Palpate scrotal contents with attention to the epididymis.
- Retract foreskin to inspect the glans.
- Have the patient or healthcare provider "milk" the urethra to make any discharge more apparent.

Females

- Separate labia to adequately visualize the vaginal orifice.
- Conduct a speculum examination to visualize the cervix and vaginal walls and to evaluate endocervical and vaginal discharges.
  » Obtain specimens as indicated.
  » In the case of primary genital herpes or vaginitis, speculum examination may be deferred until acute symptoms have subsided.
- Perform a bimanual pelvic examination to detect uterine or adnexal masses or tenderness.
  » In the case of primary genital herpes or vaginitis, bimanual examination may be deferred until acute symptoms have subsided.

Investigations

- Select the appropriate screening/investigations; see "Specific Cases and Syndromes," below.

Management

- Determine the appropriate management and follow-up; see specific cases below.
  » Many STIs are reportable — check local provincial/territorial regulations.
  » Testing and treatment for coinfections are often required.
  » Partner notification may be required.
  » Recommend that the patient abstain from unprotected intercourse during treatment or until symptoms resolve.
- For sexual assault, see Chapter 1.7.

SPECIFIC CASES AND SYNDROMES

ASYMPTOMATIC PATIENT AT RISK FOR AN STI

Investigations

- The following are recommended investigations:
  » First-catch urine and/or urethral or cervical swab for *Neisseria gonorrhoeae* and *Chlamydia trachomatis*
  » Serology for syphilis, HIV
    › Consider serology for:
      · Hepatitis A — particularly with oral/anal contact
      · Hepatitis B — if no history of vaccine
      · Hepatitis C — particularly if history of injection drug use
- Consider a Pap test for female patients.

Management

- No specific treatment is indicated at the time of testing.
- Follow-up is recommend pending test results.
- If follow-up is not guaranteed or is unlikely, treat the patient empirically for chlamydia and gonorrhea (see "Recommended Treatment of Uncomplicated Gonococcal Infections in Children and Youth," below).

URETHRITIS

- Symptoms include:
  » Urethral discharge
  » Burning on urination
  » Irritation in the distal urethra or meatus
  » Meatal erythema

Investigations

- The following are recommended investigations:
  » Urethral swab for Gram stain and culture for gonorrhea
    › NAAT where available; however, NAAT does not provide antibiotic susceptibility
  » First-catch urine for *C. trachomatis* (NAAT)

Management

- Treat the patient empirically for chlamydia and gonorrhea based on index of suspicion and prospects of follow-up (see "Recommended Treatment of Uncomplicated Gonococcal Infections in Children and Youth," below).
- Resolution of symptoms can take up to 7 days after completion of therapy.
  » Follow up with the patient if symptoms persist after this time.

- Recommend that the patient abstain from unprotected intercourse until treatment is complete.
- Treat the patient's partner(s).

CERVICITIS

- Symptoms include:
  » Mucopurulent cervical discharge
  » Cervical friability
  » Vaginal discharge
  » Strawberry cervix

Investigations

- The following are recommended investigations:
  » Vaginal or cervical swab for Gram stain
    › *N. gonorrhoeae* (culture) and *C. trachomatis* (NAAT or culture)
  » Swab of cervical lesions (if present) for HSV
  » Vaginal swab for wet mount

Management

- Treat the patient empirically for chlamydia and gonorrhea based on index of suspicion and prospects of follow-up (see "Recommended Treatment of Uncomplicated Gonococcal Infections in Children and Youth," below).
- Testing for cure 3 to 4 weeks posttreatment is recommended for persistent symptoms, pregnant adolescents, and prepubertal children, or if second-line therapy was used.
- Recommend that the patient abstain from unprotected intercourse until treatment is complete.
- Treat the patient's partner(s).

SUSPECTED PHARYNGEAL GONOCOCCAL INFECTION

- Patients may have:
  » History of oral sex
  » Sore throat
  » Tonsillar exudate
  » Cervical/tonsillar lymphadenopathy

Investigations

- Obtain a swab of the posterior pharynx and tonsillar crypts.
  » Use the swab to directly inoculate appropriate culture medium or place in transport medium.

Management

- Treat the patient for chlamydia and gonorrhea (see "Recommended Treatment of Uncomplicated Gonococcal Infections in Children and Youth," below).
- Follow-up testing by culture is recommended 3 to 4 days posttreatment or NAAT 3 to 4 weeks posttreatment.

GENITAL ULCER DISEASE

Physical Exam

- Possible pathogens and associated clinical presentation / symptoms include:
  » HSV (95% of STI-related cases of general ulcer disease [GUD])
    › Grouped vesicles evolve toward superficial circular ulcers on an erythematous base.
    › Enlarged, nonfluctuant, tender inguinal lymph nodes appear in primary infection.
    › Ulcers are painful and/or pruritic.
    › Patients experience genital pain.
    › Constitutional symptoms in primary infection are fever, malaise, and pharyngitis.
  » Primary syphilis
    › Papule evolves to painless chancre.
    › Chancre is indurated with serous exudates.
    › There is a single ulcer in 70% of cases.
    › A firm, enlarged, nonfluctuant, nontender lymphadenopathy is common.
  » Chancroid
    › Single or multiple necrotizing and painful ulcers are present.
      › 2 or more ulcers are present in 50% of cases.
    › Often, there is painful swelling and suppuration of regional lymph nodes with erythema and edema of overlying skin.
  » Lymphogranuloma venereum
    › Lymphogranuloma venereum is characterized by a single, self-limited, painless papule that may ulcerate, followed some weeks later by tender inguinal and/or femoral lymphadenopathy (mostly unilateral) and/or proctocolitis.
    › If not treated, fibrosis can lead to fistulas and strictures and/or obstruction of lymphatic drainage, causing elephantiasis.
    › Signs and symptoms are like those of urethritis.
  » Granuloma inguinale
    › Granuloma inguinale is characterized by one or multiple progressive ulcerative lesions.
      · There are 2 or more lesions in 50% of cases.
    › Lesions are highly vascular ("beefy red" appearance).
    › Lesions bleed easily on contact.
    › There are hypertrophic, necrotic, and sclerotic variants of granuloma inguinale.
    › Relapse can occur 6 to 18 months after apparently effective therapy.
    › Condition is painless.

Differential Diagnosis

- Consider non-STI–related causes on the differential diagnosis:
  » Infectious:
    › *Candida*
    › CMV
    › *Varicella* or herpes zoster
    › EBV
    › Bacterial infection (e.g., streptococcal/staphylococcal infection)
    › Parasite (e.g., scabies)
  » Noninfectious:
    › Contact dermatitis
    › Erythema multiforme
    › Autoimmune disease
    › Pyoderma gangrenosum
    › Crohn's disease
    › Carcinoma
    › Trauma
    › Idiopathic (12% to 51%)

Investigations

- Minimum testing for all cases of GUD should include a viral identification test for HSV and syphilis serology.
- Biopsies, cultures, smears, and serology should be ordered as appropriate for evaluation of all vulvar ulcers.

Management

- Obtain early referral to a physician experienced in STI-related GUDs, especially if the patient:
  » Has a history of travel
  » Is a male who has sex with males
  » Is HIV positive
  » Is immunocompromised
  » Has systemic disease
- Provide treatment at the time of presentation for genital herpes in almost all cases, especially if symptoms are typical (see "Genital Herpes," below).
  » Analgesia and laxatives may be required.
  » Urinary retention may be an indicator for hospitalization.
- Treat the patient for chancroid if the presentation warrants it; consider:
  » Ciprofloxacin 10 mg/kg to a maximum of 500 mg PO one time (cure rate of > 90%)
  » Azithromycin 20 mg/kg up to a maximum of 1 g PO one time
  » Ceftriaxone 10 mg/kg up to a maximum of 250 mg IM one time (failure is ssen in patients with HIV coinfection)

EPIDIDYMITIS

Physical Exam

- Symptoms include:
  » Unilateral testicular pain and tenderness (gradual onset)
  » Tenderness on palpation of affected side
  » Palpable swelling of epididymis

» Urethral discharge
» Hydrocele
» Erythema and/or edema of affected side
» Fever
- Sexually transmitted urethritis is a predisposing factor for epididymitis.

Differential Diagnosis

- Consider testicular torsion on the differential diagnosis (see Chapter 16.1).
  » Testicular torsion is a **surgical emergency**.
  » It is more common in patients < 20 years old.
  » It usually has a sudden onset of severe pain.
  » Consult a surgeon immediately if diagnosis is questionable.

Investigations

- The following are recommended investigations:
  » Doppler ultrasound to distinguish from testicular torsion
  » Urethral swab for Gram stain
  » Test for *Neisseria gonorrhoeae* and *Chlamydia trachomatis*
  » Microscopy and culture of midstream urine

Management

- If epididymitis is most likely caused by chlamydia or gonorrhea, manage according to guidelines in "Recommended Treatment of Uncomplicated Gonococcal Infections in Children and Youth," below.
- If it is most likely caused by enteric organisms, recommended treatment is ofloxacin 200 mg PO twice daily for 14 days.

PELVIC INFLAMMATORY DISEASE

- Pelvic inflammatory disease (PID) is an infection of the female upper genital tract and can involve any combination of the endometrium, fallopian tubes, pelvic peritoneum, and contiguous structures.
- There are approximately 100 000 cases of PID annually in Canada.
- An estimated 10% to 15% of females of reproductive age have had one episode.
- Long-term sequelae include tubal infertility, ectopic pregnancy, and chronic pelvic pain.

Physical Exam

- No single historical or physical exam finding is sensitive or specific.
- Symptoms include:
  » Lower abdominal tenderness
  » Adnexal tenderness
  » Cervical motion tenderness
  » Oral temperature > 38.3°C

Investigations

- The following are recommended investigations:
  » Complete abdominal and pelvic exam, including examination of external genitalia and speculum/bimanual exam
  » Serum beta human chorionic gonadotropin (hCG) to rule out ectopic pregnancy
  » Endocervical swabs for *N. gonorrhoeae* and *C. trachomatis*
  » Sampling of cervical lesions for HSV
  » Vaginal swabs for culture, pH testing, amine odor whiff test, normal saline and potassium hydroxide wet preparations, and Gram stain to assess for bacterial vaginosis
  » Ultrasound
    › Ultrasound can aid in diagnosis but normal ultrasound does not rule out PID.
  » Other lab investigations:
    › Complete blood count (CBC), erythrocyte sedimentation rate (ESR), C-reactive protein (CRP), endometrial biopsy
- Obtain a consultation with a colleague experienced in the treatment of PID if there are any concerns or diagnostic uncertainty.

Management

- Consider consulting a colleague who is experienced in the treatment of PID.
- Early diagnosis and management are key to maintaining fertility.
- Hospitalization may be required for youth/adolescents or if any of the following are present:
  » Physician is unable to exclude surgical emergency
  » Patient:
    › Has issues with compliance
    › Is pregnant
    › Does not respond to oral antimicrobial therapy
    › Is unable to follow or tolerate outpatient regimen
    › Is severely ill
    › Has tubo-ovarian abscess
- Treatment regimens should provide broad coverage for *N. gonorrhoeae*, *C. trachomatis*, gram-negative bacteria, and *Streptococcus*.
  » Inpatient treatment:
    › First-line treatment:
      · Cefoxitin and doxycycline
    › Second-line treatment:
      · Clindamycin and gentamicin
    › Alternatives to consider:
      · Ofloxacin or levofloxacin and metronidazole
      · Ampicillin/sulbactam and doxycycline
      · Ciprofloxacin and doxycycline with or without metronidazole

» Outpatient treatment:
  › See "Recommended Treatment of Uncomplicated Gonococcal Infections in Children and Youth," below
  › Recommend adding metronidazole for 14 days to provide anaerobic coverage

VAGINAL DISCHARGE

- The 3 most common infections with vaginal discharge are:
  » Bacterial vaginosis (BV) — not usually considered sexually transmitted
  » Vulvovaginal candidiasis — not usually considered sexually transmitted
  » Trichomoniasis — sexually transmitted
- Vaginal discharge is occasionally seen in cervicitis as a result of *N. gonorrhoeae* and/or *C. trachomatis* (see "Cervicitis," above).

- Noninfectious causes of vaginal discharge include:
  » Excessive physiologic secretions
  » Foreign bodies
  » Irritant or allergic dermatitis
  » Skin disorders such as lichen planus or psoriasis
- If on-site microscopy is not available:
  » Use complaint of vaginal discharge, history, and physical exam to determine if the patient is at risk for an STI.
    › If the patient is at risk for an STI, the patient's partner is symptomatic, or the patient presents with fever or lower abdominal tenderness, manage for *N. gonorrhoeae*, *C. trachomatis*, *T. vaginalis*, and BV.
    › If patient has none of the above features, treat for *T. vaginalis*, BV, and vulvovaginal candidiasis, and provide education and counseling.

Table 10.9.2. COMMON CAUSES OF VAGINAL DISCHARGE: THEIR DIAGNOSTIC FEATURES, INVESTIGATIONS, AND MANAGEMENT

Source: © All rights reserved. *Canadian Guidelines on Sexually Transmitted Infections.* Public Health Agency of Canada, 2013. Adapted and reproduced with permission from the Minister of Health, 2017.

	Bacterial vaginosis	Candidiasis	Trichomoniasis
Sexual transmission	• Not usually considered sexually transmitted	• Not usually considered sexually transmitted	• Sexually transmitted
Predisposing factors	• Often absent • More common if sexually active • New sexual partner • IUD use	• Often absent • More common if sexually active • Current or recent antibiotic use • Pregnancy • Corticosteroids • Poorly controlled diabetes • Immunocompromised	• Multiple partners
Symptoms	• Vaginal discharge • Fishy odor • 50% asymptomatic	• Vaginal discharge • Itch • External dysuria • Superficial dyspareunia • Up to 20% asymptomatic	• Vaginal discharge • Itch • Dysuria • 10% to 50% asymptomatic
Signs	• White or gray, thin, copious discharge	• White, clumpy, curdy discharge • Erythema and edema of vagina and vulva	• Off-white or yellow, frothy discharge • Erythema of vulva and cervix ("strawberry cervix")
Vaginal pH	• > 4.5	• < 4.5	• > 4.5
Wet mount	• PMNs • Clue cells*	• Budding yeast • Pseudohyphae	• Motile flagellated protozoa (38% to 82% sensitivity)†
Gram stain	• Clue cells* • Decreased normal flora • Predominant gram-negative curved bacilli and coccobacilli	• PMNs • Budding yeast • Pseudohyphae	• PMNs • Trichomonads
Whiff test	• Positive	• Negative	• Negative
Preferred treatment	• Metronidazole • Clindamycin	• Antifungals	• Metronidazole • Treat partner

PMNs polymorphonuclear leukocytes.

*Clue cells are vaginal epithelial cells covered with numerous coccobacilli.

†Culture is more sensitive than microscopy for *T. vaginalis*.

RECOMMENDED TREATMENT OF UNCOMPLICATED GONOCOCCAL INFECTIONS IN CHILDREN AND YOUTH

Management

General Principles

- Treat the patient concurrently for chlamydia and gonorrhea due to the high incidence of co-infection.
- A combination gonorrhea infection therapy is recommended in response to increasing antimicrobial resistance.
- Macrolide (azithromycin) is the preferred treatment for chlamydia.
  - » **Single dose, directly-observed therapy works best.**

Management in Children 9 Years of Age and Older

- Treat with:
  - » Ceftriaxone 250 mg IM (one dose) **and** azithromycin 1 g PO (one dose)
  — or —
  - » Cefixime 800 mg PO (one does) **and** azithromycin 1 g PO (one dose)
- If the patient has a history of severe allergy to cephalosporins, azithromycin 2 g PO (one dose) monotherapy can be used, but there is a risk of treatment failure.
- Doxycycline 100 mg PO twice daily for 7 days can be used in this age group as an alternative to azithromycin but is contraindicated in:
  - » Pregnant and breastfeeding females
  - » Patients for whom compliance is an issue
  - » Tetracycline-resistant strains

Management in Children Younger than 9

- Treat with:
  - » Ceftriaxone 50 mg/kg IM (one dose to a maximum of 250 mg) **and** azithromycin 20 mg/kg PO (one dose to a maximum of 1 g)
  — or —
  - » Cefixime 8 mg/kg PO twice daily (once every 12 hours) for one day (to a maximum of 400 mg/dose) **and** azithromycin 20 mg/kg PO (one dose to a maximum of 1 g)

Management in Neonates (Birth to 1 Month of Age)

- Treat with ceftriaxone 25 to 50 mg/kg IM (one dose to a maximum of 125 mg).
- Routine combination therapy with a macrolide is not recommended due to the association of macrolide therapy with pyloric stenosis.

- Initiate azithromycin therapy if infection with *C. trachomatis* is confirmed.
  - » **For disseminated infection treat with cefotaxime 50 mg/kg IV/IM every 6 hours for 10 to 14 days.**

GENITAL HERPES

Management

First Episode

- In severe cases, treat with:
  - » Acyclovir 5 mg/per kg IV over 60 minutes every 8 hours.
    - › Convert to oral therapy when substantial improvement is seen.
- In mild/moderate cases, treat with:
  - » Acyclovir 200 mg PO 5 times per day for 5 to 10 days
  — or —
  - » Famciclovir 250 mg PO 3 times a day for 5 days
  — or —
  - » Valacyclovir 1000 mg PO 2 times a day for 10 days

Note: Acyclovir 400 mg PO 2 times a day for 7 to 10 days is recommended by the U.S. Centers for Disease Control.

Recurrent Episodes

- Treat with:
  - » Valacyclovir at a dose of **either** 500 mg PO 2 times daily **or** 1 g PO once daily for 3 days
  — or —
  - » Famciclovir 125 mg PO 2 times a day for 5 days
  — or —
  - » Acyclovir 200 mg PO 5 times a day for 5 days

Note: A shorter course of acyclovir 800 mg PO 3 times a day for 2 days appears to be as efficacious as the approved 5-day regimen.

REFERENCES

Allen UD, MacDonald NE; Canadian Paediatric Society, Infectious Diseases and Immunization Committee. Sexually transmitted infections in adolescents: Maximizing opportunities for optimal care. *Paediatr Child Health.* 2014;19(8):429–439. Medline:25383001

Anaene M, Soyemi K, Caskey R. Factors associated with the overtreatment and under-treatment of gonorrhea and chlamydia in adolescents presenting to a public hospital emergency department. *Int J Infect Dis.* 2016;53:34–38. https://doi.org/10.1016/j.ijid.2016.10.009. Medline:27771470

Bonar EE, Walton MA, Caldwell MT, Whiteside LK, Barry KL, Cunningham RM. Sexually transmitted infection history among adolescents presenting to the emergency department. *J Emerg Med.* 2015;49(5):613–622. https://doi.org/10.1016/j.jemermed.2015.02.017. Medline:25952707

Goyal M, Hayes K, Mollen C. Sexually transmitted infection prevalence in symptomatic adolescent emergency department patients. *Pediatr Emerg Care.* 2012;28(12):1277–1280. https://doi.org/10.1097/PEC.0b013e3182767d7c. Medline:23187982

Goyal MK, Teach SJ, Badolato GM, Trent M, Chamberlain JM. Universal screening for sexually transmitted infections among asymptomatic adolescents in an urban emergency department: high acceptance but low prevalence of infection. *J Pediatr*. 2016;171:128–132. https://doi.org/10.1016/j.jpeds.2016.01.019. Medline:26846572

Jain N. Sexually transmitted diseases in the pediatric patient. *BCMJ*. 2004;46(3):133–138.

Lester R, Montgomery C, Arnold B, et al. British Columbia treatment guidelines: sexually transmitted infections in adolescents and adults [Internet]. Vancouver, BC: BC Centre for Disease Control; 2014 August [cited 2018 Apr 11]. Available from: http://www.bccdc.ca/resource-gallery/Documents/Communicable-Disease-Manual/Chapter%205%20-%20STI/CPS_BC_STI_Treatment_Guidelines_20112014.pdf

Public Health Agency of Canada. Section 4-1: Canadian guidelines on sexually transmitted infections – Management and treatment of specific infections – Syndromic approach [Internet]. Ottawa, ON: Government of Canada; 2013 February [cited 2018 Apr 11]. Available from: https://www.canada.ca/en/public-health/services/infectious-diseases/sexual-health-sexually-transmitted-infections/canadian-guidelines/sexually-transmitted-infections/canadian-guidelines-sexually-transmitted-infections-19.html

Public Health Agency of Canada. Section 5-6: Canadian guidelines on sexually transmitted infections – Management and treatment of specific infections – Gonococcal infections [Internet]. Ottawa, ON: Government of Canada; 2013 July [updated 2017 August; cited 2017 Mar 9]. Available from: https://www.canada.ca/en/public-health/services/infectious-diseases/sexual-health-sexually-transmitted-infections/canadian-guidelines/sexually-transmitted-infections/canadian-guidelines-sexually-transmitted-infections-34.html

Public Health Agency of Canada. Canadian guidelines on sexually transmitted infections: supplementary statement for the management and follow-up of sexual abuse in postpubertal adolescents and adults [Internet]. Ottawa, ON: Government of Canada; 2014 October [cited 2018 Apr 11]. Available from: https://www.canada.ca/en/public-health/services/infectious-diseases/sexual-health-sexually-transmitted-infections/canadian-guidelines/sexually-transmitted-infections/canadian-guidelines-sexually-transmitted-infections-14.html

Public Health Agency of Canada. Canadian guidelines on sexually transmitted infections: supplementary statement for the management and follow-up of sexual abuse in peripubertal and prepubertal children [Internet]. Ottawa, ON: Government of Canada; 2014 October [cited 2018 Apr 11]. Available from: https://www.canada.ca/en/public-health/services/infectious-diseases/sexual-health-sexually-transmitted-infections/canadian-guidelines/sexually-transmitted-infections/canadian-guidelines-sexually-transmitted-infections-15.html

Public Health Agency of Canada. Executive Summary. Report on Sexually Transmitted Infections in Canada: 2013–2014 [Internet]. Ottawa, ON: Government of Canada; 2017 April. [cited 2018 Apr 11] Available from: https://www.canada.ca/en/public-health/services/publications/diseases-conditions/report-sexually-transmitted-infections-canada-2013-14.html#s3

Public Health Agency of Canada. Canadian guidelines on sexually transmitted infections [Internet]. Ottawa, ON: Government of Canada; 2017 [updated 2018 Feb 18; cited 2018 Apr 11]. Available from: https://www.canada.ca/en/public-health/services/infectious-diseases/sexual-health-sexually-transmitted-infections/canadian-guidelines/sexually-transmitted-infections.html

Schneider K, FitzGerald M, Byczkowski T, Reed J. Screening for asymptomatic gonorrhea and chlamydia in the pediatric emergency department. *Sex Transm Dis*. 2016;43(4):209–215. https://doi.org/10.1097/OLQ.0000000000000424. Medline:26967296

Toronto Public Health. STI Treatment Reference Guide [Internet]. Toronto, ON: Peel Health and York Region Health Services; 2017 [cited 2017 Apr 1]. Available from: https://www.toronto.ca/wp-content/uploads/2017/12/9390-tph-sti-treatment-guide-2017.pdf

Uppal A, Chou KJ. Screening adolescents for sexually transmitted infections in the pediatric emergency department. *Pediatr Emerg Care*. 2015;31(1):20–24. https://doi.org/10.1097/PEC.0000000000000322. Medline:25526018

van Schalkwyk J, Yudin MH; Infectious Disease Committee. Vulvovaginitis: screening for and management of trichomoniasis, vulvovaginal candidiasis, and bacterial vaginosis. *J Obstet Gynaecol Can*. 2015;37(3):266–274. https://doi.org/10.1016/S1701-2163(15)30316-9. Medline:26001874

10.10

Cervical Lymphadenitis

Ahmed Alterkait

- Lymphadenopathy is defined as abnormal lymph nodes either due to an increase in size (> 1–1.5 cm) and/or change in consistency.
  » Lymph nodes larger than 2 cm are considered pathologic.
- Cervical lymphadenopathy is a common presentation to the emergency department (ED).
- 38% to 45% of normal children may have palpable lymph nodes on examination.
- Cervical lymphadenitis usually presents as a neck mass, which can pose a diagnostic challenge due to the large differential diagnosis (see "Differential Diagnosis," below).
  » The most common causes of cervical lymphadenitis are infectious.
  » In developing countries, tuberculosis (TB) is a cause of cervical lymphadenitis that presents a major challenge.
- Lymphadenitis is associated with symptoms such as:
  » Fever
  » Pain
  » Skin discoloration
  » Swelling
  » Abscess formation
  » Purulent discharge

Anatomy of Cervical Lymph Nodes

- The location of affected lymph nodes will help indicate the source of entry of the causative organism.
- The superficial cervical chain (superficial to the sterno-cleidomastoid) is divided into anterior (located along the anterior jugular vein) and posterior (located along the external jugular vein).
  - » Enlargement of this group of lymph nodes indicates a portal of entry through an epithelial surface such as the skin or buccal mucosa.
    - › These nodes also drain the mastoid, tissues of the neck and parotid and submaxillary lymph nodes.
- The deep cervical chain (deep to the sternocleidomas-toid) includes:
  - » Superior lymph nodes — found below the angle of the mandible
  - » Inferior lymph nodes — located at the base of the neck
- Infected lymph nodes in the superior deep cervical chain result from infections in the middle ear, oral cavity, or pharynx.

Diagnosis

Noninfectious Causes

- Noninfectious causes of lymphadenopathy are:
  - » Malignancy
    - › Lymphoma
    - › Neuroblastoma
    - › Rhabdomyosarcoma
  - » Kawasaki disease
  - » Collagen vascular disease
  - » Postvaccination
  - » Histiocytosis
  - » Immunodeficiency
    - › Leukocyte adhesion defect
    - › Chronic granulomatous disease
    - › Hyper-IgE syndrome
  - » Drugs

Infectious Causes

- The most common cause of cervical lymphadenitis is reactive hyperplasia, which is usually associated with viral infections that cause upper respiratory tract infections (URTI).
- *Staphylococcus aureus* and *Streptococcus pyogenes* (Group A *Streptococcus*) are the most common bacterial causes of local cervical lymphadenitis.
- Nontuberculous (atypical) mycobacteria are a common cause of chronic lymphadenitis in children.
- Infectious causes of cervical lymphadenitis are:
  - » Viral:
    - › Adenovirus
    - › Coxsackievirus
    - › Epstein-Barr virus (EBV) / cytomegalovirus (CMV)
    - › Herpes simplex
    - › HIV
    - › Influenza
    - › Parainfluenza
    - › Respiratory syncytial virus (RSV)
    - › Varicella
    - › Vaccine viruses:
      - · Rubella
      - · Measles
      - · Mumps
  - » Bacterial:
    - › *Staphylococcus aureus* and methicillin-resistant *Staphylococcus aureus* (MRSA)
    - › Group A *Streptococcus*
    - › Group B *Streptococcus*
    - › Anaerobes
    - › *Corynebacterium diphtheriae*
    - › *Bartonella henselae*
    - › Mycobacteria:
      - · *Mycobacterium tuberculosis*
      - · *Mycobacterium avium-intracellulare*
      - · *Mycobacterium scrofulaceum*
  - » Fungal:
    - › *Aspergillus fumigatus*
    - › *Candida* sp.
    - › Dermatophytes
    - › *Histoplasma capsulatum*
  - » Protozoan:
    - › *Toxoplasma gondii*
    - › *Leishmania* sp.

Differential Diagnosis

- In a child presenting with a neck mass, it is important to consider other causes that mimic lymphadenopathy.
  - » Neck masses can be divided into inflammatory, congenital, and traumatic.
  - » Consider the following on the differential diagnosis of neck mass in children:
    - › Mumps
    - › Thyroglossal cyst
    - › Branchial cleft cyst
    - › Sternocleidomastoid tumor
    - › Cervical rib
    - › Dermoid cyst
    - › Cystic hygroma
    - › Hemangioma
    - › Nodular goiter

History

- Collect appropriate age-related information.
  - » In newborns, unilateral cervical lymphadenitis can be caused by *Staphylococcus aureus* or group B *Streptococcus*.

» Adenitis-cellulitis syndrome may be seen in 3- to 7-week-old infants with a history of fever, poor feeding, and neck swelling with overlying cellulitis.
» The majority of cases of bacterial and atypical mycobacterial cervical lymphadenitis present in children < 5 years of age.
» More chronic causes of lymphadenitis are associated with older children and adolescents:
  › EBV, CMV
  › Toxoplasmosis
  › *Bartonella henselae*
  › Anaerobes from dental disease
• Collect information about symptoms, including:
  » Lymph node characteristics
    › Infected lymph nodes can be significantly enlarged with associated signs of inflammation, cellulitis, and high-grade fever.
    › In late stages of atypical mycobacterial infections, involved lymph nodes can become fluctuant and overlying skin will appear violaceous.
  » Involvement of other lymph node regions
    › This may indicate generalized lymphadenopathy.
  » Signs of URTI such as cough or rhinorrhea
    › These suggest a viral etiology.
  » Systemic symptoms such as fever, anorexia, weight loss, rashes, or joint pain

Symptom Duration and Acuity

• Ask about symptom duration and determine acuity.

ACUTE LYMPHADENITIS

• Acute lymphadenitis has a typical duration of 2 weeks and is caused by either a bacterial or viral infection.
• Acute lymphadenitis may be unilateral or bilateral.
  » Unilateral lymphadenitis
    › The acute presentation of unilateral lymphadenitis is more likely caused by bacterial infection, with the submandibular gland involved in more than 50% of cases.
    › It is commonly caused by *Staphylococcus aureus* or *Streptococcus pyogenes* (group A *Streptococcus*).
    › MRSA should be considered in cases unresponsive to antibiotic therapy.
  » Bilateral lymphadenitis
    › Bilateral lymphadenitis is caused by viral infection of the upper respiratory tract.
    › Group A *Streptococcus* can cause bilateral lymphadenitis associated with pharyngitis, impetigo, or scarlet fever.

SUBACUTE/CHRONIC LYMPHADENITIS

• Subacute/chronic lymphadenitis has a duration of more than 2 weeks.
  » Viral causes include EBV and CMV.
    › These can present over weeks with bilateral enlarged cervical lymph nodes or generalized lymphadenopathy.
  » Common bacterial causes include TB, atypical mycobacteria and catscratch disease (*Bartonella henselae*).
    › Presentation can be similar to unilateral acute bacterial lymphadenitis but is usually more insidious and occurs over weeks to months.
  » Chronic lymphadenitis is more often due to opportunistic infections such as HIV or a neoplastic process.

Other Factors

• Other important factors to consider on history include:
  » Dental pain, periodontal disease, and/or dental abscess
  » Exposure to animals and insect bites
    › Exposure to cats increases risk of catscratch disease, which:
      · Leads to chronic unilateral lymphadenopathy and constitutional symptoms
      · May cause suppuration of lymphadenopathy
      · Can lead to Parinaud oculoglandular syndrome (conjunctivitis and periauricular or submandibular lymphadenopathy) with ocular inoculation
    › Tularemia, brucellosis, and *Yersinia pestis* are associated with contact with animals or infected ticks and can result in regional lymphadenopathy.
  » Skin lesions, which can occur in the following infections:
    › Catscratch disease
    › Tularemia
    › Anthrax
    › Plague
    › Scrub typhus
    › African trypanosomiasis
    › Cutaneous leishmaniasis
  » Contact with sick persons
    › Viral causes of cervical lymphadenopathy are highly contagious.
    › Streptococcal pharyngitis can also be infectious.
    › Ask about contact with persons with TB symptoms or history of travel to endemic areas.
  » Constitutional symptoms associated with painless cervical (or generalized) lymphadenopathy
    › These can be a result of noninfectious causes (see "Noninfectious Causes," above).
  » Recent travel to endemic areas or rural regions
  » Recurrent infections
    › Recurrent cervical lymphadenitis is a common presentation of chronic granulomatous disease.
  » Immunization status
    › Almost all vaccine-preventable diseases can cause lymphadenitis.

Physical Exam

• Examination of the neck should assess infected lymph node characteristics, the number of lymph nodes involved, and the distribution of the involved lymph nodes.

- In bacterial cervical lymphadenitis, the lymph nodes are usually enlarged, erythematous, and tender.
- The physical exam should include an assessment of all lymph nodes regions, including axillary and inguinal lymph nodes.
- It is also important to examine the following:
  » Chest — for respiratory findings
  » Liver and spleen — to assess for organomegaly
  » Dentition — for evidence of dental disease and dental abscess
  » Pharynx — for vesicles that result from enteroviruses and to assess for signs of pharyngitis, which can be associated with group A *Streptococcus* or diphtheria
  » Conjunctiva — for conjunctivitis associated with catscratch disease or adenovirus
  » Skin — for rashes associated with viral infections, lesions, and petechiae and ecchymosis that could be associated with malignancy

Investigations

- See *Table 10.10.1* (below) for investigations related to specific viral causes of cervical lymphadenitis.

ACUTE CERVICAL LYMPHADENITIS

- Laboratory testing is usually not required to identify the causative organism.
- If lymph node is fluctuant or an abscess is confirmed, surgical drainage is indicated.
  » Send drained fluid for Gram stain and culture.
- In bacterial infections, complete blood count (CBC) will show left shift.
  » CBC may also show atypical lymphocytosis in infectious mononucleosis.
- Obtain a pharyngeal swab and culture if a group A beta-hemolytic streptococci infection is suspected.
- A blood culture is indicated if patient is toxic-looking and febrile.

SUBACUTE/CHRONIC CERVICAL LYMPHADENITIS

- Chronic presentations require more an extensive workup to rule out infectious and noninfectious causes.
- Viral serologies and liver function tests for EBV/CMV should be considered in patients with pharyngitis, bilateral lymphadenopathy, or hepatosplenomegaly.
- Infectious workup should include investigations for TB and HIV.
- Order a purified protein derivative (PPD), tuberculin skin test, and chest X-ray (CXR) for patients at risk of developing TB.
- If atypical mycobacteria are suspected, material from the lymph node should be sent for acid-fast stain, histology, and culture.
  » Histology will show noncaseating granulomas.
- Catscratch disease is diagnosed by serology or polymerase chain reaction (PCR).
- HIV serologic testing should be considered in patients with generalized lymphadenopathy and a history of opportunistic infections.

Imaging

- Imaging studies will depend on the suspected cause of the illness and the duration of symptoms.
- Plain chest radiographs are indicated:
  » For patients with respiratory symptoms
  » In cases of positive PPD test
  » To rule out malignancy
- Ultrasonography is:
  » Often helpful in differentiating types of neck masses
  » Helpful in identifying lymph nodes and collections that require surgical drainage
- Factors associated with increased risk for surgical drainage and requiring ultrasound are:
  » Patient < 1 year of age
  » Swelling duration > 3 days
  » Failure of antibiotic therapy after 24 to 48 hours

Tissue Sampling

FINE-NEEDLE ASPIRATION

- Fine-needle aspiration is diagnostic in cases of chronic/subacute cases that have failed antibiotic therapy.
- It can be performed in suppurative or fluctuant lymphadenitis to send for Gram stain, culture, and acid-fast staining.
- It can also be therapeutic in cases of bacterial fluctuant lymphadenitis.
- It is contraindicated in cases of atypical mycobacteria as it may increase the risk of developing a skin fistula, a common complication of atypical mycobacterial lymphadenitis.
- Disadvantages of fine-needle aspiration include need for sedation and difficulty with draining loculated abscesses.

EXCISIONAL BIOPSY

- Excisional biopsy is indicated in cases of chronic lymphadenopathy and suspicion of malignancy and TB.
- It is a treatment of atypical mycobacterial lymphadenitis.

Management

- The majority of cases of viral-induced cervical lymphadenopathy self-resolve and no treatment is required.
- See *Table 10.10.1* for management of common causes of cervical lymphadenitis.

Table 10.10.1. MANAGEMENT OF COMMON CAUSES OF CERVICAL LYMPHADENITIS

Infective organism	Investigations	Management
Staphylococcus aureus Group A *Streptococcus*	• CBC, inflammatory markers • Blood culture if patient is toxic-looking or immunocompromised • Ultrasound if patient is not responding to treatment or if signs of abscess • Consider lymph node needle aspiration	• PO cephalexin, cloxacillin • IV cefazolin • Amoxicillin and clavulanic acid, clindamycin, or vancomycin if MRSA suspected • Incision and drainage if abscess identified
Anaerobic bacteria	• Similar to *Staphylococcus aureus* and Group A *Steptococcus*	• Penicillin, amoxicillin and clavulanic acid, or clindamycin • Treat periodontal disease
Atypical mycobacteria	• Lymph node histology, acid-fast bacilli, and culture	• Surgical excision of infected lymph node • If surgery is not feasible, patient should be treated with a antimycobacterial regimen containing macrolides (clarithromycin or azithromycin plus ethambutol and/or rifampin)
Catscratch disease	• Serology or PCR for *Bartonella henselae*	• Self-resolving • PO antibiotics azithromycin, clarithromycin, rifampin, ciprofloxacin • Repeated node aspiration of suppurative lymph nodes

CBC complete blood count. **MRSA** methicillin-resistant Staphylococcus aureus. **PCR** polymerase chain reaction.

REFERENCES

American Academy of Pediatrics. *Red Book®: 2015 report of the committee on infectious diseases. American Academy of Pediatrics; 2015.* Section 3: Summaries of Infectious Diseases; Chapter, Diseases Caused by Nontuberculous Mycobacteria; p. 831-839.

Chiappini E, Camaioni A, Benazzo M, et al; Italian Guideline Panel for Management of Cervical Lymphadenopathy in Children. Development of an algorithm for the management of cervical lymphadenopathy in children: consensus of the Italian Society of Preventive and Social Pediatrics, jointly with the Italian Society of Pediatric Infectious Diseases and the Italian Society of Pediatric Otorhinolaryngology. *Expert Rev Anti Infect Ther.* 2015;13(12):1557–1567. https://doi.org/10.1586/14787210.2015.1096777. Medline:26558951

Darne S, Rajda T. Cervical lymphadenopathy in children-a clinical approach. *Int J Contemp Med Res.* 2016;3:1207–1210.

Golriz F, Bisset GS III, D'Amico B, et al. A clinical decision rule for the use of ultrasound in children presenting with acute inflammatory neck masses. *Pediatr Radiol.* 2017;47(4):422–428. https://doi.org/10.1007/s00247-016-3774-9. Medline:28108796

Gosche JR, Vick L. Acute, subacute, and chronic cervical lymphadenitis in children. *Semin Pediatr Surg.* 2006;15(2):99–106. https://doi.org/10.1053/j.sempedsurg.2006.02.007. Medline:16616313

Leung AK, Davies HD. Cervical lymphadenitis: etiology, diagnosis, and management. *Curr Infect Dis Rep.* 2009;11(3):183–189. https://doi.org/10.1007/s11908-009-0028-0. Medline:19366560

Leung AK, Robson WL. Childhood cervical lymphadenopathy. *J Pediatr Health Care.* 2004;18(1):3–7. https://doi.org/10.1016/S0891-5245(03)00212-8. Medline:14722499

McCulloh RJ, Alverson B. Cervical lymphadenitis. *Hosp Peds.* 2011;1(1):52–54. https://doi.org/10.1542/hpeds.2011-0016.

Peters TR, Edwards KM. Cervical lymphadenopathy and adenitis. *Pediatr Rev.* 2000;21(12):399–405. Medline:11121496

Rosenberg TL, Nolder AR. Pediatric cervical lymphadenopathy. *Otolaryngol Clin North Am.* 2014;47(5):721–731. https://doi.org/10.1016/j.otc.2014.06.012. Medline:25213279

Yaris N, Cakir M, Sözen E, Cobanoglu U. Analysis of children with peripheral lymphadenopathy. *Clin Pediatr (Phila).* 2006;45(6):544–549. https://doi.org/10.1177/0009922806290609. Medline:16893860

11.1

Conjunctivitis

April J. Kam

- Conjunctivitis is an inflammation of the conjunctivae lining the eyelids and covering the surface of the sclera.
- The etiology can be classified as:
  » Infectious
  » Irritant
  » Chemical exposure or burns
    › See Chapter 18.8 for more information on pediatric burns.
  » Allergic
- A physical exam can be challenging, especially for very young children.
- Conjunctivitis can present with unilateral or bilateral symptoms.

BACTERIAL CONJUNCTIVITIS

- The most common pathogens are *Staphylococcus aureus*, *Haemophilus influenzae*, and *Staphylococcus epidermidis*.
- Also consider specific bacterial infections in these populations:
  » Patients who are contact lens wearers — *Pseudomonas*
  » Neonates — can have vertical transmission of *Chlamydia trachomatis* and *Neisseria gonorrhoeae*

Physical Exam

- Clinical features include:
  » Bulbar conjunctiva
  » Episcleral vessels
  » Papillae in palpebral conjunctiva
  » Thick, mucopurulent discharge

Management

- Evidence suggests that antibiotics do not have a significant impact on the course of the disease.
  » Broad-spectrum topical antibiotics can be used for suspected bacterial conjunctivitis (polymyxin B, erythromycin ointment, or tobramycin ointment).
- Contact lens wearers should stop wearing lenses for the duration of the infection and be treated with fluoroquinolone.
- For neonatal infectious conjunctivitis, admit the patient to hospital, do a septic workup, and treat with intravenous antibiotics.

VIRAL CONJUNCTIVITIS

- Adenovirus is associated with epidemic keratoconjunctivitis.
  » It is highly contagious.
  » It is associated with preauricular lymphadenopathy.
- Hemorrhagic conjunctivitis is associated with adenovirus, enterovirus, and Coxsackievirus.

Physical Exam

- Clinical features include:
  » Punctate keratosis in cornea
  » Tearing
  » Redness
  » Serous discharge
  » Edema of eyelid
  » Subconjunctival hemorrhage
  » Photophobia
  » Upper respiratory tract infection (URTI) symptoms and lymphadenopathy
- If surrounding vesicles are present, herpetic eye disease should be suspected.

Management

- For suspected herpetic eye disease, obtain a referral to ophthalmology and treat with acyclovir.
- Treat patients symptomatically.

- The disease is contagious, so patients should avoid school or daycare.

ALLERGIC CONJUNCTIVITIS

- Allergic conjunctivitis can be divided into seasonal, perennial, vernal, and atopic.
  » Seasonal allergic conjunctivitis is caused by airborne pollen and is usually seen in the spring and summer.
  » Perennial allergic conjunctivitis occurs year-round.
  » Vernal allergic conjunctivitis is usually a disease of the tropics and warmer climates and is induced by nonspecific stimuli.
    › It is mediated by T-helper cells (TH-2).
  » Atopic allergic conjunctivitis is a bilateral chronic inflammation of the ocular surface and eyelid that is IgE mediated along with T-helper cells.
    › It is an allergen-induced inflammation of the conjunctiva.
    › It is a hypersensitivity reaction that is IgE mediated.

Physical Exam

- Clinical features include:
  » Itchiness
  » Chemosis
  » Tearing or clear discharge

Management

- Management of allergic conjunctivitis includes:
  » Avoidance of offending agent (if possible)
  » Artificial tears — can be used as a barrier to exposure
  » Cool compresses
  » Antihistamines
  » Mast cell stabilizers
  » Decongestants

REFERENCES

LaMattina K, Thompson L. Pediatric conjunctivitis. *Dis Mon.* 2014;60(6):231–238. https://doi.org/10.1016/j.disamonth.2014.03.002. Medline:24906667

La Rosa M, Lionetti E, Reibaldi M, et al. Allergic conjunctivitis: a comprehensive review of the literature. *Ital J Pediatr.* 2013;39(1):18. https://doi.org/10.1186/1824-7288-39-18. Medline:23497516

Sethuraman U, Kamat D. The red eye: evaluation and management. *Clin Pediatr (Phila).* 2009;48(6):588–600. https://doi.org/10.1177/0009922809333094. Medline:19357422

Wong MM, Anninger W. The pediatric red eye. *Pediatr Clin North Am.* 2014;61(3):591–606. https://doi.org/10.1016/j.pcl.2014.03.011. Medline:24852155

11.2

Chalazion and Hordeolum

April J. Kam

CHALAZION

- A chalazion is a noninfectious mass (lipogranuloma) surrounding the Meibomian gland on the eyelid.

History

- A chalazion has a longer history than, and may develop from, a hordeolum.
- Risk factors for developing a chalazion (and for recurrence) include:
  » Internal hordeolum
  » Rosacea
  » Seborrheic dermatitis
  » Blepharitis
  » Demodicosis

Physical Exam

- Chalazia may present:
  » As painless lesions
  » On an external or internal surface
  » with or without edema of the eyelid
  » with or without purulent discharge
- Diagnosis of chalazia is clinical.

Management

- Initial management is often conservative, with warm compresses and massage.
- There is little evidence supporting the use of topical antibiotics.
- Refer the patient to ophthalmology:
  » For nonresolution over several weeks

- » For consideration for specialized treatment:
  - › Intralesional triamcinolone
  - › Incision with curettage
- » To rule out malignancy, especially in cases of:
  - › Recurring lesions
  - › Lack of resolution
  - › Ulcerative changes
- Large lesions in children should be referred early to reduce the risk of amblyopia.

Complications

- A chalazion may deform the cornea, leading to astigmatism or a reduced peripheral visual field.
- Other complications include eyelid deformity, disruption of lash growth, and eyelid fistula.

HORDEOLUM (STYE)

- A hordeolum or stye is a well-defined mass at the eyelid margin often caused by a bacterial infection of an eyelash follicle.
  - » It is an infection of either:
    - › The internal meibomian sebaceous gland
    - › The external hordeolum secondary to infection or inflammation of the Zeiss or Moll sebaceous glands of the eyelid
  - » The most common bacterial source of infection is *Staphylococcus aureus*.

Physical Exam

- The hordeolum occurs at the level of the eyelash.
- It presents as a red, swollen bump that looks like a pimple.

- The mass can be tender.
- It is often self-limited to 4 to 7 days.

Management

- Conservative treatment with warm compresses is often the initial management.
- There is little evidence to support the use of topical antibiotics. but they are sometimes prescribed with coverage for *Staphylococcus* species.
- Eyelash scrubs with baby shampoo may be effective.
- If the condition persists beyond 4 weeks, surgery may be an option for uncomfortable lesions.

Complications

- A hordeolum can cause cellulitis.
- Other complications include eyelid deformity, disruption of lash growth, and eyelid fistula.

REFERENCES

Deibel JP, Cowling K. Ocular inflammation and infection. *Emerg Med Clin North Am.* 2013;31(2):387–397. https://doi.org/10.1016/j.emc.2013.01.006. Medline:23601478

Lederman C, Miller M. Hordeola and chalazia. *Pediatr Rev.* 1999;20(8):283–284. https://doi.org/10.1542/pir.20-8-283. Medline:10429150

Liang L, Ding X, Tseng SC. High prevalence of demodex brevis infestation in chalazia. *Am J Ophthalmol.* 2014;157(2):342–348.e1. https://doi.org/10.1016/j.ajo.2013.09.031. Medline:24332377

Lindsley K, Nichols JJ, Dickersin K. Interventions for acute internal hordeolum. *Cochrane Database Syst Rev.* 2013;4:CD007742. Medline:23633345

Mustafa TA, Oriafage IH. Three methods of treatment of chalazia in children. *Saudi Med J.* 2001;22(11):968–972. Medline:11744967

Sethuraman U, Kamat D. The red eye: evaluation and management. *Clin Pediatr (Phila).* 2009;48(6):588–600. https://doi.org/10.1177/0009922809333094. Medline:19357422

11.3

Hyphema

April J. Kam

- Hyphema is an accumulation of blood in the anterior chamber of the eye.
- There is a higher incidence in males than females.
- The condition is usually secondary to blunt or penetrating trauma.

- » In blunt trauma, compression of the globe results in the rupture of the ciliary blood vessels.
  - › A projectile hitting the eye can lead to stretching and displacement of the lens-iris diaphragm.
  - › Stretching can produce tears in the anterior face of the ciliary body and iris vessels.

» Penetrating trauma is direct injury to the ciliary vessels.
- Other causes of hyphema include:
  » Spontaneous occurrence
  » Retinoblastoma
  » Hematological disorders such as hemophilia, von Willebrand disease (vWD), and immune thrombocytopenia

History

- On history, collect information about:
  » Time of injury
  » Any decrease in visual acuity
  » Photophobia
  » Pain
  » Vomiting
  » Prior ophthalmological issues
  » Other head injuries
  » Prior medical history:
    › Bleeding dyscrasias
    › Sickle cell disease (SCD)

Physical Exam

- Obtain visual acuity for both eyes.
- Check for relative afferent pupillary defect.
- Measure intraocular pressure (IOP).
  » Rule out globe rupture prior to any IOP measurement.
- Conduct a slit lamp examination:
  » Look for other injuries:
    › Corneal abrasions
    › Corneal edema
    › Presence of foreign body
    › Lens subluxation
  » Look for blood in the anterior chamber, and quantify as:
    › Grade 0 — microscopic
    › Grade I — < 1/3 of anterior chamber
    › Grade II — up to 50% of anterior chamber
    › Grade III — > 50% of anterior chamber
    › Grade IV — complete (8-ball)

Management

- Restrict activity (bed rest).
- Elevate the head of the bed to 30° to 45°.

- Apply a nonpressure eyepatch.
  » Use a shield with holes in it to allow patient to have some vision.
- Obtain an ophthalmology consult.
- Provide close daily follow-up with or without hospital admission.
- Corticosteroid and cycloplegic drops are sometimes used (though there is no definitive evidence):
  » Cycloplegic drops: 1 drop of cyclopentolate given four times daily
  » Corticosteroid drops: 1 drop prednisolone 1% given four times daily
    › Use with caution in pediatric population.
- Provide analgesia.

Complications

- Complications associated with hyphema include:
  » Increased intraocular pressure
  » Corneal blood staining
  » Optic nerve damage
  » Anterior and posterior synechiae
  » Rebleeding
    › Rebleeding can cause optic nerve damage and glaucoma.
- Patients with a higher risk of complications include those with:
  » Blood in > 20% of anterior chamber
  » Rebleeding
    › The risk of rebleeding is highest in the first 4 to 7 days.
    › Patients with SCD are at increased risk for elevated intraocular pressure, optic nerve damage, and central retinal occlusion.
  » Blood not cleared beyond 3 days
  » Bleeding associated with significant trauma

REFERENCES

Agrawal R, Shah M, Mireskandari K, Yong GK. Controversies in ocular trauma classification and management: review. *Int Ophthalmol.* 2013;33(4):435–445. https://doi.org/10.1007/s10792-012-9698-y. Medline:23338232

Forbes BJ. Management of corneal abrasions and ocular trauma in children. *Pediatr Ann.* 2001;30(8):465–472. https://doi.org/10.3928/0090-4481-20010801-08. Medline:11510344

Salvin JH. Systematic approach to pediatric ocular trauma. *Curr Opin Ophthalmol.* 2007;18(5):366–372. https://doi.org/10.1097/ICU.0b013e3282ba54ac. Medline:17700228

Trief D, Adebona OT, Turalba AV, Shah AS. The pediatric traumatic hyphema. *Int Ophthalmol Clin.* 2013;53(4):43–57. https://doi.org/10.1097/IIO.0b013e3182a129fd. Medline:24088932

11.4

Orbital and Periorbital Cellulitis

April J. Kam

- The orbital septum is the anatomic distinction between orbital and periorbital cellulitis.

History

- On history, ask about:
  » Recent upper respiratory tract infection (URTI) symptoms
  » Sinus disease
  » Presence of fever
  » Dental disease or recent dental surgery

Diagnosis

Table 11.4.1. DIFFERENTIATING BETWEEN PERIORBITAL AND ORBITAL CELLULITIS

Clinical features of periorbital (preseptal) cellulitis	Clinical features of orbital (septal) cellulitis
• Eyelid pain, edema, warmth, and erythema	• Eyelid pain, edema, warmth, and erythema
• May or may not present with fever	• May or may not present with fever
• Normal visual acuity	• Decreased visual acuity
• Normal extraocular movements	• Proptosis
• Intact pupillary reflex	• Chemosis
• No proptosis	• Reduced extraocular movement
	• Pain on extraocular movement

- Orbital cellulitis can threaten sight. Look specifically for:
  » Decreased visual acuity
  » Relative afferent pupillary defect
  » Visual field changes
  » Diminished color vision

Investigations

- A clinical diagnosis can be made with periorbital cellulitis.
- Request a CT scan if orbital cellulitis is suspected.
- Request a complete blood count (CBC) with or without blood culture (low sensitivity).

PERIORBITAL (PRESEPTAL) CELLULITIS

- Periorbital cellulitis is usually seen in children < 5 years of age.
- It is a bacterial infection of the eyelid and surrounding soft tissues (anterior to the orbital septum).
- It has no globe involvement.
- It is more common than orbital cellulitis.

Pathophysiology

- There are 3 main routes of pathogen inoculation in periorbital tissue:
  1. Direct inoculation — eyelid trauma, laceration, or insect bites
  2. Contiguous spread — sinusitis, chalazia or hordeolum, dacryocystitis
  3. Hematogenous — inoculation via blood vessels from a URTI or otitis media
- Periorbital cellulitis is most commonly caused by gram-positive cocci (*Staphylococcus* and *Streptococcus* species).

Management

- Use antibiotics targeted at gram-positive organisms:
  » Cephalexin at 50 mg/kg per day divided and given three times daily
  » Amoxicillin-clavulanate at 40 mg/kg per day divided and given three times daily (based on amoxicillin component)
- Patients should be followed closely for any progression of symptoms.
- Consider decongestant spray as periorbital cellulitis is commonly associated with sinusitis.
- Patients < 2 years of age and those with a systemic illness should be admitted for intravenous antibiotics and close observation.
  » Give ceftriaxone 50 to 100 mg/kg every 24 hours.
- If the patient is methicillin-resistant *Staphylococcus aureus* (MRSA) positive or if MRSA is prevalent in the community, consider:

» Vancomycin:
› 10 mg/kg every 6 hours
— **or** —
› 40 mg/kg per day divided into 3 to 4 doses

ORBITAL (SEPTAL) CELLULITIS

- Orbital cellulitis an infection of the soft tissues posterior to the orbital septum.
- It occurs more frequently in the winter months.

Pathophysiology

- Orbital cellulitis is usually caused by a sinus infection (the ethmoid and maxillary sinuses are the most commonly affected), with erosion of the sinus process leading to the contiguous spread of the disease.
  » It can also be from a recent URTI.
- The most common causative organisms for orbital cellulitis include *Streptococcus pneumonia*, *Staphylococcus aureus*, and *Streptococcus pyogenes*.
  » The incidence of *Haemophilus influenzae* infection is markedly decreased since the introduction of the influenza vaccine.

Management

- Admit the patient to hospital and obtain an ophthalmology consult to determine if abscess drainage is required.

- Start broad spectrum intravenous antibiotics that are aimed at respiratory pathogens and anaerobes from sinuses:
  » Ceftriaxone 50 to 100 mg/kg every 24 hours
  — **or** —
  » Clindamycin 30 mg/kg per day divided into 3 to 4 doses
- If the patient is MRSA positive or if MRSA is prevalent in the community, consider:
  » Vancomycin:
    › 10 mg/kg every 6 hours
    — **or** —
    › 40 mg/kg per day divided into 3 to 4 doses

Complications

- Contiguous spread of the abscess can be life threatening, leading to:
  » Meningitis
  » Intracranial abscess
  » Cavernous sinus thrombosis

REFERENCES

Ekhlassi T, Becker N. Preseptal and orbital cellulitis. *Dis Mon.* 2017;63(2):30–32. Medline:27884386

Hauser A, Fogarasi S. Periorbital and orbital cellulitis. *Pediatr Rev.* 2010;31(6):242–249. https://doi.org/10.1542/pir.31-6-242. Medline:20516236

Prentiss KA, Dorfman DH. Pediatric ophthalmology in the emergency department. *Emerg Med Clin North Am.* 2008;26(1):181–198, vii. https://doi.org/10.1016/j.emc.2007.11.001. Medline:18249262

12.1

Stevens-Johnson Syndrome (SJS) and Toxic Epidermal Necrolysis (TEN)

David Bulir, Judy Wismer

- Stevens-Johnson syndrome (SJS) and toxic epidermal necrolysis (TEN) represent a spectrum of disease that is the result of a severe cell-mediated response leading to epidermal necrosis with detachment and mucocutaneous complications in 90% of patients.
- SJS and TEN are primarily differentiated based on the amount of body surface area (BSA) affected.
  - » SJS involves < 10% of BSA.
  - » SJS and TEN overlap involves 10% to 30% BSA.
  - » TEN involves > 30% BSA.

Epidemiology

- SJS occurs in 1 to 7 people per million per year.
- TEN occurs in 0.4 to 1.5 people per million per year.
- There is equal incidence among male and female children.

Pathophysiology

- The exact mechanism by which SJS and TEN occur is not well characterized.
- Histopathology demonstrates widespread, full-thickness epidermal detachment, which is believed to be initiated by CD8+ cytotoxic T lymphocytes.
- Approximately 75% to 95% of SJS and TEN cases are caused by medication or upper respiratory tract infections (URTIs).

Risk Factors

- Patients are at higher risk for SJS or TEN:
  - » With the rapid introduction of medication
  - » Within the first 8 weeks of starting certain medications
  - » If genetically associated with HLA-B12, HLA-B1502, HLA-5801 haplotypes, or of Han Chinese descent
  - » With systemic disease, including HIV/AIDS and systemic lupus erythematosus

- Common medications associated with the development of TEN or SJS are:
  - » Nonsteroidal anti-inflammatory drugs (NSAIDs)
  - » Sulfa antibiotics
  - » Phenobarbital
  - » Lamotrigine
  - » Carbamazepine
  - » Allopurinol
- Infections associated with the development of TEN and SJS are:
  - » *Mycoplasma pneumoniae*
  - » Cytomegalovirus (CMV)
  - » Herpes simplex virus
  - » Hepatitis A virus

Physical Exam

- Children initially present with flu-like symptoms:
  - » Fever
  - » Arthralgia
  - » Dysphagia
  - » Malaise
  - » Myalgia
- 30% of patients present with ophthalmic symptoms, including photophobia, conjunctivitis, pain, or erythematous and edematous eyelids.
- Skin and mucosal lesions begin to develop 1 to 3 days after the onset of constitutional symptoms.
  - » Lesions begin as dusky, purpuric macules, which can then form vesicles and bullae.
- After the initial phase and development of skin lesions, there is diffuse epidermal detachment.
  - » Applying tangential pressure on the skin can cause sloughing of the epidermis (a positive Nikolsky sign).
    - › A positive Nikolsky sign is nonspecific to SJS and TEN but can help narrow the diagnosis toward diseases that affect skin integrity.

- SJS and TEN typically start on the face and thorax and spread progressively in a symmetrical fashion.
  » The palms and the soles of the feet can also be early sites for the development of SJS and TEN.
- Reepithelization of the skin can take up to 3 weeks to finish and begins one week after the onset of symptoms.
- The mean duration from the onset of symptoms to maximum detachment is 8 days.

Complications

- The loss of barrier function of the skin can lead to significant complications, including:
  » Pain
  » Fluid and protein loss
  » Electrolyte imbalances
  » Bacterial infection of the skin
  » Sepsis

Investigations

- SJS and TEN can resemble other diseases such as erythema multiforme (EM), staphylococcal scalded skin syndrome (SSSS), and Kawasaki disease.
  » Unlike SJS and TEN, SSSS has no involvement of the mucous membranes.
  » Kawasaki disease (see Chapter 9.1) can be differentiated from SJS and TEN based on the following:
  » Kawasaki disease has a number of defining features which differentiate it from SJS/TEN, including the characteristic "strawberry tongue" (marked redness and prominent gustative papillae), swollen lips with vertical cracking and bleeding, and bilateral conjunctival injection.
    › Skin lesions that typically develop in Kawasaki disease are polymorphous exanthema and tend not to form vesicular or bullous lesions.
    › Ophthalmic changes seen in Kawasaki disease are nonexudative, whereas those of SJS and TEN are exudative.
    › Kawasaki disease tends to have unilateral cervical lymphadenopathy
  » The limited BSA affected and the lack of mucosal involvement can help differentiate EM from SJS and TEN.
- Skin biopsy can be used as part of the diagnosis.
- Histopathological findings from biopsy should reveal extensive apoptotic keratinocytes with full thickness dermal–epidermal separation.
- Patients currently on medication should have their medication scored using the algorithm of drug causality for epidermal necrolysis (ALDEN) to assess the likelihood that their medication may be related to the development of SJS or TEN.

Management

- Early intervention is critical.
- Upon diagnosis of SJS or TEN, it is possible to estimate prognosis using the Score of TEN (SCORTEN) criteria:

Table 12.1.1. SCORTEN CRITERIA
Adapted from Fouchard et al. (2000).

Risk factor	0 points	1 point
Age	< 40 years	> 40 years
Pulse (beats per minute)	< 120	> 120
Serum BUN (mmol/L)	< 10	> 10
Body surface area (BSA) detached	< 10%	> 10%
Serum bicarbonate (mmol/L)	> 20	< 20
Serum glucose (mmol/L)	< 14	> 14
Active malignancy	No	Yes

- Patients with SJS or TEN who score 0 or 1 on SCORTEN criteria, and whose disease has limited BSA involvement and is not rapidly progressing, may be treated in a nonspecialized medical ward.
- Patients with a SCORTEN score ≥ 2 who have > 30% BSA involvement should be transferred to a more specialized unit such as burn or ICU.
- Although the criteria may be helpful in estimating prognosis, management of the patient should be assessed on a case-to-case basis.
- The quicker the offending agent is removed, the better the prognosis; for each day the drug has been removed before the development of blisters and erosions, there is a 30% reduction in mortality.

Supportive Care

- There is limited evidence regarding the approach to treatment, but the focus is on aggressive supportive care to minimize side effects due to the loss of the barrier function of the skin and to prevent secondary infection.

Wound Care

- Perform a routine evaluation of the affected areas of skin to assess for infection.
- An early gynecologic examination should be performed on all female patients to minimize vaginal and labial sequelae such as vaginal adenosis and adhesions.
  » Use of intravaginal topical corticosteroids, suppression of the menstrual cycle, and soft vaginal molds is the mainstays for female urogenital involvement.
- There is no consensus on the treatment approach for affected skin in SJS and TEN.
- An observational study has shown that debridement versus leaving the detached skin in place as a biological dressing was associated with equivalent survival and tissue reepithelization.

- Numerous types of wound dressings have also been used successfully in the treatment of SJS and TEN but have not been compared to one another, including:
  » Nonadherent nanocrystalline gauze containing silver
  » Petrolatum-impregnated gauze
  » Biosynthetic skin substitutes such as Suprathel, Aquacel AG, and Biobrane

Ocular care

- Obtain an ophthalmology consult.
- Assess the severity of eye involvement daily using the following criteria to determine appropriate therapy:
  » None (0) — No eye involvement
    › Provide daily lubrication.
  » Mild (1) — Conjunctival hyperemia
    › Give topical broad-spectrum antibiotics and corticosteroids with lubrication.
  » Severe (2) — Ocular surface epithelial defect **or** pseudomembrane formation
    › Give topical broad-spectrum antibiotics and corticosteroids with lubrication and amniotic membrane transplantation.
  » Very severe (3) — Surface epithelial defect **and** pseudomembrane formation
    › Give topical broad-spectrum antibiotics and corticosteroids with lubrication and amniotic membrane transplantation.

Other Primary Management

FLUID AND ELECTROLYTE MANAGEMENT

- Increase fluids to account for loss of water from the denuded skin.
- One small study of 21 patients found that fluid replacement over the first 24 hours can be estimated as follows:

  2 mL/kg of body weight × % BSA of detached skin.

NUTRITION

- Ensure adequate nutrition due to increased metabolic demand (caloric requirements are similar to burn patients).

ORAL FEEDING OR NASOGASTRIC TUBE

- Use an oral feeding or nasogastric (NG) tube if necessary.
- Care should be taken when placing an NG tube to minimize trauma to affected mucosal tissue.

TEMPERATURE REGULATION

- Ensure the room is 30°C to 32°C to minimize caloric expenditure in regulating body temperature.
- Body warmers can also help keep the patient warm and minimize caloric expenditure.

PAIN MANAGEMENT

- Pain is caused by the cutaneous lesions in SJS and TEN.
- Pain management can be approached in a very similar manner as for burn patients.

Adjunctive Therapy

- There is no consensus on the use of adjunctive therapies such as systemic corticosteroids, intravenous immunoglobulin (IVIG), and cyclosporine.

SYSTEMIC CORTICOSTEROIDS

- There are no clinical trials to support the use of systemic corticosteroids in SJS and TEN.
- Limited studies have found conflicting results.
- Trials exploring the use of corticosteroids have demonstrated no improvement in mortality or morbidity; however, smaller, retrospective observation studies appear to demonstrate a potential benefit for reducing ocular complication.
- Corticosteroids may worsen SJS and TEN given the fact that patients may be at a greater risk of sepsis and may slow the reepithelialization process; however, two small trials with less than 30 patients total did not demonstrate a difference in the incidence of sepsis or prolonged time to reepithelialization.

IVIG

- Although the use of IVIG is commonly used in the management of SJS/TEN, the literature is the literature lacks high quality, randomized trials which clearly demonstrate a reduction of morbidity and mortality.
- Variables such as timing, dose, and combination with other treatments are still active areas of investigation.
- Patients with severe SJS or TEN can be treated with 3 g/kg body weight of IVIG within 24 to 48 hours of cutaneous symptoms.

CYCLOSPORINE A

- Cyclosporine A has been gaining attention as possible treatment in the management of SJS/TEN.
- A number of small studies and case reports have demonstrated that treatment with 3 to 5 mg/kg per day of cyclosporine may slow the progression of the disease and decrease mortality.
- A recent study involving 44 patients found that individuals treated with cyclosporine at 3 mg/kg per day for 10 days, then 2 mg/kg per day for 10 days, and then 1 mg/kg per day for 10 days had fewer deaths than the control group treated with supportive therapy alone.

REFERENCES
Atiyeh BS, Dham R, Yassin MF, El-Musa KA. Treatment of toxic epidermal necrolysis with moisture-retentive ointment: a case report and review of the literature. *Dermatol Surg.* 2003;29(2):185–188. Medline:12562352

Boorboor P, Vogt PM, Bechara FG, et al. Toxic epidermal necrolysis: use of Biobrane or skin coverage reduces pain, improves mobilisation and decreases infection in elderly patients. *Burns.* 2008;34(4):487–492. https://doi.org/10.1016/j.burns.2007.06.008. Medline:17919820

Cartotto R, Mayich M, Nickerson D, Gomez M. SCORTEN accurately predicts mortality among toxic epidermal necrolysis patients treated in a burn center. *J Burn Care Res.* 2008;29(1):141–146. https://doi.org/10.1097/BCR.0b013e31815f3865. Medline:18182912

Dalli RL, Kumar R, Kennedy P, Maitz P, Lee S, Johnson R. Toxic epidermal necrolysis/Stevens-Johnson syndrome: current trends in management. *ANZ J Surg.* 2007;77(8):671–676. https://doi.org/10.1111/j.1445-2197.2007.04184.x. Medline:17635282

Fouchard N, Bertocchi M, Roujeau JC, Revuz J, Wolkenstein P, Bastuji-Garin S. SCORTEN: a severity-of-illness score for toxic epidermal necrolysis. *J Invest Dermatol.* 2000;115(2):149–153. https://doi.org/10.1046/j.1523-1747.2000.00061.x. Medline:10951229

Harr T, French LE. Severe cutaneous adverse reactions: acute generalized exanthematous pustulosis, toxic epidermal necrolysis and Stevens-Johnson syndrome. *Med Clin North Am.* 2010a;94(4):727–742, x. https://doi.org/10.1016/j.mcna.2010.04.004. Medline:20609860

Harr T, French LE. Toxic epidermal necrolysis and Stevens-Johnson syndrome. *Orphanet J Rare Dis.* 2010b;5(1):39. https://doi.org/10.1186/1750-1172-5-39. Medline:21162721

Kaser DJ, Reichman DE, Laufer MR. Prevention of vulvovaginal sequelae in Stevens-Johnson syndrome and toxic epidermal necrolysis. *Rev Obstet Gynecol.* 2011;4(2):81–85. Medline:22102931

Kohanim S, Palioura S, Saeed HN, et al. Acute and chronic ophthalmic involvement in Stevens-Johnson syndrome/toxic epidermal necrolysis: a comprehensive review and guide to therapy. II. Ophthalmic Disease. *Ocul Surf.* 2016;14(2):168–188. https://doi.org/10.1016/j.jtos.2016.02.001. Medline:26882981

Lee HY, Fook-Chong S, Koh HY, Thirumoorthy T, Pang SM. Cyclosporine treatment for Stevens-Johnson syndrome/toxic epidermal necrolysis: Retrospective analysis of a cohort treated in a specialized referral center. *J Am Acad Dermatol.* 2017;76(1):106–113. https://doi.org/10.1016/j.jaad.2016.07.048. Medline:27717620

Mayes T, Gottschlich M, Khoury J, Warner P, Kagan R. Energy requirements of pediatric patients with Stevens-Johnson syndrome and toxic epidermal necrolysis. *Nutr Clin Pract.* 2008;23(5):547–550. https://doi.org/10.1177/0884533608323434. Medline:18849560

Mockenhaupt M, Viboud C, Dunant A, et al. Stevens-Johnson syndrome and toxic epidermal necrolysis: assessment of medication risks with emphasis on recently marketed drugs. The EuroSCAR-study. *J Invest Dermatol.* 2008;128(1):35–44. https://doi.org/10.1038/sj.jid.5701033. Medline:17805350

Palmieri TL, Greenhalgh DG, Saffle JR, et al. A multicenter review of toxic epidermal necrolysis treated in U.S. burn centers at the end of the twentieth century. *J Burn Care Rehabil.* 2002;23(2):87–96. https://doi.org/10.1097/00004630-200203000-00004. Medline:11882797

Rzany B, Hering O, Mockenhaupt M, et al. Histopathological and epidemiological characteristics of patients with erythema exudativum multiforme major, Stevens-Johnson syndrome and toxic epidermal necrolysis. *Br J Dermatol.* 1996;135(1):6–11. https://doi.org/10.1111/j.1365-2133.1996.tb03598.x. Medline:8776350

Sassolas B, Haddad C, Mockenhaupt M, et al. ALDEN, an algorithm for assessment of drug causality in Stevens-Johnson Syndrome and toxic epidermal necrolysis: comparison with case-control analysis. *Clin Pharmacol Ther.* 2010;88(1):60–68. https://doi.org/10.1038/clpt.2009.252. Medline:20375998

Schwartz RA, McDonough PH, Lee BW. Toxic epidermal necrolysis. Part I. Introduction, history, classification, clinical features, systemic manifestations, etiology, and immunopathogenesis. *J Am Acad Dermatol.* 2013;69(2):173.e1–173.e13, quiz 185–186. https://doi.org/10.1016/j.jaad.2013.05.003. Medline:23866878

Sotozono C, Ueta M, Nakatani E, et al; Japanese Research Committee on Severe Cutaneous Adverse Reaction. Predictive factors associated with acute ocular involvement in Stevens-Johnson syndrome and toxic epidermal necrolysis. *Am J Ophthalmol.* 2015;160(2):228–237.e2. https://doi.org/10.1016/j.ajo.2015.05.002. Medline:25979679

12.2

Common Pediatric Viral Exanthems

David Bulir, Judy Wismer

- An exanthem or exanthema is a rash that appears abruptly on multiple areas of the skin.
- An enanthem or enanthema is an eruption on a mucosal surface.
- Viral exanthems are rashes that are caused by a virus; in childhood, there are 5 diseases that are commonly responsible:
  » Measles/rubeola (measles virus)
  » Rubella (rubella virus)
  » Erythema infectiosum (parvovirus B19)
  » Roseola infantum (HHV-6/HHV-7)
  » Hand-foot-and-mouth disease (Coxsackievirus A16/A6 or enterovirus 71)
  » Chickenpox (*Varicella zoster* virus)

- Lesion may be:
  » Macule — flat lesion, no elevation or depression, < 1 cm at greatest diameter
  » Patch — flat lesion, no elevation or depression, > 1 cm at greatest diameter
  » Papule — raised, solid, palpable lesion, < 1 cm at greatest diameter
  » Plaque — raised, solid, palpable lesion, > 1 cm at greatest diameter
  » Pustule — elevated, fluid-filled lesion containing purulent fluid
  » Vesicle — elevated, fluid-filled lesion, < 1 cm at greatest diameter
  » Bulla — elevated, fluid-filled lesion, > 1 cm at greatest diameter

Table 12.2.1. COMMON VIRAL INFECTIONS AND CUTANEOUS PRESENTATION

Viral pathogen	Disease	Epidemiology	Prodrome before rash	Diagnosis	Rash features	Management	Potential complications
Measles virus	Rubeola	Nonimmune children 5 to 9 years of age	• Onset 1 to 2 days prior to rash » High-grade fever » Malaise » Conjunctivitis » Coryza » Koplik spots	• Clinical diagnosis • Serology • IgG or IgM • PCR	• **Exanthem:** erythematous maculopapular rash » Starts on the head and proceeds cephalocaudally to involve the trunk and, extremities including the palms and soles » Spreads and coalesces over a 2- to 3-day period • **Enanthem:** Koplik spots (occur during prodrome) » Found on buccal mucosa but can involve the hard and soft palate and labial mucosa » Bluish- or grayish-white spots resembling grains of salt	• Supportive management: » Nutrition and fluid intake • Fever: » Antipyretics to reduce fever • Vitamin A: » Vitamin A supplementation can reduce mortality and morbidity associated with measles. » Dosage: › < 6 months of age: 50,000 IU once daily › 6 to 11 months of age: 100,000 IU once daily › ≥12 months of age: 200,000 IU once daily • Preventing transmission: » Avoid contact with individuals susceptible to measles for approximately 5 days after rash disappears.	• More common: » Diarrhea » Otitis media » Pneumonia • Less common: » Bacterial skin infection in immunosuppressed patients » Hepatosplenomegaly » Keratitis » Encephalitis » Subacute sclerosing panencephalitis
Rubella virus	Rubella (German measles)	Nonimmune children	• Onset 1 to 5 days prior to rash » Low-grade fever » Headache » Malaise » Pharyngitis » Coryza » Lymphadenopathy › Cervical, suboccipital, and postauricular » Forchheimer spots » Arthralgia » Arthritis	• Clinical diagnosis • Serology • IgG or IgM PCR	• **Exanthem:** noncoalescing pink-reddish maculopapular rash » Spreads cephalocaudally from face to trunk and extremities over 24 hours • **Enanthem:** Forchheimer spots » Found during prodrome on soft palate » Small, red, petechial spots	• Supportive management: » Nutrition and fluid intake • Fever: » Antipyretics to reduce fever • NSAIDs: » Give for arthralgia or arthritis • Preventing transmission: » Avoid contact with individuals susceptible to rubella for 7 days after onset of rash.	• More common: » Joint effusions » Thrombocytopenia • Less common: » Encephalitis » Congenital anomalies in newborns

Viral pathogen	Disease	Epidemiology	Prodrome before rash	Diagnosis	Rash features	Management	Potential complications

Parvovirus B19	Erythema infectiosum	Children 3 to 12 years of age	• Onset 2 to 5 days prior to rash
			  » Low-grade fever
			  » Malaise
			  » Headache
			  » Pruritus
			  » Coryza
			  » Myalgia
			  » Arthralgia
			  » Arthritis
				• Clinical diagnosis
				• Serology
				• IgG or IgM
				• PCR
					• **Exanthem:**
					  » Begins with "slapped cheeks" — confluent, erythematous, edematous plaques on cheeks for 1 to 4 days
					  » Erythematous reticular rash on trunk and extremities for 5 to 9 days
					  » Note: Can also present as papular purpuric "gloves and socks" syndrome
					  » Painful and pruritic papules, petechiae, and purpura on hands and feet with oral erosions
						• Supportive management:
						  » Nutrition and fluid intake
						• Fever:
						  » Antipyretics to reduce fever
						• NSAIDs:
						  » For arthralgia or arthritis
						• Preventing transmission:
						  » Patients with normal immune system are most likely not infectious after development of exanthem, arthralgia, or arthritis.
						  » Pregnant women exposed to the virus may wish to contact their healthcare provider; there is no single recommended way to monitor pregnant women and parvovirus B19.
							• Transient aplastic crisis:
							  » Can cause transient aplastic crisis requiring transfusion in patients with underlying hematologic abnormalities
							• Chronic infection:
							  » Chronic infection is associated with individuals who are immunosuppressed or have cancer, leukemia, tissue transplant, or congenital or acquired immunodeficiency.
							  » Consider IVIG for immunocompromised patients with confirmed parvovirus B19 infection and anemia.

HHV-6/HHV-7	Roseola infantum	Children aged 6 months to 3 years of age	• Onset 3 to 7 days before rash
			  » High-grade fever
			  » Palpebral edema
			  » Cervical lymphadenopathy
			  » URTI symptoms
			  » Irritability
				• Clinical diagnosis
				• Serology
				• IgG or IgM
				• PCR
					• **Exanthem:** pink macules and papules with white halo
					  » Start on trunk and spreads over body, lasting 1 to 3 days
					• **Enanthem:** Nagayama spots
					  » Found on soft palate and uvula
					  » Small, erythematous papules
						• Supportive management:
						  » Nutrition and fluid intake
						• Fever:
						  » Antipyretics to reduce fever
						• Preventing transmission:
						  » There is no recommended period of time for exclusion of out-of-home activities.
							• Less common:
							  » Febrile seizure
							  » Aseptic meningitis
							  » Encephalitis
							  » Thrombocytopenic purpura

Coxsackievirus A16/A6 or enterovirus 71	Hand-foot-and-mouth disease	Children < 5 years of age	• Onset 1 to 2 days before rash
			  » Low-grade fever
			  » Malaise
			  » Sore throat
				• Clinical diagnosis	• **Exanthem:**
					  » Develops after enanthem
					  » Begins as bright pink macules and papules, then painful vesicles with erythematous halos, transitioning to erosions with surrounding skin being erythematous
					• **Enanthem:** erythematous erosions that resemble "canker sores" (aphthae)
					  » Occur first in mouth before spreading to hands and feet
					  » May occasionally involve buttocks, elbows, and diaper area
						• Supportive management:
						  » Nutrition and fluid intake
						• Fever:
						  » Antipyretics to reduce fever
						• Preventing transmission:
						  » There is no recommended period of time for exclusion of out-of-home activities; patients are typically most infectious during the first week of illness and continue to shed the virus for approximately 6 weeks.
						  » Good hand hygiene as the virus is spread through the fecal-oral route
							• Less common:
							  » Rhombencephalitis
							  » Acute flaccid paralysis
							  » Aseptic meningitis
							  » Pulmonary edema
							  » Heart failure
							• Note: Complications are more associated with enterovirus HFMD.

Viral pathogen	Disease	Epidemiology	Prodrome before rash	Diagnosis	Rash features	Management	Potential complications

Varicella zoster virus	Chickenpox	90% of cases occur in children < 10 years of age	• Onset 1 to 2 days before rash
			  » Low-grade fever
			  » Malaise
			  » Anorexia
			  » Pharyngitis
			  » Oral sores
				• Clinical diagnosis
				• Serology
				• IgG or IgM
				• PCR
					• **Exanthem:** vesicular rash
					  » begins as an erythematous macule, progressing rapidly to a papule, and then a vesicle over a 4-day period
					  » Vesicles can develop into pustules that typically fully crust over after 4 to 6 days, which heal and leave a temporary area of hypopigmentation where the lesion was
					• **Enanthem:** small erythematous erosions or vesicles on buccal surfaces
					  » May resemble "canker sores" (aphthae)
						• Supportive management:
						  » Nutrition and fluid intake
						• Fever:
						  » Antipyretics to reduce fever (Avoid use of ASA due to risk of Reye Syndrome)
						• Antiviral (if indicated):
						  » Antivirals are effective if given within the first 24 hours for those at risk of complications, including:
						    › Newborns
						    › Children with chronic skin disorders
						    › Children with pulmonary disorders
						    › Children on chronic steroid therapy
						• Antipruritics:
						  » Antihistamines
						  » Calamine lotion
						  » Pramoxine gel
						• Preventing transmission:
						  » Patients are considered infectious from 48 hours prior to onset of rash until all lesions have fully crusted over.
							• More common:
							  » Secondary bacterial skin infection
							• Less common:
							  » Encephalitis
							  » Reye syndrome
							  » Pneumonia
							  » Hepatitis

IgG immunoglobulin G. **IgM** immunoglobulin M. **PCR** polymerase chain reaction. **URTI** upper respiratory tract infection.

REFERENCES

Anderson LJ. Role of parvovirus B19 in human disease. *Pediatr Infect Dis J.* 1987;6(8):711–718. https://doi.org/10.1097/00006454-198708000-00003. Medline:2823211

Asano Y, Yoshikawa T, Suga S, et al. Clinical features of infants with primary human herpesvirus 6 infection (exanthem subitum, roseola infantum). *Pediatrics.* 1994;93(1):104–108. Medline:8265302

Huiming Y, Chaomin W, Meng M. Vitamin A for treating measles in children. *Cochrane Database Syst Rev.* 2005;(4):CD001479. https://doi.org/10.1002/14651858.CD001479.pub3. Medline:16235283

Hussey GD, Klein M. A randomized, controlled trial of vitamin A in children with severe measles. *N Engl J Med.* 1990;323(3):160–164. https://doi.org/10.1056/NEJM199007193230304. Medline:2194128

Lebwohl M. *Treatment of skin disease: comprehensive therapeutic strategies.* 2nd ed. Philadelphia, Pa.: Mosby/Elsevier; 2006.

McKinnon HD Jr, Howard T. Evaluating the febrile patient with a rash. *Am Fam Physician.* 2000;62(4):804–816. Medline:10969859

Perry RT, Halsey NA. The clinical significance of measles: a review. *J Infect Dis.* 2004;189(Suppl 1):S4–S16. https://doi.org/10.1086/377712. Medline:15106083

Ramdass P, Mullick S, Farber HF. Viral skin diseases. *Prim Care.* 2015;42(4):517–567. https://doi.org/10.1016/j.pop.2015.08.006. Medline:26612372

Richardson M, Elliman D, Maguire H, Simpson J, Nicoll A. Evidence base of incubation periods, periods of infectiousness and exclusion policies for the control of communicable diseases in schools and preschools. *Pediatr Infect Dis J.* 2001;20(4):380–391. https://doi.org/10.1097/00006454-200104000-00004. Medline:11332662

Straus SE, Ostrove JM, Inchauspé G, et al. NIH conference. Varicella-zoster virus infections. Biology, natural history, treatment, and prevention. *Ann Intern Med.* 1988;108(2):221–237. https://doi.org/10.7326/0003-4819-108-2-221. Medline:2829675

12.3

Impetigo

David Bulir, Chih-Ho Hong

- Impetigo is a superficial bacterial skin infection most commonly seen in children.
- Cases can occur in previously healthy skin (primary impetigo) or areas of skin with loss of barrier function (secondary impetigo).
- Impetigo is the most common bacterial skin infection in children < 6 years of age.
  - » Annual incidence is estimated at:
    - › 2.8% in children ≤ 4 years of age
    - › 1.6% in children 5 to 15 years of age
- Males and females are equally affected.
- There is an increased incidence of impetigo in:
  - » Summer months
  - » Individuals living in overcrowded conditions
  - » Children with poor personal hygiene

Pathophysiology

- Two bacteria are most commonly responsible for causing impetigo:
  1. Group A beta-hemolytic streptococci (GAS)
  2. *Staphylococcus aureus*
- Approximately 30% of individuals are colonized with *S. aureus* in the nares.
- Individuals may be able to be colonized by GAS if they are chronically exposed to carriers (e.g., living in the same household as a known carrier).
- 70% of all cases of impetigo are nonbullous impetigo, with the remaining 30% being bullous impetigo.
- Transient colonization of the skin by GAS and *S. aureus* can occur as a result of alterations in climate (temperature and humidity) or as a result of preexisting skin conditions (atopic dermatitis).
- Once attached to the skin, the bacteria can invade and cause a localized infection through the use of various virulence factors, leading to a robust inflammatory response.
- Ecthyma (an infection of the dermis) may occur as a result of continued invasion of *S. aureus* and GAS into deeper tissues, leading to ulcer formation.
  - » Bullous impetigo occurs primarily as a result of *S. aureus* infection in the skin.
    - › *S. aureus* can produce exfoliative toxins (ET-A or ET-B) that cleave desmoglein 1, a structural protein within the epidermis that mediates cellular adhesion.
    - › Subsequent bullae formation results from a robust cellular immune response and replication of the bacteria within the bullae.
    - › Unlike staphylococcal scalded skin syndrome (SSSS), the bullae contain *S. aureus*, whereas SSSS results from systemic distribution of exfoliative toxins.

History

NONBULLOUS IMPETIGO

- Lesions are most commonly located on the exposed skin surfaces of the face, primarily the nares and perioral region, and on the extremities.
- Lesions begin with a small, erythematous macule or papule that progresses to a clear, then purulent vesicle on an erythematous base measuring up to 2 cm in diameter.
  - » The fragile vesicles rupture, revealing an erosion that dries, forming a characteristic "honey-colored" adherent crust.
- Lesions may be pruritic or painful.
- Systemically, patients feel well, but may have local lymphadenopathy.
  - » Infections that progress through deeper layers of the skin increase the risk for developing ecthyma (infection of the dermis), cellulitis, osteomyelitis, septic arthritis, or septicemia.
  - » Though rare, some patients with impetigo caused by GAS can develop poststreptococcal glomerulonephritis or rheumatic fever.

BULLOUS IMPETIGO

- Bullous impetigo typically occurs more frequently in neonates but may also cause disease in older children.
- Lesions are typically located on the trunk, but can also be found in intertriginous regions, buttocks, and extremities.
  - » Unlike nonbullous impetigo, bullous impetigo may affect buccal mucosa.
- Lesions begin as small vesicles that progress to flaccid bullae up to 2 cm in diameter.
  - » The contents of the bullae are initially clear but become purulent with progression of the lesion and rupture.

» Bullae are easily ruptured, revealing a moist, erythematous base that, when dried, forms a collarette of scale with a thin, brown crust.

- Patients may also present with some systemic symptoms, including fever, weakness, and diarrhea.
  » Though rare, infants and children can develop pneumonia, lymphangitis, guttate psoriasis, SSSS, toxic shock syndrome, endocarditis, septic arthritis, osteomyelitis, or septicemia.

Differential Diagnosis

- The differential diagnosis for impetigo depends on whether the patient is suspected to have nonbullous or bullous impetigo.

NONBULLOUS IMPETIGO

- On the differential diagnosis of nonbullous impetigo, consider:
  » Atopic dermatitis
    › Patients typically have a personal or family history of atopy.
    › Lesions are pruritic and follow classical distribution according to age group (facial and extensor involvement in children).
    › Children with atopic dermatitis are at greater risk of impetigo as disruption of the skin barrier can lead to increased susceptibility and colonization.
  » Childhood discoid lupus erythematosus
    › This presents as adherent scales penetrating into hair follicles on well-defined plaques that, when peeled off the lesion, reveal a scale with a "carpet tack" appearance due to the penetration into the follicles
  » Contact dermatitis
    › Contact dermatitis is associated with exposure to an irritant/allergen prior to the development of pruritic lesions.
  » Dermatophytosis
    › Dermatophytosis presents as annular, scaly, and erythematous plaques with a slightly raised border.
  » Herpes simplex virus (HSV)
    › Lesions may resemble impetigo (**bullous and nonbullous**) since they present similarly with vesicles on an erythematous base that when ruptured reveal an erosion.
    › Lesions are typically grouped together; if lesions are recurrent, the patient will have a history of prior lesions in same anatomic location.
    › Lesions can be painful and are typically found on the lips and skin.
  » Scabies
    › Lesions are curvilinear (burrows) with associated vesicles typically around the hand web spaces.
    › Scabies is associated with nocturnal itching.
  » Varicella
    › Lesions may resemble impetigo (**bullous and nonbullous**) since they present similarly with

thin-walled vesicles on an erythematous base ("dewdrops on a rose petal") that rupture easily and form a crust when dry. However, varicella lesions quickly become pustular and then crust. Seeing lesions in various stages of evolution is typical.
    › Lesions classically start on the trunk and spread to extremities and the face.
    › Varicella is associated with fever and other systemic signs of viral infection.

BULLOUS IMPETIGO

- On the differential diagnosis of nonbullous impetigo, consider:
  » Autoimmune blistering diseases
  » Stevens-Johnson syndrome / toxic epidermal necrolysis
    › These are severe mucocutaneous reactions typically associated with recent new medication use or infection leading to separation at the epidermal-dermal junction.
  » Dermatitis herpetiformis
    › Dermatitis herpetiformis is characterized by intensely pruritic papules and vesicles in a herpetiform arrangement.
    › It is classically located on the occipital scalp, elbows, and knees.

Investigations

- The diagnosis of impetigo is typically made clinically, and treatment can be initiated regardless of further investigations.
- Culture or Gram stain of exudate or pus can be performed to identify the causative bacteria and susceptibility, especially if methicillin-resistant *Staphylococcus aureus* (MRSA) is suspected.

Management

- The primary goals in the treatment of impetigo are to minimize the spread of the disease, improve cosmesis, and hasten the healing process.
- Nonmedical interventions that help prevent the spread of the disease include:
  » Avoiding school or daycare for at least 24 to 48 hours after starting treatment
  » Routine handwashing and bathing for children < 15 years old
    › In studies, this resulted in a 34% lower incidence of impetigo.
  » Ensuring that fomites such as clothes, towels, utensils, and furniture are appropriately cleaned
  » Minimizing scratching of affected areas and keeping fingernails short to minimize excoriations
- Patients with limited skin disease are typically treated with topical medications, and more diffuse disease is treated systemically.

Topical Therapy

- Consider the following topical therapies:
  - » Mupirocin 2% ointment (Bactroban)
    - › Apply 3 times daily to the affected area for 5 days.
  - » Retapamulin 1% ointment (Altargo)
    - › Apply twice daily to the affected area for 5 days.
  - » Fusidic acid 2% ointment (Fucidin)
    - › Apply a small amount 3 to 4 times daily until resolution of the lesion.

Note: There has been increasing incidence of resistance to fusidic acid, so consider other topical therapies if local resistance has been noted.

Systemic Therapy

- Oral antibiotics are reversed for individuals who have extensive disease or ecthyma and are usually given as a 7-day course.
- Penicillin-resistant *S. aureus* is the most common causative agent in impetigo, necessitating the use of beta-lactamase resistant antimicrobials:
  - » Cloxacillin 12.5 to 25 mg/kg per day divided and given 4 times a day
  - » Cephalexin 25 to 50 mg/kg per day divided and given 3 or 4 times a day
  - » In patients ≥ 3 months of age, amoxicillin-clavulanate 50 mg/kg (based on amoxicillin component) per day divided given 3 times a day
- In patients with penicillin or cephalosporin sensitivity, consider using the following:
  - » Erythromycin (base) 40 mg/kg per day divided and given 3 or 4 times a day
  - » Clarithromycin 15 mg/kg and day divided and given 2 times a day

Note: Some strains of GAS have documented resistance to macrolides and a thorough follow-up should occur to ensure disease resolution.

- If MRSA is suspected, consider starting the patient on:
  - » Clindamycin 20 mg/kg per day divided and given 3 times a day
  - » Trimethoprim-sulfamethoxazole 8 to 12 mg/kg (trimethoprim) per day divided and given 2 times a day
  - » In patients > 8 years of age only, doxycycline 2 to 4 mg/kg per day divided and given 2 times a day

REFERENCES

Bangert S, Levy M, Hebert AA. Bacterial resistance and impetigo treatment trends: a review. *Pediatr Dermatol.* 2012;29(3):243–248. https://doi.org/10.1111/j.1525-1470.2011.01700.x. Medline:22299710

Bolognia J, Jorizzo JL, Schaffer JV, eds. *Dermatology.* 3rd ed. 2 vols. Philadelphia: Elsevier/Saunders; 2012.

Brown J, Shriner DL, Schwartz RA, Janniger CK. Impetigo: an update. *Int J Dermatol.* 2003;42(4):251–255. https://doi.org/10.1046/j.1365-4362.2003.01647.x. Medline:12694487

Cole C, Gazewood J. Diagnosis and treatment of impetigo. *Am Fam Physician.* 2007;75(6):859–864. Medline:17390597

Geria AN, Schwartz RA. Impetigo update: new challenges in the era of methicillin resistance. *Cutis.* 2010;85(2):65–70. Medline:20349679

Hanakawa Y, Schechter NM, Lin C, et al. Molecular mechanisms of blister formation in bullous impetigo and staphylococcal scalded skin syndrome. *J Clin Invest.* 2002;110(1):53–60. https://doi.org/10.1172/JCI0215766. Medline:12093888

Hartman-Adams H, Banvard C, Juckett G. Impetigo: diagnosis and treatment. *Am Fam Physician.* 2014;90(4):229–235. Medline:25250996

Jackson-Richards D, Pandya AG. *Dermatology atlas for skin of color.* New York: Springer; 2014.

Luby SP, Agboatwalla M, Feikin DR, et al. Effect of handwashing on child health: a randomised controlled trial. *Lancet.* 2005;366(9481):225–233. https://doi.org/10.1016/S0140-6736(05)66912-7. Medline:16023513

McCormick A, Fleming D, Charlton J; Royal College of General Practitioners; Office of Population Censuses and Surveys; Department of Health. *Morbidity statistics from general practice: fourth national study 1991–1992.* London: HMSO; 1995.

Rook A, Burns T. *Rook's textbook of dermatology.* Chichester, UK; Hoboken, NJ: Wiley-Blackwell; 2010.

Schachner LA, Hansen, RC, eds. *Pediatric dermatology.* 4th ed. 2 vols. New York: Mosby Elsevier; 2011.

Stevens DL, Kaplan EL, eds. *Streptococcal infections: clinical aspects, microbiology, and molecular pathogenesis.* New York: Oxford University Press; 2000.

Tong SY, Davis JS, Eichenberger E, Holland TL, Fowler VG Jr. Staphylococcus aureus infections: epidemiology, pathophysiology, clinical manifestations, and management. *Clin Microbiol Rev.* 2015;28(3):603–661. https://doi.org/10.1128/CMR.00134-14. Medline:26016486

12.4

Pediatric Eczema (Atopic Dermatitis)

David Bulir, Judy Wismer

- Pediatric eczema, also known as atopic dermatitis, is a chronic pruritic inflammatory skin disease.
- Worldwide, 5% to 20% of children are affected by pediatric eczema.
- Onset of the condition typically occurs before the age of 5.
- Females are slightly more likely than males to have atopic dermatitis (by a ratio of 1.3:1).
- 70% of patients with eczema have a family history of atopy (allergies, asthma, atopic dermatitis).

Pathophysiology
- Two main factors play into the development of eczema:
  1. Altered immunity
     › Alterations in both adaptive and innate immune response contribute to the pathogenesis of eczema.
       · Innate immune response — Patients with eczema have altered function of pattern recognition receptors TLR2 and TLR9, leading to abnormal repair, severe inflammation, and a Th2-polarized immune response in the skin.
       · Adaptive immune response — Dysfunctional barrier protection can lead to antigen penetration in the skin allowing for an IgE-mediated allergic sensitization.
  2. Altered skin barrier function
     › Barrier function of the skin is primarily mediated by the stratum corneum where cells are embedded in an extracellular matrix composed of filaggrin and lipids such as ceramides, cholesterol, and free fatty acids.
     › Transepidermal loss of water in patients with atopic dermatitis is believed to be a result of genetically impaired barrier function of the epidermis.
     › Permeability is controlled by numerous interactions between proteins, lipids and cells.

Physical Exam
- Presentation can vary depending on the age of the child, but patients typically present with dry skin and intense pruritus.
- Acute eczema has severely pruritic lesions that are typically erythematous papules and vesicles with crusting and exudates.

- Chronic eczema can be dry and scaly with excoriated erythematous papules; lichenification and fissuring may develop over time from chronic scratching.
  » Children < 2 years of age typically present with crusted, erythematous, scaly, pruritic lesions on extensor surfaces (with sparing of the diaper region), cheeks, and scalp.
  » Children 2 to 16 years of age usually also have crusted, erythematous, scaly, pruritic lesions, but they may be more lichenified depending on the patient's age at presentation.
    › Lesions are typically found on flexural surfaces such as the antecubital and popliteal fossa, wrists, ankles, face, and neck.
  » Patients may also have other cutaneous findings that are suggestive of atopic dermatitis:
    › Hertoghe's sign — thinning of the lateral aspect of the eyebrows
    › Infraorbital folds and periorbital darkening
    › Centrofacial pallor
    › Dermographism
    › Fissuring around the ear
    › Hyperlinearity of the palm

Diagnosis
- Diagnosis of atopic dermatitis is based on history and clinical features.

The UK Working Party's diagnostic criteria for atopic dermatitis
Based on Williams et al (1994).

- Patients must have pruritic skin based on history from the patient or parent **and** 3 or more of the following:
  » Involvement of flexural surfaces (popliteal and antecubital fossa), front of ankles, periorbital, and neck (cheeks if the patient is < 10 years of age)
  » History of asthma or hay fever (or a first-degree relative with atopy) in children < 4 years of age
  » Dry skin within the last year
  » Visible eczema on flexural surfaces or on cheeks/forehead for children < 4 years of age
  » Eczema that has started before the age of 2 (this criterion cannot be used if the patient is < 4 years of age)

- The severity of disease can be classified as mild, moderate, or severe.
  » Mild eczema is characterized by:
    › Minimal impact on daily activities and psychosocial well-being
    › Infrequent itching with minimal erythema
    › Few areas of dry skin
  » Moderate eczema is characterized by:
    › Moderate impact on daily activities, including sleeping and psychosocial well-being
    › Frequent itching and erythema (may have excoriations or minimal lichenification)
    › Multiple areas of dry skin
  » Severe eczema is characterized by:
    › Significant impact on daily activities, including loss of sleep and psychosocial functioning
    › Insatiable pruritus and erythema (may have excoriations, fissuring, bleeding, lichenification, and altered pigmentation)
    › Significant surface area of dry skin

Differential Diagnosis

More Common

CONTACT DERMATITIS (ALLERGIC OR IRRITANT)

- Consider the location of the rash versus typical location for atopic dermatitis.
- Enquire about exposure history to irritants and known allergens.

SEBORRHEIC DERMATITIS

- Seborrheic dermatitis presents as erythematous patches with greasy scales.
- There is typically little to no pruritus.
- There is scalp involvement.

PSORIASIS

- Psoriasis involves the diaper area.
- It presents as well-demarcated erythematous patches and plaques with little scaling.

INFECTIOUS DISEASES

- Consider the following infectious diseases on the differential diagnosis:
  » Dermatophyte infection
    › Dermatophyte infection presents as one to many scaly, well-demarcated plaques with central clearing.
    › There is variable pruritus.
  » Impetigo
    › Impetigo presents as well-demarcated erythematous patches with blisters and/or honey-yellow crusting; see Chapter 12.3.

» Scabies
  › Scabies involves skin folds and the diaper area.
  › It presents with vesicopustules on the palms and soles of the feet.

Less Common

ZINC DEFICIENCY

- Zinc deficiency presents as scaly, erythematous patches or plaques around the anus and mouth.

HYPER-IGE SYNDROME

- Eczematous rash and pustules occur within the first week after birth.
- Patients will have high serum IgE.
- Other signs of Hyper-IgE syndrome are:
  » Recurrent staphylococcal infections of the skin, sinuses, and lungs
  » Eosinophilia

WISKOTT-ALDRICH SYNDROME

- The Wiskott-Aldrich syndrome rash is identical to atopic dermatitis.
- It occurs in the first weeks of life in boys.
- Patients are thrombocytopenic.

OMENN SYNDROME

- Patients with omenn syndrome presents with:
  » Erythroderma (reddening of the skin) and desquamation
    › The rash is widespread and scaly.
  » Chronic diarrhea
  » Lymphadenopathy, hepatosplenomegaly

Management

- Ensure skin hydration.
  » Use emollients (creams or ointments) to maintain skin hydration (Grade A, Level I).
  » Apply emollients at least 2 times per day after bathing or handwashing.
  » Try to apply emollients an hour before or after applying topical corticosteroids.

Topical Corticosteroids (Grade A, Level I)

- Topical corticosteroids, in addition to emollients, are the mainstay treatment for eczema.
  » When choosing a topical corticosteroid, choose the most effective steroid that is the least potent.
  » Consider patient preference for greasier (ointment) versus less greasy (cream) formulations.
  » Consider the location of the area being treated.
    › For areas of thin skin where atrophy is a concern (e.g., face, neck, and skin-fold regions), consider a less-potent steroid.
    › On face and skin folds, limit treatment to low potency 1% hydrocortisone cream.

» Limit higher-potency corticosteroid use to no more than 2 weeks.

» Evidence exists that demonstrates similar efficacy for once daily versus twice daily application; however, twice daily application is the most generally recommended and used in clinical practice.

- For patients with mild disease, consider lower potency corticosteroid cream or ointment such as desonide 0.05% cream (low potency) or ointment (low to medium potency).

- For patients with moderate disease, consider a medium to high potency corticosteroid cream or ointment such as:

» Mometasone furoate 0.1% cream (medium potency) or ointment (high potency)

» Betamethasone valerate 0.1% cream or ointment (both medium potency)

- For patients with severe disease, consider a high to very high potency corticosteroid cream or ointment.

» Limit the use of these steroids to no more than 2 weeks:

› Fluocinonide 0.05% cream or ointment (both high potency)

› Clobetasol propionate 0.05% cream or ointment (both very high potency)

- Monitor the patient for side effects and treatment efficacy (Grade A, Level I).

» Children have a higher body surface to weight ratio, resulting in a larger amount of corticosteroid being absorbed for the same amount applied, and as a result, they are more susceptible to side effects.

» Cutaneous skin changes may occur with long-term use, including:

› Telangiectasias
› Striae
› Purpura
› Skin atrophy

» Systemic side effects are rare but are associated with higher potency corticosteroids and could potentially lead to hypothalamic-pituitary-adrenal axis suppression; however, there are no specific recommendations for monitoring this.

Topical Calcineurin Inhibitors (Grade A, Level I)

- Topical calcineurin inhibitors are noncorticosteroid anti-inflammatory inhibitors of T cell activation, which decreases inflammation.

- Consider using a topical calcineurin inhibitor when:

» Patient is recalcitrant to corticosteroids
» Sensitive areas are involved (e.g., face, skin folds, anogenital region)
» Patient has corticosteroid-induced atrophy
» Patient has had long-term, uninterrupted topical corticosteroid use

- Topical calcineurin inhibitors should be applied twice daily.

- Tacrolimus 0.03% ointment and pimecrolimus 1% cream are indicated for use in patients ≥ **2 years of age.**

- Tacrolimus 0.1% ointment is indicated for patients ≥ **15 years of age.**

- Evidence from clinical trials have demonstrated the efficacy and safety of tacrolimus 0.03% ointment and pimecrolimus 1% cream in children < 2 years of age (Grade A, Level I).

- Consider using topical calcineurins 2 to 3 times per week to prevent recurrence of disease (Grade A, Level I).

Antimicrobials

- Patients with eczema are at risk for developing skin infections due to altered barrier function of the skin, especially *S. aureus*.

- Children with moderate to severe disease may benefit from dilute bleach baths with intranasal mupirocin ointment (Grade B, Level I).

» Dilute 120 mL of 6% bleach in 40 gallons of lukewarm water, and soak for 5 to 10 minutes.

» A recent meta-analysis has concluded that bleach baths can help reduce the severity of atopic dermatitis; however, bleach baths were no more effective then plain water baths.

Other Therapy with Consultation

- Consider:
» Phototherapy
› Use of phototherapy is not suitable for young children and infants.
» Systemic immunosuppressive therapies:
› Cyclosporine
· Use of oral cyclosporine is not recommended for atopic dermatitis in young children and infants.
· Consider using oral cyclosporine in older children and adolescents who have significant impairment in quality of life and severe disease that has had limited response to topical corticosteroids.
· Use of oral cyclosporine in North America is considered off-label; give 2.5 to 5 mg/kg per day divided into 2 doses daily for 6 weeks.
· After 6 weeks and with significant clinical improvement, consider stopping cyclosporine and beginning topical corticosteroids and emollients.
› Methotrexate
· Use of methotrexate is off-label for atopic dermatitis; however, significant improvement has been seen in children with severe disease.

› Azathioprine
  · Use of azathioprine is off-label for atopic dermatitis; however, significant improvement has been seen in children with severe disease.
› Dupilumab
  · Dupilumab is a promising treatment currently being investigated for safety and efficacy in the pediatric population; however, it is currently approved for the treatment of atopic dermatitis in adults.
  · Dupilumab is a monoclonal antibody administered by injection which targets two cytokines central to the pathogenesis of atopic dermatitis.
» Probiotics
  › Use of a synbiotic (a combination oral fructo-oligosaccharide with *L. salivarius*) has shown significant improvement in reducing the severity of disease in children with severe atopic dermatitis.
  › Earlier meta-analyses have previously demonstrated lack of efficacy for probiotics in reducing the severity of eczema.

Complications

- Complications of eczema include:
  » *Staphyloccocus aureus* infection — secondary skin infections due to loss of barrier function of the skin
  » Eczema herpeticum — widespread infection or reactivation of herpes simplex virus, typically in severe atopic dermatitis
  » Molluscum contagiosum — atopic dermatitis is associated with an increased risk of molluscum contagiosum infection in children and adolescents

REFERENCES

Chopra R, Vakharia PP, Sacotte R, Silverberg JI. Efficacy of bleach baths in reducing severity of atopic dermatitis: a systematic review and meta-analysis. *Ann Allergy Asthma Immunol.* 2017;119(5):435–440. https://doi.org/10.1016/j.anai.2017.08.289

Eichenfield LF, Boguniewicz M, Simpson EL, et al. Translating atopic dermatitis management guidelines into practice for primary care providers. *Pediatrics.* 2015;136(3):554–565. https://doi.org/10.1542/peds.2014-3678. Medline:26240216

Eichenfield LF, Hanifin JM, Luger TA, Stevens SR, Pride HB. Consensus conference on pediatric atopic dermatitis. *J Am Acad Dermatol.* 2003;49(6):1088–1095. https://doi.org/10.1016/S0190-9622(03)02539-8. Medline:14639390

Eichenfield LF, Tom WL, Berger TG, et al. Guidelines of care for the management of atopic dermatitis: section 2. Management and treatment of atopic dermatitis with topical therapies. *J Am Acad Dermatol.* 2014;71(1):116–132. https://doi.org/10.1016/j.jaad.2014.03.023. Medline:24813302

Eichenfield LF, Tom WL, Chamlin SL, et al. Guidelines of care for the management of atopic dermatitis: section 1. Diagnosis and assessment of atopic dermatitis. *J Am Acad Dermatol.* 2014;70(2):338–351. https://doi.org/10.1016/j.jaad.2013.10.010. Medline:24290431

Galli E, Neri I, Ricci G, et al. Consensus Conference on Clinical Management of Pediatric Atopic Dermatitis. *Ital J Pediatr.* 2016;42(1):26. https://doi.org/10.1186/s13052-016-0229-8. Medline:26936273

Haeck IM, Knol MJ, Ten Berge O, van Velsen SG, de Bruin-Weller MS, Bruijnzeel-Koomen CA. Enteric-coated mycophenolate sodium versus cyclosporin A as long-term treatment in adult patients with severe atopic dermatitis: a randomized controlled trial. *J Am Acad Dermatol.* 2011;64(6):1074–1084. https://doi.org/10.1016/j.jaad.2010.04.027. Medline:21458107

Lauffer F, Ring J. Target-oriented therapy: emerging drugs for atopic dermatitis. *Expert Opin Emerg Drugs.* 2016;21(1):81–89. https://doi.org/10.1517/14728214.2016.1146681. Medline:26808004

Raimer SS. Managing pediatric atopic dermatitis. *Clin Pediatr (Phila).* 2000;39(1):1–14. https://doi.org/10.1177/000992280003900101. Medline:10660813

Sidbury R, Davis DM, Cohen DE, et al; American Academy of Dermatology. Guidelines of care for the management of atopic dermatitis: section 3. Management and treatment with phototherapy and systemic agents. *J Am Acad Dermatol.* 2014;71(2):327–349. https://doi.org/10.1016/j.jaad.2014.03.030. Medline:24813298

Sidbury R, Tom WL, Bergman JN, et al. Guidelines of care for the management of atopic dermatitis: section 4. Prevention of disease flares and use of adjunctive therapies and approaches. *J Am Acad Dermatol.* 2014;71(6):1218–1233. https://doi.org/10.1016/j.jaad.2014.08.038. Medline:25264237

Silverberg JI. Atopic dermatitis: an evidence-based treatment update. *Am J Clin Dermatol.* 2014;15(3):149–164. https://doi.org/10.1007/s40257-014-0062-z. Medline:24464934

Weidinger S, Novak N. Atopic dermatitis. *Lancet.* 2016;387(10023):1109–1122. https://doi.org/10.1016/S0140-6736(15)00149-X. Medline:26377142

Williams HG, Jburney PG, Hay RJ, Archer CB, Shipley MJ, Ahunter JJ, Bingham EA, Finlay AY, Pembroke AC, CGraham-Brown RA, Atherton DA, Lewis-Jones MS, Holden CA, Harper JI, Champion RH, Poyner TF, Launer J, David TJ. The UK Working Party's diagnostic criteria for atopic dermatitis. *Brit J of Derm.* 1994;131(3):383–396. https://doi.org/10.1111/j.1365-2133.1994.tb08530.x

12.5

Neonatal Rashes

David Bulir, Channy Muhn, Judy Wismer

ERYTHEMA TOXICUM NEONATORUM

- Erythema toxicum neonatorum (ETN) is a self-limiting rash found in newborns.
- It is also referred to as erythema neonatorum allergicum, as it is a noninfectious, inflammatory skin condition.
- The condition is idiopathic and asymptomatic.
- It is estimated to affect 15% of 20% of newborns.
- ETN may have a slightly higher rate of incidence in males.

Risk factors

- Risk factors for developing ETN are:
  » Later gestational age
  » Term birth
  » First pregnancy
  » Vaginal delivery

Pathophysiology

- Histology reveals inflammatory infiltrates around hair follicles consisting primarily of eosinophils and numerous inflammatory mediators (NOS1–3, IL-1, IL-9, eotaxin, Psoriasin).
- ETN is found only on skin surfaces with hair follicles, suggesting that the hair follicle provides a nidus for local invasion of new, developing skin flora.

Diagnosis

- Diagnosis of ETN is clinical.
- It typically presents within the first 24 to 48 hours of life and resolves within 5 to 7 days.
- Lesions are found only on areas of the body with hair follicles, not on the palms of the hands, soles of the feet, or penis.
- Lesions may start with erythematous macules and papules of varying size, which then rapidly progress to papules or pustules with an erythematous base.

Differential Diagnosis

- Consider the following on the differential diagnosis:
  » Transient neonatal pustular melanosis

  › Transient neonatal pustular melanosis can be differentiated from ETN based on the presence of hyperpigmented macules, scaling of the erythematous macules, and pustules without an erythematous base.
  » Neonatal acne (neonatal cephalic pustulosis)
  › Neonatal acne typically occurs around 3 weeks of age.
  › It is characterized by inflammatory papules and pustules without a comedonal lesion and distributed over the face and occasionally the scalp.
  » Miliaria pustulosa
  › This is a nonfollicular associated rash caused by the obstruction of sweat glands leading to a localized inflammatory response and erythematous pustules.

Investigations

- No investigations are required; diagnosis is clinical.
- Cultures from pustules are negative for fungi, bacteria, and viruses.
- Microscopy with a Wright-stained smear of pustule contents will reveal numerous eosinophils and occasional neutrophils.

Management

- ETN self-resolves within 5 to 7 days.

SEBORRHEIC DERMATITIS IN THE INFANT

- Seborrheic dermatitis is a common skin condition that occurs in all age groups.
- It is characterized by greasy and yellow plaques with or without erythema on areas associated with an abundance of sebaceous glands (i.e., central face, scalp, external ears, and intertriginous regions).
- Seborrheic dermatitis occurs in approximately 70% of infants at 3 months of age; the rate of occurrence decreases thereafter.
- There is no significant difference in prevalence between males and females.

Pathophysiology

- The exact mechanism is unknown, but the following factors are believed to play a role:
  » The lipid-dependent yeast *Malassezia*
    › *Malassezia* is necessary but not sufficient for seborrheic dermatitis.
    › Pruritus, erythema, and scaling are believed to be the result of *Malassezia* invading the stratum corneum and secreting lipases that produce free fatty acids.
    › The free fatty acids trigger an inflammatory process, causing hyperproliferation within the stratum corneum and also leading to altered barrier function by inhibiting corneocyte differentiation.
  » Maternal androgens
    › Maternal androgens may stimulate the growth of sebaceous glands, leading to excessive sebum production and providing a nidus for *Malassezia* infection.

Diagnosis

- Seborrheic dermatitis has 2 main presentations in the newborn and infant.
  1. The most common presentation is "cradle cap."
    › Cradle cap is an asymptomatic accumulation of greasy, yellow scales on the scalp (vertex and frontal area) and is typically not erythematous.
    › Scales are also found on other parts of the body, including:
      · Face
      · Forehead
      · Behind the ears
      · Eyebrows
      · Eyelids
      · Cheeks (including nasolabial folds)
      · Diaper area
      · Trunk (especially around umbilicus)
      · Intertriginous regions
  2. Lesions may also appear as scaly, salmon-pink, erythematous plaques.
- The condition causes little to no pruritus; the child behaves normally, feeds well, and has no irritability.

Differential Diagnosis

- On differential diagnosis, consider:
  » Atopic dermatitis (see Chapter 12.4)
    › Atopic dermatitis is intensely pruritic.
    › Lesions are typically poorly demarcated.
    › Family history is positive for atopy.
    › Lesions are usually localized to cheeks, scalp, and extensor surfaces.
  » Langerhans cell histiocytosis
    › This may resemble seborrheic dermatitis or diaper rash with ulcerations and erosions.

» Both seborrheic dermatitis and Langerhans cell histiocytosis may be self-limiting; seborrheic dermatitis typically has a much shorter course of disease.
    › Other cutaneous manifestations include brown to purple papules or nodules, and oral lesions (e.g., mucosal ulcers).
    › It can be differentiated based on a biopsy.
  » Diaper dermatitis or "diaper rash"
    › Diaper rash occurs in moist environments where there is friction.
    › Skin folds are typically spared, but occasionally diaper rash also occurs in the context of a *Candida* infection that appears "beefy" red in color, with superficial erosions that involve skin folds.
    › Occasionally, small papular or pustular lesions may occur on the edge or just outside of the bulk of the rash.
  » Psoriasis
    › Lesions develop on flexor or diaper areas with typically shiny, silvery scales and well-demarcated, erythematous plaques.
  » Tinea capitis
    › Tinea capitis is a scaly dermatitis of the scalp with mild to moderate inflammation and hair loss (may be difficult to assess).
    › Tinea infections are rare in infants.
    › It can be differentiated via other conditions using a potassium hydroxide test and fungal cultures.

Investigations

- Seborrheic dermatitis is a clinical diagnosis.
- A thorough history and examination can help differentiate seborrheic dermatitis in the newborn from other conditions with scaly lesions.
- If there are concerns that the infection is fungal, potassium hydroxide examination and fungal cultures can be used; however, treatment for many suspected skin fungal infections of the newborn are similar to that for seborrheic dermatitis.

Management

- Management of seborrheic dermatitis involves a watchful waiting approach as most cases are self-limiting and resolve over weeks to months.
  » Conservative management is the mainstay of treatment while the seborrheic dermatitis is resolving.
- The application of emollients (e.g., baby oil, mineral oil, vegetable oil, or white petrolatum) and/or frequent shampooing with mild baby shampoo can help loosen scales on the scalp.
  » After shampooing or application of the emollients, physical removal of the scales can be attempted with gentle brushing using a soft toothbrush or fine comb.

- In persistent or more severe presentations, consider:
  - » 1% hydrocortisone cream applied once daily for up to 7 days
  — or —
  - » Ketoconazole 2% cream or shampoo twice per week for 2 weeks
- Intertriginous areas typically have a superimposed *Candida* infection.
  - » These regions should be treated with ketoconazole 2% cream applied once daily for 1 to 2 weeks, plus the application of a topical cream or ointment containing zinc oxide and/or petrolatum to limit skin maceration.

TRANSIENT NEONATAL PUSTULAR MELANOSIS

- Transient neonatal pustular melanosis is a benign, self-limited skin condition.
- It affects approximately 2.2% to 3.4% of infants and occurs equally in both sexes.
- There is a higher incidence among infants of African descent (4.4%) compared to Caucasian infants (0.2% to 0.6%).
- Transient neonatal pustular melanosis is also more common in full-term infants.

Pathophysiology

- The exact pathophysiology behind transient neonatal pustular melanosis is not widely understood.
- Histological examination of transient neonatal pustular melanosis lesions shows polymorphic neutrophils with occasional eosinophils.
- There is a possible overlap between erythema toxicum neonatorum (ETN) and transient neonatal pustular melanosis.
  - » This is believed to possibly represent a spectrum of a disease termed "sterile transient neonatal pustulosis."

Physical Exam

- The neonate is systemically well.
- Lesions are found all over the body, though they are less commonly found on the palms and soles.
- Transient neonatal pustular melanosis consists of 3 different types of lesions that progress in a stepwise fashion (all 3 can be seen at the same time):
  1. Sterile pustules on a healthy, nonerythematous base
     - › This typically resolves over a period of 48 hours if present after birth.
     - › Pustules in the early stages are quite fragile and often rupture *in utero* or while the infant is being cleaned in the delivery suite.
  2. Erythematous macules with collarette of scale

  3. Hyperpigmented macules
     - › Macules gradually fade over a period of weeks to months.

Differential Diagnosis

- On differential diagnosis, consider:
  - » ETN
    - › ETN is characterized by small, erythematous papules that do not develop postinflammatory hyperpigmentation.
  - » Milia
    - › Milia is characterized by small, firm, white, non-fragile, keratin-filled papules.
  - » Miliaria
    - › Miliaria is characterized by clear vesicles or pustules that develop in the context of increased body temperature (hyperthermia).
  - » Candidiasis
    - › Candidiasis is characterized by pustules with a "beefy" red erythema, sometimes with erosions or ulcerations in more severe infections.
  - » Acropustulosis
    - › Acropustulosis is characterized by pustules, not present at birth, primarily located on the palms and soles.
  - » Neonatal herpes simplex virus (HSV)
    - › Lesions are vesicular, typically not present at birth, and occur in the context of fever, irritability, and pain.

Investigations

- Transient neonatal pustular melanosis is a clinical diagnosis.

Management

- No treatment is necessary; lesions disappear over a period of weeks to months.

INCONTINENTIA PIGMENTI

- Incontinentia pigmenti, also called Bloch-Sulzberger syndrome, is an inherited skin disorder.
  - » It is an X-linked dominant disease caused by mutations in the *IKBKG/NEMO* gene, an inhibitor of NF-kB, leading to disordered regulation of inflammation, cellular survival, and immune response.
- The disease is nearly always lethal in males at the prenatal stage, meaning that the disease almost exclusively affects females.
- In addition to cutaneous manifestations of the disease, individuals may also have ocular or neurological manifestations.
- Incontinentia pigmenti affects approximately 1 in 40 000 to 50 000 infants.

Pathophysiology

- In approximately 90% of incontinentia pigmenti cases, the disease is caused by mutations in the *IKBKG/ NEMO* gene, with the remaining 10% caused by duplications, substitutions, and deletions.
  - » Since *IKBKG/NEMO* is a regulatory subunit of IkK (an NF-kB inhibitor), mutations in the *IKBKG/ NEMO* gene prevent activation of NF-kB, causing a cell to not appropriately generate a prosurvival/ proinflammatory response to tumor necrosis factor (TNF).
  - » Activation of the receptor TNF-R1 by TNF-alpha downstream signaling leads to a proapoptotic response.
- The varying severity of disease in incontinentia pigmenti may be the result of X-inactivation.
  - » X-inactivation is a random process that occurs during embryogenesis, and the chromosome that is inactivated in each cell depends on the tissue type.

Diagnosis

- Cutaneous lesions are the hallmark of incontinentia pigmenti.
- These lesions may be present at birth or a few months after birth.

Lesion Stages

- The lesions manifest in 4 distinct stages:
  - » Stage 1 — Vesiculo-bullous
    - › Stage 1 occurs at 0 to 4 months of age.
    - › Tense vesicular or pustular lesions with an erythematous base appear at or around the time of birth along Blaschko lines on the torso and extremities, lasting for a few months.
      - · Blaschko lines are nonvisible lines in the skin believed to represent the migration pathways of embryonic cells.
    - › Differential diagnosis for stage 1:
      - · Congenital herpes simplex
      - · Varicella
      - · Staphylococcal or streptococcal bullous impetigo
      - · Dystrophic epidermolysis bullosa
      - · Epidermolysis bullosa simplex
  - » Stage 2 — Verrucous, "wart-like"
    - › Stage 2 may occur over varying lengths of time.
    - › Lesions begin to transition into a wart-like stage and start to become more crusted and papular in nature.
    - › Some variability has been noted in patients with incontinentia pigmenti in that not all develop wart-like lesions.
    - › Stages 1 and 2 may be associated with eosinophilia as a result of abnormal *IKBKG/NEMO* mutations leading to abundant eotaxin production.

- › Differential diagnosis for stage 2:
  - · Simple warts
  - · Molluscum contagiosum
- » Stage 3 — Hyperpigmentation
  - › Stage 3 occurs from about 6 months of age into adolescence / early adulthood.
  - › It is characterized by the development of brown to gray-brown macules.
  - › The pigmented macules may occur in varying arrangements, from linear to swirling patterns or a combination of both.
  - › In most patients, these lesions usually resolve by adolescence, but a small percentage of patients develop stage 4 cutaneous findings.
- » Stage 4 — Hypopigmentation and atrophy
  - › Stage 4 may be accompanied by alopecia.
  - › It is associated with the development of linear hypopigmented macules or patches after the previous hyperpigmented lesions fade.
  - › Differential diagnosis of stage 4:
    - · Vitiligo
    - · Piebaldism
    - · Hypomelanosis of Ito

Other Cutaneous Changes

- Other cutaneous changes can also occur in incontinentia pigmenti:
  - » Alopecia
    - › Alopecia may occur during any stage of skin lesion development.
    - › Hair changes may also occur — hair may become thin, lusterless, wiry, and coarse.
  - » Nail changes
    - › Dystrophic changes similar to fungal infection may occur.
    - › These typically begin in stage 2 or later.
  - » Central nervous system (CNS) manifestations
    - › 30% of patients with incontinentia pigmenti have some form of CNS abnormality:
      - · Seizures
      - · Intellectual and learning disabilities
      - · Structural abnormalities
  - » Ophthalmologic manifestations
    - › The most common ophthalmologic finding is retinal hypervascularization leading to retinal detachment if left untreated.
    - › Various ophthalmologic abnormalities have been noted in patients with incontinentia pigmenti, including:
      - · Optic atrophy
      - · Abnormal retinal pigmentation
      - · Microphthalmia
      - · Strabismus
      - · Cataracts

Table 12.5.1 DIAGNOSTIC CRITERIA FOR INCONTINENTIA PIGMENTI

Major criteria			Minor criteria (supportive evidence)
Criterion	**Stage**	**Clinical findings**	
Typical incontinentia pigmenti skin lesions distributed along Blaschko lines	Stage 1 — Vesiculo-bullous	Erythema and blistering	• Dental anomalies • Ocular anomalies • CNS anomalies • Alopecia or abnormal hair • Abnormal nails • Palate anomalies • Nipple and breast anomalies • Multiple miscarriages of male fetuses • Typical skin pathohistological findings
	Stage 2 — Verrucous	Hypertrophic rash	
	Stage 3 — Hyperpigmentation	Hyperpigmentation	
	Stage 4 — Hypopigmentation and atrophy	Hypopigmentation and alopecia	

Diagnostic Criteria

- A diagnosis of incontinentia pigmenti can be made with the presence of any single major criteria.
- Minor criteria are used to support the diagnosis, and if no minor criteria are present, then the likelihood of incontinentia pigmenti should be reconsidered.

Investigations

- Genetic testing can be done to establish the diagnosis of incontinentia pigmenti.
  - » Diagnosis can be made with the identification of a heterozygous pathogenic variant of *IKBKG/NEM*.
  - » Common testing methods include targeted mutation analysis to identify a common deletion of 11.7-kb in *IKBKG*, or deletion and sequence analysis, or deletion and duplication analysis.

Management

- Treatment of patients with incontinentia pigmenti requires a multidisciplinary approach, involving the appropriate disciplines that can address the abnormalities that have been identified.
- Address skin lesions (dermatology).
  - » Stages 1 and 2 are the stages at which treatment or supportive care is usually required.
  - » The blisters that form in stage 1 should be managed like any other blisters.
    - › Do not open and avoid causing trauma to the blisters.
    - › Provide appropriate wound dressing.
    - › There is some evidence supporting the use of topical corticosteroids.
    - › If blisters show signs of infection, consider starting local or systemic antibiotics.
  - » The hypertrophic rash that develops in stage 2 can cause difficulty with movement of the extremities and hands.
    - › Consider the use of emollients and topical retinoids to reduce hypertrophic rash.

- Address seizures resulting from CNS abnormalities.
  - » A limited number of studies have demonstrated the use of high-dose corticosteroids for the treatment of seizures in incontinentia pigmenti that do not respond to anticonvulsants.

LANGERHANS CELL HISTIOCYTOSIS

- Langerhans cell histiocytosis is a rare disease associated with the infiltration of histiocytes containing bean-shaped nuclei into nearly every organ except the heart and kidneys.
  - » In addition to the infiltration of histiocytes, lymphocytes, macrophages, and eosinophils can be found in the cutaneous lesions.
- Langerhans cell histiocytosis is most common in children 1 to 3 years of age.
- It is slightly more common in males than females.
- The incidence is approximately 3 to 5 cases per 1 000 000 children.
- Langerhans cell histiocytosis can be associated with single- or multisystem disease.
  - » 55% of patients have single-system disease, whereas 45% have multisystem disease.
  - » Approximately 40% of patients have skin involvement at the time of diagnosis.
  - » Children with skin-only Langerhans cell histiocytosis are usually < 1 year of age and have a better prognosis compared to multisystem disease.

Pathophysiology

- The exact cause of Langerhans cell histiocytosis is unknown, but there are 2 different theories.
  1. Reactive inflammatory disease
  2. Myeloproliferative neoplastic disease
     - › More recent evidence seems to support Langerhans cell histiocytosis being a myeloproliferative neoplastic disease as approximately 75% of lesions from Langerhans cell histiocytosis patients contain two mutations in cancer-associated proto-oncogenes.

- Unlike the name of the disease, the cells responsible for Langerhans cell histiocytosis are not derived from the skin Langerhans cell but are myeloid dendritic cells with surface markers CD1a and CD207, which are the same markers found on skin Langerhans cells.

Physical Exam

- Langerhans cell histiocytosis can manifest specifically with skin lesions or in combination with multisystem disease.
- A thorough evaluation and follow-up of a child presenting with skin-only disease should be undertaken to ensure that the disease is truly limited to the skin.
- The main skin presentations in Langerhans cell histiocytosis involve brown to purplish papules, an eczematous rash, and oral lesions.
  » The brown to purplish papules are also called congenital self-healing reticulohistiocytosis.
    › The lesions in Langerhans cell histiocytosis can be found anywhere on the body, with approximately 25% of newborns with Langerhans cell histiocytosis having a solitary lesion, and the remaining having multiple lesions.
    › The papules typically develop a central ulceration.
    › No active treatment is usually required, but the patient should be closely monitored and evaluated for recurrence or cutaneous lesions, or if the skin lesions were an early presentation of systemic disease.
    › An erythematous papular rash may develop on the back, groin, abdomen, and head.
      · The rash on the back, groin, and abdomen may resemble a candidal diaper rash.
- Neonates with Langerhans cell histiocytosis may appear to have a protracted course of "cradle cap" (seborrheic dermatitis) that may also involve the postauricular area.
- Both types of lesions may also be ulcerative and may lead the clinician to think the lesions are of bacterial or fungal origin.
- Lesions of the mouth include gingivitis, ulcers, and early tooth eruption in infants.

Investigations

- The diagnosis of Langerhans cell histiocytosis is based on tissue biopsy.
  » Biopsy shows presence of histiocytes with surface markers of CD1a and CD207 (also known as langerin) in abnormal clusters.

Management

- Upon diagnosis of Langerhans cell histiocytosis, the Histiocyte Society recommends the following baseline evaluation:
  » Hemoglobin, white blood cell (WBC) and differential count, platelet count
  » Total protein, albumin, bilirubin, alanine transaminase (ALT), aspartate transaminase (AST), alkaline phosphatase, gamma-glutamyl transferase (GGT)
  » Blood urea nitrogen (BUN), creatinine, electrolytes
  » Ferritin
  » International normalized ratio (INR) / prothrombin time (PT), partial thromboplastin time (PTT), fibrinogen
  » Early morning urine specific gravity and osmolality
  » Abdominal ultrasound for size and structure of liver and spleen
  » Chest X-ray (CXR)
  » Skeletal radiograph survey
- In a small study of 19 patients, it was found that skin-only lesions can spontaneously resolve within 1 month to approximately 2 years, with a mean time to resolution of 12 months.
- Presently, there is no standard of care for the treatment of skin-limited Langerhans cell histiocytosis.
- Various chemotherapeutic agents and immunomodulators have been used in the treatment of Langerhans cell histiocytosis.
- Given the high incidence of spontaneous regression, some clinicians prefer to watch and wait and to treat the condition only if there is associated morbidity.

NEONATAL HERPES SIMPLEX VIRUS

- Infection of the neonate with HSV typically happens during the intrapartum period, though intrauterine or postpartum infections can occur.
- The incidence of neonatal herpes infections varies widely across the world.
- In Canada, the incidence is approximately 6 infections per 100 000 live births.
  » 63% of cases in Ontario are caused by HSV-1, and the remaining 37% are caused by HSV-2.
- The most common route of exposure is intrapartum exposure, with approximately 75% to 85% of cases occurring through exposure in asymptomatic or recently infected women.
  » Remaining cases of neonatal HSV infection occur during intrauterine or postnatal exposure.

Pathophysiology

Infectivity

- Intrauterine HSV infections occur through two main mechanisms of infection.
- Fetal exposure can occur transplacentally via the chorionic villi or through prolonged premature rupture of the membranes.
  » Maternal primary infection with associated viremia

or an ascending HSV infection presents additional risk factors for the development of neonatal HSV.

- Postnatal transmission can occur through maternal or nonmaternal contacts from individuals with herpes labialis.
- Intrapartum HSV infections occur as a result of direct exposure to HSV from the cervix, vagina, vulva, or perianal areas.

Viral Infection

- Infection can be caused by either HSV-1 or HSV-2, which are from the herpesvirus family.
- HSV infections occur as either acute or recurrent disease.

ACUTE INFECTION

- For an acute infection to start, HSV must come in contact with abraded skin or a mucosal surface.
- Epithelial cells are the primary site of HSV replication in the skin.
- Surface glycoproteins on HSV are responsible for initial binding to the host cell and membrane fusion.
- Upon fusion of the HSV membrane to the host cell, the viral capsid is released into the cytosol, where it travels along the cytoskeleton to the nucleus where it interacts with nuclear pore complexes.
- As a result of the infection in epithelial cells, acantholysis occurs, causing a loss of cohesion between keratinocytes and leading to vesicle formation.

RECURRENT AND LATENT INFECTIONS

- HSV can establish a latent neuronal infection when a virion or viral capsid travels to the sensory ganglia via retrograde intraaxonal flow.
  » Animal models have also shown the possibility of neuronal infection as a result of viremia and not retrograde HSV transport to the sensory ganglia.
- Once at the sensory ganglia, a latent infection is established the help of latency-associated transcript RNA, which also blocks apoptosis, promoting survival.
- Upon viral reactivation, the virus replicates in the sensory ganglia, and the newly formed virus then travels in an anterograde motion along the neuron to infect epithelial cells.

Diagnosis

- Intrauterine HSV infection can cause:
  » Fetal demise
  » Hydrops fetalis
  » Pneumonitis
  » Myocarditis
  » Hepatosplenomegaly
  » Chorioretinitis
  » Encephalitis

  » Cataracts
  » Growth and mental retardation
  » Hemolytic anemia
  » Vesicles on the skin
  » Skin scarring
  » Microcephaly
  » Hydranencephaly
- Neonatal HSV manifests in 3 different ways:
  1. Skin, eye, and mucous membrane (SEM) infection
     › Neonatal HSV infection leads to SEM-only infections in approximately 45% of cases.
     › SEM infections are associated with progression to either CNS or disseminated HSV infection up to 6 weeks of age.
     › Skin lesions appear as vesicular lesions with an erythematous base that cluster or coalesce.
     › Early symptoms of eye involvement may include excessive tearing, erythematous conjunctiva, and irritability or pain.
       · Infection of the cornea and conjunctiva (keratoconjunctivitis) may lead to permanent eye damage and visual impairment.
       · Patients may also present with periorbital vesicular lesions.
     › Ulcerative lesions of the oropharynx (mouth, tongue, and palate) may develop.
  2. Localized CNS HSV
     › ~33% of neonates with HSV infections will develop CNS manifestations.
     › They can occur anytime within the first 6 weeks of life but more commonly occurs in the first 2 to 3 weeks after birth.
     › CNS involvement manifests as:
       · Irritability
       · Failure to thrive
       · Temperature instability
       · Full anterior fontanelle
       · Lethargy
       · Generalized or focal seizures
       · Tremor
  3. Disseminated HSV
     › 25% of neonates develop a disseminated, sepsis-like condition.
     › This is typically diagnosed in the second week of life, though nonspecific signs may be present during early manifestations of the disease, including:
       · Hyper- or hypothermia
       · Lethargy
       · Irritability
       · Respiratory distress
       · Abdominal findings (distention, ascites, hepatomegaly)
     › Disseminated HSV infection can cause multiorgan dysfunction, leading to death in over 80% of untreated cases.

> Organ systems involved include:
>   - Liver — hepatitis with abnormal liver enzymes, direct hyperbilirubinemia, liver failure, ascites
>   - Respiratory — respiratory failure, pneumonia, hemorrhagic pneumonitis with or without effusion
>   - CNS (as described above)
>   - Cardiac — myocarditis, myocardial dysfunction
>   - Kidney — dysfunction and failure
>   - Adrenal — dysfunction
>   - Gastrointestinal (GI) — necrotizing enterocolitis
>   - Hematologic — bone marrow suppression (thrombocytopenia and neutropenia), disseminated intravascular coagulation

Investigations

- Neonatal HSV can present with nonspecific symptoms that resemble sepsis, meningitis, and enterovirus infection.
- If HSV infection is suspected in the neonate, the following samples should be collected for detection via nucleic acid amplification, viral culture, or enzyme immunoassay (EIA) and direct fluorescent antibody (DFA) if indicated:
  » Surface swabs
    › Mouth, nasopharynx, conjunctivae, rectum
  » Cerebral spinal fluid (CSF) via lumbar puncture
  » Skin scrapings or swabs of any skin lesions
  » Whole blood or plasma
  » Amniotic testing — consider if in utero HSV infection is suspected
- A thorough laboratory investigation should be undertaken, including:
  » Complete blood count (CBC) with differential and platelets
  » Blood culture
  » CSF cell count, protein, glucose, and culture
  » Total and direct bilirubin, ammonia, and liver transaminases
- Request neuroimaging, CXR, eye examination, electroencephalogram (EEG; if CNS involvement is suspected), and abdominal ultrasound (if indicated).

Management

- In addition to supportive therapy, treatment with antivirals is indicated for all forms of neonatal HSV infection.
- Acyclovir treatment has drastically reduced 1-year mortality:
  » From 85% to 29% for disseminated infection
  » From 50% to 4% for CNS infections
- In addition to reducing mortality, antivirals prevent the progression of SEM HSV infections to both CNS or disseminated disease by approximately 60%.

- Acyclovir therapy should be started when HSV infection is suspected in the neonate.
  » All forms of neonatal HSV infection should be treated with acyclovir 20 mg/kg IV every 8 hours (Grade 1A evidence).
  » The duration of treatment is different between SEM disease or CNS and disseminated HSV disease.
    › Treat patients for SEM disease for 14 days when CNS and disseminated HSV disease have been ruled out.
    › CNS and disseminated HSV disease need to be treated for at least 21 days and treatment continued until lumbar puncture is negative for HSV DNA.
- Ocular manifestations of the disease require ophthalmologic consultation and treatment in addition to the use of acyclovir.
  » Give topical ophthalmic solution 1% trifluridine, 0.1% idoxuridine, or 0.15% ganciclovir.

REFERENCES

Allen CE, Ladisch S, McClain KL. How I treat Langerhans cell histiocytosis. *Blood*. 2015;126(1):26–35. https://doi.org/10.1182/blood-2014-12-569301. Medline:25827831

Bodemer C. Incontinentia pigmenti and hypomelanosis of Ito. *Handb Clin Neurol*. 2013;111:341–347. https://doi.org/10.1016/B978-0-444-52891-9.00040-3. Medline:23622185

Cohen S. Should we treat infantile seborrhoeic dermatitis with topical antifungals or topical steroids? *Arch Dis Child*. 2004;89(3):288–289. https://doi.org/10.1136/adc.2003.048058. Medline:14977719

El Demellawy D, Young JL, de Nanassy J, Chernetsova E, Nasr A. Langerhans cell histiocytosis: a comprehensive review. *Pathology*. 2015;47(4):294–301. https://doi.org/10.1097/PAT.0000000000000256. Medline:25938350

Emile JF, Abla O, Fraitag S, et al.; Histiocyte Society. Revised classification of histiocytoses and neoplasms of the macrophage-dendritic cell lineages. *Blood*. 2016;127(22):2672–2681. https://doi.org/10.1182/blood-2016-01-690636. Medline:26966089

Gandra NR, Reddy HB, Katta TP. Cutaneous changes in neonates in the first 72 hours of birth: an observational study. *Curr Pediatr Rev*. 2017;13(2):136–143. https://doi.org/10.2174/1573396313666170216120230. Medline:28215177

Ghosh S. Neonatal pustular dermatosis: an overview. *Indian J Dermatol*. 2015;60(2):211. Medline:25814724

Grois N, Pötschger U, Prosch H, et al.; DALHX- and LCH I and II Study Committee. Risk factors for diabetes insipidus in langerhans cell histiocytosis. *Pediatr Blood Cancer*. 2006;46(2):228–233. https://doi.org/10.1002/pbc.20425. Medline:16047354

Kapur P, Erickson C, Rakheja D, Carder KR, Hoang MP. Congenital self-healing reticulohistiocytosis (Hashimoto-Pritzker disease): ten-year experience at Dallas Children's Medical Center. *J Am Acad Dermatol*. 2007;56(2):290–294. https://doi.org/10.1016/j.jaad.2006.09.001. Medline:17224372

Kaya TI, Tursen U, Ikizoglu G. Therapeutic use of topical corticosteroids in the vesiculobullous lesions of incontinentia pigmenti. *Clin Exp Dermatol*. 2009;34(8):e611–e613. https://doi.org/10.1111/j.1365-2230.2009.03301.x. Medline:19489863

Minić S, Trpinac D, Obradović M. Incontinentia pigmenti diagnostic criteria update. *Clin Genet*. 2014;85(6):536–542. https://doi.org/10.1111/cge.12223. Medline:23802866

Minkov M. Multisystem Langerhans cell histiocytosis in children: current treatment and future directions. *Paediatr Drugs*. 2011;13(2):75–86. https://doi.org/10.2165/11538540-000000000-00000. Medline:21351807

Monteagudo B, Labandeira J, Cabanillas M, Acevedo A, Toribio J. Prospective study of erythema toxicum neonatorum: epidemiology and predisposing factors. *Pediatr Dermatol.* 2012;29(2):166–168. https://doi.org/10.1111/j.1525-1470.2011.01536.x. Medline:22066938

Morgan AJ, Steen CJ, Schwartz RA, Janniger CK. Erythema toxicum neonatorum revisited. *Cutis.* 2009;83(1):13–16. Medline:19271565

Narayanan MJ, Rangasamy S, Narayanan V. Incontinentia pigmenti (Bloch-Sulzberger syndrome). *Handb Clin Neurol.* 2015;132:271–280. https://doi.org/10.1016/B978-0-444-62702-5.00020-2. Medline:26564087

Newman B, Hu W, Nigro K, Gilliam AC. Aggressive histiocytic disorders that can involve the skin. *J Am Acad Dermatol.* 2007;56(2):302–316. https://doi.org/10.1016/j.jaad.2006.06.010. Medline:17097374

O'Connor NR, McLaughlin MR, Ham P. Newborn skin: Part I. Common rashes. *Am Fam Physician.* 2008;77(1):47–52. Medline:18236822

Rayala BZ, Morrell DS. Common skin conditions in children: noninfectious rashes. *FP Essent.* 2017;453:18–25. Medline:28196317

Reginatto FP, De Villa D, Cestari TF. Benign skin disease with pustules in the newborn. *An Bras Dermatol.* 2016;91(2):124–134. https://doi.org/10.1590/abd1806-4841.20164285. Medline:27192509

Reginatto FP, De Villa D, Muller FM, et al. Prevalence and characterization of neonatal skin disorders in the first 72h of life. *J Pediatr (Rio J).* 2017;93(3):238–245. https://doi.org/10.1016/j.jped.2016.06.010. Medline:27875703

Simko SJ, Garmezy B, Abhyankar H, et al. Differentiating skin-limited and multisystem Langerhans cell histiocytosis. *J Pediatr.* 2014;165(5):990–996. https://doi.org/10.1016/j.jpeds.2014.07.063. Medline:25441388

Swinney CC, Han DP, Karth PA. Incontinentia pigmenti: a comprehensive review and update. *Ophthalmic Surg Lasers Imaging Retina.* 2015;46(6):650–657. https://doi.org/10.3928/23258160-20150610-09. Medline:26114846

Wananukul S, Chindamporn A, Yumyourn P, Payungporn S, Samathi C, Poovorawan Y. Malassezia furfur in infantile seborrheic dermatitis. *Asian Pac J Allergy Immunol.* 2005;23(2-3):101–105. Medline:16252839

Zuniga R, Nguyen T. Skin conditions: common skin rashes in infants. *FP Essent.* 2013;407:31–41. Medline:23600337

13.1

Epiglottitis

Camila de Lima, Kevin Chan

- Epiglottitis is a cellulitis of supraglottic structures, including the epiglottis, aryepiglottic folds, and posterior lingual surface and surrounding soft tissues.
- As the supraglottic edema increases, the epiglottis is forced posteriorly, causing progressive obstruction of the airway.
- Epiglottitis classically affects children 2 to 7 years of age.
  » Cases in children < 1 year of age have been reported.
  » In the postvaccination era, the mean age of onset has shifted from 3 years of age to 6 to 12 years of age.
- In the prevaccination era, 75% to 90% of cases were caused by *Haemophilus influenzae* type B (Hib).
  » Since the vaccine became available, the incidence of epiglottitis/supraglottitis in children < 5 years of age has significantly decreased.
  » In the United States, a study showed a decrease in incidence from 41 cases in 1987 to 1.3 per 100 000 children in 1997.
  » Hib is still considered the most common infectious cause of epiglottitis in children.
    › Epiglottitis can occur even in fully immunized children, possibly due to some degree of vaccination failure.
  » Epiglottitis is now also associated with a variety of organisms:
    › Bacterial organisms:
      · Nontypeable *H. influenza* (likely the second most common pathogen), *H. parainfluenzae*, *Staphylococcus aureus*, *S. pneumonia*, group A *Streptococcus* (GAS), *Moraxella catarrhalis*, *Pseudomonas* species, *Klebsiella* species
    › Fungal organisms:
      · *Candida* species
    › Viral organisms (with or without bacteria superinfection):
      · Herpes simplex virus (HSV), parainfluenza, *Varicella zoster*, Epstein-Barr virus (EBV)

- Although the age of onset has shifted, the presentation of epiglottitis remains essentially the same as in prevaccination days.
- Risk factors include incomplete or lack of immunization, as well as an immunocompromised state.
- The risk of death is < 1% and usually occurs prior to or just after arrival to the ED, due to acute airway obstruction.

History

- Patients have a rapidly progressive inflammation of the epiglottis and surrounding tissue.
- Classic presentation includes:
  » Severe anxiety, sore throat, dysphagia, high fever, and difficulty handling oral secretions
    -The latter is due to severe odynophagia.
  » Speech that may be altered due to pain or soft tissue swelling, resulting in a muffled "hot potato" voice
  » Tripod position (sitting in an upright position, leaning forward and supported by both hands, with the chin up and an open mouth)
  » Rapidly progressive respiratory distress
    › In a study of chart reviews (1957 to 1977) for patients who had presented with acute epiglottitis, 73% presented with symptoms lasting < 12 hours.
    › Most develop notable illness over 24 hours.

Note: Not all signs and symptoms are present in all cases.

Diagnosis

- Diagnosis is made by direct visualization of the supraglottic region, which is best done via emergency endoscopy in the operating room with spontaneous breathing.
- Proper equipment is required:
  » Adequately sized endotracheal tubes

259

» Rigid bronchoscopes
» Tracheostomy supplies
- Typical findings are edema and erythema of the supraglottic features (epiglottis, arytenoids, aryepiglottic folds).
- An orotracheal tube should be placed in order to obtain samples from the supraglottic region for culture and sensitivity.
- Blood cultures and investigations can also be done at this time.
- Concomitant infections such as pneumonia, otitis media, cellulitis, or even meningitis can be present.

Differential Diagnosis
- Epiglottitis and croup resemble each other but have some notable clinical differences.
  » Both are associated with stridor.
  » Cough without drooling is more suggestive of croup, while the opposite is true for epiglottitis.
  » Hoarseness is also more associated with croup, while refusal to lie down is more associated with epiglottitis.
- Differential diagnosis should also include:
  » Thermal injury
  » Caustic ingestion
  » Foreign-body aspiration
  » Retropharyngeal abscess
  » Angioneurotic edema
  » Anaphylaxis
  » Inhalation injury

Investigations
- White blood cell (WBC) count is usually elevated, with a neutrophilic predominance / left shift.
- Neck radiographs should be obtained if respiratory distress is deemed to be mild.
  » These can confirm diagnosis as well as rule out croup, retropharyngeal abscess, or foreign body.
  » The single best exposure is lateral neck with hyperextension during inspiration.
  » Classic findings on neck radiograph are:
    › Round, thick epiglottis ("thumb sign")
    › Loss of the vallecular air space
    › Thickening of aryepiglottic folds
  » Anteroposterior (AP) view may show a normal subglottic area compared to the stenosis usually seen with croup.

Management
- The patient's degree of respiratory distress needs to be assessed.
  » If significant compromise is present, the airway should be secured, and no further diagnostic workup should be pursued.

› Intubation in a controlled setting is the preferred method.
  · Intubation may require direct fiberoptic bronchoscopy (see "Diagnosis," above).
  · Use an endotracheal tube (ETT) that is 0.5 to 1 size smaller than usual for the age/weight of the child.
» Provide oxygen if patient is hypoxemic.
  › This may need to be done via bag valve mask ventilation.
» Prepare for a difficult intubation.
  › A clinician with advanced airway skills should be present.
  › An anesthesiologist, otorhinolaryngologist (ENT), or emergency department (ED) / critical care physician may also be included.
» If oxygen saturation is not maintained (pulse oximetry below the high-80s):
  › One trial of endotracheal intubation (preferably with video laryngoscope or direct laryngoscopy) may be attempted
    · If intubation fails, the next step is cricothyroidotomy.
  › Supraglottic airway devices, such as a laryngeal mask, should not be used
» If oxygen saturation is maintained, intubation attempt should be done in the operating room (OR).
- Before the introduction of the Hib vaccine, protocols existed in which OR personnel and an appropriate physician with bronchoscopic skills would be notified rapidly on recognition of a critical airway. The child would stay with the parent or caregiver and be escorted into the OR in the caregiver's arms, with no interventions initiated until inhalational anesthesia was begun.
- Occasionally, an older patient may not require intubation and can be managed with supplemental oxygen, antibiotics, and close monitoring in an intensive care setting.
- If the child is anxious, diagnostic investigations can be delayed, including phlebotomy.
  » Increased anxiety may worsen respiratory distress and lead to complete obstruction of the airway.
  » Also delay attempt to look at the oropharynx, which can elicit local trauma.
- If the child has minimal to moderate distress, the goal is to improve oxygenation and reduce inflammation.
  » Provide oxygen if the patient is hypoxemic.
  » Keep the patient calm.
    › Laboratory tests should be avoided in most cases.
  » Cool mist may reduce the viscosity of secretions (though no large studies have been conducted to determine the efficacy of this).
  » Administer racemic epinephrine nebulizations to reduce subglottic edema (which may be or may not be present).

> › The benefit of this is not currently established.
> › It should not be attempted if anxiety is likely to worsen.
> » Neck X-rays may be attempted, especially if diagnosis is unclear.

Medication

- Antibiotics should be started once the airway is secured and cultures obtained.
  » Aim to cover the most common pathogens, including:
    › *Haemophilus influenzae* (type b as well as nontypeable)
    › *Streptococcus pneumoniae*
    › GAS
    › *Staphylococcus aureus*
  » Give empiric therapy with oxacillin or a third-generation cephalosporin such as:
    › Cefotaxime 150 to 200 mg/kg per day divided and given every 6 hours
  » In areas where there is increased prevalence of community-acquired methicillin-resistant *S. aureus* (MRSA) or penicillin-resistant pneumococci, treatment should include clindamycin or vancomycin.
  » Other sources recommend broad spectrum antibiotics, effective against beta-lactamase–producing *H. influenzae*.
    › Consider second- or third-generation cephalosporins (e.g., cefuroxime, ceftriaxone, or ampicillin/sulbactam)
  » The optimal length of therapy is not known; most clinicians treat for 7 to 10 days depending on patient response.
  » Antibiotics should be adjusted as culture and sensitivity results become available.
- Glucocorticoids have not been shown to be beneficial in patients with epiglottitis and therefore are not actively recommended.
- Rifampin prophylaxis is recommended for household and daycare contacts at a dose of 20 mg/kg (maximum 600 mg) once daily for 4 days.

Postintubation Management

- Patients should be monitored in intensive care setting until there is evidence of clinical improvement.
  » Patients should be kept sedated so as to minimize trauma from movement.
- Development of an audible air leak around the endotracheal tube suggests that extubation may be attempted.

- Alternatively, flexible laryngoscopy can be used to monitor improvement of the subglottic swelling and guide extubation.
- Some physicians advocate for pretreatment with dexamethasone at 1 to 2 mg/kg in divided doses every 6 hours, beginning 12 to 24 hours before extubation.
  » This is thought to decrease the incidence of postextubation stridor.
- At the time of extubation, appropriate personnel and equipment should be readily available.
- Studies from the 1980s showed a mean duration of intubation between 30 and 72 hours.
  » Most patients are successfully extubated after 24 to 48 hours.
- Those who fail extubation should be reintubated with a smaller endotracheal tube and possibly given dexamethasone.
  » Endoscopic evaluation of the airway may be prudent to rule out necrotizing tracheobronchitis, tracheal stenosis, or a subglottic cyst.

REFERENCES

Baines DB, Wark H, Overton JH. Acute epiglottitis in children. *Anaesth Intensive Care.* 1985;13(1):25–28. Medline:3977063

Cherry JD. Epiglottitis (supraglottitis). In: Feigin RD, Cherry JD, Demmler-Harrison GJ, Kaplan SL, editors. *Textbook of pediatric infectious diseases,* 6th ed. Philadelphia: Saunders, 2009. p. 244–253.

Cohen SR, Chai J. Epiglottitis: twenty-year study with tracheotomy. *Ann Otol Rhinol Laryngol.* 1978;87(4 Pt 1):461–467. https://doi.org/10.1177/000348947808700402. Medline:686588

Hammer J. Acquired upper airway obstruction. *Paediatr Respir Rev.* 2004;5(1):25–33. https://doi.org/10.1016/j.prrv.2003.09.007. Medline:15222951

Loftis L. Acute infectious upper airway obstructions in children. *Semin Pediatr Infect Dis.* 2006;17(1):5–10. https://doi.org/10.1053/j.spid.2005.11.003. Medline:16522499

Losek JD, Dewitz-Zink BA, Melzer-Lange M, Havens PL. Epiglottitis: comparison of signs and symptoms in children less than 2 years old and older. *Ann Emerg Med.* 1990;19(1):55–58. https://doi.org/10.1016/S0196-0644(05)82143-2. Medline:2297156

Rotta AT, Wiryawan B. Respiratory emergencies in children. *Respir Care.* 2003;48(3):248–258, discussion 258–260. Medline:12667275

Shah RK, Roberson DW, Jones DT. Epiglottitis in the Hemophilus influenzae type B vaccine era: changing trends. *Laryngoscope.* 2004;114(3):557–560. https://doi.org/10.1097/00005537-200403000-00031. Medline:15091234

Sobol SE, Zapata S. Epiglottitis and croup. *Otolaryngol Clin North Am.* 2008;41(3):551–566, ix. https://doi.org/10.1016/j.otc.2008.01.012. Medline:18435998

Stroud RH, Friedman NR. An update on inflammatory disorders of the pediatric airway: epiglottitis, croup, and tracheitis. *Am J Otolaryngol.* 2001;22(4):268–275. https://doi.org/10.1053/ajot.2001.24825. Medline:11464324

Tibballs J, Watson T. Symptoms and signs differentiating croup and epiglottitis. *J Paediatr Child Health.* 2011;47(3):77–82. https://doi.org/10.1111/j.1440-1754.2010.01892.x. Medline:21091577

13.2

Epistaxis

Rahim Valani

- Epistaxis accounts for 1% to 2% of emergency department (ED) visits.
- The peak rate of incidence occurs between 3 and 8 years of age.
  - » Epistaxis affects 30% of children < 5 years of age.
  - » By age 10, up to 60% of children will have had at least 1 episode of epistaxis.
  - » Epistaxis is rare in children < 2 years of age.

Etiology

- The most common cause of epistaxis is trauma, such as nose rubbing, blowing, or digital trauma.
- Nasal bacterial colonization has been implicated in cases of idiopathic epistaxis.
  - » Low-grade inflammation leads to crusting and angiogenesis.
  - » Irritation from digital trauma / excoriation to the area results in bleeding from friable vessels.
- Other causes include:
  - » Upper respiratory tract infections (URTIs)
  - » Lack of humidity / dry environment
  - » Medications — specifically decongestants and corticosteroids
  - » Foreign body insertion
  - » Drug use — snorting of cocaine or other substances
  - » Postoperative causes — usually nasal or sinus surgery
- Recurrent idiopathic epistaxis is defined as repeated but self-limiting bleeding with no identifiable cause.
  - » Pediatric patients are more susceptible to recurrent idiopathic epistaxis due to:
    - › Extensive vascular supply to the nasal mucosa
    - › Recurrent respiratory tract infections
      - · Nosebleeds are more common in the winter months for this reason.
- For recurrent epistaxis, further investigation may be warranted; look for:
  - » Nasopharyngeal tumor
  - » Bleeding disorders (see Chapter 8.3)
  - » Vascular abnormalities — hereditary hemorrhagic telangiectasia, juvenile nasal angiofibroma, hemangioma
  - » Underlying malignancy — acute leukemia
- Epistaxis in children < 2 years of age is extremely rare and may need further workup to rule out a more ominous etiology, such as:
  - » Bleeding disorders and malignancies

- » Chlamydia rhinitis neonatorum
- » Trauma, usually resulting from a fall directly onto the nose
  - › Always have a high index of suspicion for nonaccidental trauma (NAT).

Pathophysiology

- Blood supply to the nasal cavity arises from anastomoses between the internal and external carotid arteries.
- Bleeding is defined as either anterior or posterior, with the maxillary sinus ostium serving as the demarcation between the two.
  - » The majority of nosebleeds are anterior (80% to 90%).
    - › They arise from Little's area or Kiesselbach's plexus.
  - » Posterior bleeds are rare and need aggressive management.
    - › They originate from branches of the sphenopalatine artery at Woodruff's plexus.

History

- On history, the physician should ask about:
  - » The onset and duration of symptoms
    - › Bleeding becomes a concern if it is ongoing for > 30 minutes.
  - » Estimated amount of blood loss
  - » Other signs or symptoms that may help identify the etiology, such as:
    - › Recent URTI
    - › Digital trauma
    - › Prior history of epistaxis
    - › Family history of bleeding disorder
    - › Other sites of bleeding
    - › Other systemic diseases
  - » First aid conducted at home:
    - › Any items inserted into the nose, such as tissue
    - › Medications given to help stop bleeding

Management

- Manage ABCs.
  - » If the patient is hemodynamically unstable, resuscitate them with IV fluids and packed red cells as needed.
- Spray a topical decongestant (e.g., oxymetazoline) into each naris for vasoconstriction and apply direct pressure for 5 to 15 minutes.

» Have the patient sit with head upright or leaning slightly forward.
- Identify the source of the bleeding.
  » Clear the nose of clots and blood by asking the patient to blow their nose gently or suctioning the nose to identify the site of bleeding.
  » If an anterior site of bleeding cannot be located, inspection with an endoscope (if skilled) is warranted.

ANTERIOR BLEED

Management

- Perform chemical cautery with silver nitrate.
  » Avoid prolonged or bilateral nasal cauterization due to the risk of septal damage.
- Apply thrombogenic agents, such as:
  » Gelatin (Gelfoam) or collagen (Surgicel) sponge
  » Tranexamic acid
    › This is an antifibrinolytic agent that hinders the bonding of plasminogen and plasmin with fibrin.
    › An injectable solution is applied to a nasal pledget and inserted so as to have contact with Little's area.
- Apply nasal tampon or packing.
  » Bleeding is stopped via direct pressure.
  » Balloon devices that ease insertion are now available.
  » Packing is removed in 48 to 96 hours (consult with otorhinolaryngologist [ENT]).
  » Consider bilateral packing for more extensive bleeds.

Disposition

- On discharge, provide the patient and caregivers with discharge instructions.
  » Applying moisturizing ointments is the simplest option.
    › Apply to nares twice daily.
  » Avoid blowing the nose too hard.
  » Avoid picking or rubbing the nose.
- Consider nonselective beta-blockers in patients with primary recurrent idiopathic epistaxis.
  » One option is propranolol 1.5 to 2 mg/kg per day PO divided and given 3 times daily for 2 to 4 weeks.
  » There is no difference in recurrence rates when compared to silver nitrate cautery.
- Topical antibacterial treatment has not been found to provide any benefit.

POSTERIOR BLEED

Management

- Have the patient moved to a resuscitation area.
- Manage ABCs.
- Provide IV access.
  » Administer a normal saline bolus of 20 mL/kg if the patient is hemodynamically unstable.
  » The patient may require a packed cell transfusion 5 mL/kg.
- Obtain an urgent ENT consult.
- Place posterior nasal packing with a Foley catheter or epistaxis balloon.
  » This allows for rapid hemostasis while awaiting ENT.
  » The patient may need intubation and sedation for airway control.

Complications

- There is a risk of toxic shock syndrome / sinusitis due to packing.
  » Consider antibiotic therapy:
    › Amoxicillin-clavulanate 40 mg/kg (based on amoxicillin component) given twice daily

Investigations

- Order bloodwork:
  » Complete blood count (CBC)
  » Coagulation profile — if ongoing bleeding or recurrent episodes
  » Group and screen / type and cross for packed red blood cells (PRBCs) — needed for transfusion

REFERENCES

Ahmed AE, Abo El-Magd EA, Hasan GM, El-Asheer OM. A comparative study of propranolol versus silver nitrate cautery in the treatment of recurrent primary epistaxis in children. *Adolesc Health Med Ther.* 2015;6:165–170. https://doi.org/10.2147/AHMT.S84806. Medline:26457059

Davies K, Batra K, Mehanna R, Keogh I. Pediatric epistaxis: epidemiology, management & impact on quality of life. *Int J Pediatr Otorhinolaryngol.* 2014;78(8):1294–1297. https://doi.org/10.1016/j.ijporl.2014.05.013. Medline:24882453

DeLaroche AM, Tigchelaar H, Kannikeserwan N. A rare but important entity: epistaxis in infants. *J Emerg Med.* 2017;52(1):89–92. Medline:27712897

Kamble P, Saxena S, Kumar S. Nasal bacterial colonization in cases of idiopathic epistaxis in children. *Int J Pediatr Otorhinolaryngol.* 2015;79(11):1901–1904. https://doi.org/10.1016/j.ijporl.2015.08.041. Medline:26384831

Korkmaz M, Çetinkol Y, Korkmaz H, Batmaz T. Nasal bacterial colonization in bacterial epistaxis: the role of topical antibacterial treatment. *Balkan Med J.* 2016;33(2):212–215. https://doi.org/10.5152/balkanmedj.2015.151239. Medline:27403392

Patel N, Maddalozzo J, Billings KR. An update on management of pediatric epistaxis. *Int J Pediatr Otorhinolaryngol.* 2014;78(8):1400–1404. https://doi.org/10.1016/j.ijporl.2014.06.009. Medline:24972938

Pfaff JA, Moore GP. Otolaryngology. In: Walls R, et al, editors. *Rosen's emergency medicine.* 9th ed. Elsevier; 2018. p. 820–832.

Simmen DB, Jones NS. Epistaxis. In: Flint PW, et al, editors. *Cummings otolaryngology.* 6th ed. Elsevier; 2015. p. 678–90.

Stoner MJ, Dulaurier M. Pediatric ENT emergencies. *Emerg Med Clin North Am.* 2013;31(3):795–808. https://doi.org/10.1016/j.emc.2013.04.005. Medline:23915604

Yoon PJ, Scholes MA, Friedman NR. Ear, nose, and throat. In: Hay WW Jr, Levin MJ, Deterding RR, Abzug MJ, editors. *CURRENT diagnosis & treatment pediatrics.* 23rd ed. New York, NY: McGraw-Hill; 2016. Available from: https://accessmedicine.mhmedical.com/content.aspx?bookid=1795&sectionid=125740558

OTORHINOLARYNGOLOGY EMERGENCIES

13.3

Pharyngitis

Marina I. Salvadori

- Acute pharyngitis is one of the most common infectious illnesses in children.
- It accounts for 1% to 2% of all emergency department (ED) visits.
- Pharyngitis most commonly has a viral etiology.
  » About 20% to 25% of clinical pharyngitis in children and adolescents is caused by Group A *Streptococcus* (GAS), which is the only usual pathogen that requires therapy.
  » Accurate diagnosis of streptococcal pharyngitis is important for the prevention of acute rheumatic fever and of suppurative complications (e.g., peritonsillar abscess, cervical lymphadenitis, and mastoiditis).

GROUP A STREPTOCOCCAL PHARYNGITIS

Diagnosis

- No clinical features reliably differentiate between GAS pharyngitis and viral pharyngitis, though viral pharyngitis can be presumed when there is rhinorrhea, oral ulcers, hoarseness, or cough.
- Clinical scoring systems were not designed for use in children and are only 30% to 50% accurate, so should **not** be used.
- If there are no overt features of viral pharyngitis, do either a rapid antigen detection test or a throat swab.
- The rapid antigen detection test is highly specific, and antibiotics should be prescribed if the test is positive.
  » This test has a sensitivity of 86% and specificity of 95%.
- If the rapid antigen detection test is negative or unavailable, a throat swab should be taken.
- Avoid testing or treatment in the following groups:
  » Children < 2 years of age
    › Children of this age group rarely get GAS pharyngitis, so need not be routinely tested unless there are other factors involved, such as a family member with the disease.
  » Asymptomatic individuals
- Many adolescents have painful pharyngitis with exudate and fever.

- It is usually worth doing a monospot test to diagnose acute mononucleosis so that antibiotics can be avoided (see "Infectious Mononucleosis," below).

Management

- All children with laboratory-confirmed acute GAS pharyngitis should be treated.
- Every GAS is susceptible to penicillin and cephalexin; resistance to penicillin has never been described.
- Repeat or follow-up cultures are not indicated and should not be done.
- If a patient has apparent recurrent GAS infections, be aware that up to 20% of children are asymptomatic GAS carriers.

Antibiotic Therapy

- First-line antibiotic therapy is:
  » Amoxicillin 50 mg/kg per day given 3 times a day
  — **or** —
  » Penicillin 50 mg/kg per day divided and given twice a day for 10 days
- If the patient is allergic to penicillin, give:
  » Cephalexin 50 mg/kg per day divided and given 3 times a day for 10 days
    › Give the first dose of cephalexin in the ED.
- The clinician can consider clindamycin or a macrolide, but resistance is common.
  » Consider clarithromycin 15 mg/kg per day divided and given twice a day.

Analgesia

- All pediatric patients should be assessed for pain.
- The recommended treatment is acetaminophen or ibuprofen.
- Consider corticosteroids for severe pain or hypertrophic ("kissing") tonsils as they are associated with more rapid pain relief in some studies.

PERITONSILLAR ABSCESS (QUINSY)

- The most common complication of GAS pharyngitis is peritonsillar abscess.
- A peritonsillar abscess occurs beside the tonsil in the peritonsillar space.

Physical Exam

- Symptoms include acute, severe, unilateral sore throat (worse on the affected side) as well as fever, neck pain, and dysphagia.
- The patient may appear distressed, with the following:
  » Drooling
  » Trismus (lockjaw)
  » Muffled voice ("hot potato voice")
  » Deviation of the uvula
  » Localized swelling or fluctuance
  » Tenderness (when touched with a tongue depressor)
  » Cervical lymphadenitis
- The peripheral white blood cell count is frequently elevated.

Investigations

- Peritonsillar abscess is difficult to distinguish from peritonsillar cellulitis.
  » CT scan is the preferred diagnostic test, with a sensitivity of 100% and specificity of 75%.
  » Clinical diagnosis of peritonsillar abscess is reported to have a sensitivity of 78% and specificity of 50%.
  » Intraoral ultrasound can be helpful but is operator dependent.
- Blind needle aspiration is not recommended.
  » Only 70% of abscesses are in the superior pole, which is where most physicians who perform a needle aspiration are comfortable.
- Pus should be sent for routine and anaerobic culture.

Management

- Manage via drainage of the abscess.
  » This can be done either by needle aspiration or by formal incision and drainage.
  » Obtain an otorhinolaryngology (ENT) consult.
- The decision about whether to treat peritonsillar abscess on an inpatient or an outpatient basis depends on patient factors, including:
  » Age of the patient
  » Level of pain
  » Need for IV hydration
  » Airway monitoring
- The choice of antibiotic varies but should include coverage for beta-lactamase–producing bacteria and anaerobes.
  » For beta-lactamase coverage, choices include:
    › Amoxicillin-clavulanate 50 mg/kg per day (based on amoxicillin component)
    › Cefuroxime 30 mg/kg per day divided and given twice a day
- Anaerobic coverage can include clindamycin:
  » 40 mg/kg per day IV administered every 6 to 8 hours
  — or —

» 30 mg/kg per day PO divided and given 3 times a day
  › Give clindamycin orally unless the patient cannot take medication orally.

Complications

- Left untreated, peritonsillar abscess can lead to:
  » Airway obstruction
  » Aspiration of pus from a ruptured abscess
  » Extension of the infection into the deep tissues of the neck and mediastinum

RETROPHARYNGEAL ABSCESS

- Another complication of pharyngitis is retropharyngeal abscess.
- Retropharyngeal abscess is a deep tissue infection of the neck that occurs between the posterior pharyngeal wall and the prevertebral fascia.
- The abscess is commonly a polymicrobial infection with mixed aerobic and anaerobic organisms.

Physical Exam

- Symptoms of retropharyngeal abscess include:
  » Fever
  » Severe sore throat
  » Drooling
  » Dysphagia
  » Torticollis
  » Stridor (rare)
- It is more common in children < 5 years of age.

Investigations

- Consider lateral soft tissue neck radiography.
  » Widening of the soft tissue prevertebral space on radiography may indicate retropharyngeal abscess.
- CT scan of the neck with contrast is the imaging of choice.
  » It helps distinguish between retropharyngeal abscess and cellulitis.

Management

- Obtain an ENT consult.
  » If the abscess is > 20 mm, it will need surgical drainage.
  » If the abscess is < 20 mm, consider IV antibiotics for 48 hours and then reassess.
- Give IV antibiotics.
  » There are many choices; antibiotic therapy can include a third-generation cephalosporin and clindamycin.

Complications

- Complications arise from extension of the abscess or infection into the different tissue planes:

» Posterior — prevertebral space, discitis, osteomyelitis, and epidural abscess
» Anterior — airway compromise
» Lateral — carotid artery and jugular vein complications (hemorrhage, thrombosis)
» Mediastinitis
» Lemierre syndrome

INFECTIOUS MONONUCLEOSIS

- The most common cause of infectious mononucleosis is the Epstein-Barr virus (EBV).

Physical Exam

- Patients present with fever, pharyngitis, cervical adenopathy, and fatigue.
- Young children are often asymptomatic.
- Patients may also present with:
  » Abdominal pain
  » Hepatomegaly
  » Splenomegaly
  » Nausea and/or vomiting
  » Hepatitis
    › This may occur in up to 75% of cases with elevated alanine transaminase (ALT) but no jaundice.
  » Rash
    › Rash is especially seen in patients taking a penicillin-family antibiotic.
- In adolescents, the presence of adenopathy, palatine petechiae, splenomegaly, or atypical lymphocytes increases the likelihood of mononucleosis.

Diagnosis

- A quick ED diagnosis can be done with heterophile antibody testing, though this is a nonspecific test, and the younger the patient, the less accurate the test is.
  » Heterophile antibody testing identifies about 85% of adolescents with EBV-induced mononucleosis.
- 40% of children < 4 years of age will have a false-negative monospot.
- An absolute increase in atypical lymphocytes, especially during the second week of illness, is characteristic.
- Heterophile antibody testing is also not specific for EBV and can be positive in many other conditions, including other infections, autoimmune diseases, and malignancies.

Management

- Management is largely symptomatic.
- Corticosteroids may be used, but the role of corticosteroids in patients with mononucleosis is still debated; the main benefit is pain control.

Complications

- Hematologic complications occur in 25% to 50% of patients.
  » These are usually mild and self-limiting.
  » Complications include anemia, thrombocytopenia, neutropenia.
- Neurologic complications occur in 1% to 5% of patients.
  » Neurologic complications include Guillain-Barré syndrome (GBS), facial palsies, aseptic meningitis.
- Splenic rupture occurs in < 1% of patients.
  » There are no specific guidelines to recommend when a patient can return to playing sports after splenomegaly.
  » If there are no symptoms or palpable splenomegaly, then a reasonable, conservative wait time would be a minimum of 3 weeks before returning to sports.
- Airway compromise occurs in 1% of cases.
- EBV is also one of the major infectious causes of hemophagocytic lymphohistiocytosis (HLH).

REFERENCES

Cohen JF, Bertille N, Cohen R, Chalumeau M. Rapid antigen detection test for group A streptococcus in children with pharyngitis. *Cochrane Database Syst Rev.* 2016;7:CD010502. Medline:27374000

Ebell MH, Call M, Shinholser J, et al. Does this patient have infectious mononucleosis? The rational clinical examination systematic review. *JAMA.* 2016;315(14):1502–1509. https://doi.org/10.1001/jama.2016.2111. Medline:27115266

Hoffmann C, Pierrot S, Contencin P, Morisseau-Durand MP, Manach Y, Couloigner V. Retropharyngeal infections in children: treatment strategies and outcomes. *Int J Pediatr Otorhinolaryngol.* 2011;75(9):1099–1103. https://doi.org/10.1016/j.ijporl.2011.05.024. Medline:21705095

Putukian M, O'Connor FG, Stricker P, et al. Mononucleosis and athletic participation: an evidence-based subject review. *Clin J Sport Med.* 2008;18(4):309–315. https://doi.org/10.1097/JSM.0b013e31817e34f8. Medline:18614881

Rezk E, Nofal YH, Hamzeh A, Aboujaib MF, AlKheder MA, Al Hammad MF. Steroids for symptom control in infectious mononucleosis. *Cochrane Database Syst Rev.* 2015;(11):CD004402. Medline:26558642

Scott PM, Loftus WK, Kew J, et al. Diagnosis of peritonsillar abscess infections: a prospective study of ultrasound, computerized tomography, and clinical diagnosis. *J Laryngol Otol.* 1999;13:229–232. Medline:10435129

Shulman ST, Bisno AL, Clegg HW, et al; Infectious Diseases Society of America. Clinical practice guideline for the diagnosis and management of group A streptococcal pharyngitis: 2012 update by the Infectious Diseases Society of America. *Clin Infect Dis.* 2012;55(10):e86–e102. https://doi.org/10.1093/cid/cis629. Medline:22965026 *Erratum in: Clin Infect Dis.* 2014;58(10):1496. https://doi.org/10.1093/cid/cis629

van Driel ML, De Sutter AIM, Habraken H, Thorning S, Christiaens T. Different antibiotic treatments for group A streptococcal pharyngitis. *Cochrane Database Syst Rev.* 2016;9:CD004406. Medline:27614728

Wing A, Villa-Roel C, Yeh B, Eskin B, Buckingham J, Rowe BH. Effectiveness of corticosteroid treatment in acute pharyngitis: a systematic review of the literature. *Acad Emerg Med.* 2010;17(5):476–483. https://doi.org/10.1111/j.1553-2712.2010.00723.x. Medline:20536799

13.4

Otitis Media and Otitis Externa

Christopher Skappak, Marina I. Salvadori

OTITIS MEDIA

Note: This chapter is not intended to address children with craniofacial abnormalities, those who are immune compromised, those with tympanostomy tubes, or children with recurrent acute otitis media.

- Otitis media is a common pediatric condition with 80% of children having 1 episode by age 10.
- 50% of Canadian households with children between the ages of 2 and 3 reported at least 1 ear infection per year.
  - » 75% of children experience at least 1 ear infection before starting school.
- It is one of the most common conditions for which children receive antibiotics.
- Acute otitis media (AOM) generally occurs concurrently or after a viral respiratory tract infection, with 35% of viral upper respiratory tract infections (URTIs) being complicated by middle-ear effusions.

Risk Factors

- Risk factors can be divided into host and environmental factors.
  - » Host factors:
    - › Unimmunized child
    - › Younger age
    - › Atopy
    - › Craniofacial deformity (e.g., cleft palate, Down syndrome)
    - › Ethnicity (Indigenous ancestry)
    - › Immunodeficiency
  - » Environmental factors:
    - › Increased exposure to viral illness (e.g., daycare, siblings, crowded living conditions)
    - › Lower socioeconomic status
    - › Pacifier use
    - › Exposure to tobacco use / smoking

Pathophysiology

- The eustachian tube is responsible for draining mucus and secretions, as well as clearing bacteria from the middle ear into the nasopharynx.
- Infants and children have shorter and more horizontal tubes than adults.
- Viral infections are associated with eustachian tube dysfunction.
- Bacteria associated with AOM are:
  - » *Streptococcus pneumoniae*
  - » *Haemophilus influenzae*
  - » *Moraxella catarrhalis*
  - » Group A *Streptococcus* (GAS)

Physical Exam

- Older children usually present with a history of rapid onset ear pain.
- Young children may tug, rub, or hold the affected ear.
- Nonspecific symptoms include fever; crying; and sleep, behavior, or appetite disturbance.
- Most patients have had an antecedent viral URTI.
- Common clinical symptoms of AOM are:
  - » Otalgia (ear pain)
  - » Decreased appetite
  - » Decreased hearing
  - » Difficulty sleeping
  - » Ear tugging
  - » Fever
  - » Irritability
  - » Nausea
  - » Vomiting
- Rare clinical symptoms associated with complicated AOM are:
  - » Altered level of consciousness
  - » Failure of ipsilateral eye abduction
  - » Facial droop
  - » Headache
  - » Hearing loss
  - » Lethargy
  - » Mastoid tenderness

Diagnosis

- Physical examination of the tympanic membrane is key to an accurate diagnosis of AOM.
- Cerumen removal is required in 30% of children in order to visualize the tympanic membrane.

- Otoscopy findings associated with AOM include:
  » Bulging tympanic membrane
    › This is highly predictive of AOM (95% sensitivity and 85% specificity).
  » Cloudy or yellow tympanic membrane
  » Impaired mobility of the tympanic membrane
    › Pneumatic otoscopy has the best sensitivity and specificity for the diagnosis of middle ear effusion but is rarely employed by front-line clinicians.
  » Hemorrhagic or erythematous tympanic membrane
    › This demonstrates poor predictability for AOM.
  » Middle ear effusion
    › This is a required diagnostic criterion for AOM.
    › Signs include air-fluid levels and loss of bony landmarks.
  » Perforated tympanic membrane with purulent drainage
    › This is highly associated with bacterial infections.
    › Drainage must be distinguished from acute otitis externa (AOE).
    › Drainage occurs in the absence of tympanostomy tubes.

Management

- All children with AOM should be assessed for pain and recommended acetaminophen or ibuprofen.
- In recent years, the use of antibiotics for AOM has been controversial.
  » Children who have a bulging tympanic membrane, high fever, symptoms lasting > 48 hours, or who look unwell, as well as those with a perforated tympanic membrane and purulent drainage should be treated with antibiotics.
  » If the patient is > 6 months of age with mild symptoms, fever < 39°C, illness lasting < 48 hours, and reliable caregivers, antibiotics can be withheld and the patient observed; if the patient worsens clinically or has not improved in 48 hours, antibiotics should be given.

Antibiotic Therapy

- First-line therapy is amoxicillin 75 to 90 mg/kg per day divided and given 2 or 3 times daily.
- If the patient has a penicillin allergy, consider:
  » Cefprozil 30 mg/kg per day divided and given twice daily
  — **or** —
  » Cefuroxime 30 mg/kg per day divided and given twice daily
    › Consider giving a first dose of cefprozil or cefuroxime in the emergency department (ED) and observing the patient.
- If therapy is not effective after 2 to 3 days, or if amoxicillin has been taken in the last 30 days, consider:
  » Amoxicillin-clavulanate

  › Dosage is weight based:
    · < 35 kg: 45 to 60 mg/kg per day (based on amoxicillin component) divided and given 3 times daily
    · > 35 kg: 500 mg (based on amoxicillin component) given 3 times daily
- For AOM with purulent conjunctivitis:
  » Consider *Haemophilus influenzae* and *Moraxella catarrhalis* as etiology
  » Give amoxicillin-clavulanate
- For children who are vomiting or cannot tolerate oral medication, use:
  » Ceftriaxone 50 mg/kg IM for 3 days
- The duration of antibiotic therapy is dependent on age.
  » Children < 2 years of age should be given 10 days of antibiotics.
  » Current guidelines suggest children > 2 years of age can have 5 days of antibiotics; however, a recent, well-designed trial showed that 10 days was beneficial in all age groups.
    › This remains controversial.

Complications

- Complications of AOM include:
  » Mastoiditis — acute pain, tenderness, and swelling over the mastoid bone with forward protrusion of the ear
    › Consult ENT.
    › Obtain a CT scan.
  » Labyrinthitis
  » Meningitis
  » Sinus venous thrombosis

OTITIS EXTERNA

- Otitis externa is a diffuse inflammation of the external ear canal that may also involve the pinna and tympanic membrane.
- The hallmark sign is tenderness of the tragus, pinna, or both that is often intense and disproportionate to what is expected on visual inspection.
  » Pulling or manipulation of the pinna or tragus causes intense pain.
- It most often occurs in the summer with water exposure and is known as "swimmer's ear."
- Assess the patient for factors that will modify management:
  » Perforated tympanic membrane
  » Tympanostomy tube
  » Diabetes
  » Immune compromise
  » Prior radiotherapy

Management

- Manage pain with oral analgesia (acetaminophen or ibuprofen).
- Topical preparations are the drugs of choice.
  - » Quinolone drops are the first choice.
  - » There is no need for systemic antibiotics unless there is extension of the infection outside the ear canal or specific host factors that would indicate the need for systemic therapy.
- Prescribe ciprofloxacin otic drops for children > 1 year of age at a dose of 4 drops twice daily for 7 days.
  - » Enhance the delivery of topical drops with aural toilet and ear wick as needed.
- If the tympanic membrane is perforated, **do not use** ototoxic drugs (aminoglycosides, alcohol, neomycin/polymyxin); use quinolone otic drops.
- If there is no response within 72 hours, the patient needs to be reassessed.

REFERENCES

Bowatte G, Tham R, Allen KJ, et al. Breastfeeding and childhood acute otitis media: a systematic review and meta-analysis. *Acta Paediatr.* 2015;104(467):85–95. https://doi.org/10.1111/apa.13151. Medline:26265016

Coyte PC, Croxford R, Asche CV, To T, Feldman W, Friedberg J. Physician and population determinants of rates of middle-ear surgery in Ontario. *JAMA.* 2001;286(17):2128–2135. https://doi.org/10.1001/jama.286.17.2128. Medline:11694154

Hoberman A, Paradise JL, Rockette HE, et al. Shortened antimicrobial treatment for acute otitis media in young children. *N Engl J Med.* 2016;375(25):2446–2456. https://doi.org/10.1056/NEJMoa1606043. Medline:28002709

Le Saux N, Robinson JL; Canadian Paediatric Society, Infectious Diseases and Immunization Committee. Management of acute otitis media in children six months of age and older. *Paediatr Child Health.* 2016;21(1):39–44. https://doi.org/10.1093/pch/21.1.39. Medline:26941560

Lieberthal AS, Carroll AE, Chonmaitree T, et al. The diagnosis and management of acute otitis media. *Pediatrics.* 2013;131(3):e964–e999. https://doi.org/10.1542/peds.2012-3488. Medline:23439909

Nokso-Koivisto J, Marom T, Chonmaitree T. Importance of viruses in acute otitis media. *Curr Opin Pediatr.* 2015;27(1):110–115. https://doi.org/10.1097/MOP.0000000000000184. Medline:25514574

Rosenfeld RM, Schwartz SR, Cannon CR, et al. Clinical practice guideline: acute otitis externa. *Otolaryngol Head Neck Surg.* 2014;150(1 Suppl):S1–S24. https://doi.org/10.1177/0194599813517083. Medline:24491310

Schilder AG, Chonmaitree T, Cripps AW, et al. Otitis media. *Nat Rev Dis Primers.* 2016;2:16063. https://doi.org/10.1038/nrdp.2016.63. Medline:27604644

Shaikh N, Hoberman A, Paradise JL, et al. Development and preliminary evaluation of a parent-reported outcome instrument for clinical trials in acute otitis media. *Pediatr Infect Dis J.* 2009;28(1):5–8. https://doi.org/10.1097/INF.0b013e318185a387. Medline:19077917

Thomas EM. Recent trends in upper respiratory infections, ear infections and asthma among young Canadian children. *Health Rep.* 2010;21(4):47–52. Medline:21269011

Urschel S. Otitis media in children with congenital immunodeficiencies. *Curr Allergy Asthma Rep.* 2010;10(6):425–433. https://doi.org/10.1007/s11882-010-0143-x. Medline:20740389

OTORHINOLARYNGOLOGY EMERGENCIES

14.1

Acute Gastroenteritis

Rahim Valani

- Gastroenteritis is a common presenting problem in the emergency department (ED).
  - » 1 in 8 Canadians (all age groups) get sick each year from contaminated food.
- Patients present with nausea/vomiting and associated diarrhea.
- The most common organisms in Canada that cause gastroenteritis are:
  - » Norovirus
  - » Listeria
  - » *Salmonella*
  - » *Escherichia coli* O157
  - » *Campylobacter*
- Outbreaks of food poisoning can be:
  - » Sporadic — localized or solitary cases
  - » Outbreaks — more common in developed countries due to centralized food processing
  - » Seasonal — viral gastroenteritis infections are more common in winter months
- Vomiting or diarrhea can also be a manifestation of nongastrointestinal (non-GI) pathology such as testicular torsion (see Chapter 16.1) or otitis media (see Chapter 13.4).
  - » Always consider a non-GI etiology when patients present with such symptoms.

Pathophysiology

- Transmission is usually from ingestion of the pathogen, such as:
  - » Eating contaminated food (e.g., due to poor handling or washing, or inadequate cooking)
  - » Fecal-oral transmission with hands or fomites
- In order for the pathogen to cause disease, it needs to overcome the natural defenses of the patient:
  - » Gastric acid — fasting gastric pH < 4 is toxic to most enteropathogens
    - › Use of proton pump inhibitors (PPIs) makes the person more susceptible.

- » Bowel motility — ongoing movement of the bowels decreases the chance of pathogen adherence to the lumen or absorption of toxins
- » Natural colonic flora
- » Local antibodies
- The bacteria or associated toxins affect the bowel mucosa, resulting in diarrhea that can be either:
  - » Secretory — excessive secretion usually due to enterotoxins, resulting in watery diarrhea
  - » Inflammatory — changes in intestinal mucosa that can result in bloody diarrhea
- The incubation period can provide clues to the suspected organism (see *Table 14.1.1*).

Table 14.1.1. INCUBATION PERIOD WITH SUSPECTED ORGANISMS

Incubation period	Suspected organisms
< 1 hour	Scromboid poisoning, puffer fish
> 1 week	*Giardia lamblia, Entamoeba histolytica*
> 3 weeks	*Giardia lamblia, Entamoeba histolytica, Yersinia enterocolitica*

History

- On history, ask about:
  - » Frequency of vomiting and bowel movements
  - » Presence of fever
  - » Rash
  - » Recent travel or camping
    - › Enterotoxigenic *E. coli* is the most common cause of traveler's diarrhea worldwide.
  - » Recent hospitalization
  - » Localized pain
    - › Consider other causes such as regional enteritis, appendicitis, or intussusception.
  - » Well water use
  - » Food ingested over the past few days (see *Table 14.1.2* for suspected etiology based on sources):
    - › Restaurant / street food

- › Seafood
- › Raw meat
- › Unpasteurized milk
- » Contact with others who have similar symptoms (e.g., daycare outbreaks)
- » Recent antibiotic use
- » Blood in stools:
  - › Hemolytic uremic syndrome (HUS)
  - › *Clostridium difficile* colitis
  - › Enterotoxigenic cause
- » Any neurologic symptoms
  - › Consider the following toxins in patients with neurologic symptoms:
    - · Ciguatera
    - · Paralytic shellfish
    - · Neurotoxic shellfish
    - · Puffer fish

Table 14.1.2. SUSPECTED ETIOLOGY BASED ON SOURCE

Source	Suspected pathogens
Milk	• *Campylobacter jejuni* • *Yersinia enterocolitica* • *Salmonella* • *Shigella* • *Listeria monocytogenes*
Contaminated water	• *Giardia lamblia* • Norwalk virus • *E. coli*
Eggs, poultry	• *Salmonella* • *Campylobacter jejuni*
Raw meat	• *E. coli*
Raw fish, shellfish	• *Vibrio parahaemolyticus* • Paralytic shellfish • Neurotoxic shellfish • Norwalk virus
Improperly home-canned foods	• *Clostridium botulinum*
Unrefrigerated or improperly refrigerated meats, egg/potato salad, cream, custard	• *Staphylococcus aureus*
Fried rice, gravies	• *Bacillus cereus*

Physical Exam

- Pay close attention to the patient's vital signs and hydration status.
  - » If signs of severe dehydration are present, do not delay fluid resuscitation.
- Check for peritoneal signs to rule out other causes.
- Examine the patient for rashes.

Investigations

- Investigations are not routinely needed.
- Consider bloodwork:
  - » Complete blood count (CBC)

- » Electrolytes
- » Renal function tests
- Consider cultures (if bacteremia is suspected or if patient is toxic-looking):
  - » Blood culture and sensitivity tests
  - » Stool culture for ova and parasites
  - » *C. difficile* toxin if patient has recently used antibiotics

Management

- Assess the patient's ABCs.
- If patient is obtunded or in shock:
  - » Check blood sugar
    - › If patient is hypoglycemic, give up to 5 mL/kg of 10% dextrose solution and reassess.
  - » For patients with moderate to severe dehydration or patients in shock, administer a bolus of 20 mL/kg normal saline or 5% normal saline.
    - › If there are any concerns for HUS, start with 10 mL/kg and reassess frequently.
  - » Look for other causes of vomiting/diarrhea such as intussusception.

Hydration

- Oral rehydration is preferred.
  - » Administer ondansetron 0.15 mg/kg via oral dissolvable tablet (ODT) or IV to a maximum of 8 mg to help with oral rehydration intake.
  - » Caution with patients with cardiac issues as ondansetron has been shown to prolong the QT interval.
- Encourage slow, frequent feeds with an electrolyte-balanced solution (oral rehydration solution).

Antimotility Agents

- Avoid antimotility agents (e.g., loperamide) because of the numerous side effects and contraindications.
- Antimotility agents are not recommended for use in children.
- They may worsen *Salmonella*, *Shigella*, and Shiga toxin–producing *E. coli*.

Probiotics and Antibiotics

- Probiotics, when used with hospitalized patients, decrease the mean duration of hospital stays by 1.12 days.
- Antibiotics are not routinely recommended.

VIRAL ETIOLOGY

- Viral causes of gastroenteritis are usually self-limiting.
- The most common viral causes are:
  - » Rotavirus
    - › Rotavirus affects 90% of children by the age of 3 years.

› It is the most common cause of infectious diarrhea in the winter months.
› A vaccine is available in Canada.
  · The Canadian Pediatric Society position statement recommends vaccination for all infants except those who are immunocompromised or predisposed to intussusception.
  · The risk of intussusception with vaccine is estimated to be 1 to 3 per 100 000.
» Enteric adenovirus
» Norovirus
- Patients present with vomiting and secretory diarrhea.
- Treat symptomatically (see "Management," above).

BACTERIAL ETIOLOGY

- Clinical features suggestive of a bacterial versus viral pathogen include:
» > 10 bowel movements per day or ongoing for > 4 days
» Blood in the stool
» Fever of 39.5°C or higher
» Unwell appearance
» Presence of polymorphonuclear leukocytes (PMNs) in the stool
- The 5 most common bacterial causes of gastroenteritis are:
» *Salmonella*
» *Shigella*
» *Yersinia*
» *Campylobacter*
» *E. coli*

SALMONELLA

- The risk of *Salmonella* is higher with consumption of:
» Poultry — the most common source of *Salmonella*
» Raw eggs
» Unpasteurized milk or milk products
» Raw fruits and vegetables
- *Salmonella* can result in bacteremia, meningitis, osteomyelitis, and endocarditis.
- Patients with sickle cell disease (SCD) have increased risk for osteomyelitis from *Salmonella*.
- *Salmonella* is usually not treated with antibiotics unless:
» Patient is a neonate
» Patient is toxic looking
» Patient has typhoid fever

SHIGELLA

- There is a high risk of *Shigella* infection with consumption of:
» Foods that have been "handled" — salads, meats
» Foods potentially exposed to polluted water — oysters, shellfish, vegetables

- *Shigella* is usually self-limited, so no antibiotics are prescribed.
- The toxin may lead to central nervous system (CNS) irritation causing meningismus; cerebrospinal fluid (CSF) analysis is normal.
- Patient may have a high band count.

YERSINIA

- *Yersinia* is an invasive infection of the terminal ileum and mesenteric nodes.
- Abdominal pain and diarrhea last longer than in other infections (close to 2 weeks).
- 5% to 10% of patients develop a rash and arthritis.

CAMPYLOBACTER

- *Campylobacter* is common among campers.
- There is a high risk of *Campylobacter* infection with consumption of:
» Raw or undercooked meat
» Raw eggs
» Unpasteurized milk or milk products
» Raw vegetables
» Shellfish
- Complications include:
» Reactive arthritis
» Guillain-Barré syndrome
» Mesenteric adenitis and ileocolitis
» Meningitis

E. COLI

- There is a high risk of *E. coli* infection from contaminated food or water.
- *E. coli* 0157 is associated with improperly cooked hamburger.
- Shiga-like toxin is cytotoxic to intestinal vascular endothelial cells, resulting in hemorrhagic colitis.
- Complications include:
» HUS
» Thrombotic thrombocytopenic purpura
- Treatment is not recommended as there is a potentially increased risk of HUS.

PARASITIC INFECTIONS

- The most common protozoan infections are caused by:
» *Entamoeba histolytica*
» *Giardia lamblia*
» *Cryptosporidium*

ENTAMOEBA HISTOLYTICA

- Characteristic colonic ulcerations are caused by invasive trophozoites.

- *Entamoeba histolytica* can result in hepatic infection causing hepatomegaly and jaundice.
- Liver abscess may be present in 1% to 5% of cases.
- Complications include:
  » Perforation
  » Ameboma
  » Stricture
  » Hemorrhage from direct invasion
  » Intussusception
  » Abscess

GIARDIA LAMBLIA

- *Giardia lamblia* infection is usually from contaminated water (contaminated municipal supplies or backpackers/hikers consuming water from rivers, etc.).
- It can present as an asymptomatic infection.
- All patients with *Giardia* should be treated (even if asymptomatic).

CRYPTOSPORIDIUM

- *Cryptosporidium* is resistant to chlorine disinfection and can survive for several days in swimming pools / recreational parks.
- Stool samples do not contain blood or leukocytes.
- Consider this in HIV patients who have a CD4 count < 100 cells/μL.
- *Cryptosporidium* infection can result in biliary tract infections causing:
  » Sclerosing cholangitis
  » Acalculous cholecystitis

TRAVELER'S DIARRHEA

- The most common cause worldwide of traveler's diarrhea is enterotoxigenic *E. coli*.
- Other causes include:
  » *Campylobacter jejuni*
  » *Salmonella*
  » *Giardia lamblia*
  » *Vibrio parahaemolyticus*
  » Norwalk virus
- Diarrhea commonly occurs within 2 to 3 days of arrival at a foreign destination.
- It is caused by food or water contaminated by feces (either uncooked or improperly cooked food and untreated water or ice).
- Most cases are short lived, lasting 3 to 5 days.

SCOMBROID POISONING

- Scombroid poisoning usually occurs within an hour of ingestion.

- It most commonly results from eating spoiled tuna, bonito, mackerel, yellow jack, bluefish, or mahi-mahi.
  » Histidine in the muscles of the fish is converted to histamine by bacteria.
  » The process can be stopped with appropriate refrigeration.
- Scombroid poisoning presents similarly to an allergic reaction, with flushing, urticaria, paresthesia, cramps, and diarrhea.
- Symptoms last for several hours.
- Management is supportive.
  » Scombroid poisoning responds well to antihistamines.

CIGUATERA POISONING

- Ciguatera poisoning is caused by ingesting certain marine fish — barracuda, amberjack, sea bass, grouper, and snapper — that have been contaminated by ciguatoxin.
  » Ciguatoxin is not inactivated by cooking the fish (it is heat and acid stable).
- Patients present with:
  » GI symptoms — abdominal pain, nausea, vomiting, diarrhea
  » Neurologic symptoms — paresthesia, reversal of hot-cold sensations, weakness, and headache
- Symptoms can persist for months.
- Management is supportive.

REFERENCES

Brillman JC, Quenzer RW. *Infectious disease in emergency medicine.* 2nd ed. Philadelphia: Lippincott Raven; 1998.

Cohen J, Powderly WG, Opal SM, et al. *Infectious diseases.* 3rd ed. Maryland Heights, MO: Mosby Elsevier; 2010.

Feigin RD, Cherry JD, Demmler-Harrison GJ, Kaplan SL. *Feigin and Cherry's textbook of pediatric infectious diseases.* 6th ed. Philadelphia: Saunders Elsevier; 2009.

Fleisher GR, Ludwig S. *Textbook of pediatric emergency medicine.* 6th ed. Philadelphia: Lippincott Williams & Wilkins; 2010.

Freedman SB, Ali S, Oleszczuk M, Gouin S, Hartling L. Treatment of acute gastroenteritis in children: an overview of systematic reviews of interventions commonly used in developed countries. *Evid Based Child Health.* 2013;8(4):1123–1137. https://doi.org/10.1002/ebch.1932. Medline:23877938

Le Saux N; Canadian Pediatric Society Infectious Diseases and Immunization Committee. Position Statement. Recommendations for the use of rotavirus vaccine in infants. *Paediatr Child Health.* 2017;22(5):290–294.

Public Health Agency of Canada. A–Z infectious diseases [Internet]. Ottawa, ON: Government of Canada; 2016 Oct 7 [cited May 2017]. Available from: https://www.canada.ca/en/public-health/services/infectious-diseases/a-infectious-diseases.html#es

U.S. Food and Drug Administration. Foodborne illnesses: what you need to know [Internet]. Silver Spring, MD: U.S. Food and Drug Administration; updated 2018 Jan 12 [cited May 2017]. Available from: https://www.fda.gov/food/resourcesforyou/consumers/ucm103263.htm

GASTROINTESTINAL EMERGENCIES

14.2

Acute Peritonitis

Rahim Valani

APPENDICITIS

- Appendicitis has an estimated lifetime risk of 7% to 8%, with the peak rate of incidence occurring in the second decade of life.
  - » The median age is 10 to 11 years.
- The exact etiology of appendicitis is unknown.

Pathophysiology

- A luminal obstruction from stool, appendicolith, lymphoid tissue, or neoplasm increases luminal pressure, leading to diminished blood supply and tissue necrosis.
- 30% of patients present with perforated appendix.

Diagnosis

- Appendicitis most commonly presents with periumbilical pain that migrates and localizes to the right lower quadrant (LR 1.9–3.1).
- Patients may have nausea, vomiting, and diarrhea, as well as a fever.
- Consider the following diagnostic signs and tests:
  - » Rovsing's sign — right lower quadrant pain when the left lower quadrant is palpated
  - » Obturator sign — pain with flexion and internal rotation of the right hip
  - » Psoas sign — pain with flexion of the hip against resistance
  - » Dunphy's sign — pain with cough
  - » Markle test — right lower quadrant pain when patient stands on toes and makes a jarring landing onto the heels
- Clinical scoring systems are helpful as clinical decision guidelines for identifying what to image and what to investigate further.
  - » The two most common scoring systems — the Alvarado and pediatric appendicitis scoring systems — are summarized in *Table 14.2.1*.
- Imaging studies that aid in the diagnosis of appendicitis can be found in *Table 14.2.2*.

Table 14.2.1. SENSITIVITY, SPECIFICITY, AND CRITERIA FOR THE ALVARADO AND PEDIATRIC APPENDICITIS SCORING PREDICTOR

	Alvarado	**Pediatric Appendicitis Score**
Sensitivity	72% to 93%	82% to 100%
Specificity	49% to 98%	65% to 96%
Criteria	• Migration of pain • Anorexia • Nausea/vomiting • Right lower quadrant tenderness • Rebound tenderness • Fever • Leukocytosis (WBC > 10 × 10⁹/L) • Neutrophilia > 75%	• Migration of pain • Anorexia • Nausea/vomiting • Cough/hop/percussion tenderness in right lower quadrant • Fever • Leukocytosis (WBC > 10 × 10⁹/L) • Neutrophilia > 75%

WBC white blood cell.

Table 14.2.2. IMAGING MODALITIES FOR DIAGNOSING APPENDICITIS

Imaging	Comments	Validity	Diagnostic criteria
X-ray	• Rarely useful		• Appendicolith (seen in < 5% of cases) • Loss of psoas shadow • Small bowel obstruction • Localized air fluid levels
Ultrasound	• Imaging of choice • Involves no radiation	• Sensitivity 88% • Specificity 94%	**For the appendix:** • ≥ 6–7 mm • Aperistaltic • Noncompressible • Hyperemia • Appendicolith • Target appearance (distinct wall layers) **Secondary findings:** • Periappendiceal fluid • Echogenic prominent pericecal fat
CT scan	• High accuracy	• Sensitivity 95% • Specificity 95% • NPV of 98.7%	**For the appendix:** • Enlarged diameter (> 7 mm) • Nonopacified lumen • Significant wall enhancement (with IV contrast) **Secondary findings:** • Periappendiceal fat stranding • Free fluid in right lower quadrant

NPV negative predictive value.

Management

- The management of appendicitis is primarily operative, so consider early surgical consultation.
- If the patient is unstable or septic:
  » Administer fluid resuscitation with a normal saline bolus of 20 mL/kg.
  » Give empiric antibiotics (as with stable patients, below)
  » Consult surgery immediately
- If the patient is stable:
  » Give appropriate parenteral analgesia
  » Obtain imaging studies to make the diagnosis
  » Give antibiotics:
    › Ceftriaxone 50 to 75 mg/kg IV every 24 hours
    › Metronidazole 15 to 30 mg/kg per day divided and given every 8 hours

Operative Management

- Laparoscopic appendectomy is the most common surgical method.
  » Delays < 24 hours have not been associated with increased rate of perforation, abscess formation, or gangrene.
    › Delaying appendectomy avoids emergency late-night operations and allows for safer surgery the following day.
    › Early appendectomy has not been shown to prevent complications compared to delayed appendectomy for patients with phlegmon or abscess.
- Nonoperative treatment is considered safe in select patients, but further studies are needed to determine the safety of this management choice.
  » Nonoperative treatment is effective as initial treatment in 97% of children with acute uncomplicated appendicitis.
  » The recurrence rate of appendicitis is 14%.

COMPLICATIONS

- Complications of surgical repair include:
  » Direct bowel injury
  » Bleeding from appendiceal artery
  » Postoperative abscess (0% to 1%)
    › With perforated appendix, the rate of abscess rises to 15% to 20%.
  » Wound infection (2%)
  » Postoperative ileus/obstruction (1.3%)
  » Venous thromboembolism (< 0.1%)

INTUSSUSCEPTION

- Intussusception is the telescoping of one proximal portion of bowel into the adjacent bowel.
- It is most common in children aged 3 months to 5 years.
  » Peak incidence is in children 5 to 11 months of age.
  » 90% of cases occur before 2 years of age.

- Intussusception is most commonly ileocolic (80% to 95% of cases).
- It is the most common cause of bowel obstruction in children < 5 years of age.
- The old rotavirus vaccine had an eight-fold increased incidence of intussusception; the new-generation vaccine has not been shown to have the same effect.
- The condition can be divided into primary or secondary intussusception:
  » Primary intussusception
    › There is, in general, no pathologic lead point (possibly Peyer's patches in terminal ileum).
    › Primary intussusception constitutes the majority of cases.
  » Secondary intussusception
    › Pathologic lead points are seen in up to 10% of cases and usually in older children (secondary intussusception).
    › Common lead points include:
      · Meckel's diverticulum
      · Henoch-Schönlein purpura
      · Lymphoma
      · Intestinal polyps

Pathophysiology

- The intussusceptum and associated mesentery are dragged into the intussuscipiens, resulting in:
  » Venous and lymphatic obstruction/congestion
  » Bowel edema
  » Ischemic bowel
  » Perforation and peritonitis

Diagnosis

- Patients classically present with colicky abdominal pain that is intermittent, usually occurring every 15 to 30 minutes.
  » Bilious vomiting occurs if an obstruction is present.
- The presence of "red currant jelly" stools signifies bowel ischemia.
- The classic triad of colicky abdominal pain, a palpable mass, and bloody stools is seen in < 40% of patients.
- Conduct imaging investigations.
  » Findings on plain X-rays include:
    › Paucity of gas in the right lower quadrant
    › Rim/target sign (echogenic mucosa, hypoechoic muscularis, and echogenic serosa)
    › Abdominal mass
    › Small bowel obstruction
    › Lateralization of the ileum
  » Ultrasound has 98% to 100% sensitivity, and may show:
    › Target or donut sign
    › Pseudokidney sign
  » Fluoroscopic enema can be both diagnostic and therapeutic, but is contraindicated if patient has peritonitis, perforation, or bowel necrosis.

Management

- Most ileoileal intussusceptions resolve spontaneously.
- Reduction is required if the intussusception is ileocolic.

Hydrostatic or Pneumatic Enema Reduction

- Hydrostatic or pneumatic enema reduction has a 1% complication rate for perforation.
- Intussusception recurs in 10% of patients, with most occurring in the first 48 hours after reduction.
  » Using dexamethasone as an adjunct may reduce risk of recurrence.

Surgical Reduction

- Surgical reduction is indicated if:
  » Reduction failed with enema
  » Peritonitis is present
  » There is evidence of a pathologic lead point

INCARCERATED INGUINAL HERNIA

- Inguinal hernias are a common referral for pediatric surgery.
- The rate of incidence is estimated to be 0.8% to 4% of the pediatric population.
  » There is an increased incidence of up to 30% in pre-term infants.
- Incarcerated inguinal hernias are usually due to indirect inguinal hernias.
  » Indirect inguinal hernias are lateral to the inferior epigastric vessels.
  » They are more common in males that females (5:1) and are due to failure of the processus vaginalis to close.
- 60% of cases are right sided.

Pathophysiology

- Incarcerated inguinal hernias are due to entrapment of the peritoneal contents into the inguinal hernia.
- An inguinal hernia is said to be incarcerated when it is irreducible.
- A strangulated hernia is irreducible and involves vascular compromise.

Diagnosis

- Patients may present with:
  » Irritability with inconsolable crying when inguinal hernia is incarcerated
  » Nausea/vomiting
  » Fever
  » Presence of an inguinal bulge on examination
  » Extremely tender bulge that is irreducible, and/or has skin discoloration suggestive of strangulated hernia
- Conduct an imaging study.
  » Ultrasound has 98% sensitivity.

Management

- Attempt reduction in the ED with appropriate sedation and analgesia.
  » 70% to 95% of incarcerated inguinal hernia are successfully reduced.
- If reduction is unsuccessful or hernia is strangulated, consult surgery.
  » Operative repair can be either open or laparoscopic.

REFERENCES

Abdulhai SA, Glenn IC, Ponsky TA. Incarcerated pediatric hernias. *Surg Clin North Am.* 2017;97(1):129–145. https://doi.org/10.1016/j.suc.2016.08.010. Medline:27894423

Charles T, Penninga L, Reurings JC, Berry MC. Intussusception in children: a clinical review. *Acta Chir Belg.* 2015;115(5):327–333. https://doi.org/10.1080/00015458.2015.11681124. Medline:26559998

Cheng Y, Xiong X, Lu J, Wu S, Zhou R, Cheng N. Early versus delayed appendicectomy for appendiceal phlegmon or abscess. *Cochrane Database Syst Rev.* 2017;6(6):CD011670. Medline:28574593

Craig S, Dalton S. Diagnosing appendicitis: what works, what does not and where to go from here? *J Paediatr Child Health.* 2016;52(2):168–173. https://doi.org/10.1111/jpc.12998. Medline:26437742

Georgiou R, Eaton S, Stanton MP, Pierro A, Hall NJ. Efficacy and safety of nonoperative treatment for acute appendicitis: a meta-analysis. *Pediatrics.* 2017;139(3):e20163003. https://doi.org/10.1542/peds.2016-3003. Medline:28213607

Gluckman S, Karpelowsky J, Webster AC, McGee RG. Management for intussusception in children. *Cochrane Database Syst Rev.* 2017;6(6):CD006476. Medline:28567798

Linnaus ME, Ostlie DJ. Complications in common general pediatric surgery procedures. *Semin Pediatr Surg.* 2016;25(6):404–411. https://doi.org/10.1053/j.sempedsurg.2016.10.002. Medline:27989365

López JJ, Deans KJ, Minneci PC. Nonoperative management of appendicitis in children. *Curr Opin Pediatr.* 2017;29(3):358–362. https://doi.org/10.1097/MOP.0000000000000487. Medline:28306630

Padilla BE, Moses W. Lower gastrointestinal bleeding & intussusception. *Surg Clin North Am.* 2017;97(1):173–188. https://doi.org/10.1016/j.suc.2016.08.015. Medline:27894426

Rentea RM, Peter SD, Snyder CL. Pediatric appendicitis: state of the art review. *Pediatr Surg Int.* 2017;33(3):269–283. https://doi.org/10.1007/s00383-016-3990-2. Medline:27743024

Sanchez TR, Corwin MT, Davoodian A, Stein-Wexler R. Sonography of abdominal pain in children: appendicitis and its common mimics. *J Ultrasound Med.* 2016;35(3):627–635. https://doi.org/10.7863/ultra.15.04047. Medline:26892821

Smith J, Fox SM. Pediatric abdominal pain: an emergency medicine perspective. *Emerg Med Clin North Am.* 2016;34(2):341–361. https://doi.org/10.1016/j.emc.2015.12.010. Medline:27133248

Yang W-C, Chen C-Y, Wu H-P. Etiology of non-traumatic acute abdomen in pediatric emergency departments. *World J Clin Cases.* 2013;1(9):276–284. Medline:24364022

14.3

Constipation

Mohamed Eltorki, Rahim Valani

- Acute constipation is defined as impaction of stool in the rectum that is palpable either on abdominal examination or a digital rectal exam.
- Approximately 20% of all patients presenting to the emergency department (ED) with acute abdominal pain are assigned a diagnosis of constipation.
- Functional gastrointestinal disorders, and constipation in particular, reduce overall quality of life and are correlated with anxiety and impaired mental and physical functioning.
- Constipation affects children of all ages but is more common in:
  » Infants transitioning from a liquid to a solid diet
  » Toddlers who are toilet training
  » School-aged children

Diagnosis

- Diagnosis should be based solely on history and physical examination.
- The Rome IV diagnostic criteria are a set of validated criteria used to diagnose functional gastrointestinal disorders.
  » 2 of the following criteria must be occurring at least once per week for a minimum of 1 month with insufficient criteria for irritable bowel syndrome:
    › ≤ 2 defecations in the toilet per week
    › ≥ 1 instance of fecal incontinence per week in toilet-trained children
    › History of retentive posturing or excessive volitional stool retention
    › History of painful or hard bowel movements
    › Presence of a large fecal mass in the rectum
    › History of large-diameter stools that can obstruct the toilet
    › Symptoms that cannot be explained by another medical condition
- Irritable bowel syndrome (IBS) is a closely related and underdiagnosed disorder in children.
  » The cardinal feature of IBS is abdominal pain between bowel movements that, unlike constipation, does not improve with defecation.
  » The onset of abdominal pain is often associated with a change in frequency of defecation or the consistency of stool.

» In the subset of cases where the change in stool is to firm or hard and less frequent, the only difference from constipation would be the pattern of abdominal pain.
» A treatment trial targeting constipation symptoms is often needed prior to making the diagnosis of IBS.

History Features Suggestive of an Alternative Diagnosis

- Delayed meconium passage (90% of infants pass meconium in the first 24 hours of life) or constipation starting in the first month of life is:
  » Associated with a higher incidence of organic etiology
  » Very suspicious for the following if associated with failure to thrive:
    › Lower gastrointestinal (GI) obstruction
    › Meconium plug syndrome
    › Hirschsprung disease
    › Hypothyroidism
    › Cystic fibrosis
- Bilious vomiting is suggestive of an alternative diagnosis.

Table 14.3.1. X-RAY FINDINGS OF PATHOLOGIC CONDITIONS THAT MAY MIMIC FUNCTIONAL CONSTIPATION

Pathology	Incidence	X-ray findings
Duodenal atresia	1:5000	• Double bubble sign
Jejunal atresia	1:3000	• Air fluid levels
Malrotation with midgut volvulus	1:6000*	• Corkscrew finding on upper GI series • Ultrasound finding of abnormal relationship of SMA and SMV
Necrotizing ileus	2.4:1000	• Pneumatosis intestinalis

*For symptomatic patients

SMA superior mesenteric artery. **SMV** superior mesenteric vein.

Physical Examination Features Suggestive of an Alternative Diagnosis

- Failure to thrive may indicate:
  » Hirschsprung disease
  » Cystic fibrosis
  » Hypothyroidism
  » Malignancy

- Fever and/or abdominal pain may indicate:
  » Hirschsprung enterocolitis
  » Appendicitis
  » Urinary tract infection / pyelonephritis
- Severe abdominal distension may indicate:
  » Hirschsprung disease
  » Neuroblastoma or abdominal masses with bowel obstruction
  » Cystic fibrosis
  » Hypothyroidism
- Sacral dimple; tuft of hair on spine; poor lower limb tone; decreased lower extremity strength, tone, and reflex; and absent anal or cremasteric reflex may indicate:
  » Tethered spinal cord
  » Spinal cord tumor
  » Myelomeningocele
- Mood disturbance, restricted dietary intake, and developmental delays may indicate:
  » Autism
  » ADHD
  » Anorexia nervosa
  » Depression/anxiety
- Extreme fear or anxiety on anal inspection and/or anal scars may indicate:
  » Child abuse (see Chapter 1.7)

Investigations

- Investigations should be guided by history and physical examination to exclude other medical conditions that cause constipation.
- Consider the following investigations if there is suspicion of organic etiology after a careful history and physical examination:
  » Electrolytes
    › Rule out hypokalemia or hypercalcemia.
  » Hyperthyroidism
    › Check thyroid stimulating hormone (TSH).
  » Abdominal X-rays
    › Look for signs of obstruction.
  » Rectal examination
    › Check for:
      · Stool in the ampulla.
      · Explosive stool on withdrawal of finger
      · Tight anal sphincter
- In functional constipation, evidence does not support:
  » Routine use of ultrasound or colonic transit time for diagnosis of constipation
  » Routine laboratory testing for hypothyroidism or celiac disease in the absence of any supportive clinical features
  » Abdominal X-rays for diagnosis of constipation
    › Abdominal X-rays are misleading or normal 87% of the time.

  › 50% of patients with major abdominal diagnoses have normal X-rays.
  › An association exists between abdominal X-ray use and misdiagnosis of constipation.
    · Misdiagnosis often occurs as a result of confirmation bias when X-ray is used inappropriately as a "rule-in" test for constipation.
  › Use of abdominal X-rays for constipation should be limited to patients in which abdominal examination is difficult or impossible.

Management

- Enemas give quick relief of impaction but are invasive.
  » High-dose polyethylene glycol (PEG) has a similar effect to enemas after 3 to 5 days of treatment but with a higher incidence of incontinence.
  » If impaction is not causing anxiety or stress, oral treatment with PEG is preferred.
  » Following disimpaction, all children need to be on maintenance therapy for a period of 2 to 6 months.
- Common enemas used to treat constipation are:
  » Saline enemas
    › Saline enemas are safest for children with underlying medical conditions.
  » Fleet (phosphate) enemas
    › Fleet enemas should be used cautiously with children who have known calcium homeostasis disorders (parathyroid disease, vitamin D deficiency) or GI / genitourinary (GU) issues due to the risk of severe hypocalcemia.
- Common laxatives used to treat constipation include osmotic or stimulant laxatives.
  » Because they have fewer side effects, osmotic laxatives are preferred.
    › PEG is the most effective osmotic laxative when compared to other laxatives.
      · It is very well tolerated with minimal side effects.
      · It is tasteless and dissolves quickly in fluid.
      · Dose for disimpaction is 1 to 1.5 g/kg for 5 days.
      · Dose for maintenance is 0.4 to 1 g/kg for 2 to 6 months.
      · There is no actual ceiling dose; titrate to effect of 1 soft bowel movement daily.
      · PEG is not well studied in infants < 1 year of age.
    › Lactulose is a good alternative when PEG is not available or for infants.
      · Administer lactulose 5 to 10 mL/day.
      · Lactulose has a safe profile in infants.
      · Sodium picosulfate is a stimulant laxative that can intermittently be added to PEG 3350 as a rescue for persistent constipation.

Special Treatment Considerations

- If constipation is associated with toilet training:
  » Stop toilet training efforts until treatment is effective

» Continue maintenance therapy until toilet training skills are acquired
- In infants with a short, uncomplicated history of constipation, sorbitol-based juices like prune or apple juice can be used.
- Infant glycerin tips can be used to relieve impaction in infants
- Mineral oil is contraindicated in infants due to risk of aspiration pneumonitis.

SEVERE FECAL IMPACTION
- Admit patients to hospital and administer a PEG electrolyte solution wash-out PO or through a nasogastric (NG) tube at a rate of 20 mL/kg per hour to a maximum of 1 L/hour for 4 hours.
- Manual finger disimpaction should always be done under procedural sedation and reserved for severe cases.
- Indications for reference to gastroenterology or pediatrics include:
  » Constipation with any alarming clinical features
  » Failed therapy with osmotic and stimulant laxatives
  » Multiple presentations to the ED with acute impaction
  » Patients requiring admission to the hospital for management of constipation

HIRSCHSPRUNG DISEASE
- The incidence of Hirschsprung disease is 1.5 to 2.8 per 10 000 births.
- Familial occurrence in 5% to 20% of cases suggests a genetic basis for the condition.
- Patients can have varying length of aganglionosis:
  » 80% are short segment (confined to the rectosigmoid colon)
  » 15% are long segment (extends proximal to the sigmoid colon)
  » 5% have total colon and possible small bowel involvement

Diagnosis
- Hirschsprung disease presents in 1 of 3 ways:
  1. Neonatal period:
     › Delayed meconium passage
     › Abdominal distention
     › Bilious vomiting
     › Cecal or appendix perforation
  2. Chronic constipation:
     › Usually begins after being weaned off breast milk
     › Failure to thrive
     › Abdominal distention
     › Requires frequent enemas
     › Fecal soiling
  3. Enterocolitis:
     › 10% of patients present with fever and abdominal distention
     › Major risk of perforation

Physical Examination
- See "Physical Examination Features Suggestive of an Alternate Diagnosis," above.
- Other findings include:
  » Abdominal mass
  » Tight anal canal during rectal exam followed by explosive stool

Investigations
- Biopsy of distal rectal mucosa and submucosa shows:
  » Absence of ganglion cells
  » Hypertrophied submucosal nerves
  » Abnormal acetylcholinesterase enzyme staining pattern
- Anorectal manometry has a sensitivity of 91% and specificity of 94%.
- X-rays show:
  » Fecal loading
  » Dilated proximal colon with empty rectum
- Water-soluble contrast enema:
  » Shows a narrow rectosigmoid segment with a transition zone
  » Has a sensitivity of 7% and specificity of 97%

Management
- Consider an enema if the patient has severe discomfort or has not had a bowel movement for a few days.
- For enterocolitis:
  » Give nothing by mouth (NPO)
  » Provide IV hydration
     › Consider a normal saline bolus if there are signs of dehydration or sepsis.
  » Use NG intubation for decompression
  » Administer antibiotics
  » Obtain an immediate surgical consult
- If surgical management is required:
  » Use the pull-through procedure — the removal of the aganglionic segment and reconnection of the bowel to the anus.

Complications
- Patients may have long-term issues associated with Hirschsprung disease:
  » Dysmotility syndrome — may require ongoing laxative use
  » Soiling effects — enterocolitis can present post–surgical repair

GASTROINTESTINAL EMERGENCIES

REFERENCES

Alper A, Pashankar DS. Polyethylene glycol: a game-changer laxative for children. *J Pediatr Gastroenterol Nutr.* 2013;57(2):134–140. https://doi.org/10.1097/MPG.0b013e318296404a. Medline:23591910

Caperell K, Pitetti R, Cross KP. Race and acute abdominal pain in a pediatric emergency department. *Pediatrics.* 2013;131(6):1098–1106. https://doi.org/10.1542/peds.2012-3672. Medline:23690514

Freedman SB, Thull-Freedman J, Manson D, et al. Pediatric abdominal radiograph use, constipation, and significant misdiagnoses. *J Pediatr.* 2014;164(1):83–88.e2. Medline:24128647

Gfroerer S, Rolle U. Pediatric intestinal motility disorders. *World J Gastroenterol.* 2015;21(33):9683–9687. https://doi.org/10.3748/wjg.v21.i33.9683. Medline:26361414

Harrington L, Schuh S. Complications of Fleet enema administration and suggested guidelines for use in the pediatric emergency department. *Pediatr Emerg Care.* 1997;13(3):225–226. https://doi.org/10.1097/00006565-199706000-00014. Medline:9220514

Hyams JS, Di Lorenzo C, Saps M, Shulman RJ, Staiano A, van Tilburg M. Functional disorders: children and adolescents. *Gastroenterology.* 2016;150(6):1456–1468.e2. Medline:27144632

Ismail EA, Al-Mutairi G, Al-Anzy H. A fatal small dose of phosphate enema in a young child with no renal or gastrointestinal abnormality. *J Pediatr Gastroenterol Nutr.* 2000;30(2):220–221. https://doi.org/10.1097/00005176-200002000-00025. Medline:10697146

Koloski NA, Talley NJ, Boyce PM. The impact of functional gastrointestinal disorders on quality of life. *Am J Gastroenterol.* 2000;95(1):67–71. https://doi.org/10.1111/j.1572-0241.2000.01735.x. Medline:10638561

Langer JC. Hirschsprung disease. *Curr Opin Pediatr.* 2013;25(3):368–374. https://doi.org/10.1097/MOP.0b013e328360c2a0. Medline:23615177

Primavera G, Amoroso B, Barresi A, et al. Clinical utility of Rome criteria managing functional gastrointestinal disorders in pediatric primary care. *Pediatrics.* 2010;125(1):e155–e161. https://doi.org/10.1542/peds.2009-0295. Medline:20008416

Rothrock SG, Green SM, Hummel CB. Plain abdominal radiography in the detection of major disease in children: a prospective analysis. *Ann Emerg Med.* 1992;21(12):1423–1429. https://doi.org/10.1016/S0196-0644(05)80053-8. Medline:1443835

Rowan-Legg A; Canadian Paediatric Society, Community Paediatrics Committee. Managing functional constipation in children. *Paediatr Child Health.* 2011;16(10):661–670. Medline:23204909

Tabbers MM, DiLorenzo C, Berger MY, et al; European Society for Pediatric Gastroenterology, Hepatology, and Nutrition; North American Society for Pediatric Gastroenterology. Evaluation and treatment of functional constipation in infants and children: evidence-based recommendations from ESPGHAN and NASPGHAN. *J Pediatr Gastroenterol Nutr.* 2014;58(2):258–274. https://doi.org/10.1097/MPG.0000000000000266. Medline:24345831

14.4

Upper and Lower Gastrointestinal Bleeding

Joanne Delaney, Kevin Chan

- Upper gastrointestinal (UGI) bleeding is defined as bleeding that arises from a lesion proximal to the ligament of Treitz at the duodenojejunal flexure.
- UGI bleeding most commonly presents with one of:
  » Hematemesis (vomiting bright red blood or coffee-ground–like material)
  » Melena (black, tarry stools)
  » Hematochezia (bright red blood from the rectum, bloody stools)
    › This is an occasional finding, typically seen in younger children and suggestive of rapid bleeding time.
- Lower GI bleeding arises from a lesion distal to the ligament of Treitz and most commonly presents as hematochezia.
- The incidence of gastrointestinal (GI) bleeds in children is not well established.
- GI bleeds are the presenting complaint for 0.2% of children visiting the emergency department (ED).
- The rate of incidence is 6% to 25% for critically ill children in the intensive care unit.

Etiology

- Etiology varies with age (see *Table 14.4.1*).

Table 14.4.1. CAUSES OF UPPER AND LOWER GASTROINTESTINAL BLEEDING BY AGE GROUP

	Upper GI tract	Lower GI tract

Neonates	• Swallowed maternal blood
	• Vitamin K deficiency
	• Stress gastritis / ulcers
	• Congenital vascular or intestinal anomalies
	• Reflux esophagitis
	• Coagulopathy, secondary to:
	  » Infection
	  » Liver failure
	  » Factor deficiency
		• Swallowed maternal blood
		• Vitamin K deficiency
		• Anorectal fissure
		• Milk protein intolerance
		• Infectious colitis
		• Necrotizing enterocolitis
		• Malrotation/volvulus
		• Hirschsprung enterocolitis
		• Vascular malformations
		• Coagulopathy

Table 14.4.1 continues on next page.

	Upper GI tract	Lower GI tract
Infants and toddlers	• Esophageal varices • Mallory-Weiss tear • Stress gastritis / ulcers • Gastric/duodenal ulcer • Reflux esophagitis • Bowel obstruction • Swallowed nasopharyngeal blood (e.g., postepistaxis) • Coagulopathy	• Anorectal fissure • Milk protein intolerance • Infectious colitis • Nodular lymphoid hyperplasia • Coagulopathy • Intussusception • Infectious colitis • Early-onset IBD
Older children and adolescents	• Swallowed nasopharyngeal blood (e.g., postepistaxis) • Esophageal varices • Hemorrhagic gastritis • Gastric/duodenal ulcer • Mallory-Weiss tear • Gastritis • Reflux esophagitis • Eosinophilic esophagitis • Pill esophagitis • Foreign body ingestion	• Infectious colitis • IBD • Meckel's diverticulum • Hemolytic-uremic syndrome • Henoch-Schönlein purpura (IgA vasculitis) • Juvenile polyps • Hemorrhoids

IBD inflammatory bowel disease.

Diagnosis

- Assess the patient's ABCs.
- Hemodynamic instability is suggested by:
  - » Tachycardia
  - » Hypotension
  - » Orthostatic changes in heart rate and/or blood pressure
- If the patient is unstable, resuscitation must be provided before pursuing diagnostic tests.
- A gastroenterologist and surgeon should be notified of any acute unstable GI bleed.
- In a stable patient, confirm the presence of blood (see Table 14.4.2).

Table 14.4.2. SUBSTANCES COMMONLY MISTAKEN FOR BLOOD

Hematemesis	Hematochezia	Melena
• Swallowed maternal blood • Food dyes • Nasopharyngeal bleeding	• Ampicillin • Food dyes • Menstruation • Hematuria	• Iron, lead • Beets, spinach, blueberries • Licorice, chocolate • Charcoal, dirt

APPROACH TO UPPER GASTROINTESTINAL BLEEDING

History

- On history, physician should ask about:
  - » The time course of the bleeding event
  - » The estimated amount of blood loss
  - » The estimated rate of bleeding
    - › Bright red hematemesis suggests brisk bleeding rate.
    - › "Coffee-ground" emesis indicates slower rate of bleeding.
    - › Melena can be a result of UGI bleeding or proximal lower GI bleeding.
    - › Hematochezia may be seen in a massive, brisk UGI bleed.
  - » Associated symptoms, especially:
    - › Recent epistaxis
    - › Recent forceful vomiting
    - › Recent history of choking episode
    - › Abdominal or epigastric pain/discomfort
    - › Odynophagia
    - › Jaundice, easy bruising, or bleeding
  - » History of dyspepsia, reflux, dysphagia, abdominal pain, or weight loss
  - » Drug history, including:
    - › Nonsteroidal anti-inflammatory drugs (NSAIDs), corticosteroids, and ibuprofen — may cause ulceration
    - › Tetracycline or bisphosphonates — may lead to pill esophagitis
  - » History of alcohol consumption, and of binge-drinking episodes in particular
  - » Underlying chronic disease, especially liver disease or bleeding disorder
  - » Family history of liver disease or bleeding disorder

Physical Exam

- Assess the patient's ABCs, including vital signs.
- Evaluate the patient's general appearance for the presence of pallor or jaundice.
- Note the presence of:
  - » Bruising, petechiae, or mucosal bleeding
  - » Vascular malformations (hemangiomas, telangiectasias)
- Perform a nasopharyngeal examination to locate a possible bleeding source.
- Perform an abdominal examination for pain, distention, and hepatosplenomegaly.
- Note any stigmata of chronic liver disease and/or portal hypertension.

Investigations

- Order laboratory tests:
  - » Complete blood count (CBC)
  - » International normalized ratio (INR), partial thromboplastin time (PTT)
  - » Liver function tests
  - » Electrolytes, renal function
  - » Cross-match, type, and screen — in cases of severe bleeding

- Apt-Downey test — in infants, to establish whether blood is maternal or infant
- Order imaging studies.
  » Abdominal flat plate X-ray should be performed:
    › If foreign body ingestion is suspected
    › In any infant with acute hematochezia, to evaluate for:
      · Intestinal obstruction
      · Ischemic bowel disease
  » Abdominal ultrasound should be performed:
    › If variceal bleeding is suspected in a severe UGI bleed
    › To evaluate the patient for suspected liver disease or portal hypertension
- An upper endoscopy should be performed:
  » Within 24 to 48 hours for acute, severe UGI bleeding — earlier if bleeding is uncontrollable
  » In children with low-grade hemorrhage if bleeding is recurrent or persistent **or** if there is no obvious cause on history or physical exam for bleeding
  » Note that:
    › Patients should be hemodynamically stable prior to procedure.
    › Pediatric patients will typically require sedation or general anesthesia.
- Consider other investigations.
  » There may be a role for angiography or radionucleotide imaging if the endoscopy does not identify a source of bleeding.

Initial Management

- If the patient is hemodynamically stable, the volume of blood is small, and the source of bleeding is evident on history:
  » Provide supportive care
  » Observe the patient for further bleeding
  » Provide pharmacologic management
    › Consider an oral proton pump inhibitor (PPI) (omeprazole, lansoprazole, or esomeprazole).
- If the patient is hemodynamically unstable and/or the volume of blood is large:
  » First establish IV access and replace blood volume with a crystalloid fluid bolus
    › Consider early blood transfusion.
  » Administer nasogastric (NG) or orogastric (OG) lavage with water or normal saline
    › The return of "coffee-ground" or bright red blood suggests UGI bleeding.
    › A negative lavage does not rule out a UGI bleed if bleeding has already stopped or if the lesion is beyond the pylorus.
    › This intervention will facilitate endoscopy and decrease aspiration risk by removing blood, clots, and other particulate matter.

- Provide pharmacologic management (see *Table 14.4.3*):
  › IV proton-pump inhibitor — pantoprazole or esomeprazole
  › IV histamine-2 receptor antagonist (H2RA) — ranitidine
  › Consider octreotide if bleeding is poorly controlled by the above measures and is thought to be secondary to varices

Table 14.4.3. MEDICATIONS COMMONLY USED TO CONTROL UPPER GI BLEEDING

Medication	Dosage
Pantoprazole (IV)	• Patient weight 5 to 15 kg: 1 dose 2 mg/kg IV, then 0.2 mg/kg per hour IV • Patient weight 15 to 40 kg: 1 dose 1.8 mg/kg IV, then 0.18 mg/kg per hour • Patient weight >40 kg: 1 dose 80 mg IV, then 8 mg/h IV • Dose limit 80 mg/dose; maximum rate 8 mg/hr
Ranitidine (IV)	• 1 mg/kg IV divided and given every 6 hours
Octreotide (IV) — for severe bleeding, especially from varices	• 1 mcg/kg IV bolus, then 1 to 2 mcg/kg per hour; increase infusion rate every 8 hours; maximum rate 4 mcg/kg per hour

Disposition

- Consider hospitalizing the patient for observation if:
  » The patient is < 1 year of age
  » Blood loss is significant
  » Portal hypertension is suspected

Table 14.4.4. KEY FEATURES OF COMMON CAUSES OF UPPER GI BLEEDING

Condition	Key features
Swallowed maternal blood	• Seen in breastfeeding babies • Mother may have a history of cracked or bleeding nipples
Vitamin K deficiency	• Seen in babies who did not receive vitamin K prophylaxis at birth • Enquire about location of birth
Coagulopathy	• May present with bleeding from other sites, such as oozing from umbilical stump, prolonged bleeding after blood tests, or intracranial hemorrhage in a full-term baby
Mallory-Weiss tear	• History of recent forceful or excessive vomiting or coughing
Foreign body	• History of choking episode or ingestion (may have occurred days to weeks prior to presenting with bleeding)
Peptic ulcer disease	• Following use of NSAIDs or in the context of critical illness • May be associated with *Helicobacter pylori* or other infectious causes
Pill esophagitis	• Presents with hematemesis preceded by odynophagia • Associated with NSAIDs, tetracycline, and bisphosphonates
Variceal bleeding	• History of liver disease and/or portal hypertension • If no history, check for splenomegaly and thrombocytopenia

NSAIDs nonsteroidal anti-inflammatory drugs.

APPROACH TO LOWER GASTROINTESTINAL BLEEDING

History

- On history, ask about:
  - » Duration of bleeding
  - » Quantity of blood
  - » Color of blood
  - » Consistency of stool and presence or absence of diarrhea
  - » Fever, contact with sick individuals, and history of travel
  - » Abdominal pain
  - » Rectal pain and/or pain with defecation
  - » Chronic constipation or diarrhea
  - » Recent dietary changes — especially transition to cow's milk
  - » Growth history
  - » History of weight loss
  - » History of constitutional symptoms
  - » History of recent, large-volume epistaxis
  - » Drug history — especially recent NSAID use
  - » Past medical history and known chronic illnesses

Physical Exam

- Assess the patient's ABCs and vital signs.
- Evaluate the patient's general appearance for the presence of pallor or jaundice.
- Note the presence of bruising, petechiae, or mucosal bleeding.
- Perform a nasopharyngeal examination to locate a possible bleeding source.
- Perform an oral examination to determine the presence of oral ulcers.
- Perform an abdominal examination for pain, distention, and hepatosplenomegaly.
- Inspect the perianal area for fissures, skin tags, and fistulas.
- Perform a digital rectal exam.
  - » Evaluate for rectal polyps.
  - » Note whether there is an explosive expulsion of stool with the removal of digit (squirt sign).

Investigations

- Order laboratory tests:
  - » CBC
  - » Electrolytes, renal function tests
  - » Coagulation studies
  - » Liver function tests
  - » Cross-match, type, and screen — in cases of severe bleeding
  - » Fecal occult blood test — to confirm presence of blood
  - » Stool — send for viruses, bacterial culture, and/or presence of *C. difficile* toxin if patient has diarrhea
- Perform colonoscopy.
  - » Colonoscopy is indicated for any pediatric patient with unexplained rectal bleeding persisting > 2 weeks or in those with evidence of inflammation suggestive of inflammatory bowel disease (IBD).
- Perform other investigations dependent on presentation.
  - » If there is high suspicion for intussusception:
    - › Air- or water-soluble contrast enema can be diagnostic and therapeutic
  - » If there is high suspicion for intestinal ischemia:
    - › CT scan
  - » If ischemia has been ruled out:
    - › Consider technetium-99m pertechnetate nuclear scan (Meckel scan) to evaluate for Meckel diverticulum

Differential Diagnosis

Table 14.4.5. THE DIFFERENTIAL DIAGNOSIS OF LOWER GI BLEEDING

Condition	Key features
Anal fissures	• History of painful defecation, constipation, or diarrhea • Easily diagnosed on visual inspection of the perianal area
NEC	• Acute presentation, often with abdominal distention and signs of neonatal sepsis • Typically seen in premature infants, especially if receiving enteral nutrition • Hallmark on X-ray is pneumatosis intestinalis (gas in the bowel wall)
Milk- or soy-induced colitis	• Well-appearing child with history of loose, bloody stools • Most often seen in formula-fed babies • May present at transition from breast milk to formula or cow's/soy milk
Hirschsprung disease	• History of chronic constipation • May present with acute obstruction • Bleeding on presentation in 25% of cases • Diagnosis suggested by positive squirt sign (explosive expulsion of stool with digital rectal exam)
Hirschsprung enterocolitis (toxic megacolon)	• Rectal bleeding in patients with known Hirschsprung disease • This is a medical emergency requiring rectal decompression and antibiotic therapy
Intussusception	• Severe, colicky abdominal pain that awakens child from sleep • May see "red currant jelly" stool or frank blood
Meckel's diverticulum	• Painless rectal bleeding (chronic or acute) • Requires technetium-99m pertechnetate nuclear scan for diagnosis
Hemolytic-uremic syndrome	• Infectious colitis with Shiga-like toxin, followed 5 to 10 days later by acute renal injury, hemolytic anemia, and thrombocytopenia
Henoch-Schönlein purpura (IgA vasculitis)	• Gross or occult GI bleeding preceded by palpable purpura, abdominal pain, and diffuse arthralgia

Table 14.4.5 continues on next page.

Condition	Key features
Inflammatory bowel disease	• Typical presentation consists of bloody diarrhea, abdominal pain, and fever • Usually on a background of chronic diarrhea and weight loss or poor growth
Infectious colitis	• Usually presents as bloody diarrhea with abdominal pain and tenesmus, with or without fever • May be associated with recent travel, ingestion of uncooked foods, or antibiotic use (*Clostridium difficile*) • Most common pathogens include *Escherichia coli*, *Salmonella*, *Shigella*, *Campylobacter*, and *C. difficile*

NEC necrotizing enterocolitis.

Disposition

- Consider hospitalization if the patient is hemodynamically unstable.
- Outpatient investigations may be appropriate for stable patients.

REFERENCES

Ament ME. Diagnosis and management of upper gastrointestinal tract bleeding in the pediatric patient. *Pediatr Rev.* 1990;12*(4)*:107–116. https://doi.org/10.1542/pir.12-4-107. Medline:2235773

Boyle JT. Gastrointestinal bleeding in infants and children. *Pediatr Rev.* 2008;29*(2)*:39–52. https://doi.org/10.1542/pir.29-2-39. Medline:18245300

Flynn DM, Booth IW. Investigation and management of gastrointestinal bleeding in children. *Curr Paediatr.* 2004;14*(7)*:576–585. https://doi.org/10.1016/j.cupe.2004.09.001

Fox VL. Gastrointestinal bleeding in infancy and childhood. *Gastroenterol Clin North Am.* 2000;29*(1)*:37–66, v. https://doi.org/10.1016/S0889-8553(05)70107-2. Medline:10752017

Hussey S, Kelleher KT, Ling SC. Emergency management of major upper gastrointestinal hemorrhage in children. *Clin Pediatr Emerg Med.* 2010;11*(3)*:207–216. https://doi.org/10.1016/j.cpem.2010.06.003

Neidich GA, Cole SR. Gastrointestinal bleeding. *Pediatr Rev.* 2014;35*(6)*:243–253, quiz 254. https://doi.org/10.1542/pir.35-6-243. Medline:24891598

Teach SJ, Fleisher GR. Rectal bleeding in the pediatric emergency department. *Ann Emerg Med.* 1994;23*(6)*:1252–1258. https://doi.org/10.1016/S0196-0644(94)70350-7. Medline:8198299

14.5

Gastroesophageal Reflux Disease (GERD)

Fahad Masud, Rahim Valani

- Gastroesophageal reflux (GER) is the passage of gastric contents into the esophagus, a normal process in infants, children, and adults.
- Gastroesophageal reflux disease (GERD) indicates GER resulting in symptoms or complications, especially:
  » Vomiting — the expulsion of refluxed gastric contents from the mouth
  » Regurgitation — the passage of refluxed gastric contents into the oral pharynx
- Most patients will have at least 1 of the following symptoms:
  » Vomiting
  » Chronic cough
  » Epigastric pain
  » Feeding difficulties
  » Failure to thrive — if condition is severe
  » Bronchospasm
- Sandifer syndrome is caused by severe reflux that is expressed as posturing, with arching of the back and abdominal muscle wall contractions.

Pathophysiology

- Reflux is the result of relaxation of the lower esophageal sphincter (LES).
  » This is transient in healthy infants and children.
- Gastric distension associated with larger feeds and delayed gastric emptying causes increased frequency of LES relaxation.
- Impaired esophageal clearance and mucosal defense lead to esophagitis.
- Neurologically impaired children have decreased basal LES tone.

Differential Diagnosis

- Extraintestinal causes may be:
  » Infectious — sepsis, meningitis, gastroenteritis, urinary tract infection (UTI), otitis media (OM)
  » Anatomic — intestinal malrotation, pyloric stenosis
  » Central nervous system (CNS)–related — increased intracranial pressure (ICP), migraines, drugs
  » Respiratory — pneumonia, posttussive emesis

» Renal — obstructive uropathy, renal insufficiency
» Cardiac — congestive heart failure (CHF)
» Oncologic — malignancies
» Toxin-related
» Pregnancy-related
» Psychosocial/behavioral — overfeeding, self-induced vomiting/regurgitation
- Gastrointestinal (GI) causes may be:
  » Infectious — gastroenteritis, peritonitis, appendicitis, hepatitis
  » Inflammatory — GER, gastric outlet inflammation, peptic ulcer disease (PUD), celiac disease, eosinophilic gastroenteritis/esophagitis, food allergy/intolerance, pancreatitis, inflammatory bowel disease (IBD)
  » Mechanical — congenital anomaly, malrotation and volvulus, intussusception, foreign body / bezoar, meconium ileus, hernia
  » Motility-related — achalasia, pseudo-obstruction, Hirschsprung disease, gastroparesis
  » Other — anorexia, cyclic vomiting syndrome

Table 14.5.1. CLINICAL PRESENTATION OF GASTROESOPHAGEAL REFLUX (GER)

Infants		Children and Adolescents	
GI	**Extraintestinal**	**GI**	**Extraintestinal**
• Regurgitation • Feeding difficulties • Hematemesis	• Failure to thrive • Wheezing • Stridor • Persistent cough • Apnea • Irritability • Sandifer syndrome	• Heartburn • Vomiting • Regurgitation • Feeding difficulties • Dysphagia • Chest pain • Hematemesis	• Persistent cough • Wheezing • Laryngitis • Stridor • Chronic asthma • Recurrent pneumonia • Dental erosions • Anemia

Investigations

- In infants, a thorough history and physical examination are sufficient to diagnose GER; further investigations are not necessary.
- Further investigations should, however, be done:
  » For patients with suspected complications related to GERD
  » To investigate other causes of vomiting
- Empiric treatment with a positive response in patients who have classic GERD symptoms is diagnostic.

Chest X-rays

- Chest X-rays (CXRs) are not specific.
- CXRs show incidental findings of hiatal hernia of a dilated esophagus.

Upper GI Series

- An upper GI series demarcates anatomy and identifies anatomical causes of vomiting.
- It is not used to diagnose GERD, but rather rule out other causes of vomiting and reflux.

Esophageal pH Monitoring

- Esophageal pH monitoring measures frequency and duration of reflux via transnasal catheter with pH probe.
- It is useful for assessing the association between GER and symptoms.
- It is limited in that it cannot detect nonacid reflux or complications related to GER.

Esophagogastroduodenoscopy

- Esophagogastroduodenoscopy (EGD) allows direct visualization and biopsy of upper GI tract.
- EGD can determine the presence of esophagitis and other complications of GER.
- EGD is limited in that:
  » It requires sedation
  » There is a poor correlation between endoscopic appearance and histopathology
  » It does not rule out extraintestinal manifestations of GERD

Scintigraphy

- Scintigraphy is a gastric emptying scan using technetium-99 (^{99}Tc).
- It has low sensitivity (15% to 59%) and moderate specificity (83% to 100%) for diagnosing GERD.
- Scintigraphy is not recommended to diagnose or manage reflux.

Management

Conservative Management

- In infants:
  » Normalize feeding volumes
  » Increase calorie concentration of feed and reduce volume
  » Use thickened formula
  » Elevate the head
  » Use hypoallergenic formula
- In children and adolescents:
  » Modify diet to avoid caffeine, spicy food, and chocolate
  » Avoid large meals, and meals soon before lying down
  » Suggest weight loss if patient is obese
  » Eliminate alcohol and tobacco

GASTROINTESTINAL EMERGENCIES

Complications

Table 14.5.2. COMPLICATIONS OF GASTROESOPHAGEAL REFLUX

Esophageal complications	Extraintestinal complications
• Esophagitis	• Aspiration
• Barrett esophagus	• Bronchospasms
• Strictures	• Pneumonia
• Food aversion	• Dental caries

Pharmacotherapy

ANTACIDS

- Antacids buffer gastric contents.
- Use short-term for intermittent GER in children and adolescents; chronic therapy is not recommended.
- Antacids are used to neutralize gastric acids.
- Use caution: infants treated with aluminum-containing antacids show significantly increased plasma aluminum.
- Antacid use in infants is not well studied; better/safer approaches are available.

HISTAMINE-2 RECEPTOR ANTAGONIST (H2RA)

- Use ranitidine 4 to 10 mg/kg per day PO, divided and given every 8 to 12 hours.
- H2RA decreases acid production by binding to histamine-2 receptors on gastric parietal cells.
- H2RA is a common first-line therapy in infants.
- Significant improvement of reflux esophagitis with esophageal healing is seen with H2RA therapy.
- Side effects may include increased irritability, head banging, and headaches in some infants.
- It causes tachyphylaxis with chronic use.

PROTON PUMP INHIBITORS (PPIS)

- PPIs work by irreversibly blocking the proton pump (H^+-K^+ ATPase), the final step in parietal acid secretion.
- PPIs are more effective than H2RAs.
- PPIs are administered daily before meals; optimal acid suppression takes several days.
- They are not approved in children < 1 year of age.
- Side effects include headaches, diarrhea, constipation, and nausea in up to 15% of children.
- In neonates, there is a high carriage rate of *Candida* and increased rates of necrotizing enterocolitis (NEC).
- Consider lansoprazole.
  - » If patient weighs < 30 kg, dose at 15 mg PO once daily.
  - » If patient weighs > 30 kg, dose at 30 to 60 mg PO once daily.

PROKINETIC AGENTS

- Metoclopramide is given as 0.1 to 0.2 mg/kg per dose given four times daily for a maximum of 12 weeks.
  - » Complications include tardive dyskinesia.
- Prokinetic agents stimulate rapid emptying of the stomach.
- They are used in children who have evidence of delayed gastric emptying.
- Each medication carries potential adverse effects and are therefore **not recommended** for the treatment of GERD.

SURFACE AGENTS

- Surface agents adhere to lesions and protect the esophageal mucosal surface.
- There is inadequate data to determine safety and efficacy in pediatric patients.

Surgical Management

- The main indications for surgery include:
  - » Poor response to medical management
  - » Significant complications such as:
    - › Failure to thrive
    - › Pulmonary disease from reflux
    - › Esophageal strictures
    - › Barrett esophagus
  - » Neurologically impaired children

REFERENCES

Blanco FC, Davenport KP, Kane TD. Pediatric gastroesophageal reflux disease. *Surg Clin North Am.* 2012;92(3):541–558, viii. https://doi.org/10.1016/j.suc.2012.03.009. Medline:22595708

Lightdale JR, Gremse DA; Section on Gastroenterology, Hepatology, and Nutrition. Gastroesophageal reflux: management guidance for the pediatrician. *Pediatrics.* 2013;131(5):e1684–e1695. https://doi.org/10.1542/peds.2013-0421. Medline:23629618

Malfertheiner P, Hallerbäck B. Clinical manifestations and complications of gastroesophageal reflux disease (GERD). *Int J Clin Pract.* 2005;59(3):346–355. https://doi.org/10.1111/j.1742-1241.2005.00370.x. Medline:15857335

Stockman J III. A global, evidence-based consensus on the definition of gastroesophageal reflux disease in the pediatric population. *Yearbook of Pediatrics.* 2011;2011:133–137. https://doi.org/10.1016/S0084-3954(09)79678-2

Sullivan JS, Sundaram SS. Gastroesophageal reflux. *Pediatr Rev.* 2012;33(6):243–253, quiz 254. https://doi.org/10.1542/pir.33-6-243. Medline:22659255

Vandenplas Y. Gastroesophageal reflux. In Guandalini S, Dhawan A, Branski D, editors. *Textbook of pediatric gastroenterology, hepatology and nutrition: a comprehensive guide to practice.* New York: Springer: 2016. p. 105–130.

Vandenplas Y, Rudolph CD, Di Lorenzo C, et al; North American Society for Pediatric Gastroenterology Hepatology and Nutrition; European Society for Pediatric Gastroenterology Hepatology and Nutrition. Pediatric gastroesophageal reflux clinical practice guidelines: joint recommendations of the North American Society for Pediatric Gastroenterology, Hepatology, and Nutrition (NASPGHAN) and the European Society for Pediatric Gastroenterology, Hepatology, and Nutrition (ESPGHAN). *J Pediatr Gastroenterol Nutr.* 2009;49(4):498–547. Medline:19745761

14.6

Foreign Body Aspiration or Ingestion

Katrina F. Hurley

Risk Factors

- Foreign body ingestion or aspiration is common in young children due to the following risk factors:
  - » Lack of teeth
  - » Poor mastication
  - » Lack of attention to the task of eating
  - » Oral exploration — they put everything in their mouths
- Some risk characteristics for ingestion or aspiration in adolescents include:
  - » Piercings and simulated piercings (magnets)
  - » Experimentation
  - » Impulsivity
  - » Substance use (altered mental status)
  - » Transporting objects by mouth (e.g., headscarf pins)
- ADHD and developmental delay increase the risk for self-inserted/ingested foreign bodies or trauma.
- Always have a high index of suspicion for children with a history of choking, vomiting, chest or neck pain, or dysphagia.

FOREIGN BODY ASPIRATION

- The most commonly aspirated items are food related.
  - » In the United States, nuts (41%) and seeds (8%) are the most commonly aspirated foods.
- Commonly aspirated nonorganic items include headscarf pins and pen tops.
- Items associated with fatal aspiration include:
  - » Hot dogs
  - » Candy
  - » Nuts and seeds
  - » Grapes
  - » Balloons
- The patient's history may include sudden coughing or choking episodes, stridor, wheezing, and difficulty breathing.
- Bronchial foreign bodies originate from the oral cavity.
  - » Nasal aspiration of foreign bodies is very rare.
- Aspirated items more commonly end up in the bronchial tree in children (vs upper airway obstruction, which is more common in adults).

- Although the right main stem bronchus is steeper than the left, the carina is more often positioned to the left of the trachea, making the distribution of bronchial foreign bodies more even (right vs left) in children compared to adults.
  - » Case studies report bilateral bronchial foreign bodies in 1% to 3% of patients.
- The "classic" triad of symptoms occurs in less than one-third of patients:
  - » Coughing
  - » Wheezing
  - » Unilaterally decreased breath sounds
- Up to 20% of bronchial foreign bodies are asymptomatic.

Diagnosis

- Plain radiography allows the identification of radio-opaque foreign bodies and complications (e.g., pneumonia, barotrauma).
- Inspiratory and expiratory films can be used to assess the relative change in lung volumes.
  - » Hyperinflation is seen in 34% of cases.
  - » Atelectasis occurs in 20% of cases.
- Decubitus films have a sensitivity of 27% and specificity of 67%.
- Multidetector CT scan has a sensitivity of 94% and specificity of 95%.
- The gold standard for diagnosis remains endoscopy.
  - » Fluoroscopy is an option, but proceed directly to endoscopy if the level of suspicion is high.

Management

- First responders can do back blows and/or chest thrusts.
- Use direct laryngoscopy plus Magill forceps to remove a foreign body from the oropharynx.
- Obtain an airway if necessary using:
  - » Endotracheal intubation with selective ventilation of the unaffected side
  - » Surgical or needle cricothyrotomy
- Perform endoscopic removal of the foreign body in a controlled setting.

Complications

- Note that delayed diagnosis increases the risk of complications.
- Complications include:
  » Airway obstruction
  » Hyperinflation
  » Barotrauma, such as:
    › Pneumothorax
    › Pneumomediastinum
  » Fistula (tracheoesophageal, bronchopleural)
  » Granulomatous tissue
  » Bleeding from:
    › Friable tissue due to local trauma / pressure necrosis
    › Erosions into vasculature
  » Pneumonia, abscess
  » Foreign body migration

FOREIGN BODY INGESTION (SWALLOWED)

- Patients may present with drooling, refusal to eat, chest pain, or vomiting.
- Commonly swallowed objects, such as the following, are usually radio-opaque:
  » Coins
  » Batteries
  » Toys
  » Jewelry
- High-risk objects that require immediate attention include:
  » Magnets
  » Button batteries (> 20 mm in diameter)
  » Sharp objects (e.g., needles)
- Most esophageal foreign bodies in children are lodged in the upper esophagus.
  » Anatomical locations where foreign bodies can get hung up in the esophagus are:
    › Upper esophagus (cricopharyngeus muscle at C6)
    › Thoracic inlet
    › Level of the carina
    › Aortic arch
    › Lower esophageal sphincter
    › Anatomically different areas such as a tracheo-esophageal fistula or scar
- The anatomical relationship between the esophagus and the trachea means that it is possible for an esophageal foreign body to compromise the airway.
- From the stomach onward, a foreign body can become lodged at the following locations:
  » Pylorus
  » Duodenal sweep (a fixed retroperitoneal structure that may restrict the length of a rigid object that can pass)
  » Meckel's diverticulum
  » Ileocecal valve
  » Anal sphincter

Diagnosis

- A hand-held metal detector can be used to identify whether a swallowed metallic object is above or below the diaphragm.
- Plain radiography (orthogonal views) is usually sufficient to localize a swallowed object if it is radio-opaque.
- A coin in the upper esophagus can be differentiated from a coin in the airway by its orientation.
  » Esophageal coins are oriented in the coronal plane, whereas tracheal coins are oriented in the anteroposterior plane due to the rigid tracheal rings.
- To differentiate a coin from a button battery on radiography, remember that a button battery is bilaminar (double ring or halo is visible on the round view with a visible step-off on the lateral view of the battery).

Management

- Most objects that pass into the stomach are able to pass through the remainder of the gastrointestinal (GI) tract without difficulty.
  » Exceptions include:
    › Sharp objects
    › Objects > 5 cm in length
    › More than 1 magnet
    › Water beads — ingestion of superabsorbent beads has been reported to cause intestinal obstruction
- Foreign body removal should be done within 4 to 6 hours of ingestion.
  » Relatively **asymptomatic** esophageal coins can be observed in consultation with the endoscopist for 16 to 24 hours and then reimaged.
    › Up to 30% will pass spontaneously.
  » Coins in the lower one-third of the esophagus are more likely to pass spontaneously than those located more proximally.
  » Persistent esophageal coins will require endoscopic removal.
- The following require urgent consultation:
  » Any evidence of airway compromise
  » Esophageal obstruction (inability to swallow secretions, drooling, wheezing)
  » Inability to swallow fluids
  » Esophageal foreign body present for > 4 hours or unknown duration
  » Esophageal button battery
  » Sharp or long (> 5 cm) object in the esophagus or stomach
  » More than 1 high-powered magnet (e.g., neodymium)
  » Signs of intestinal perforation or obstruction

- Parents should be instructed to monitor the patient's stool.
- The North American Society for Pediatric Gastroenterology, Hepatology and Nutrition (NASPGHAN) recommends serial X-rays every 1 to 2 weeks to document the passage of a coin until it is cleared.
  » Coins retained for 2 to 4 weeks may be electively removed endoscopically.
- Consider whole bowel irrigation for lead pellet ingestion to prevent lead poisoning.
- Specific recommendations about button batteries and magnets are described below.
- Complications from ingested foreign bodies can occur at any level of the GI tract.
- Delay in diagnosis increases the risk of the following complications:
  » Bleeding
  » Pressure necrosis
  » Obstruction
  » Perforation
  » Mediastinitis
  » Sepsis
  » Tracheoesophageal fistula

BUTTON BATTERIES

- Button batteries are easily accessed from electronic devices that do not have a child protection battery cover or screw.
- Identified risk factors for button battery ingestion include:
  » < 6 years of age (peak is between 1 and 3 years of age)
  » Male children
- 1.3% of button battery ingestions have clinically significant complications.
- Injuries from button batteries are due to:
  » Electrical discharge (hydrogen ions)
    › Even "dead" batteries have sufficient residual voltage to cause damage.
  » Leakage of caustics (alkaline) from battery
    › This results in liquefactive necrosis and severe tissue damage.
  » Pressure necrosis
  » Heavy-metal poisoning (a remote possibility — last reported in 2004)
    › Mercury and lithium are possible toxins.

Diagnosis

- Plain radiography (orthogonal views) is sufficient to localize a button battery.
- To differentiate a coin from a button battery on radiography, note that a button battery is bilaminar (double ring or halo is visible on the round view with a visible step-off on the lateral view of the battery).

Management

- Urgent consultation with an endoscopist should be obtained when a button battery is identified in the esophagus regardless of the duration since ingestion or the presenting symptoms.
- Button batteries that pass into the stomach are likely to pass through the remainder of the GI tract without sequelae.

Complications

- Missed diagnoses are common due to nonspecific presentation or mistaking the battery for a coin and managing the condition conservatively.
- Complications include:
  » Perforation
  » Tracheoesophageal fistula
  » Stricture
  » Bleeding — reported to occur up to 1 month after battery removal
  » Vascular-enteric fistula
- Complications can also occur after the battery is removed, so follow-up is important (i.e., injuries can extend after battery removal).
- Risk factors for worse outcomes include:
  » Ingestion of battery > 20 mm in diameter
  » Age < 4 years
  » Ingestion of more than 1 battery
  » Unwitnessed ingestion or unknown time of ingestion
  » Misdiagnosis at first presentation
  » Delayed battery removal

MAGNETS

- A significant increase in magnet exposures has been documented.
- Rare earth magnets are 10 to 20 times more powerful than ferrite magnets.
- Magnets are strong enough to attract one another through body tissues, leading to necrosis and perforation.
- Although there has been a recall of Buckyballs (small neodymium magnets), more than 2.5 million sets were sold, so they are commonly available.

Diagnosis

- Plain radiography (orthogonal views) is sufficient to localize a swallowed magnet.

Management

- Do not delay endoscopic consultation in patients with multiple magnets identified on radiography.
- Consultation is still advisable when a single magnet has been ingested.
  » Patients may be managed expectantly with close follow-up.

REFERENCES

Abbas MI, Oliva-Hemker M, Choi J, et al. Magnet ingestions in children presenting to US emergency departments, 2002-2011. J Pediatr Gastroenterol Nutr. 2013;57(1):18–22. https://doi.org/10.1097/MPG.0b013e3182952ee5. Medline:23575300

Bamber AR, Pryce J, Ashworth M, Sebire NJ. Fatal aspiration of foreign bodies in infants and children. Fetal Pediatr Pathol. 2014;33(1):42–48. https://doi.org/10.3109/15513815.2013.846446. Medline:24144502

Bhargava R, Brown L. Esophageal coin removal by emergency physicians: a continuous quality improvement project incorporating rapid sequence intubation. CJEM. 2011;13(1):28–33. https://doi.org/10.2310/8000.2011.100298. Medline:21324294

Boufersaoui A, Smati L, Benhalla KN, et al. Foreign body aspiration in children: experience from 2624 patients. Int J Pediatr Otorhinolaryngol. 2013;77(10):1683–1688. https://doi.org/10.1016/j.ijporl.2013.07.026. Medline:23962764

Harris CS, Baker SP, Smith GA, Harris RM. Childhood asphyxiation by food: a national analysis and overview. JAMA. 1984;251(17):2231–2235. https://doi.org/10.1001/jama.1984.03340410039029. Medline:6708272

Jackson J, Randell KA, Knapp JF. Two year old with water bead ingestion. Pediatr Emerg Care. 2015;31(8):605–607. https://doi.org/10.1097/PEC.0000000000000520. Medline:26241717

Jatana KR, Litovitz T, Reilly JS, Koltai PJ, Rider G, Jacobs IN. Pediatric button battery injuries: 2013 task force update. Int J Pediatr Otorhinolaryngol. 2013;77(9):1392–1399. https://doi.org/10.1016/j.ijporl.2013.06.006. Medline:23896385

Kaushal P, Brown DJ, Lander L, Brietzke S, Shah RK. Aspirated foreign bodies in pediatric patients, 1968–2010: a comparison between the United States and other countries. Int J Pediatr Otorhinolaryngol. 2011;75(10):1322–1326. https://doi.org/10.1016/j.ijporl.2011.07.027. Medline:21840609

Kramer RE, Lerner DG, Lin T, et al; North American Society for Pediatric Gastroenterology, Hepatology, and Nutrition Endoscopy Committee. Management of ingested foreign bodies in children: a clinical report of the NASPGHAN Endoscopy Committee. J Pediatr Gastroenterol Nutr. 2015;60(4):562–574. https://doi.org/10.1097/MPG.0000000000000729. Medline:25611037

Lifschultz BD, Donoghue ER. Deaths due to foreign body aspiration in children: the continuing hazard of toy balloons. J Forensic Sci. 1996;41(2):247–251. https://doi.org/10.1520/JFS15422J. Medline:8871384

Litovitz T, Whitaker N, Clark L, White NC, Marsolek M. Emerging battery-ingestion hazard: clinical implications. Pediatrics. 2010;125(6):1168–1177. https://doi.org/10.1542/peds.2009-3037. Medline:20498173

Özcan K, Özcan Ö, Muluk NB, Cingi C, Durukan K. Self-inserted foreign body and attention-deficit/hyperactivity disorder: evaluated by the Conners' Parent Rating Scales-Revised. Int J Pediatr Otorhinolaryngol. 2013;77(12):1992–1997. https://doi.org/10.1016/j.ijporl.2013.09.020. Medline:24139587

Qureshi AA, Lowe DA, McKiernan DC. The origin of bronchial foreign bodies: a retrospective study and literature review. Eur Arch Otorhinolaryngol. 2009;266(10):1645–1648. https://doi.org/10.1007/s00405-008-0885-4. Medline:19084983

Schalamon J, Haxhija EQ, Ainoedhofer H, Gössler A, Schleef J. The use of a hand-held metal detector for localisation of ingested metallic foreign bodies: a critical investigation. Eur J Pediatr. 2004;163(4-5):257–259. https://doi.org/10.1007/s00431-004-1401-5. Medline:14762711

Sersar SI. Radiopaque foreign body inhalations. Asian Cardiovasc Thorac Ann. 2012;20(3):320–323. https://doi.org/10.1177/0218492312440431. Medline:22718722

Strickland M, Rosenfield D, Fecteau A. Magnetic foreign body injuries: a large pediatric hospital experience. J Pediatr. 2014;165(2):332–335. https://doi.org/10.1016/j.jpeds.2014.04.002. Medline:24836391

Waltzman ML, Baskin M, Wypij D, Mooney D, Jones D, Fleisher G. A randomized clinical trial of the management of esophageal coins in children. Pediatrics. 2005;116(3):614–619. https://doi.org/10.1542/peds.2004-2555. Medline:16140701

Walz PC, Scholes MA, Merz MN, Elmaraghy CA, Jatana KR. The internet, adolescent males, and homemade blowgun darts: a recipe for foreign body aspiration. Pediatrics. 2013;132(2):e519–e521. https://doi.org/10.1542/peds.2012-3340. Medline:23878050

Wright CC, Closson FT. Updates in pediatric gastrointestinal foreign bodies. Pediatr Clin North Am. 2013;60(5):1221–1239. https://doi.org/10.1016/j.pcl.2013.06.007. Medline:24093905

15.1

Jaundice in the Newborn Period

Rodrick Lim

- Newborn hyperbilirubinemia is frequently encountered.
  - » It is defined as a total serum bilirubin (TSB) of > 86 μmol/L.
- Jaundice is extremely common in full-term newborns.
  - » It is caused by the deposition of unconjugated bilirubin on the skin and mucosa.
  - » 60% of full-term newborns have jaundice in the first week of life.
  - » 2% develop a TSB concentration > 340 μmol/L.
  - » It is the most common reason for readmission to hospital.
- The Canadian Paediatric Surveillance Program (CPSP) reviewed full-term infants over a 2-year period (2002–2004) who had either a critical hyperbilirubinemia or required an exchange transfusion.
  - » The most common causes were ABO incompatibility and glucose-6-phosphate dehydrogenase (G6PD) deficiency.
  - » Approximately 4 in 10 000 live births develop severe hyperbilirubinemia.
  - » Approximately 1 in 10 000 of live births develop complications from severe hyperbilirubinemia.
- Many countries have screening and programs in place that identify and arrange follow-up for infants screened for hyperbilirubinemia in hospital and prior to discharge.

Pathophysiology

- Bilirubin is the final product of heme degradation.
  - » It is bound to albumin and carried to the liver, where it is conjugated.
  - » Conjugated bilirubin can be excreted via bile.
- The mechanisms that lead to unconjugated hyperbilirubinemia can be divided into:
  - » Increased bilirubin production
    - › Conversion to adult hemoglobin
    - › Increased blood cell load
    - › Lysis
  - » Decreased conjugation
    - › Enzyme deficiencies
    - › Prematurity
  - » Impaired excretion
    - › Ileus or delayed meconium passage
    - › Sepsis
    - › Asphyxia

History

- On presentation to the ED, triage should easily identify infants at risk for sepsis or jaundice.
  - » These patients should be reviewed early to ensure appropriate management.
- A thorough history should be taken from the parent or caregiver to identify any risk factors or predispositions, including but not limited to:
  - » Prenatal, antenatal, and neonatal history, including gestational age
  - » Timing of onset of jaundice (< 24 hours after birth is more likely to be pathologic)
  - » Presence of isoimmune hemolytic disease
  - » Family history of blood dyscrasias (e.g., G6PD) or older sibling who had hyperbilirubinemia
  - » Ethnicity — Asian and Indigenous populations
  - » Maternal age
  - » Cephalohematoma
  - » Dehydration
  - » Sepsis
  - » Changes in an infant's feeding or alertness, and irritability

Risk Factors

- Risk factors for hyperbilirubinemia can be divided into:
  - » Patient factors
    - › Increased red blood cell load
      - · Significant bruising during birth

- Polycythemia
- Delayed cord clamping
- Twin-twin transfusion syndrome
  › Medications
  › TORCH infections
  › Prematurity
  › Male
» Maternal factors
  › ABO and Rh incompatibility
  › Medications
  › Gestational diabetes
  › Ethnicity — Asian and Indigenous populations
» Other
  › Older sibling who had jaundice

Physical Exam

- A thorough physical exam should be undertaken, including but not limited to:
  » Vital signs
    › Check for fever via rectal temperature.
      · Febrile patients will require a full septic workup and antibiotics (see Chapter 2.4 for details on pediatric fever).
  » Weight (naked)
    › Calculate percentage weight loss from birth weight.
  » Hydration status, along with level of alertness
  » Presence of bruising or cephalohematoma
  » Assessment of the presence of neurologic signs of bilirubin encephalopathy
    › Symptoms of severe bilirubin encephalopathy include hypertonia, retrocollis, arching, opisthotonos, or high-pitched cry.
  » Examination of abdomen for presence of hepatomegaly, bowel distention, or presence of ileus

Investigations

- Once the initial assessment is complete, and the patient is stabilized, promptly initiate bloodwork, including:
  » Unconjugated and total serum bilirubin levels
  » Direct Coombs test (direct antigen test)
  » Complete blood count (CBC)
  » G6PD — consider in high-risk populations or patients with a family history of G6PD deficiency
- Review the thyroid screening test usually performed at birth.

Management

- Follow ABCs for immediate management.
- Ensure the infant is not at risk of sepsis.
  » There is a different treatment algorithm for patients at risk of sepsis (see Chapter 2.4).
- Initiate phototherapy prior to the availability of blood results in patients with clinically significant jaundice

who have risk factors (e.g., positive Coombs test) or who show early signs of bilirubin encephalopathy.
- Initiate phototherapy according to the Canadian Pediatric Society or American Academy of Medicine phototherapy tables, based on age, gestational age, and appearance.
  » Phototherapy should be "intensive," defined as therapy given via devices capable of delivering greater than 30 μW/cm² per nanometer.
- Ensure excellent exposure of skin but note that noninterruption of breastfeeding is currently recommended.
- Dehydrated patients should receive intravenous fluids.
  » Infants receiving phototherapy who have a high risk of progressing to exchange transfusion should receive PO or IV fluids.
- Obtain an intensive care consultation.
  » Patients above thresholds should be transferred or admitted to a center capable of exchange transfusion.
- Consider IV gamma globulin.

Complications

- Acute encephalopathy (kernicterus) is a rare but potentially devastating complication of hyperbilirubinemia and is largely preventable.
- The emergency department (ED) approach to jaundice aims at detecting infants at risk for complications and initiating timely management.

Disposition

- Patients not requiring phototherapy should be reevaluated in 24 to 48 hours.

REFERENCES

American Academy of Pediatrics, Provisional Committee for Quality Improvement and Subcommittee on Hyperbilirubinemia. Practice parameter: management of hyperbilirubinemia in the healthy term newborn. *Pediatrics*. 1994;94*(4 Pt 1)*:558–565. Medline:7755691

Barrington KJ, Sankaran K; Canadian Paediatric Society, Fetus and Newborn Committee. Guidelines for detection management and prevention of hyperbilirubinemia in term and late preterm newborn infants (35 or more weeks gestation). *Paediatr Child Health*. 2007;12(Suppl B):1B–12B.

Bhutani VK; Committee on Fetus and Newborn, American Academy of Pediatrics. Phototherapy to prevent severe neonatal hyperbilirubinemia in the newborn infant 35 or more weeks of gestation. *Pediatrics*. 2011;128*(4)*:e1046–e1052. https://doi.org/10.1542/peds.2011-1494. Medline:21949150

Centers for Disease Control and Prevention (CDC). Jaundice and kernicterus. Atlanta (GA): CDC; 2015 [cited 2016 Nov 11]. Available from: https://www.cdc.gov/ncbddd/jaundice/

National Institute for Health and Clinical Evidence (NICE). Jaundice in newborn babies under 28 days. London (UK): National Institute for Health and Clinical Excellence; 2010 [cited 2016 Nov 13]. Available from: https://www.nice.org.uk/guidance/cg98

Province of Ontario. Clinical pathway handbook for hypebilirubinemia in term and late pre-term infants (≥35 weeks). Toronto (ON): Provincial Council for Maternal and Child Health & Ministry of Health and Long-term Care; 2013 [cited 2016 Nov 13]. Available from: http://www.health.gov.on.ca/en/pro/programs/ecfa/docs/qbp_jaundice.pdf

15.2

Congenital Diaphragmatic Hernia

Jennifer Y. Lam, Mary E. Brindle

- The incidence of congenital diaphragmatic hernia (CDH) is 1 in 2000 to 5000 births.
- Having a first-degree relative with CDH is a risk factor.
- 80% of CDH defects are left-sided and 20% are right-sided; bilateral defects are rare.
- Associated anomalies are seen in up to 50% of infants with CDH, including chromosomal anomalies, cardiac defects, and neural tube defects.

Pathophysiology

- The exact cause of CDH is unknown.
- The diaphragm develops from 4 distinct components:
  1. The anterior central tendon from the septum transversum
  2. The dorsolateral portions from the pleuroperitoneal membranes
  3. The dorsal crura from the esophageal mesentery
  4. The muscular portion from the thoracic intercostal muscle groups
- Delay or failure of muscular fusion in the posterolateral diaphragm between weeks 4 and 10 of gestation is thought to predispose the individual to herniation and the development of CDH.
  » Genetic and environmental exposures that disrupt the differentiation of mesenchymal cells may also play a role in the development of CDH.
- Herniation of the abdominal viscera into the chest causes compression and impairs lung development, which contributes to pulmonary hypoplasia.
- Pulmonary vascular development follows airway development, and a reduction in arterial branching leads to muscular hyperplasia and resultant pulmonary hypertension.
- Although effects are more severe on the ipsilateral lung, the contralateral lung is also affected.

Diagnosis

- Up to 90% of cases are diagnosed on prenatal ultrasound usually by 24 weeks of gestation.
- Findings include:
  » Bowel loops in the chest
  » Echogenic chest mass
  » Absent or intrathoracic gastric bubble
  » Polyhydramnios

- Risk factors for a poor prognosis include liver herniation and small relative lung volumes reflected by either a low lung-to-head ratio on ultrasound or low fetal lung volumes on MRI.
  » Both modalities are most accurate when looked at as an observed:expected ratio (corrected for gestational age).
- Postnatal confirmation of the CDH diagnosis by chest X-ray (CXR) will show bowel loops in the chest.
  » Gastric bubble location can be confirmed by placing an orogastric tube.
  » Other CXR findings include:
    › Lobar compression
    › Shifting of the cardiac silhouette to the contralateral chest
    › Decreased or absent air-containing intra-abdominal bowel
  » If right-sided, the liver may be the only herniated organ and will be seen as a large intrathoracic soft tissue mass on the X-ray.
- CDH may closely resemble a cystic lung malformation.
  » If diagnosis is in doubt, an ultrasound may aid in differentiation between potential diagnoses.
- Echocardiography should be performed early to detect associated cardiac anomalies and to assess the degree of pulmonary hypertension; it may be repeated as necessary to assess and guide ongoing treatment of pulmonary hypertension.

Physical Exam

- The spectrum of respiratory symptoms varies from immediate respiratory distress to delay of symptoms for 24 to 48 hours to late presentation years into life.
- Symptoms include:
  » Tachypnea
  » Chest wall retractions
  » Grunting
  » Cyanosis
  » Pallor
  » Scaphoid abdomen
- The degree of respiratory distress is generally related to the degree of pulmonary hypoplasia and pulmonary hypertension.
- Symptoms of a bowel obstruction may accompany

CDH presentation but are more frequently seen in delayed presentations of CDH.

Management

- CDH is a physiologic emergency, **not** usually a surgical emergency, so treatment is aimed at resuscitation and stabilization of pulmonary hypertension prior to surgical correction of the defect.
- Initial resuscitation includes:
  » Prompt endotracheal intubation (avoid blow-by oxygen and bag valve mask ventilation to prevent further gastric distension)
  » Placement of a Salem sump nasogastric (NG) tube to decompress the stomach and confirm the diagnosis
  » Placement of an umbilical venous catheter for resuscitation
    › A preductal (i.e., right radial) arterial catheter should be placed to guide further therapy.

Ventilation

- Principles of ventilation include low-pressure ventilation to avoid barotrauma, permissive hypercapnia, and spontaneous respiration.
- Ventilation is initiated with simple pressure support with the goals of:
  » Peak inspiratory pressure < 22 cm H_2O
  » Rate of 40 to 60 breaths per minute
  » Preductal O_2 saturation of > 85%
  » $PaCO_2$ < 65 mmHg
- Parameters may be adjusted to ensure appropriate oxygenation, stable blood pressure, normal lactate, and no acidosis.
- High-frequency oscillator ventilation can be considered if preductal O_2 saturations of > 85% cannot be achieved while keeping peak inspiratory pressure < 25 cm H_2O or if $PaCO_2$ rises above 65 mmHg.
  » High-frequency jet ventilation is an alternative strategy.
- Lung recruitment strategies should be avoided as this could cause barotrauma/volutrauma to the hypoplastic lungs.
- There is no overall benefit in the use of surfactant, and its use is currently not recommended.
- Paralysis with neuromuscular blocking agents is generally not needed and should be avoided.
  » If necessary, a short-acting agent such as rocuronium should be used.

Cardiovascular Support

- Cardiovascular support with inotropes and vasopressors may be required to minimize right and left ventricular dysfunction and to provide afterload reduction to help reduce pulmonary hypertension.

- Aim for normal systemic blood pressure with avoidance of excessive tachycardia.
- Agents include milrinone, as well as dopamine, dobutamine, and epinephrine.
- Persistent severe pulmonary hypertension is associated with decreased survival.
  » Vasodilators may be required to treat pulmonary hypertension.
    › Include inhaled nitric oxide and sildenafil.
  » Prostaglandins may be used to keep the ductus arteriosus patent to offload the right ventricle.
- Extracorporeal membrane oxygenation (ECMO) can be considered in patients who fail to respond to conventional and high-frequency ventilation strategies.
  » Indications for ECMO include:
    › Inability to maintain adequate oxygenation
    › Persistent metabolic acidosis
    › Refractory hypotension
    › Elevated airway pressures
  » ECMO exclusion criteria include:
    › Lethal chromosomal anomalies
    › Significant congenital anomalies
    › Weight < 2 kg
    › Intracranial hemorrhage
    › Gestational age < 34 weeks

Surgical Management

- Optimal timing for surgical correction of the defect is unknown.
- Criteria for readiness for repair have been published but are at the discretion of the surgeon and may not always be achievable preoperatively.
- Criteria for repair include:
  » Stability on conventional ventilation for 24 hours and FiO_2 < 50%
  » Hemodynamic stability — patient is off inotropes/vasopressors or on stable infusions
  » Optimization of right ventricular function with resolution/stability of pulmonary hypertension
  » Lactate < 3
  » Adequate urine output > 2

Complications

- Improved survival rates (approximately 60% to 90%) are accompanied by increased recognition of morbidity.
- Recurrence of the defect and reherniation occur in approximately 2% to 22% of cases.
  » Risk factors include a large defect, the necessity of prosthetic material for closure, and ECMO use (patch closure and ECMO use are surrogates of a large defect).
  » Reherniation typically occurs in the medial aspect.
  » Acute reherniation can be associated with an

incarcerated and/or strangulated stomach/bowel; volvulus may also be present.

» Reherniation may be completely asymptomatic or may present with respiratory compromise or intestinal obstruction with or without vascular compromise.

» Diagnosis is made by CXR, with or without a CT scan.

» Treatment is dependent on the stability of the patient; nasogastric (NG) tube placement may be required for decompression and emergent surgery referral in the case of compromised viscera.

PULMONARY COMPLICATIONS

- Pulmonary issues are the most common, including chronic lung disease, bronchopulmonary dysplasia, impaired pulmonary function, reactive airway disease, and recurrent infections.

» Recurrent episodes of pneumonia occur in up to 30% of CDH survivors.

» These patients have increased risk of morbidity associated with respiratory syncytial virus (RSV) infection.

› RSV prophylaxis is recommended.

» A high proportion of patients will have evidence of bronchospasm and wheezing and be diagnosed with asthma.

» Pulmonary function tests are abnormal and may demonstrate obstructive, restrictive, or combined airway disease in most patients for the first 2 to 3 years of life.

› As the child grows, pulmonary function gradually improves, reaching near-normal exercise capacity by adolescence and adulthood.

» Postoperative chylothorax is a very rare presentation to the emergency department (ED).

› It presents as pleural effusion that usually develops shortly after the initiation of an enteral diet.

› It is mostly treated nonoperatively with a medium-chain triglyceride diet and pleural drainage for symptom control, with or without octreotide.

· There is no definitive evidence to support the use of octreotide.

› Pleurodesis, thoracic duct embolization, and thoracic duct ligation are potential invasive strategies for treating a postoperative chylothorax that does not respond to nonoperative therapy.

- Pulmonary hypertension resolves by 3 weeks of life in about 50% of patients.

» Long-term effects of transient pulmonary hypertension are unknown.

» Early pulmonary hypertension is usually associated with bidirectional or right-to-left shunting through a patent ductus arteriosus, flattening of the intraventricular septum, and tricuspid regurgitation.

» Persistent pulmonary hypertension can impact survival, and late deaths have occurred.

› The changes of long-term pulmonary hypertension are documented by right axis deviation on ECG and right ventricular hypertrophy on echocardiogram.

› Prolonged pulmonary hypertension can lead to cardiac failure.

GASTROINTESTINAL COMPLICATIONS

- Gastrointestinal (GI) morbidity includes gastroesophageal reflux disease (GERD), intestinal obstruction, and growth and nutritional problems leading to failure to thrive.

» GERD occurs in 20% to 80% of infants with CDH repair.

› Patients should be started on medical therapy (see Chapter 14.5).

› Up to 20% of infants will require antireflux surgery for severe GERD.

› Long-term effects of GERD in the CDH population are poorly studied, but one study reports esophagitis in up to 54% of adults who underwent neonatal CDH repair.

» Intestinal obstruction can occur in 10% to 20% of patients due to a number of potential causes.

› Intestinal obstruction may occur as a result of adhesions.

› Abnormal intestinal rotation may predispose a subset of patients to obstruction from midgut volvulus.

› It can result from reherniation of the abdominal viscera into the chest.

› Prolonged intestinal paralysis caused by critical illness in the neonatal period, and increased intraabdominal pressure and hypoperfusion, may also contribute to hypomotility of the bowel.

» Multiple factors contribute to growth difficulties and failure to thrive, including increased caloric requirements, GERD, and oral aversion.

› Many patients require gastrostomy tube feeds for supplementation.

OTHER COMPLICATIONS

- Patch infection may occur when a patch is used to close the CDH.

» Patch infection is a rare but serious complication that requires broad-spectrum antibiotics, patch removal, and diaphragmatic reconstruction.

- Musculoskeletal deformities including pectus excavatum and scoliosis are common after the repair of a large CDH.

» Treatment may include bracing or surgical repair if severe deformities exist.

- Neurodevelopmental abnormalities can occur in patients with CDH as either an associated anomaly or as an acquired neurologic insult resulting from neonatal hypoxemia.

  » Abnormalities include impaired motor and cognitive skills, language problems, and progressive sensorineural hearing loss.

LATE-PRESENTING CDH

- 5% to 20% of all CDH cases are late presenting.
  » These cases can present any time after the first month of life, with most presenting at around 1 year of age.
- The wide range of presenting symptoms and relative scarcity of the condition cause diagnostic difficulties.
  » Cases can range from being asymptomatic to have sudden acute or chronic symptoms.
    › Left-sided CDH tends to present with more acute symptoms associated with sudden herniation of a large volume of abdominal viscera.
    › Right-sided CDH tends to present with more chronic symptoms as the liver prevents large volumes of abdominal viscera from herniating.
    › 5% to 10% of late-presenting CDH cases are asymptomatic and are identified incidentally on imaging done for other reasons.
  » Symptoms can be respiratory, gastrointestinal, or both.
    › Younger patients more commonly present with respiratory issues, whereas older patients present with gastrointestinal symptoms.
- Late-presenting CDH is rarely associated with pulmonary hypoplasia or other defects (chromosomal anomalies or cardiac or neural tube defects).
  » Herniation of the abdominal viscera into the chest likely occurs as a relatively late event in pregnancy or even in the postnatal period.
    › This supposition is supported by the fact that up to 16% of patients diagnosed with a late-presenting CDH had a previous normal chest radiograph.
- As with neonatal CDH, a CXR remains the most important investigation for diagnosis of late-presenting CDH.
  » Approximately 50% of cases are diagnosed based on a single CXR.
  » Diagnostic X-ray findings include intrathoracic radiolucent structures with mediastinal shift (if the bowel is herniated).
    › Solid organ herniation increases the risk of radiologic misdiagnosis.
    › Misinterpretation of initial imaging occurs in > 25% of patients.
    › Placement of an NG tube can identify an intrathoracic stomach and help improve diagnostic certainty.
    › Upper GI fluoroscopy and/or a CT scan can help with diagnosis in patients with diagnostic uncertainty.

  › Misdiagnosis of the CDH as pneumothorax or pleural effusion can lead to chest tube insertion and iatrogenic perforation of herniated organs.
- Management of late-presenting CDH is dependent on the presenting symptoms.
  » Asymptomatic patients and those with chronic symptoms with no evidence of bowel compromise or gastric volvulus may be appropriate for elective repair.
  » Acute and sudden presentation and symptoms suggestive of compromise of the herniated viscera will require the following:
    › Immediate NG tube placement for decompression
    › Emergent surgical referral for operative repair
      · High morbidity and mortality is seen when delay of treatment occurs in patients with ischemia related to gastric volvulus and/or a strangulated bowel.

REFERENCES

Bagłaj M. Late-presenting congenital diaphragmatic hernia in children: a clinical spectrum. *Pediatr Surg Int.* 2004;20(9):658–669. https://doi.org/10.1007/s00383-004-1269-5. Medline:15349741

Bagłaj M, Dorobisz U. Late-presenting congenital diaphragmatic hernia in children: a literature review. *Pediatr Radiol.* 2005;35(5):478–488. https://doi.org/10.1007/s00247-004-1389-z. Medline:15778858

Bagolan P, Morini F. Long-term follow up of infants with congenital diaphragmatic hernia. *Semin Pediatr Surg.* 2007;16(2):134–144. https://doi.org/10.1053/j.sempedsurg.2007.01.009. Medline:17462566

Chiu P, Hedrick HL. Postnatal management and long-term outcome for survivors with congenital diaphragmatic hernia. *Prenat Diagn.* 2008;28(7):592–603. https://doi.org/10.1002/pd.2007. Medline:18551724

Hedrick HL, Adzick NS. Congenital diaphragmatic hernia in the neonate [Internet]. Post TW (editor), UpToDate, Waltham, MA: UptoDate Inc.; 2016 Aug 1 [cited 2016 Sept 5]. Available from: https://www.uptodate.com/contents/congenital-diaphragmatic-hernia-in-the-neonate

Hedrick HL, Adzick NS. Congenital diaphragmatic hernia: prenatal diagnosis and management [Internet]. Post TW (editor), UpToDate, Waltham, MA: UptoDate Inc.; 2016 Apr 5 [cited 2016 Sept 5]. Available from: https://www.uptodate.com/contents/congenital-diaphragmatic-hernia-prenatal-diagnosis-and-management

Howlett A, Tierney A, Vorhies E, et al. AHS congenital diaphragmatic hernia guideline [Internet]. Edmonton, AB: Alberta Health Services; 2016 June 17 [cited 2016 Aug 18]. Available from: https://myahs.ca/insite/assets/policy/clp-calgary-childrens-health-neonatology-congenital-diaphragmatic-hernia-2-c-11.pdf

Nayak HK, Maurya G, Kapoor N, Kar P. Delayed presentation of congenital diaphragmatic hernia presenting with intrathoracic gastric volvulus: a case report and review. *BMJ Case Rep.* 2012;2012 Nov 28:bcr2012007332. https://doi.org/10.1136/bcr-2012-007332. Medline:23195824

Peetsold MG, Heij HA, Kneepkens CMF, Nagelkerke AF, Huisman J, Gemke RJ. The long-term follow-up of patients with a congenital diaphragmatic hernia: a broad spectrum of morbidity. *Pediatr Surg Int.* 2009;25(1):1–17. https://doi.org/10.1007/s00383-008-2257-y. Medline:18841373

Stolar CJH, Dillon PW. Congenital diaphragmatic hernia and eventration. In: Coran AG, editor. *Pediatric surgery.* Philadelphia, PA: Saunders; 2012. p. 809–824. https://doi.org/10.1016/B978-0-323-07255-7.00063-5

Tsao K, Lally KP. Congenital diaphragmatic hernia and eventration. In: Holcomb GW III, Murphy JP, editors. *Ashcraft's pediatric surgery.* Philadelphia, PA: Saunders; 2010.p. 304–321. https://doi.org/10.1016/B978-1-4160-6127-4.00024-0

16.1

Testicular Torsion

Tim Lynch

- Testicular torsion has an estimated incidence of 4 in 100 000 boys aged 18 and under.
- It can occur at any age but typically occurs in boys between 12 and 16 years of age, peaking at age 13.
- Neonatal torsion is often representative of antenatal compromise of the testicle.

Pathophysiology

- Twisting of the spermatic cord that results in ischemia and infarction of the testicle may also present in the perinatal period due to lack of fixation of the testicle in the scrotum.
- Bell-clapper deformity is often found during surgical exploration and is often bilateral — the testicle can rotate within the tunica vaginalis because the posterior testicle is not fixed to the scrotum and has a horizontal lie.
  » This is seen in 12% of males with testicular torsion; of those, 40% of cases are bilateral.
- Complications include infertility.
- Initial evaluation depends on the patient's history and the physical exam.

History

- On history, gather information about:
  » Acute onset of testicular pain and/or swelling or abdominal pain
  » Unrelenting pain (abdominal/testicular)
  » Associated nausea/vomiting
  » Swelling of the scrotum or change in the position of the testicle

Physical Exam

- Patients may present with the following:
  » Unilateral tender testicle
  » Abnormal lie of the testicle (transverse orientation)
  » High-riding testicle
  » Enlarged testicle
  » Absence of cremasteric reflex
    › The presence of the cremasteric reflex does not rule out torsion.
    › Sensitivity is 100% but specificity is 66%.
- It may occasionally be possible to palpate a twist in the spermatic cord.
- Adolescents will often minimize or deny their symptoms.
- Examination of the external genitalia should always be included in patients with abdominal pain.
- Neonates often present with a painless scrotal mass.

Risk Factors

- Past history of testicular pain may indicate possible intermittent torsion with detorsion.
- Patients with cryptorchidism / undescended testicles are at an increased risk of torsion.

Investigations

- Obtain an urgent surgical consultation with imaging if clinical suspicion of torsion is high.
  » Salvage rates are often decreased due to delays in obtaining imaging.
- There are 2 main imaging modalities for diagnosis of testicular torsion:
  1. Doppler ultrasound
    › Ultrasound may show absent or decreased blood flow.
    › Doppler ultrasound has a sensitivity of 90% to 97%, a specificity of 99%, and a false positive rate of 1%.
  2. Radionuclide imaging
    › Radionuclide imaging is not easily obtainable.
    › A Doppler ultrasound is more accessible at many centers.

Differential Diagnosis

- Consider the following on the differential diagnosis:
  » Spermatic cord torsion
  » Torsion of appendix testis
    › This presents with a "blue dot" sign (tender, blue nodule on the upper pole).
  » Torsion of epididymis
  » Hernia
  » Hydrocele/varicocele
  » Trauma
  » Epididymitis/orchitis

Management

- If there is high suspicion of testicular torsion based on the patient's history and physical exam, consult surgery or urology for an immediate surgical exploration.
  » The salvage rate window is 4 to 8 hours.
- Manual detorsion is not recommended unless there is a delay in obtaining surgical exploration.
  » Manual detorsion is best done by a surgeon and is considered a temporizing measure.
  » The concept is like opening a book such that the affected testicle is rotated at least 360° in a medial to lateral fashion or outward toward the patient's thigh.
  » The patient will have immediate relief of pain.
- An orchidopexy is performed if the testicle is viable.
- An orchiectomy is performed if the testicle is not viable.
- Surgery should include exploration of the contralateral testicle with prophylactic, contralateral orchidopexy.

Prognosis

- Tissue loss is directly proportional to the duration of ischemia.
- Salvage rates are time sensitive:
  » < 6 hours — 90% salvage rate
  » >12 hours — 50% salvage rate
  » >24 hours — < 10 % salvage rate (most likely not salvageable)
- A prior orchidopexy does not preclude future torsion.
- Neonatal torsion salvage rates are extremely low.

REFERENCES

Bowlin PR, Gatti JM, Murphy JP. Pediatric testicular torsion. *Surg Clin North Am.* 2017;97(1):161–172. https://doi.org/10.1016/j.suc.2016.08.012. Medline:27894425

Jefferies MT, Cox AC, Gupta A, Proctor A. The management of acute testicular pain in children and adolescents. *BMJ.* 2015;350:h1563. https://doi.org/10.1136/bmj.h1563. Medline:25838433

Kapoor S. Testicular torsion: a race against time. *Int J Clin Pract.* 2008;62(5):821–827. https://doi.org/10.1111/j.1742-1241.2008.01727.x. Medline:18412935

Ludvigson AE, Beaule LT. Urologic emergencies. *Surg Clin North Am.* 2016;96(3):407–424. https://doi.org/10.1016/j.suc.2016.02.001. Medline:27261785

Molokwu CN, Somani BK, Goodman CM. Outcomes of scrotal exploration for acute scrotal pain suspicious of testicular torsion: a consecutive case series of 173 patients. *BJU Int.* 2011;107(6):990–993. https://doi.org/10.1111/j.1464-410X.2010.09557.x. Medline:21392211

Waldert M, Klatte T, Schmidbauer J, Remzi M, Lackner J, Marberger M. Color Doppler sonography reliably identifies testicular torsion in boys. *Urology.* 2010;75(5):1170–1174. https://doi.org/10.1016/j.urology.2009.07.1298. Medline:19913882

16.2

Priapism

Shawn Mondoux

- Priapism is defined as a prolonged, penile erection lasting > 4 hours without sexual stimulation.
- Patients' chief complaint is penile swelling and pain.
  » This is typically caused by inflammatory response and ischemia.
- Risk of ischemia increases after 4 hours of sustained erection.
- If treatment fails, consult urology for consideration of a surgical shunt.
  » Sickle cell patients may receive plasmapheresis for treatment of sustained priapism.

LOW-FLOW PRIAPISM

- Low-flow priapism is also known as ischemic or veno-occlusive priapism.
  » Low-flow priapism is very painful — the equivalent of compartment syndrome of the penis.
  » It is the most common type of priapism.
  » It is the most concerning type of priapism as it carries a much higher risk of ischemia.
  » It is caused by decreased venous outflow from the penis.
    › This results in hypoxia, acidosis, and glucopenia.
    › Smooth muscle dysregulation and necrosis ensue with prolonged duration of ischemia.

Risk Factors

- Risk factors for low-flow priapism in children include:
  » Leukemia
  » Hemoglobinopathies
    › Sickle cell disease (SCD) — Up to 42% of male children with sickle cell disease will have at least 1 episode of priapism.
    › Thalassemia
  » Less-common causes
    › Kawasaki disease
    › Hypercoagulable states
    › Alcohol abuse
    › Side effects of medications (e.g., SSRIs, phenothiazines, antihypertensives, anticoagulants, and drugs of abuse)
    › Parenteral nutrition

Management

- Manage symptoms.
  » Early and appropriate pain control is very important.
  » See Chapter 8.2 on the management of patients with SCD.
- Control pain.
  » Systemic opiate therapy should be considered in priapism patients; consider IV morphine at 0.1 to 0.15 mg/kg.
  » In the case of dorsal penile nerve block:
    › Use sterile technique
    › Use lidocaine without epinephrine and perform a field block at the base of the penis
      · Consider the use of bupivacaine (Marcaine) for a sustained block.
- Perform aspiration.
  » Notify the urology team if available.
  » Aspiration is performed after appropriate penile anesthesia.
  » Insert a 19G to 21G angiocatheter or butterfly into the corpus cavernosum and attempt withdrawal of blood (at the 3 o'clock or 9 o'clock position to avoid the dorsal neurovascular bundle).
    -Aspirate until the shaft is soft.
  » If there is no resolution, irrigate each side with normal saline.
    › Instill 3 to 8 mL in each cavernosum.
    › Let the saline permeate the corpus cavernosum for 3 to 5 minutes, then withdraw the instilled fluid.
    › Perform irrigation up to 3 times.
  » The above methodology relieves approximately 30% of cases.
- Inject alpha-adrenergic agonist.
  » Inject alpha-1 selective adrenergic agonists if the above method fails.

  » Instill 0.25 mL to 0.5 mL of phenylephrine solution (100 mcg/mL in normal saline).
  » This can be repeated every 5 minutes.
    › It should be done while the patient is on a cardiac monitor.
  » Attempt aspiration after each injection.
  » These patients should be admitted for observation.

STUTTERING (RECURRENT) PRIAPISM

- Stuttering priapism has the highest risk of muscle necrosis.
- It is classically seen in patients with SCD.

Management

- Stuttering priapism is usually self-limiting.
  » See Chapter 8.2 on the management of patients with SCD.
  » If prolonged, consider aspiration as with ischemic (low-flow) priapism.

HIGH-FLOW PRIAPISM

- High-flow priapism is also known as nonischemic priapism.
  » It is generally painless acutely but may lead to stagnation, hypoxia, and ischemia.
  » Penile vascular inflow is greater than outflow.
  » It is typically associated with trauma (penile artery laceration with increased arterial inflow) or spinal trauma (corporal engorgement).

TRAUMATIC PRIAPISM

- Trauma management should take priority while considering early consultation with a pediatric urologist.
- Conservative treatment is usually recommended as the first line.
  » 60% to 70% of cases resolve spontaneously, but long-term sequelae are frequent.
- Other options include arteriography with embolization.

REFERENCES

McCollough M, Sharieff G. Genitourinary and renal tract disorders. *Rosen's emergency medicine*. 8th ed. p 2205–2206.

McGrath NA, Howell JM, Davis JE. Pediatric genitourinary emergencies. *Emerg Med Clin North Am*. 2011;29(3):655–666. https://doi.org/10.1016/j.emc.2011.04.003. Medline:21782080

Muneer A, Ralph D. Guideline of guidelines: priapism. *BJU Int*. 2017;119(2):204–208. https://doi.org/10.1111/bju.13717. Medline:27860090

Shigehara K, Namiki M. Clinical management of priapism: a review. *World J Mens Health*. 2016;34(1):1–8. https://doi.org/10.5534/wjmh.2016.34.1.1. Medline:27169123

GENITOURINARY EMERGENCIES

16.3

Vulvovaginitis

Marcia Edmonds

- Vaginitis is defined as inflammation of the vagina, and vulvitis is inflammation of the vulva. They may present separately or in combination.
- Vulvitis may present with pruritus, tenderness, dysuria, and erythema of the vulva.
- In prepubertal patients, vaginitis usually presents with discharge and/or bleeding.
- In postpubertal patients, vaginitis usually presents with a change in normal discharge or vaginal discomfort.
- It is necessary to distinguish the normal discharge that occurs in infancy and with the onset of puberty (usually thin and mucoid) from the pathological discharge of vaginitis.

History

- On history, collect information about the following:
  - » Duration of symptoms
  - » Discharge, if any, and:
    - › Color and odor of discharge
    - › Amount of discharge
  - » Bleeding
  - » Itching or burning in the perineum
  - » Dysuria
  - » Specific clothing:
    - › Nylon tights
    - › Wearing a swimsuit for long periods
    - › Tight jeans, stockings, or tights
  - » Hygiene:
    - › Wiping front to back / back to front
    - › Use of soaps or bubble baths
  - » Other symptoms:
    - › Recent diarrhea
    - › Dermatological conditions
  - » Type of laundry detergent used
  - » Use of fabric softeners
  - » Use of home remedies to treat symptoms
  - » Insertion of a foreign body (e.g., toilet paper, beads, other items)
  - » Other infections in the family:
    - › Respiratory symptoms
    - › Gastroenteritis
  - » History of sexual abuse

Physical Exam

- In prepubertal and postmenarchal patients who are never sexually active, an external genital exam should be performed, and swabs should be taken of the discharge.
- In prepubertal patients, in most cases, a parent or caregiver should remain in the room for the examination.
  - » Use the frog-leg position or the knee-chest position on the examination table or parent's lap to facilitate the exam.
  - » Gentle lateral traction on the labia majora, with a cough or deep breathing, will allow visualization of the lower part of the vagina and is frequently sufficient to visualize a foreign body.
  - » For a suspected pelvic mass or in certain cases of abdominal pain, a rectovaginal exam may be performed.
- Examine the perineum to assess:
  - » General hygiene
  - » Evidence of vaginal discharge
  - » Hymenal anomalies
  - » Other skin lesions
  - » Signs of trauma
  - » Excoriations

Pathophysiology

- 75% of vulvovaginitis cases are nonspecific.
  - » Vaginal cultures reveal normal flora.
  - » Clinical presentation includes a small amount of discharge and mild erythema.
- Anatomical features predisposing the prepubertal patient to vulvovaginitis include:
  - » Small labia minora tissue
  - » Lack of vulvar fat pads
  - » Lack of pubic hair
  - » Short distance between vagina and anus
  - » Small hymenal opening
- Physiologic factors predisposing the prepubertal patient to vulvovaginitis include:
  - » Thin, atrophic skin due to lack of estrogen
  - » Atrophic mucosa
  - » Neutral/alkaline pH

- Etiology of specific causes can be broken down into:
  » Infection caused by:
    › *Candida*
      · *Candida* is rare in prepubertal girls unless there is recent antibiotic use, diaper wearing, diabetes, or immunocompromise.
    › Sexually transmitted diseases
      · In sexually active adolescents, always consider sexually transmitted diseases, most commonly gonorrhea and chlamydia (see Chapter 10.9).
      · Always consider sexual abuse as potential cause (see Chapter 1.7).
    › *Trichomonas*
      · *Trichomonas* may be seen in infants (from maternal transmission) and may present in babies with thin vaginal discharge in the first few weeks or months of life.
      · In adolescents, it may present with frothy yellow discharge or nondescript symptoms.
    › Enteric bacteria (*E. coli*, *Yersinia*, *Shigella*)
    › Respiratory pathogens (Group A *Streptococcus* [GAS], *Streptococcus pneumoniae*)
    › Pinworms
      · Pinworm infection is characterized by intense vulvar and perianal pain with pruritus, usually nocturnal.
      · Ask about siblings with similar symptoms.
  » Noninfectious vulvovaginitis caused by:
    › Foreign body
    › Trauma
    › Systemic illness — Kawasaki disease, Crohn's disease
    › Vulvar skin disease — atrophic dermatitis, psoriasis, lichen sclerosus
    › Trauma — playground equipment, bikes, sexual abuse
    › Vulvar irritation — scratching, masturbation

Investigations

- If pinworms are suspected, inspection of the perianal area at night with a flashlight or the application of clear plastic tape to the perianal region first thing in the morning may be used to detect ova.
- Culture and sensitivity swabs of vaginal secretions may be used in prepubertal patients to identify streptococcal vaginitis, *Shigella*, and other pathogens, with specific swabs to exclude *Neisseria gonorrhoeae*.
- Instillation and aspiration of a small amount of saline may be helpful in collecting samples for wet mount and cultures.
- Trichomoniasis (in infants or adolescents) can be diagnosed using either immunoassay or nucleic acid amplification testing and can be collected with a cotton swab.
- In a sexually active adolescent, perform a speculum examination to collect swabs from the vagina and cervix, and assess for other lesions.

- Bacterial vaginosis typically presents with a homogeneous, white, adherent discharge. A wet preparation may be used to identify bacterial vaginosis and trichomoniasis but has limited accuracy.
  » Specific antigen detection tests are more accurate but may not be available.
- The presence of red, irritated vaginal epithelium with a thick, white, adherent discharge may indicate yeast infection.
  » Hyphae may be seen on a potassium hydroxide preparation or on Gram-stained specimens, but sensitivity is poor, so patient should be treated for a yeast infection if it is suspected based on symptoms and examination.
- If ulcerations are seen on examination, inquire about pain, recurrences, systemic symptoms, and oral ulcerations.
  » Painful ulcerations should have viral testing done for herpes and are usually sexually transmitted but can sometimes be caused by autoinoculation from other body sites.
  » Bacterial, viral, and fungal testing, as well as biopsy may be needed in unclear cases.

Management

- For nonspecific vulvovaginitis:
  » Avoid tight-fitting clothes
  » Remove swimsuit immediately after activity
  » Avoid bubble baths
  » Use milder laundry detergent
  » Wear cotton underwear
  » Use a short course of a mild topical steroid for itchiness
  » Try barrier creams such as Vaseline

Management of Specific Causes

FOREIGN BODY

- The most common foreign body is toilet paper.
- If a foreign body is visualized or suspected, gentle flushing using saline through a small feeding tube or Foley catheter may help remove it.

SEXUALLY TRANSMITTED INFECTION

- Swab and/or culture results are needed to guide treatment.
- Refer to Chapter 10.9.

SUSPECTED OR CONFIRMED GROUP A *STREPTOCOCCUS* INFECTION

- Treat with either penicillin or amoxicillin.

PINWORMS

- In children > 2 years of age use mebendazole 100 mg PO (one dose).
  » Dose can be repeated in 3 weeks.

TRICHOMONAS

- Use oral metronidazole.
  - » For patients < 45 kg, give metronidazole 15 mg/kg per day divided twice daily for 7 days (to a maximum of 1 g per day).
  - » For patients > 45 kg, give metronidazole 500 mg PO twice daily for 7 days.
- Partner treatment in sexually active adolescents enhances cure rate.

BACTERIAL VAGINOSIS.

- Use metronidazole (topical or oral) but note that recurrences are common.

REFERENCES

Government of Canada. Section 4-8: Canadian guidelines on sexually transmitted infections—management and treatment of specific syndromes—vaginal discharge. Ottawa (ON): Public Health Agency of Canada; 2013 [cited 2016 Nov 6]. Available from: http://www.phac-aspc.gc.ca/std-mts/sti-its/cgsti-ldcits/section-4-8-eng.php

Van Eyk N, Allen L, Giesbrecht E, et al. Pediatric vulvovaginal disorders: a diagnostic approach and review of the literature. *J Obstet Gynaecol Can.* 2009;31(9):850–862. https://doi.org/10.1016/S1701-2163(16)34304-3. Medline:19941710

van Schalkwyk J, Yudin MH; Infectious Disease Committee. Vulvovaginitis: screening for and management of trichomoniasis, vulvovaginal candidiasis, and bacterial vaginosis. *J Obstet Gynaecol Can.* 2015;37(3):266–274. https://doi.org/10.1016/S1701-2163(15)30316-9. Medline:26001874

Zuckerman A, Romano M. Clinical recommendation: vulvovaginitis. *J Pediatr Adolesc Gynecol.* 2016;29(6):673–679. https://doi.org/10.1016/j.jpag.2016.08.002. Medline:27969009

16.4

Abnormal Uterine Bleeding and Dysmenorrhea

Marcia Edmonds

ABNORMAL UTERINE BLEEDING

- Recent guidelines suggest that abnormal uterine bleeding (AUB) replace the previous nomenclature (i.e., dysfunctional uterine bleeding, menorrhagia, menometrorrhagia, and others).
- Descriptions are usually based on the cyclicity and quantity of menstrual flow.
  - » This may be difficult to quantify accurately (i.e., attempt to quantify volume, regularity, frequency, and duration).
- The patient's experience and the impact of the condition on the patient's function and quality of life are paramount to management in stable patients.
- 85% of cycles during the first year postmenarche are anovulatory.

Pathophysiology

- Changes in the endometrium depend on the phase of the menstrual cycle.
  - » In the **proliferative phase**, the endometrium thickens in response to estrogen.
  - » In the **secretory phase**, the endometrium develops further with progesterone.
  - » In the **menstrual phase**, a drop in progesterone and estrogen levels causes prostaglandin release and vasospasm of endometrial vasculature, resulting in sloughing of the endometrium.
- Uterine bleeding can be classified as ovulatory, nonovulatory, or other.
  - » Ovulatory uterine bleeding presents with regular intervals of menses but is characterized by heavier bleeding than normal.
    - › Bleeding may be associated with primary coagulopathies, thrombocytopenia, or anticoagulation use.
    - › Up to 40% of adolescents presenting to the emergency department (ED) with heavy menstrual bleeding may have an underlying bleeding disorder.
    - › Bleeding may be associated with endometritis (postpartum or postinstrumentation).
    - › Associated structural abnormalities include fibroids and adenomyosis.
    - › Often, no underlying cause is found.
  - » Nonovulatory uterine bleeding usually occurs with polycystic ovarian syndrome (PCOS).
    - › It may be associated with hirsutism, acne, insulin resistance, and acanthosis nigricans.
    - › Heavy menstrual bleeding is experienced by 12% to 37% of adolescents, usually secondary to an immature hypothalamic-pituitary-ovarian axis in the first year or more after menarche.

» Other bleeding may be associated with medications, including:
  › Contraceptives
  › SSRIs
  › Corticosteroids
  › Antipsychotics

History

- Determine the amount and frequency of menses.
- Assess whether the condition is likely to be ovulatory or nonovulatory.
  » Ovulatory bleeding is more likely if there are regular premenstrual symptoms and increasing time since menarche.
- Ask the patient about:
  » Symptoms suggestive of anemia
  » Sexual and reproductive history, especially the risk of pregnancy or STIs
  » History suggestive of a bleeding disorder, such as:
    › Family history
    › Onset of heavy bleeding with menarche
    › Easy bleeding or bruising (thrombocytopenia is the most common hematologic disorder causing heavy menstrual bleeding)
  » History suggestive of endocrine disease, such as thyroid dysfunction, PCOS, adrenal dysfunction, hyperprolactinemia, and hypothalamic dysfunction.
  » Other symptoms of note, such as:
    › Vaginal discharge or odor
    › Pelvic pain

Physical Exam

- Start with the ABCs of resuscitation.
  » If the patient is unstable, consider the need for volume replacement and blood product administration.
- Assess the patient's overall appearance, signs of anemia, and the possibility of an underlying systemic disorder (endocrine, coagulopathy, or other).
- Evaluate the lower genitourinary tract.
  » Perform an internal exam in sexually active patients to confirm whether bleeding is cervical or from another site.
  » Perform an external genital exam in patients who have never been sexually active to confirm that bleeding is vaginal and that no obvious structural abnormalities are present.

Investigations

- Always obtain a pregnancy test in patients of child-bearing age.
- Order bloodwork:
  » Complete blood count (CBC)
  » Coagulation studies, as indicated:
    › International normalized ratio (INR)
    › Partial thromboplastin time (PTT) in acute phase

» Coagulopathy workup
  › Consider screening for hemophilia and von Willebrand disease.
- Request imaging.
  » Ultrasound may be helpful if there are concerns of pregnancy or structural abnormality.

Management

- For acute heavy bleeding:
  » Stabilize the patient with fluids and blood product replacement as indicated
    › Consider vaginal packing if hemorrhaging is severe.
  » Rule out pregnancy and confirm the source of bleeding (uterine vs other)
    › Give IV conjugated estrogens (Premarin) 25 mg every 6 hours.
    › Give tranexamic acid 1 g IV or PO every 6 hours.
  » Obtain a gynecologic consultation
    › Surgical management has a very rare role in heavy bleeding in adolescents.
- For less severe bleeding, outpatient management may include:
  » Oral estrogens, usually in the form of a combined oral contraceptive (COC)
    › COCs (or contraceptive patch or vaginal ring) decrease bleeding up to 50% and improve dysmenorrhea.
    › Aim for high-dose estrogen pill, 35 to 50 mcg ethinyl estradiol or equivalent for the first 5 days (2 to 4 pills daily for 5 days), then once daily to finish the package.
    › Estrogens cause nausea, so the patient will likely also need treatment for nausea while on high-dose estrogen.
  » Nonsteroidal anti-inflammatory drugs (NSAIDs)
    › NSAIDs may be helpful as they are shown to decrease menstrual blood loss by 33% to 55% in ovulatory bleeding.
    › They work best if started the day prior to onset of menses and continued for 3 to 5 days.
    › They also improve dysmenorrhea.
  » Referral of select patients for a levonorgestrel-released IUD (increasing use in adolescents) or injectable progestin as an outpatient

DYSMENORRHEA

- Dysmenorrhea is defined as painful menstruation.
- Most adolescents will present with primary dysmenorrhea, where the pain cannot be attributed to a specific pelvic abnormality (rather than secondary dysmenorrhea, where a specific cause such as endometriosis or pelvic inflammatory disease is found).

GENITOURINARY EMERGENCIES

Pathophysiology

- Dysmenorrhea is related to prostaglandin synthesis in endometrial tissue.
- The prevalence of dysmenorrhea increases with age and is strongly associated with ovulatory cycles.

History

- Symptoms typically include cramping and lower abdominal pain, usually at about the time of the start of bleeding.
- There may be associated back or thigh pain, headache, nausea, vomiting, and diarrhea.
- Symptoms usually resolve within 48 hours.
- Dysmenorrhea that starts with the patient's first cycles is more likely to be associated with structural abnormalities.
  » Also consider complete obstruction of the genital tract in patients complaining of cyclical dysmenorrhea symptoms in the absence of bleeding.

Physical Exam

- Physical exam is usually normal.
  » Look for signs of:
    › Pelvic inflammatory disease
    › Partial outflow obstruction

Investigations

- Rule out pregnancy.
- Consider a CBC and sexually transmitted infection (STI) testing.
- Obtain a pelvic ultrasound as needed.

Management

- First-line treatment of dysmenorrhea is NSAIDs, which provide reasonable to excellent pain relief in approximately half of patients.
- COCs are usually quite effective; low-dose pills are recommended.
- For patients with severe, recurrent symptoms despite above treatments, refer to gynecology for consideration for further investigations.
  » Patients may need laparoscopy or other treatments, including levonorgestrel-releasing IUD or depot medroxyprogesterone acetate.

_____

REFERENCES

American College of Obstetricians and Gynecologists. ACOG Committee Opinion No. 392, December 2007. Intrauterine devices and adolescents. *Obstet Gynecol.* 2007;110:1493–1495. https://doi.org/10.1097/01.AOG.0000291575.93944.1a. Medline:18055754

Lefebvre G, Pinsonneault O, Antao V, et al; SOGC. Primary dysmenorrhea consensus guideline. *J Obstet Gynaecol Can.* 2005;27(12):1117–1130. https://doi.org/10.1016/S1701-2163(16)30395-4. Medline:16524531

Leminen H, Hurskainen R. Tranexamic acid for the treatment of heavy menstrual bleeding: efficacy and safety. *Int J Womens Health.* 2012;4:413–421. Medline:22956886

Lethaby A, Duckitt K, Farquhar C. Non-steroidal anti-inflammatory drugs for heavy menstrual bleeding. *Cochrane Database Syst Rev.* 2013;(1):CD000400. Medline:23440779

Marjoribanks J, Ayeleke RO, Farquhar C, Proctor M. Nonsteroidal anti-inflammatory drugs for dysmenorrhoea. *Cochrane Database Syst Rev.* 2015;(7):CD001751. Medline:26224322

Singh S, Best C, Dunn S, et al; Clinical Practice – Gynaecology Committee. Abnormal uterine bleeding in pre-menopausal women. *J Obstet Gynaecol Can.* 2013;35(5):473–475. https://doi.org/10.1016/S1701-2163(15)30939-7. Medline:23756279

Wong CL, Farquhar C, Roberts H, Proctor M. Oral contraceptive pill for primary dysmenorrhoea. *Cochrane Database Syst Rev.* 2009;(4):CD002120. Medline:19821293

16.5

Amenorrhea

Marcia Edmonds

- Amenorrhea is either primary or secondary.
  » Primary amenorrhea is defined as the failure to start menstruation by the age of 16, in the presence of normal growth and secondary sexual characteristics.
    › The most common cause is gonadal dysgenesis, which is due to the absence or depletion of ovarian follicles within the first few years of life.
  » Secondary amenorrhea is the absence of menstruation for 3 to 6 months after the establishment of regular cycles, in the absence of pregnancy.
    › It is most commonly due to chronic hyperandrogenic anovulation (polycystic ovary syndrome [PCOS]).
- Normal menstrual cycles require normal functioning of the hypothalamus, pituitary gland, and ovaries, as well as a uterus and patent outflow tract.

Etiology

- The etiology of amenorrhea can be categorized as:
  - » Anatomic — either congenital or acquired
  - » Endocrine

Anatomic Causes of Amenorrhea

- About 20% of cases of primary amenorrhea are due to reproductive tract abnormalities. These patients have normal secondary sexual characteristics but fail to start menstruation.
- Congenital anatomical causes of amenorrhea include:
  - » Agenesis of the uterus or vagina
  - » Absence of Müllerian duct system
  - » Obstruction of the menstrual outflow tract at the level of the cervix, vagina, or hymen
    - › Patients may present with cyclical pain and/or a mass due to collection of menstrual blood above the obstruction.
  - » Androgen insensitivity syndrome
- Acquired anatomical causes of amenorrhea include:
  - » Cervical stenosis or obstruction
  - » Asherman syndrome — intrauterine adhesions, usually from retained products of conception, endometritis, or prior curettage

Endocrine Causes of Amenorrhea

- Hypothalamic causes of amenorrhea include:
  - » Gonadotropin-releasing hormone (GnRH) deficiency
    - › This may be associated with anosmia with or without midline facial defects (e.g., cleft palate), skeletal abnormalities, and renal agenesis (Kallmann syndrome).
  - » Hypothalamic amenorrhea related to stress, low weight, anorexia, or excessive exercise
- Pituitary causes include:
  - » Empty sella syndrome
  - » Tumors, including prolactinomas
  - » Deficiency in GnRH receptors
  - » Follicle-stimulating hormone (FSH) gene mutations
- Ovarian causes include:
  - » Gonadal dysgenesis — the depletion of follicles prior to puberty
    - › This is most commonly due to Turner syndrome (45,XO karyotype)
  - » Primary ovarian failure — may be due to:
    - › Autoimmune ovarian failure
    - › Chemotherapy
    - › Radiation therapy
- Other causes include:
  - » Hypothyroidism
  - » PCOS

History

- The history will provide clues as to the etiology of the amenorrhea. Collect information about:
  - » Age of thelarche, menarche, and adrenarche
  - » Sexual activity
  - » Chronic illnesses
  - » Prior therapy (e.g., chemotherapy)
  - » Head trauma
  - » Weight changes
  - » Headaches or visual changes
  - » Hirsutism or virilization symptoms
  - » Medications, including contraceptive use

Investigations

- In many cases, the cause may be apparent on history and physical exam.
- Always rule out pregnancy in any female of child-bearing age.
- Most cases of primary and secondary amenorrhea can be investigated and managed by primary care or outpatient referral to a specialist.
- For patients presenting with secondary amenorrhea due to extreme low body weight:
  - » Determine the cause of weight loss (e.g., eating disorder, extreme exercising, severe stress, or chronic medical condition)
  - » Ensure clinical stability
    - › Patient may need to be admitted
  - » Check electrolytes
- In select situations, it may be appropriate to initiate imaging of the brain and/or lower genital tract in cases of primary amenorrhea.
- Consider thyroid-stimulating hormone (TSH), FSH, luteinizing hormone (LH) and/or prolactin levels.

Management

- Management is largely dependent on the underlying cause of the amenorrhea.
- In the emergency department (ED), the most important causes to rule out are:
  - » Pregnancy and its complications
  - » Anorexia nervosa with severe electrolyte abnormalities
  - » Lower genital tract obstruction (if patient presents with severe pain)
- Other causes can usually be managed on an outpatient basis.
- Obtain a primary care or specialist referral as indicated.

REFERENCES

Deligeoroglou E, Athanasopoulos N, Tsimaris P, Dimopoulos KD, Vrachnis N, Creatsas G. Evaluation and management of adolescent amenorrhea. *Ann N Y Acad Sci.* 2010;1205(1):23–32. https://doi.org/10.1111/j.1749-6632.2010.05669.x. Medline:20840249

Goodman NF, Cobin RH, Futterweit W, Glueck JS, Legro RS, Carmina E; American Association of Clinical Endocrinologists (AACE); American College of Endocrinology (ACE); Androgen Excess and PCOS Society (AES). American Association of Clinical Endocrinologists, American College of Endocrinology, and Androgen Excess and PCOS Society disease state clinical review: guide to the best practices in the evaluation and treatment of polycystic ovarian syndrome – part 1. *Endocr Pract.* 2015;21(11):1291–1300. https://doi.org/10.4158/EP15748.DSC. Medline:26509855

Gordon CM, Kanaoka T, Nelson LM. Update on primary ovarian insufficiency in adolescents. *Curr Opin Pediatr.* 2015;27(4):511–519. https://doi.org/10.1097/MOP.0000000000000236. Medline:26087426

Klein DA, Poth MA. Amenorrhea: an approach to diagnosis and management. *Am Fam Physician.* 2013;87(11):781–788. Medline:23939500

Misra M. Neuroendocrine mechanisms in athletes. *Handb Clin Neurol.* 2014;124:373–386. https://doi.org/10.1016/B978-0-444-59602-4.00025-3. Medline:25248600

Practice Committee of American Society for Reproductive Medicine. Current evaluation of amenorrhea. *Fertil Steril.* 2008;90(5 Suppl):S219–S225. https://doi.org/10.1016/j.fertnstert.2008.08.038. Medline:19007635

16.6

Penile Emergencies

Rahim Valani

- The most common cause of penile injuries in infants is secondary to circumcision.
- Assess patients for:
  » Inability to void
  » Presence of fever
  » Prior penile injuries or infection
  » History of trauma
- Penile injuries can be embarrassing, especially for adolescents.
- Inform parents and the patient about the need to examine the genitalia.

PHIMOSIS

- Normal physiologic phimosis exists at birth.
  » By 3 years of age, 90% of foreskins can be retracted.
- Persistent phimosis is due to a stenosed prepuce.
- Phimosis arises from forcefully retracting the prepuce over the glans.
- It can also be the result of recurrent balanitis, balanoposthitis, and urinary tract infections.
- Patients present with pain and the inability to void.

Management

- Medical management involves:
  » Use of topical steroid cream
  » Use of sedation and placement of a Foley catheter to prevent urinary retention when foreskin is sealed off

- Surgical management involves:
  » Creation of a dorsal or ventral slit to preserve the prepuce
  » Circumcision

PARAPHIMOSIS

- Paraphimosis is caused by the retraction of the prepuce proximal to the glans for a prolonged period.
- Edema of the glans is due to the constricting effect of the retracted tissue and can ultimately result in glans necrosis due to arterial insufficiency.
- The patient presents with pain and swelling of the penile shaft and glans distal to the constriction.

Management

- The goal is to return the foreskin to its normal position and allow the edema to recede.
- Ensure the patient is comfortable and cooperative.
  » Topical or parenteral analgesia may be required.
- Apply manual compression of the glans while reducing the edematous skin.
- Placing ice packs or a compression bandage on the glans prior to reduction may help.
- Surgical management involves:
  » Consideration of a surgical consultation if there is concern for significant ischemia to the glans or after failed attempts
  » Multiple punctures to the foreskin — may be required to drain the edema
  » Creation of a dorsal slit to relieve pressure

BALANOPOSTHITIS

- Balanitis is cellulitis that is confined only to the glans.
- Balanoposthitis is when both the glans and foreskin are involved.
- The patient presents with swollen and erythematous glans.
- The patient may also complain of dysuria.

Management

- Management involves:
  » Oral antibiotics — amoxicillin at 50 mg/kg divided and given 3 times per day
  » Steroid cream — 0.5% hydrocortisone cream
    › Steroid cream is to be avoided if there is suspicion of fungal infection.
  » Warm soaks two or three times daily
- Prescribe an antifungal cream if satellite lesions are present that suggest a fungal cause.

CIRCUMCISION INJURIES

- The complication rate for circumcisions varies from 0.2% to 3%.
- The most common complications are:
  » Bleeding
    › Bleeding can usually be controlled with direct pressure to the area.
    › Cauterize the area with silver nitrate sticks; avoid dabbing directly on the urethra.
    › Placement of a suture may be necessary if bleeding is ongoing.
      · Consider consultation with urology.
  » Infection
    › Use topical or oral antibiotics.
  » Partial amputation
    › This usually occurs from incorporation of the frenulum into a Mogen clamp.
      › Consult urology; if the preserved glans is brought in, it may be possible to reattach it.
  » Necrosis
    › Necrosis is caused by overuse of cautery during the circumcision.
    › Consult urology.

ZIPPER INJURIES

- This type of injury is caused by penile entrapment in a zipper.
- Any part of the penis can be entrapped — foreskin, glans, or shaft.

Management

- Consider analgesia as needed.
- The simplest way to free the penis is to cut the median bar of the zipper and release the teeth.
- Apply mineral oil to allow the penile tissue to slide through the teeth.

REFERENCES

Clifford ID, Craig SS, Nataraja RM, Panabokke G. Paediatric paraphimosis. *Emerg Med Australas.* 2016;28(1):96–99. https://doi.org/10.1111/1742-6723.12532. Medline:26781045

Gearhart JP. *Pediatric urology.* Totowa, NJ: Humana Press; 2002.

Ludvigson AE, Beaule LT. Urologic emergencies. *Surg Clin North Am.* 2016;96(3):407–424. https://doi.org/10.1016/j.suc.2016.02.001. Medline:27261785

Lukacs S, Tschobotko B, Mazaris E. A new nonsurgical technique for managing zipper injuries. *Eur J Emerg Med.* 2014;21(4):308–309. https://doi.org/10.1097/MEJ.0000000000000073. Medline:23995667

Moreno G, Corbalán J, Peñaloza B, Pantoja T. Topical corticosteroids for treating phimosis in boys. *Cochrane Database Syst Rev.* 2014;Sep 2(9). https://doi.org/10.1002/14651858.CD008973.pub2.

Tintinalli JE. *Tintinalli's emergency medicine: a comprehensive study guide.* 7th ed. New York: McGraw Hill; 2011.

Wein AJ. *Campbell-Walsh urology.* 9th ed. Philadelphia: Saunders Elsevier; 2007.

17.1

Hemolytic Uremic Syndrome

Archna Shah, Andrew Dixon

- Hemolytic uremic syndrome (HUS) is one of the most common causes of acquired acute renal failure in young children.
  - » Incidence of typical HUS is estimated at 2 to 6 per 100 000 children.
  - » HUS accounts for 25% of all acute renal injury in children.
- HUS is characterized by a triad of:
  - » Microangiopathic hemolytic anemia
  - » Thrombocytopenia
  - » Acute renal failure

Pathophysiology

- Capillary and endothelial damage leads to localized thrombosis and damage to vessels.
- Thrombocytopenia results from platelet aggregation at the damaged endothelium.
- Microangiopathic hemolytic anemia results from mechanical damage as red blood cells (RBCs) pass through damaged and thrombotic microvasculature.
- Kidney damage results from decreased perfusion from thrombosis formation.
- Thrombotic thrombocytopenia purpura (TTP) is similar to HUS but includes central nervous system (CNS) involvement and fever with more gradual onset (more common in adults).

Etiology

- HUS is traditionally classified into diarrhea positive (D+ HUS) or diarrhea negative (D- HUS).
  - » Unreliable reporting of diarrheal prodrome has led to new recommendations to classify HUS as typical (tHUS) and atypical (aHUS).

TYPICAL HUS

- Typical HUS (or D+ HUS) is more common (90% of cases) and usually has an infectious cause:
  - » Shiga toxin–producing bacteria
    - › Most commonly, these are enterohemorrhagic *E. coli* O157:H7 and *Shigella dysenteriae* type 1.
    - › Bacteria are found in undercooked meat, unpasteurized milk, cheese, lettuce, spinach, swimming pools, lakes, petting zoos, and contaminated water supply.
    - › Bacteria can be spread by person-to-person contact.
  - » *Streptococcus pneumoniae*
  - » Influenza A
  - » HIV

ATYPICAL HUS

- Atypical HUS (or D- HUS) encompasses HUS caused by various other triggers and is less common (10% of cases).
- The cause of atypical HUS may be:
  - » Genetic
    - › The most common genetic cause is a defect in one of the factors that are supposed to stop complement activation at the C3-level in the alternate pathway, preventing uncontrolled activation of terminal complement components C5 to C9 (membrane attack complex).
    - › Other genetic causes include:
      - · Complement factor H deficiency (the most common mutation involved with atypical HUS)
      - · Membrane cofactor protein mutation
      - · Complement factor I mutation
      - · Familial autosomal recessive or autosomal dominant
    - › Most genetic forms do not have diarrhea as a symptom.
    - › Complement will be low.
    - › Treat atypical HUS with genetic etiology with fresh frozen plasma (FFP) and sometimes plasma exchange.

- Medication related:
  - Calcineurin inhibitor (cyclosporine, tacrolimus)
  - Cytotoxic, chemotherapy (cisplatin, VEGF inhibitors, tyrosine kinase inhibitors)
  - Antibacterial agents (quinine)
  - Antiviral medications (valacyclovir)
  - Antiplatelet agents (clopidogrel, ticlopidine)
  - Oral contraceptives
- Associated with systemic disease with microvascular injury:
  - Systemic lupus erythematosus (SLE)
  - Antiphospholipid-antibody syndrome
  - Complication of bone marrow transplant
  - Malignant hypertension
  - Primary glomerulopathy
  - HELLP syndrome

Physical Exam

- HUS occurs most commonly in preschool- and school-aged children.
- Diarrhea is present in most cases.
  - Most patients (two-thirds of cases) have bloody diarrhea.
  - The other symptoms of HUS usually start on day 5 to 8 of illness, when diarrhea is starting to resolve.
- The other symptoms of HUS are:
  - Microangiopathic hemolytic anemia:
    - Pallor
    - Weakness
    - Lethargy from anemia
    - Jaundice from hemolysis
  - Thrombocytopenia:
    - Petechiae and bleeding from thrombocytopenia
  - Renal involvement:
    - Hematuria
    - Proteinuria
    - Oliguria
    - Anuria from renal insufficiency
  - Dehydration or fluid overload depending on stage of presentation
    - Dehydration is an early presentation from gastroenteritis.
    - Fluid overload presents because of renal insufficiency.
  - Pneumonia (if etiology is *Streptococcus pneumoniae*)
  - Cardiac involvement:
    - Cardiomyopathy
    - Myocarditis
    - High-output cardiac failure
  - Central nervous system (CNS) involvement
    - There is severe CNS involvement in < 20% of cases with seizures and encephalopathy.
    - CNS involvement is caused by focal ischemia secondary to microvascular thrombosis.
    - Patients may be irritable and/or lethargic.
  - Gastrointestinal (GI) involvement:
    - Inflammatory colitis
    - Ischemic enteritis
    - Bowel perforation
    - Intussusception
    - Liver injury (hepatosplenomegaly or elevated transaminases)
    - Pancreatitis

Investigations

- Microangiopathic anemia is characterized by:
  - Low hemoglobin (50–90 g/L)
  - Smear showing schistocytes, burr cells, helmet cells
  - Negative Coombs test **except** with pneumococcus-induced HUS
- Thrombocytopenia is characterized by:
  - Low platelet count (< 150×10^9/L)
  - Bone marrow showing normal number of megakaryocytes
    - This indicates that thrombocytopenia is from excessive platelet destruction.
- Initiate laboratory studies:
  - Coagulation studies
    - Prothrombin time (PT) / partial thromboplastin time (PTT) are usually normal.
    - Patients may have elevated D-dimer levels.
    - Normal coagulation distinguishes HUS from sepsis and DIC.
  - Electrolytes
    - Hyperkalemia results from rapid cell break down.
  - Renal function
    - Increased blood urea nitrogen (BUN) and creatinine are present.
  - Liver function
    - Studies show elevated lactate dehydrogenase, bilirubin, and transaminases.
  - Urinalysis
    - Studies show hematuria, proteinuria, and cast cells.
  - Stool cultures
    - Cultures are often negative in typical (D+) HUS.
    - Newer methods of isolating Shiga-like toxin using enzyme-linked immunosorbent assay (ELISA) or polymerase chain reaction (PCR) are more successful.
  - Genetic evaluation
    - Initiate if there is no history of diarrhea prodrome.
    - Complement is often low.
    - Patients are at risk of recurrence and severe prognosis.

Management

- Supportive care is the mainstay of treatment in the emergency department (ED). Patients will usually need to be admitted and require a nephrology consultation.
  - » Supportive care is the same for all HUS patients regardless of etiology.
- If family members also have diarrhea, order CBC, BUN, and creatinine, and follow the patient clinically.

Supportive Care

FLUID AND ELECTROLYTE MANAGEMENT

- There is a delicate balance between correcting dehydration and potential for fluid overload.
- Reassess fluid balance, weight, vital signs, and laboratory workups frequently.
- Fluid management is guided by renal function (creatinine/BUN) and urine output.

RENAL REPLACEMENT THERAPY AND URINE OUTPUT

- If oliguria is present, consider furosemide 0.5 to 1 mg/kg to maintain urine output.
- If oliguria/anuria persists, manage fluids carefully to avoid fluid overload.
- Patients will urgently need peritoneal dialysis.
- General indications for acute renal replacement therapy (RRT) in acute renal injury include:
  - » Oligoanuria
  - » Fluid overload
  - » Severe azotemia
  - » Electrolyte abnormalities
  - » Acidosis
  - » Nutritional support
- Plasmapheresis has not been shown to be of benefit in pediatric patients with typical HUS.

CORRECTION OF ELECTROLYTE ABNORMALITIES AND ACIDOSIS

- Watch for hyperkalemia.

HYPERTENSION CONTROL

- Administer calcium channel blockers:
  - » Nifedipine 0.25 mg/kg (not to exceed 3 mg/kg per day; maximum 120 mg/day)
  - » Amlodipine 0.1 mg/kg (or 2.5 to 5 mg once daily; maximum 10 mg)
- If the patient has severe hypertension, then consider IV options with:
  - » Esmolol 100 to 500 mcg/kg per min
  - » Sodium nitroprusside 0.5 to 4 mcg/kg per minute (maximum infusion rate 10 mcg/kg per minute)

BLOOD TRANSFUSION

- Consider blood transfusion if:
  - » Hemoglobin <60 g/L
  - » Hematocrit < 18%

ANTIBIOTICS

- Antibiotics are not routinely recommended (see "Contraindicated Therapies in HUS," below).
- Treatment of pneumococcal disease **is** recommended.

Contraindicated Therapies in HUS

- **Do not** use platelets because they are immediately consumed and can potentially worsen the disease.
  - » Platelets are only indicated with active bleeding or during an invasive procedure.
- Antibiotic therapy directed against the infectious agent in associated diarrhea does **not** change the course of the disease and can make the disease worse by causing bacterial lysis and increasing toxin release.

Prognosis

- For typical (D+) HUS, expect:
  - » < 5% mortality
  - » 50% of patients to need dialysis
  - » Most patients to recover renal function completely
  - » 5% of patients to remain dependent on dialysis
  - » 20% to 30% of patients to have chronic renal insufficiency
- For atypical (D-) HUS, expect:
  - » A more severe prognosis
  - » Pneumococcal-related mortality of 20%
  - » Familial forms to be progressive or to relapse with poor prognosis
- Follow-up is required if a patient with typical HUS has hypertension, any level of renal insufficiency, or residual urinary abnormality persisting a year after an episode of typical HUS.

REFERENCES

Alberta Health. Alberta public health notifiable disease management guidelines: hemolytic uremic syndrome [Internet]. Edmonton (AB): Government of Alberta; 2015. Available from: https://open.alberta.ca/dataset/aa5a3267-41c0-41c1-8a68-bb27838cc8ae/resource/4ffbd9de-b780-42ce-acd7-fd9ccb825488/download/Guidelines-Haemolytic-Uremic-Syndrome-2015.pdf

American Academy of Pediatrics. *Escherichia coli* diarrhea. In: Pinchering LK, editor. *Red book: 2012 report of the Committee on Infectious Disease.* 29th ed. Elk Grove Village, IL: American Academy of Pediatrics; 2012: p. 324–328.

Ariceta G, Besbas N, Johnson S, et al; European Paediatric Study Group for HUS. Guideline for the investigation and initial of 9-negative hemolytic uremic syndrome. *Pediatr Nephrol.* 2009;24(4):687–696. https://doi.org/10.1007/s00467-008-0964-1. Medline:18800230

Berger E, Langlois V. Nephrology. In: Dipchand A, Friedman J, editors. *The HSC handbook of pediatrics.* 11th ed. Toronto: Elsevier Saunders; 2009. p. 603–36.

Burns RA, Kaplan RL. Renal and electrolyte emergencies. In: Shaw KN, Bachur RG, editors. *Fleisher & Ludwig's textbook of pediatric emergency medicine.* 7th ed. Philadelphia, PA: Wolters Kluwer Health; 2015.

Dhull RS, Baracco R, Jain A, Mattoo TK. Pharmacologic treatment of pediatric hypertension. *Curr Hypertens Rep.* 2016;18(4):32. https://doi.org/10.1007/s11906-016-0639-4. Medline:27048353

Grisaru S. Management of hemolytic-uremic syndrome in children. *Int J Nephrol Renovasc Dis.* 2014;7:231–239. https://doi.org/10.2147/IJNRD.S41837. Medline:24966691

Grisaru S, Midgley JP, Hamiwka LA, Wade AW, Samuel SM. Diarrhea-associated hemolytic uremic syndrome in southern Alberta: a long-term single-centre experience. *Paediatr Child Health.* 2011;16(6):337–340. Medline:22654544

Karpman D, Loos S, Tati R, Arvidsson I. Haemolytic uraemic syndrome. *J Intern Med.* 2017;281(2):123–148. Medline:27723152

Lalani A, Valani R. Hematologic emergencies: hemolytic uremic syndrome. In: Lalani A, Schneeweiss S, editors. *The Hospital for Sick Children handbook of pediatric emergency medicine.* Mississauga, ON: Jones and Bartlett; 2008.

Proulx F, Sockett P. Prospective surveillance of Canadian children with the haemolytic uraemic syndrome. *Pediatr Nephrol.* 2005;20(6):786–790. https://doi.org/10.1007/s00467-005-1843-7. Medline:15834619

Salvadori M, Bertoni E. Update on hemolytic uremic syndrome: diagnostic and therapeutic recommendations. *World J Nephrol.* 2013;2(3):56–76. https://doi.org/10.5527/wjn.v2.i3.56. Medline:24255888

Scheiring J, Rosales A, Zimmerhackl LB. Clinical practice. Today's understanding of the haemolytic uraemic syndrome. *Eur J Pediatr.* 2010;169(1):7–13. https://doi.org/10.1007/s00431-009-1039-4. Medline:19707787

Van Why SK, Anver ED. Hemoyltic-uremic syndrome. In: Kliegman RM, Stanton BF, Schor NF, St. Geme III JW, Behrman RE, editors. *Nelson textbook of pediatrics.* 19th ed. Philadelphia, PA: Elsevier Saunders; 2011. p. 1791–1793.

17.2

Nephrotic Syndrome

Archna Shah, Andrew Dixon

Epidemiology

- Nephrotic syndrome is mainly a pediatric disorder with an estimated incidence of 2 to 7 per 100 000 children per year.
- It is more common in male children, with a 2:1 ratio of males to females.
- The condition is characterized by proteinuria, hypoalbuminemia, and edema.
  » Proteinuria is characterized by urine protein > 40 mg/m² per hour or a ratio > 2 of spot protein (mg) to creatinine (mg).
  » Hypoalbuminemia is the state of having serum albumin < 30 g/L.
  » Edema, usually periorbital, is present.
- 90% of patients have primary (idiopathic) nephrotic syndrome, which includes:
  » Minimal change nephrotic syndrome
    › Minimal change nephrotic syndrome represents approximately 85% of patients.
    › It is the most common form of the disease in children aged 18 months to 6 years.
    › More than 90% of cases respond to steroids.
  » Focal segmental glomerulosclerosis (FSGS)
    › FSGS represents approximately 10% of patients.
    › It is more common in older children.
    › 20% of cases respond to steroids.
    › Patients can have relapses following infection and reactions to bee stings, insect bites, and poison ivy.
  » Mesangial proliferation

- 10% of cases are secondary to systemic or glomerular diseases, such as:
  » Systemic lupus erythematosus (SLE)
  » Henoch-Schönlein purpura
  » Diabetes
  » Infections — HIV, hepatitis B, malaria, toxoplasmosis, syphilis
  » Malignancy — leukemia, lymphoma
  » Drugs — nonsteroidal anti-inflammatory drugs (NSAIDs), gold, penicillamine, lithium, interferon, pamidronate, heroin
  » Immune/allergic conditions — food allergens, bee stings
- Congenital nephrotic syndrome is diagnosed in the first 3 months of life.
  » It usually has a genetic cause.
  » It can be related to congenital infections.
  » It can also be associated with syndromes (e.g., Pierson syndrome, Galloway-Mowat syndrome).

Pathophysiology

- Increased permeability of the glomerular capillary wall leads to proteinuria and hypoalbuminemia.
- Nephrotic syndrome consists of:
  » Heavy proteinuria
  » Hypoalbuminemia — primarily from the loss of albumin in the urine
  » Edema — decreased plasma oncotic pressure from the loss of serum albumin, causing water to extravasate into the interstitial space

RENAL EMERGENCIES

» Hyperlipidemia — hypoalbuminemia stimulates generalized synthesis of liver proteins resulting in high concentrations of cholesterol, triglycerides, and lipoproteins

History

- General symptoms are:
  » Failure to thrive
  » Anorexia
  » Fatigue
  » Nausea
  » Abdominal discomfort
  » Diarrhea
- Other symptoms include:
  » Edema, which may be:
    › Periorbital (often the initial finding, mistaken as allergic reaction)
    › Facial
    › Pedal
    › Ascites
    › Scrotal or labial
  » Respiratory distress
    › Respiratory distress is the result of pleural effusion or pulmonary edema.
  » Hypertension
    › The cause of edema is decreased intravascular volume, leading to renal hypoperfusion and stimulation of the renin-angiotensin-aldosterone (RAA) system.
    › Aldosterone increases reabsorption of sodium, particularly at the level of the distal segments of the nephron, which can lead to hypertension.
  » Microscopic hematuria
    › Microscopic hematuria occurs in 20% to 30% of patients.

Physical Exam

- Look for signs of intravascular volume depletion:
  » Tachycardia
  » Peripheral vasoconstriction
  » Oliguria
- Determine respiratory status.
  » Dyspnea or tachypnea is characteristic only if there is a pleural effusion and pulmonary edema.
- Measure blood pressure.
  » Blood pressure can be elevated due to:
    › Hypoperfusion of renal system (thus stimulating the RAA system)
    › Renal vein thrombosis
  » Blood pressure can be low due to intravascular volume depletion.
- Check recent fluid balance:
  » Diuretic use

» Urine output
» GI losses
- Initiate an abdominal exam.
  » Look for signs of ascites.
  » Abdominal pain or guarding may indicate spontaneous bacterial peritonitis.

Investigations

- The diagnostic criteria of nephrotic syndrome are:
  » Hypoalbuminemia: serum albumin < 30 g/L
  » Proteinuria: urine protein > 40 mg/m^2 per hour
- Initiate a urine dipstick test.
  » The urine dipstick test mainly detects albumin among the various proteins in urine.
  » It is sensitive to albumin concentrations as low as 15 mg/dL.
  » False negative can be seen with:
    › Dilute urine (specific gravity < 1.005)
    › Acidic urine (pH < 4.5)
    › Proteins other than albumin
  » False positive may occur with:
    › Highly concentrated urine (specific gravity > 1.015)
    › pH > 7.0
    › Gross hematuria
    › Contamination with an antiseptic agent
  » If urine specific gravity < 1.010 and urine dipstick shows trace for proteins, the sample is positive for proteins.
  » If urine specific gravity > 1.015 and urine dipstick shows 1+ for proteins, the sample is positive for proteins.
- Initiate urinalysis:
  » Protein (mg) : creatinine (mg) ratio
    › On a random urine sample, this should be < 20 mg/mmol.
    › Spot urine protein:creatinine ratio is abnormal if it is > 0.5 in children < 2 years of age or > 0.2 in children > 2 years of age.
      · A ratio of > 1 is suspicious for nephrotic range proteinuria.
      · A ratio > 2 is suggestive of nephrotic range proteinuria.
  » Protein level on a 24-hour urine collection
    › Discard the first morning void, then collect for 24 hours, including first morning void of the next day.
      · Levels are normal at 0 to 4 mg/m^2 per hour.
      · Proteinuria levels are 4 to 40 mg/m^2 per hour.
      · Nephrotic levels are > 40 mg/m^2 per hour.
  » Assessments for the presence of other abnormalities
    › Hematuria (microscopic in 20% of patients)
    › Glucosuria

- Investigate renal function:
  » Electrolytes
    › Serum sodium is decreased due to:
      · Hyperlipidemia
      · Retention of water caused by hypovolemia and increased secretion of antidiuretic hormone
    › Total calcium value may be low because of hypo-albuminemia; ionized calcium concentration is normal.
  » Creatinine
    › Creatinine is usually normal but may be raised if intravascular volume is depleted.
  » Urea
    › Urea may be elevated depending on the degree of renal impairment.
- Cholesterol and triglycerides are elevated.
- Complement levels are usually normal.
  » Abnormal complement levels are helpful in determining secondary causes.
    › SLE is characterized by low C_3 and C_4.
    › Postinfectious glomerular nephritis is characterized by low C_3 and normal C_4.

Management

- Involve the nephrology team to determine appropriate therapy and follow-up.
- Restrict fluid to insensible loss (400 mL/m^2) plus ongoing losses.
- Restrict sodium intake.
- Optimize dietary protein.
- Measure weight daily.

Prednisone

- Prednisone can be initiated without diagnostic renal biopsy because most patients respond.
- Dose at 60 mg/m^2 per day (2 mg/kg per day) for 4 to 6 weeks.
  » The maximum daily dose is 80 mg as a single dose or divided into 2 to 3 doses.
  » Anticipate a response in 7 to 10 days; 80% to 90% respond within 4 weeks.
  » Dose for 4 weeks, then taper and discontinue over 1 to 2 months.
- Remission is defined as 3 consecutive days with no protein or only trace protein on urinalysis.
- If the patient is steroid resistant (defined as proteinuria that continues after 8 weeks), then refer them for biopsy

Albumin and Diuretics

- Indications for albumin infusion are:
  » Symptomatic hypovolemia
  » Peritonitis
  » Severe edema or respiratory distress from pleural effusions
- Aggressive diuresis can lead to intravascular depletion and thrombotic events — use with caution.
- IV 25% albumin (0.5–1 g/kg per dose every 6 to 12 hours, infused over 2 to 4 hours) followed by Lasix (1 to 2 mg/kg) is often necessary when fluid restriction and diuretics do not work.
  » The effect is temporary because the rise in albumin will lead to increased urine excretion.
  » Patient must be monitored for side effects:
    › Intravascular overload
    › Hypertension
    › Pulmonary edema

Biopsy

- Biopsy is **not** required for the diagnosis of most cases.
- Biopsy **is** required if the clinical features listed below are present:
  » Persistent proteinuria after 8 weeks of steroids
  » < 1 year of age or > 8 years of age
  » Low complement
  » Presence of features not typical for nephrotic syndrome such as hematuria, hypertension, or renal insufficiency

Note: If the above features are present, the diagnosis of minimal change nephrotic syndrome is unlikely.

Relapse Management

- In the case of relapse, repeat steroids at a dose of 60 mg/m^2 per day (2 mg/kg per day to 80 mg daily maximum) in single morning doses until remission (i.e., no protein in urine for 3 consecutive days), then change to alternating days (dose as above) and taper.
- Consider other treatments and consult nephrology if:
  » There is no response to initial course of steroids
  » There is no response to prednisone during relapse
  » Patient experiences frequent relapses
  » Significant side effects develop from steroids, such as growth failure
- Patients who relapse frequently and those who are steroid resistant may benefit from an alkylating agent such as cyclophosphamide (2 mg/kg per day), generally given for 8 to 12 weeks.
  » Consult nephrology for further management.
- Other relapse management options include:
  » Cyclosporin
  » Tacrolimus
  » Mycophenolate

Complications

THROMBOEMBOLIC COMPLICATIONS

- Thromboembolic complications occur in 2% to 5% of cases and include:
  - » Deep vein thrombosis, pulmonary embolus, renal vein thrombosis, sagittal sinus thrombosis
  - » Increased prothrombotic factors (fibrinogen, thrombocytosis, hemoconcentration, relative immobilization) and decreased fibrinolytic factors (antithrombin III, protein S, and protein C lost in the urine)
- Prophylactic anticoagulation is **not** recommended unless a thrombotic event has occurred.
- Avoid diuretic and indwelling catheters to reduce thromboembolic risk.
- Use caution with femoral venous access because of thromboembolic risk.

INFECTIONS

- Infections occur from encapsulated organisms, and complications include:
  - » Urine loss of immunoglobulins and factor B (which contributes to opsonization of bacteria), decrease in IgG synthesis, and impaired T cell function
  - » Spontaneous bacterial peritonitis (rate 2% to 6%)
    - › *Streptococcus pneumoniae* is the most common cause.
    - › *E. coli* accounts for 25% to 50% of cases and presents with fever, abdominal distension, abdominal pain, and diarrhea or ileus.
  - » Sepsis, pneumonia, cellulitis, meningitis, and urinary tract infection (UTI)
- Vaccination has reduced infections from *S. pneumoniae* substantially and increased the relative frequency of gram-negative organisms.
- Avoid live vaccines while patient is on steroids (immunosuppressive therapy).

OTHER COMPLICATIONS

- Other possible complications include:
  - » Acute renal failure from hypovolemia
    - › This is reversed when the intravascular volume is expanded by albumin infusion and diuresis is induced by furosemide.
  - » Respiratory distress caused by pleural effusion or pulmonary edema

Prognosis

- 30% to 40% of patients relapse, but this rate decreases as the child gets older.
- Those who respond quickly to steroids and have no relapse in the first 6 months are less likely to relapse.
- Patients are unlikely to develop chronic kidney disease if they are steroid responsive.
- If a patient is steroid resistant (most likely focal segmental glomerulosclerosis, or FSGS), they will likely develop progressive renal failure leading to dialysis or transplant.
- Recurrent nephrotic syndrome develops in 30% to 50% of transplanted FSGS.

REFERENCES

Andolino TP, Reid-Adam J. Nephrotic syndrome. *Pediatr Rev.* 2015;36(3):117–125, quiz 126, 129. https://doi.org/10.1542/pir.36-3-117. Medline:25733763

Berger E, Langlois V. Nephrology. In: Dipchand A, Friedman J, editors. *The HSC handbook of pediatrics.* 11th ed. Toronto: Elsevier Saunders; 2009. p. 603–36.

Burns RA, Kaplan RL. Renal and electrolyte emergencies. In: Shaw KN, Bachur RG, editors. *Fleisher & Ludwig's textbook of pediatric emergency medicine.* 7th ed. Philadelphia, PA: Wolters Kluwer Health; 2015.

Eddy AA, Symons JM. Nephrotic syndrome in childhood. *Lancet.* 2003;362(9384):629–639. https://doi.org/10.1016/S0140-6736(03)14184-0. Medline:12944064

Gipson DS, Massengill SF, Yao L, et al. Management of childhood onset nephrotic syndrome. *Pediatrics.* 2009;124(2):747–757. https://doi.org/10.1542/peds.2008-1559. Medline:19651590

Gordillo R, Spitzer A. The nephrotic syndrome. *Pediatr Rev.* 2009;30(3):94–104, quiz 105. https://doi.org/10.1542/pir.30-3-94. Medline:19255123

Lennon R, Watson L, Webb NJ. Nephrotic syndrome in children. *Paediatr Child Health.* 2010;20(1):36–42. https://doi.org/10.1016/j.paed.2009.10.001

Pais P, Anver ED. Nephrotic syndrome. In: Kliegman RM, Stanton BF, Schor NF, St. Geme III JW, Behrman RE, editors. *Nelson textbook of pediatrics.* 19th ed. Philadelphia, PA: Elsevier Saunders; 2011. https://doi.org/10.1016/B978-1-4377-0755-7.00521-2

Thull-Freedman J. Renal emergencies: nephrotic syndrome. In: Lalani A, Schneeweiss S, editors. *The Hospital for Sick Children handbook of pediatric emergency medicine.* Mississauga, ON: Jones and Bartlett; 2011. p. 228–30.

18.1

Head Injury

Carlos R. Alvarez-Allende, Mary E. Brindle

- Traumatic brain injury (TBI) is a leading cause of death in the 0 to 14 year age group.
- Approximately 85% of brain injuries are classified as mild.
- Nonaccidental trauma (NAT) is associated with 80% of severe and fatal TBIs (see Chapter 1.7).
- Many brain injuries in children can be prevented by the proper use of vehicle restraints, helmets, and increased vigilance.
- Head injuries can be categorized into extraaxial injuries and intraaxial injuries:
  » Extraaxial injuries:
    › Epidural hematoma
    › Subdural hematoma
    › Subarachnoid hemorrhage
  » Intraaxial injuries:
    › Diffuse axonal injury
      · Diffuse axonal injuries are caused by angular or rotational forces having a shearing effect on neurons.
    › Contusion
    › Cerebral edema

Pathophysiology

- Consider the following physiological parameters:
  » Cerebral perfusion pressure (CPP)
    › The calculation for CPP is:
      · Mean arterial pressure (MAP) – intracranial pressure (ICP) = CPP
    › The ideal CPP in adults is 70 mmHg.
    › Children are able to tolerate lower CPP (30 to 40 mmHg) due to increased elasticity of the cranial vault.
  » Cerebral blood flow (CBF)
    › CBF is maintained through autoregulation.
      · Autoregulation is disrupted by trauma, hypoxia, and hypercarbia.

  › In order to maintain CBF, systolic blood pressure must range between 60 and 150 mmHg.

Diagnosis

- All trauma patients should be initially evaluated with a systematic approach; follow the protocols of advanced trauma life support (ATLS).
  » Primary survey — remember "ABCDE":
    › **A**irway
    › **B**reathing
    › **C**irculation
    › **D**isability
    › **E**xposure
  » Once the primary survey is completed and the patient stabilized, a secondary survey is performed, consisting of:
    › A complete neurological examination
    › The determination of the patient's score Glasgow Coma Scale (GCS; see "Glasgow Coma Scale," below)
- Clinical findings seen in patients with TBI include:
  » Altered mental status
  » Loss of consciousness
  » Skull fracture
  » Emesis
  » Headache
  » Neurologic deficit

Glasgow Coma Scale

- Patients should have a score classified as mild, moderate, or severe on the GCS.
  » Mild — GCS 13 to 15
  » Moderate — GCS 9 to 12
  » Severe — GCS < 9

Table 18.1.1. GLASGOW COMA SCALE*

Adapted from Teasdale and Jennett (1974) and Teasdale, Jennett, Brennan, McElhinney, and Allen (2014).

> 5 years old		< 5 years old	
Response	**Score**	**Response**	**Score**
Eye opening		**Eye opening**	
Opens eyes spontaneously	4	Opens eyes spontaneously	4
Opens eyes to verbal stimuli	3	Opens eyes to verbal stimuli	3
Opens eyes to painful stimuli	2	Opens eyes to painful stimuli	2
Does not open eyes	1	Does not open eyes	1
Best verbal response		**Best verbal response**	
Oriented and converses	5	Talks normally	5
Confused and converses	4	Words only	4
Uses inappropriate words	3	Vocal sounds but no words	3
Makes incomprehensible sounds	2	Cries only	2
Makes no sounds	1	Makes no sounds	1
Best motor response		**Best motor response**	
Obeys commands	6	Moves spontaneously or obeys commands	6
Localizes pain	5	Localizes to stimuli	5
Withdraws from pain	4	Withdraws from pain	4
Flexion response to pain	3	Flexion response to pain	3
Extension response to pain	2	Extension response to pain	2
Makes no movements	1	Makes no movements	1

*There have been additional modifications to the GSC or interpretations of the GCS to account for varying age ranges less than 5 years (at birth, 6 months of age, 6–12 months of age, 1–2 years of age, and 2–5 years of age). For more information, see "How is the Glasgow Coma Scale modified for children?" at http://www.glasgowcomascale.org/.

Investigations

- Head CT scan is the imaging standard for the evaluation of TBI in the acute setting.
  » CT scan allows evaluation of extra- and intraaxial injury, herniation, and fractures.
- All patients with moderate and severe head trauma should be evaluated with a head CT scan.
- Patients with minor head injuries should have a head CT scan if they present with the signs and symptoms listed below (i.e., if they are at high risk):
  » Focal neurologic deficit
  » Suspicion of an open or depressed skull fracture
  » 2 hours after injury GCS < 15
  » Persistent irritability in young children (< 2 years of age)
  » High risk of bleeding (coagulation disorders)
- Relative indications for a head CT scan:
  » GCS < 14
  » Signs of basilar skull fracture

  » Clinical deterioration while being observed in the ED (4 to 6 hours)
  » Seizures at the time of injury or after
  » High-energy injury mechanism
  » Suspicion of NAT
- A repeat head CT scan should be performed in cases in which there is a change in the neurologic exam.
- MRI should be reserved for:
  » Patients in whom the findings in the head CT scan do not correlate with the clinical picture of the patient
  » Patients who present with subacute injuries with associated neurocognitive deficit
- Consider obtaining a neurosurgical consultation for the timing and planning of subsequent imaging.

Management

MINOR TRAUMATIC BRAIN INJURY

- Asymptomatic patients can be discharged when the following criteria are met:
  » Normal neuroimaging
  » Linear, nondisplaced skull fracture
  » No suspicion or concern for NAT
- Consider a neurocognitive evaluation before discharge and as an outpatient.

MODERATE TO SEVERE TRAUMATIC BRAIN INJURY

- The mainstay of management is to prevent and minimize secondary injury.
- The goals of therapy include:
  » MAP according to age group (note that there is variability in these recommendations):
    › Infants and toddlers (0–2 years of age): 60 mmHg
    › Children (2–10 years of age): 70 mmHg
    › Adolescents (10–18 years of age): 80 mmHg
  » ICP < 20 mmHg in children and adolescents; < 15 mmHg for infants and toddlers
  » CPP:
    › Infants and toddlers (0–2 years of age): > 40 mmHg
    › Children (2–10 years of age): > 50 mmHg
    › Adolescents (10–18 years of age): > 70 mmHg

Note: An increase in mortality has been observed in patients in whom the CPP goal is not achieved.

- The following are recommended initial interventions:
  » Intubate children with GCS < 8
  » Maintain adequate ICP levels
  » Admit patient to the PICU
  » Obtain a neurosurgery consult

Management of elevated ICP

- For first-line treatment:
  - » Elevate head of bed to 30°
  - » Maintain head position at midline
  - » Prevent hypoxia ($pO_2 > 60$ mmHg)
  - » Maintain normocapnea (35 to 40 mmHg)
  - » Maintain normothermia (36.5°C to 37.5°C)
  - » Provide adequate sedation and analgesia
- For second-line treatment, consider:
  - » A hypertonic (3%) saline infusion — a 6 to 10 mL/kg bolus followed by 0.1 to 1 mL/kg per hour infusion
    - › Maintain serum osmolarity < 360 mOsm/L.
    - › Maintain serum sodium < 150 mmol/L.
  - » Mannitol — 0.25 to 1 g/kg
    - › Use with caution — serum osmolarity > 320 mOsm/L increases risk of renal injury.
  - » Mechanical decompression
    - › Consider intraventricular catheter for ICP monitoring and cerebrospinal fluid (CSF) removal.
    - › Consider lumbar drain for CSF removal.
    - › Consider decompressive craniectomy.
- For third-line treatment, consider:
  - » Therapeutic hypothermia
    - › Decrease temperature to 32°C to 33°C in cases of refractory increased ICP.
    - › Hypothermia for long periods (48 to 72 hours) followed by slow rewarming (0.5°C to 1°C every 3 to 4 hours) may reduce mortality.
  - » Barbiturate coma
  - » Electroencephalogram (EEG)
    - › Monitor activity for 24 to 48 hours due to increased risk (up to 30%) of clinical and subclinical seizures.
- There is no role for the administration of corticosteroids in pediatric patients with severe TBI.
- Seizure activity increases ICP and metabolic activity, which can cause secondary brain injury.
  - » Consider the use of prophylactic anticonvulsants in the setting of severe TBI.

Prognosis

- Severe TBI has a mortality of approximately 20%.
- Poor outcomes are associated with:
  - » High-energy injury
  - » Persistently high ICP
  - » Presence of chest/abdominal injury
  - » Edema and shifting on initial imaging
- Long-term effects can be seen in intelligence, behavior, language, attention span, and memory after a severe TBI.
- TBI as a result of NAT is associated with higher morbidity and mortality, approaching 40%.

REFERENCES

Abend NS, Wusthoff CJ, Goldberg EM, Dlugos DJ. Electrographic seizures and status epilepticus in critically ill children and neonates with encephalopathy. *Lancet Neurol.* 2013;12(12):1170–1179. https://doi.org/10.1016/S1474-4422(13)70246-1. Medline:24229615

Adelson PD, Wisniewski SR, Beca J, et al; Paediatric Traumatic Brain Injury Consortium. Comparison of hypothermia and normothermia after severe traumatic brain injury in children (Cool Kids): a phase 3, randomised controlled trial. *Lancet Neurol.* 2013;12(6):546–553. https://doi.org/10.1016/S1474-4422(13)70077-2. Medline:23664370

Alderson P, Roberts I. Corticosteroids for acute traumatic brain injury. *Cochrane Database Syst Rev.* 2005;(1):CD000196. Medline:15674869

Allen BB, Chiu YL, Gerber LM, Ghajar J, Greenfield JP. Age-specific cerebral perfusion pressure thresholds and survival in children and adolescents with severe traumatic brain injury. *Pediatr Crit Care Med.* 2014;15(1):62–70. https://doi.org/10.1097/PCC.0b013e3182a556ea. Medline:24196011

Arbuthnot MK, Mooney DP, Glenn IC. Head and cervical spine evaluation for the pediatric surgeon. *Surg Clin North Am.* 2017;97(1):35–58. https://doi.org/10.1016/j.suc.2016.08.003. Medline:27894431

Bishop NB. Traumatic brain injury: a primer for primary care physicians. *Curr Probl Pediatr Adolesc Health Care.* 2006;36(9):318–331. https://doi.org/10.1016/j.cppeds.2006.05.004. Medline:16996420

Bodanapally UK, Sours C, Zhuo J, Shanmuganathan K. Imaging of traumatic brain injury. *Radiol Clin North Am.* 2015;53(4):695–715. https://doi.org/10.1016/j.rcl.2015.02.011. Medline:26046506

Chambers IR, Kirkham FJ. What is the optimal cerebral perfusion pressure in children suffering from traumatic coma? *Neurosurg Focus.* 2003;15(6):1–8. https://doi.org/10.3171/foc.2003.15.6.3. Medline:15305839

Deans KJ, Minneci PC, Lowell W, Groner JI. Increased morbidity and mortality of traumatic brain injury in victims of nonaccidental trauma. *J Trauma Acute Care Surg.* 2013;75(1):157–160. https://doi.org/10.1097/TA.0b013e3182984acb. Medline:23940862

Dias MS, Lillis KA, Calvo C, Shaha SH, Li V. Management of accidental minor head injuries in children: a prospective outcomes study. *J Neurosurg.* 2004;101(1 Suppl):38–43. Medline:16206970

Farrell C; Canadian Paediatric Society, Acute Care Committee. Management of the paediatric patient with acute head trauma. *Paediatr Child Health.* 2013;18(5):253–258. https://doi.org/10.1093/pch/18.5.253

Hartwell JL, Spalding MC, Fletcher B, O'mara MS, Karas C. You cannot go home: routine concussion evaluation is not enough. *Am Surg.* 2015;81(4):395–403. Medline:25831187

Hill EP, Stiles PJ, Reyes J, Nold RJ, Helmer SD, Haan JM. Repeat head imaging in blunt pediatric trauma patients: is it necessary? *J Trauma Acute Care Surg.* 2017;82(5):896–900. https://doi.org/10.1097/TA.0000000000001406. Medline:28248802

Keenan HT, Runyan DK, Marshall SW, Nocera MA, Merten DF, Sinal SH. A population-based study of inflicted traumatic brain injury in young children. *JAMA.* 2003;290(5):621–626. https://doi.org/10.1001/jama.290.5.621. Medline:12902365

Kim JJ, Gean AD. Imaging for the diagnosis and management of traumatic brain injury. *Neurotherapeutics.* 2011;8(1):39–53. https://doi.org/10.1007/s13311-010-0003-3. Medline:21274684

National Clinical Guideline Centre (UK). *Head injury: triage, assessment, investigation and early management of head injury in children, young people and adults.* London; UK: National Institute for Health and Care Excellence; 2014.

Parsons S, Gilleland J. AHS guidelines for the management of severe traumatic brain injury [Internet]. Aug 2016. Available from: https://myahs.ca/insite/assets/picuc/tms-picuc-physician-trauma-brain-trauma-foundation-tbi.pdf

Teasdale G, Jennett B. Assessment of coma and impaired consciousness: a practical scale. *Lancet.* 1974;2(7872):81–84. *doi:*10.1016/S0140-6736(74)91639-0. *PMID* 4136544.

Teasdale G, Jennett B, Brennan P, McElhinney E, Allen D. How is the Glasgow coma scale modified for children? [Internet]. Glasgow: Glasgow Coma Scale; 2014. Available from: http://www.glasgowcomascale.org/faq/#faq-2

TRAUMA

18.2

Cervical Spine Injury

Rahim Valani

- The incidence of cervical spine injury (CSI) is estimated to be 1% to 4% of all pediatric trauma admissions to the emergency department (ED).
- For small children with nonaccidental trauma (NAT) or inflicted trauma, the incidence of cervical spine trauma is 15%.
- The type of injury varies based on age.
- Younger children tend to have injuries higher on the cervical spine (C2 to C3), whereas adolescents usually have injuries to the lower area (C5 to C6):
  » ≥2 years of age — 74% of injuries occur between the occiput and C2
  » 2 to 7 years of age — 78% of injuries occur on or between the occiput and C2
  » 8 to 15 years of age — 53% of injuries are subaxial (C3 to C7)
- Associated mortality depends on the level of injury:
  » 23% mortality for upper CSI
  » 4% mortality for lower CSI
- The incidence of CSI is twice as high in males compared to females.
- Differences in the pediatric cervical spine compared to the adult cervical spine results in decreased overall incidence of CSI, but also unique injuries.
- Characteristics of the pediatric cervical spine as compared to the adult cervical spine are as follows:
  » Cervical spine ligaments are lax
    › Consequently, there is a predisposition to rotatory movement of the cervical spine without tearing of the ligaments.
  » Cervical vertebrae are shallower and more horizontal
  » Head is disproportionately large
  » There is a steeper angle between the odontoid and facets
  » There is anterior wedging of the vertebral bodies
  » Uncinate process is absent
  » Pseudosubluxation
- The most common mechanisms of injury resulting in CSI are:
  » Motor vehicle accidents (most common)
  » Pedestrian struck by car
  » Bicycle riding accidents
  » Falls
  » Violence

- » Sports injuries
    › Diving has the highest risk overall in sports injuries.
    › The odds ratio for sports-related CSI is based on the type of organized sport (see *Table 18.2.1*).

Table 18.2.1. ODDS RATIO OF CERVICAL SPINE INJURY BASED ON THE TYPE OF ORGANIZED SPORTING ACTIVITY

Organized sport	Odds ratio of cervical spine injury
Gymnastics/cheerleading	6.4
Hockey	3.2
Football	2.8

Risk Factors

- Based on the mechanism of injury and clinical exam on arrival, risk factors associated with CSI are:
  » Altered mental status
  » Focal neurological deficit
  » Neck pain
  » Torticollis
  » Significant torso trauma
  » High-risk motor vehicle crash
- Risk factors specific for children < 3 years of age are:
  » Glasgow Coma Scale (GSC) overall score of < 14 (see *Table 18.1.1*)
  » GCS eye score of 1
  » Motor vehicle crash
  » Age > 2 years

Physical Exam

- Manage the patient as per Advanced Trauma Life Support (ATLS) protocols.
- Specific findings can help determine the site and type of injury.
  » Impaired respiratory drive occurs in injuries that are C5 or higher.
  » Hypotension without associated bradycardia is seen in patients who have lost their sympathetic tone.
  » Sensory impairment:
    › Impaired ability to feel pain/temperature may indicate anterior cord injury.
    › Impaired proprioception and ability to feel vibration may indicate posterior cord injury.

> Complete sensory loss is associated with cord transection.
» Motor impairment may indicate posterior/lateral cord injury.
- Check plantar reflexes to identify upper motor neuron lesions.
- Neck tenderness increases the likelihood of the patient having a CSI.
- Check for decreased range of motion of the cervical spine / torticollis.

Investigations

- NEXUS and the Canadian C-spine rules are helpful for adult patients, but the validity of these is uncertain in the pediatric population.
- Investigations should include:
  » X-rays
    › Plain films are 73% to 90% sensitive for bony cervical injuries.
    › Lateral view picks up approximately 80% of injuries.
  » CT scan
    › CT scan is 100% sensitive for bony cervical spine injury.
    › It can miss up to 4% of ligamentous injuries.
    › Benefits of CT scan imaging of the cervical spine include:
      · Yields the highest rate of detecting cervical spine injuries
      · Earlier time to diagnosis
      · More cost-effective
      · Fewer repeated imaging studies are required
      · No risk of sedation compared with MRI
    › The increased risk of cancer is small but significant:
      · Males: 100 additional cancer cases per 100,000 CT neck scans
      · Females: 700 additional cancer cases per 100,000 CT neck scans
    › The physician can diminish this risk by reducing the radiation dose of the CT scan and by optimizing parameters.
  » MRI
    › MRI is 100% sensitive for cervical spine injury (bone, ligament, and cord).

AXIAL INJURIES (C1 TO C3)

- Axial injuries are usually see in children < 8 years of age.
- They are most commonly due to atlantoaxial rotatory subluxation (see "Atlantoaxial Rotatory Subluxation," below).

- The normal rotation of the cervical spine is up to 90 degrees, with 60% of this rotation arising from the atlantoaxial joint.
- An axial injury may be a:
  » C1 fracture (Jefferson fracture)
    › C1 fractures are due to axial load.
    › They are usually stable unless the ligaments are disrupted.
    › The atlanto-dens interval is > 5 mm.
    › The lateral mass overhang of C1 over C2 is > 6.9 mm (rule of Spence).
  » C2 dens fracture:
    › Type I — superior portion of dens from avulsion of alar ligament
    › Type II — base of the neck
    › Type III — extends to the body of C2
  » Subluxation of C2 on C3
    › This injury is seen in children < 7 years old.
    › Use the Swischuk line and absence of prevertebral soft tissue swelling to distinguish subluxation from pseudosubluxation.
      · The Swischuk line is the line from the anterior aspect of the posterior arch of C1 to the anterior aspect of the posterior arch of C3.
      · If C2 is > 2 mm from this line, then it is true subluxation.

SUBAXIAL INJURIES

- Depending on the mechanism, subaxial injuries can result in:
  » Compression fractures
    › Compression fractures are usually from axial loading.
    › They are stable and heal with conservative treatment.
  » Burst fractures
    › Burst fractures are usually from axial loading.
    › Retropulsed fragments can injure the spinal cord.
    › They usually require surgical management.
  » Teardrop fractures
    › Teardrop fractures are avulsion fractures of the vertebral body.
    › They are from hyperflexion or hyperextension.
    › Management depends on type of injury and stability.
  » Unilateral or bilateral facet dislocation
    › These injuries are usually from hyperflexion and rotation.
    › Management is usually conservative unless the patient has neurological findings.

TRAUMA

ATLANTOAXIAL ROTATORY SUBLUXATION

- For more information about atlantoaxial rotatory subluxation, see also Chapter 6.7.
- Patients present with torticollis and decreased neck range of motion.
  - » Patients are unable to move neck to a neutral position.
  - » Patients hold head in slight flexion with the chin rotated to the contralateral side.
- This type of injury is common in patients < 13 years of age.
- Mechanism / predisposing factors include:
  - » The role of synovial folds that can be trapped, resulting in fixation after subluxation
  - » Certain congenital conditions (e.g., Down syndrome, achondroplasia, Larsen syndrome, Klippel-Feil syndrome)
  - » Severe trauma
  - » Infection — recent upper respiratory tract infection (URTI)
  - » Recent head and/or neck surgery
  - » Grisel syndrome — subluxation of atlantoaxial joint due to inflammation of adjacent tissue
- Patients usually do not have any neurologic deficits.

Diagnosis

- Diagnosis is clinical.
  - » There is palpable deviation of C2 spinous process in the same direction as the head is rotated.
  - » The ipsilateral sternocleidomastoid muscle may spasm in attempt to reduce the deformity.
  - » The patient is unable to counter-rotate the head past midline.
  - » There is a bulge in the back wall of the pharynx (from anterior displacement of the arch of C1).

Investigations

- Initiate radiological investigations.
  - » X-rays are not helpful due to the head tilt.
    - › Open-mouth odontoid may show asymmetry of the lateral masses in relation to the odontoid.
  - » CT scan is the imaging of choice.
    - › Limit radiation by focusing cuts from occiput to C3.
  - » MRI is helpful in evaluating the integrity of the ligaments.

Management

- Two classification systems are used to help identify the stability of the subluxation and management (see *Table 18.2.2*).

Table 18.2.2. CLASSIFICATION SCHEMES FOR ATLANTOAXIAL ROTATORY SUBLUXATION

Type	Fielding and Hawkins	Pand and Li
I	• Pure rotatory fixation without anterior subluxation • Most common type • Atlantoaxial ligaments are intact	• Most severe • C1 and C2 are locked
II	• Disrupted transverse ligament • 3 to 5 mm anterior displacement of the anterior arch of C1 in relation to the odontoid	• Reduced angle of C1 on C2 with forced reduction • C1 cannot cross over C2
III	• 5 mm anterior displacement of the arch of C1	• C1 can cross over C2 with forced rotation
IV	• Rotatory fixation with posterior displacement • Usually seen in patients with congenital anomalies or concomitant fractures	• Diagnostic gray zone • Rotational dynamics of C1 and C2 lie between normal and type III injury

- Management of atlantoaxial rotatory subluxation may involve:
  - » Medical management:
    - › Treating underlying pathology
    - › Nonsteroidal anti-inflammatory drugs (NSAIDs)
    - › Physical therapy
  - » Closed manual reduction:
    - › Cervical traction with muscle relaxants and analgesia
      - · A closed manual reduction can be attempted under dynamic imaging, followed by cervical immobilization.
  - » Surgical management
    - › Surgical management is usually reserved for:
      - · Unstable deformities
      - · Progressive neurological symptoms
      - · Significant structural deformities

REFERENCES

Babcock L, Olsen CS, Jaffe DM, Leonard JC; Cervical Spine Study Group for the Pediatric Emergency Care Applied Research Network (PECARN). Cervical spine injuries in children associated with sports and recreational activities. [epub ahead of print]. *Pediatr Emer Care*; 2016.

Baerg J, Thirumoorthi A, Vannix R, Taha A, Young A, Zouros A. Cervical spine imaging for young children with inflicted trauma: expanding the injury pattern. *J Pediatr Surg.* 2017;52(5):816–821. https://doi.org/10.1016/j.jpedsurg.2017.01.049. Medline:28190553

Fielding JW, Hawkins RJ. Atlanto-axial rotatory fixation. (Fixed rotatory subluxation of the atlanto-axial joint). *J Bone Joint Surg Am.* 1977;59(1):37–44. https://doi.org/10.2106/00004623-197759010-00005. Medline:833172

Hikino K, Yamamoto LG. The benefit of neck computed tomography compared with its harm (risk of cancer). *J Trauma Acute Care Surg.* 2015;78(1):126–131. https://doi.org/10.1097/TA.0000000000000465. Medline:25539213

Kinon MD, Nasser R, Nakhla J, Desai R, Moreno JR, Yassari R, Bagley CA. Atlantoaxial rotatory subluxation: a review for the pediatric emergency physician. *Pediatr Emerg Care.* 2016;32(10):710–716. https://doi.org/10.1097/PEC.0000000000000817. Medline:27749670

Leonard JC. Cervical spine injury. *Pediatr Clin North Am.* 2013;60(5):1123–1137. https://doi.org/10.1016/j.pcl.2013.06.015. Medline:24093899

Nigrovic LE, Rogers AJ, Adelgais KM, et al; Pediatric Emergency Care Applied Research Network (PECARN) Cervical Spine Study Group. Utility of plain radiographs in detecting traumatic injuries of the cervical spine in children. *Pediatr Emerg Care.* 2012;28(5):426–432. https://doi.org/10.1097/PEC.0b013e3182531911. Medline:22531194

Parent S, Mac-Thiong J-M, Roy-Beaudry M, Sosa JF, Labelle H. Spinal cord injury in the pediatric population: a systematic review of the literature. *J Neurotrauma.* 2011;28(8):1515–1524. https://doi.org/10.1089/neu.2009.1153. Medline:21501096

Somppi LK, Frenn KA, Kharbanda AB. Examination of pediatric radiation dose delivered after cervical spine trauma. *Pediatr Emer Care*; 2017.

Tat ST, Mejia MJ, Freishtat RJ. Imaging, clearance, and controversies in pediatric cervical spine trauma. *Pediatr Emerg Care.* 2014;30(12):911–915, quiz 916–918. https://doi.org/10.1097/PEC.0000000000000298. Medline:25469605

18.3

Thoracic and Lumbar Spine Injury

Carlos R. Alvarez-Allende, Mary E. Brindle

- Spine fractures represent 1% to 3% of all pediatric fractures.
- Pediatric spine fractures comprise 2% to 5% of all spine trauma.
  - » 1% of spine trauma cases are confined to the pediatric thoracic and lumbar spine.
- 20% of pediatric spinal injury occurs in the thoracolumbar region.
  - » The thoracic area (T2 to T10) is the most common site of injury, followed by the lumbar area (L2 to L5).
- Injuries show a bimodal peak of incidence, peaking in:
  - » Children < 5 years of age
  - » Children > 10 years of age
- The mechanism of injury varies by age group.
  - » In children 0 to 9 years of age, the most common mechanisms are:
    - › Motor vehicle accidents (50%)
    - › Child abuse (20%)
    - › Falls (15%)
  - » In older children (> 10 years of age) and adolescents the most common mechanisms are motor vehicle accident (40%), followed by falls and sports-related injuries.
  - » The number of thoracic and lumbar fractures increases proportionally with age due to maturity of the spine.

Diagnosis

- All trauma patients should be initially evaluated with a systematic approach; follow the protocols of advanced trauma life support (ATLS).
  - » Primary survey — remember ABCDE:
    - › **A**irway
    - › **B**reathing
    - › **C**irculation
    - › **D**isability
    - › **E**xposure
  - » Once the primary survey is completed and the patient stabilized, a secondary survey is performed, involving:
    - › A complete neurological examination
    - › The determination of the patient's score on the Glasgow Coma Scale (GCS) (see *Table 18.1.1*).
- Clinical findings seen in patients with spinal injury include:
  - » Point tenderness along the spine
  - » Swelling
  - » Ecchymosis
  - » Palpable defect or deformity along the spinous process
  - » Seatbelt sign, associated with thoracic and lumbar fractures
  - » Loss of sensation
  - » Decreased motor function
- Findings in cases of spinal or neurogenic shock include:
  - » Loss of sympathetic tone
  - » Injuries above T6
  - » Bradycardia
  - » Hypotension
  - » Unresponsiveness to fluid resuscitation
- If the patient is unconscious, assume a spinal injury until a complete assessment is performed.

Investigations

- No Canadian guidelines exist for imaging spinal injuries.
- Imaging should be specific to the level of injury or neurologic deficit.

TRAUMA

- Thoracic and lumbar spine imaging should be performed when there is deemed to be a high risk of injury.
- Consider the following imaging studies:
  - » X-ray
    - › Most bony injuries can be identified with plain radiographs (anteroposterior [AP] and lateral views).
  - » CT scan
    - › CT scan is the ideal imaging study for evaluating the thoracolumbar spine after patient is stabilized.
    - › It allows identification of occult fractures and soft tissue injuries.
  - » MRI
    - › MRI is preferable for detecting ligamentous injury and assessing stability.
    - › It is the imaging study of choice for patients with normal radiographs and suspicion of injury.
    - › MRI findings correlate with patient outcomes.

Management

- The mainstay of initial management is spinal immobilization.
  - » It is performed in the prehospital setting.
  - » The entire spinal axis must be immobilized.
  - » In the absence of a cervical collar, blocks and tape are effective substitutes for immobilization.
  - » Children < 8 years of age need special consideration.
    - › Due to their larger heads, patients will be in flexion when placed on the backboard.
      - · Align the spine with an occiput recess or elevation of the torso.
- Ensure the prevention of secondary spinal injury.
  - » Maintain adequate tissue perfusion and oxygenation.
  - » Provide cardiovascular support as needed in the setting of multisystem injury.
  - » In cases of neurogenic shock, after euvolemic resuscitation, start vasopressor therapy to maintain spinal cord perfusion.
- There is no role for the administration of corticosteroids in pediatric patients with spinal injury.
- Most spinal injuries can be managed conservatively.
  - » Consider surgical intervention in the setting of neurological deterioration, failed reduction, compression of the cord due to bone fragments, disc herniation, or enlarging hematoma.

Prognosis

- Outcomes following spinal cord injury are directly related to the level and severity of the injury.
  - » Complete spinal cord injuries show limited return of function, but full recovery is not achieved.
- Outcomes are variable in the thoracic region depending on the mechanism of injury.

Table 18.3.1. THORACOLUMBAR INJURY CLASSIFICATION AND SEVERITY SCORE
Adapted from Lee et al. (2005).

		Score	Mode of investigation
Neurological status	Intact	0	Physical examination
	Nerve root injury	2	
	Complete cord injury	2	
	Incomplete cord injury	3	
	Cauda equina	3	
Injury morphology	Compression	1	X-ray
	Burst	2	CT scan
	Translation/rotation	3	
	Distraction	4	
Posterior ligament integrity	Intact	0	MRI
	Suspected/indeterminate	2	
	Injured	3	
Management (surgical vs conservative)	Conservative	0–3	—
	Surgeon's discretion	4	
	Surgical	> 4	

- Most lumbar spine fractures in the pediatric population are stable and present no neurologic deficit.
- Long-term outcomes have been studied in multiple cohort studies.
  - » 33.3% of patients noted back pain without neurologic deficit.
  - » Complete recovery was seen in 75% of patients with incomplete spinal cord injury.

COMPRESSION FRACTURES

- Compression fractures are the most common thoracolumbar fractures in the pediatric population.
  - » They occur due to the wedge shape of the vertebral body and the kyphosis of the spine.
- Such fractures are associated with low-energy trauma such as falls and sports-related injuries.
  - » They are often the result of an axial compression load in flexion.
  - » The posterior column remains intact.
- The loss of 50% or greater of the original vertebral body height should prompt evaluation of the posterior ligament with MRI.
- Consider conservative management for stable fractures with minimal height loss.
- The nonoperative treatment of unstable fractures can be managed with a TLSO therapy brace for 6 to 8 weeks.

BURST FRACTURES

- Burst fractures comprise 15% to 20% of all vertebral body fractures.
- This type of fracture is associated with high-energy trauma.
  - » They are often the result of an axial compression load without flexion.
  - » These fractures are characterized by disruption of the anterior and middle columns.
    - › The nucleus pulposus is driven into the vertebral body.
- Burst fractures are considered unstable.
- Neurologic injury is associated with retropulsion of the posterior vertebral body.
- A CT scan should be the initial imaging modality.
  - » CT scan allows for assessment of bony injury and compression of the spinal canal.
- An MRI can be used to assess the patient's posterior ligament stability, spinal cord, and nerve roots.
- Fractures with neurologic compromise require urgent decompression and stabilization.
- Stable fractures without neurologic deficit can be managed with use of a TLSO therapy brace for 8 to 12 weeks.

VERTEBRAL APOPHYSIS FRACTURE

- Vertebral apophysis fractures occur most commonly at L4 or L5.
- This type of fracture is associated with lifting heavy objects, falls, and twisting motions.
  - » It is caused by disruption of the endplate of the vertebral body.
  - » Overweight patients are at increased risk of this type of fracture.
- Patients present with back pain, radiculopathy, and claudication.
- CT scan is the preferred modality for diagnosis.
- Manage the fracture with posterior laminar decompression at the level of the injury to relieve symptoms.

SEATBELT INJURY

- Seatbelt injury most commonly occurs at the level of L2 and L3.
  - » The rib cage protects the thoracic spine from horizontal displacement.
- This type of injury is associated with high-energy trauma.
  - » It is a flexion-distraction injury.
  - » The anterior vertebral body acts as a flexion fulcrum due to deceleration.

- 50% of patients present with intraabdominal injuries, such as:
  - » Nutcracker syndrome — a crush injury of the head of the pancreas, duodenum, and left renal vein
  - » Mesenteric injury, bowel perforation, and Chance fracture

SCIWORA

- SCIWORA is defined as "spinal cord injury without radiographic abnormalities."
- The most common mechanisms are motor vehicle accidents and sports-related injuries.
- The thoracic spine is only affected in 13% of cases; the lumbar spine is rarely affected.
- The 5 most common patterns seen on MRI in order of severity are:
  1. Complete cord disruption due to severe flexion
  2. Major cord hemorrhage, > 50% hemorrhage
  3. Minor cord hemorrhage, ≤ 50% hemorrhage
  4. Edema only
  5. No MRI abnormalities
- Conservative management includes 12 weeks of bracing and avoidance of strenuous physical activity.
- The reported mortality of patients with SCIWORA is 2%.
- Up to 50% of patients can present with delayed progressive neurologic deterioration, which can be seen up to 4 days later.

REFERENCES

Arkader A, Warner WC Jr, Tolo VT, Sponseller PD, Skaggs DL. Pediatric Chance fractures: a multicenter perspective. *J Pediatr Orthop.* 2011;31(7):741–744. https://doi.org/10.1097/BPO.0b013e31822f1b0b. Medline:21926870

Buldini B, Amigoni A, Faggin R, Laverda AM. Spinal cord injury without radiographic abnormalities. *Eur J Pediatr.* 2006;165(2):108–111. https://doi.org/10.1007/s00431-005-0004-0. Medline:16235053

Cirak B, Ziegfeld S, Knight VM, Chang D, Avellino AM, Paidas CN. Spinal injuries in children. *J Pediatr Surg.* 2004;39(4):607–612. https://doi.org/10.1016/j.jpedsurg.2003.12.011. Medline:15065038

Clark P, Letts M. Trauma to the thoracic and lumbar spine in the adolescent. *Can J Surg.* 2001;44(5):337–345. Medline:11603746

d'Amato C. Pediatric spinal trauma: injuries in very young children. *Clin Orthop Relat Res.* 2005;432:34–40. https://doi.org/10.1097/01.blo.0000156006.20089.85. Medline:15738801

Daniels AH, Sobel AD, Eberson CP. Pediatric thoracolumbar spine trauma. *J Am Acad Orthop Surg.* 2013;21(12):707–716. Medline:24292927

Deans KJ, Minneci PC, Lowell W, Groner JI. Increased morbidity and mortality of traumatic brain injury in victims of nonaccidental trauma. *J Trauma Acute Care Surg.* 2013;75(1):157–160. https://doi.org/10.1097/TA.0b013e3182984acb. Medline:23940862

Dogan S, Safavi-Abbasi S, Theodore N, et al. Thoracolumbar and sacral spinal injuries in children and adolescents: a review of 89 cases. *J Neurosurg.* 2007;106(6 Suppl):426–433. Medline:17566397

Erfani MA, Pourabbas B, Nouraie H, Vadiee I, Vosoughi AR. Results of fusion and instrumentation of thoracic and lumbar vertebral fractures in children: a prospective ten-year study. *Musculoskelet Surg.* 2014;98(2):107–114. https://doi.org/10.1007/s12306-014-0313-4. Medline:24469706

TRAUMA

Farrell CA, Hannon M, Lee LK. Pediatric spinal cord injury without radiographic abnormality in the era of advanced imaging. *Curr Opin Pediatr.* 2017;29(3):286–290. https://doi.org/10.1097/MOP.0000000000000481. Medline:28306628

Henrys P, Lyne ED, Lifton C, Salciccioli G. Clinical review of cervical spine injuries in children. *Clin Orthop Relat Res.* 1977;129:172–176. https://doi.org/10.1097/00003086-197711000-00020. Medline:608271

Herkowitz HN, Garfin SR, Eismont FJ, et al. *Rothman-Simeone: the spine.* 5th ed. Philadelphia: Saunders-Elsevier; 2006.

Knox J. Epidemiology of spinal cord injury without radiographic abnormality in children: a nationwide perspective. *J Child Orthop.* 2016;10(3):255–260. https://doi.org/10.1007/s11832-016-0740-x. Medline:27209042

Lee JY, Vaccaro AR, Lim MR, Öner FC, Hulbert RJ, Hedlund R, Fehlings MG, Arnold P, Harrop J, Bono CM, Anderson PA, Anderson DG, Harris MB, Brown AK, Stock GH, Baron EM. Thoracolumbar injury classification and severity score: a new paradigm for the treatment of thoracolumbar spine trauma. *J Orthop Sci.* 2005;10(6):671–675. https://dx.doi.org/10.1007%2Fs00776-005-0956-y

Mortazavi MM, Dogan S, Civelek E, et al. Pediatric multilevel spine injuries: an institutional experience. *Childs Nerv Syst.* 2011;27(7):1095–1100. https://doi.org/10.1007/s00381-010-1348-y. Medline:21110031

Piatt JH Jr. Pediatric spinal injury in the US: epidemiology and disparities. *J Neurosurg Pediatr.* 2015;16(4):463–471. https://doi.org/10.3171/2015.2.PEDS1515. Medline:26114993

Sayama C, Chen T, Trost G, Jea A. A review of pediatric lumbar spine trauma. *Neurosurg Focus.* 2014;37(1):E6. https://doi.org/10.3171/2014.5.FOCUS1490. Medline:24981905

Singla AA, Singla AA. Seatbelt syndrome with superior mesenteric artery syndrome: leave nothing to chance! *J Surg Case Rep.* 2015;2015(11):rjv148. https://doi.org/10.1093/jscr/rjv148. Medline:26564612

Slotkin JR, Lu Y, Wood KB. Thoracolumbar spinal trauma in children. *Neurosurg Clin N Am.* 2007;18(4):621–630. https://doi.org/10.1016/j.nec.2007.07.003. Medline:17991587

Sovio OM, Bell HM, Beauchamp RD, Tredwell SJ. Fracture of the lumbar vertebral apophysis. *J Pediatr Orthop.* 1985;5(5):550–552. https://doi.org/10.1097/01241398-198509000-00008. Medline:2931450

Srinivasan V, Jea A. Pediatric thoracolumbar spine trauma. *Neurosurg Clin N Am.* 2017;28(1):103–114. https://doi.org/10.1016/j.nec.2016.07.003. Medline:27886872

Thomas JG, Boatey J, Brayton A, Jea A. Neurogenic claudication associated with posterior vertebral rim fractures in children. *J Neurosurg Pediatr.* 2012;10(3):241–245. https://doi.org/10.3171/2012.5.PEDS1247. Medline:22768967

Vialle LR, Vialle E. Pediatric spine injuries. *Injury.* 2005;36(Suppl 2):S104–S112. https://doi.org/10.1016/j.injury.2005.06.021. Medline:15993111

Yen CH, Chan SK, Ho YF, Mak KH. Posterior lumbar apophyseal ring fractures in adolescents: a report of four cases. *J Orthop Surg (Hong Kong).* 2009;17(1):85–89. https://doi.org/10.1177/230949900901700119. Medline:19398801

18.4

Chest Trauma

Natalie L. Yanchar

- Thoracic injuries are the second most common cause of trauma mortality (second to traumatic brain injuries).
  » 5% to 15% of children seen in a trauma center will have a thoracic injury.
- The most common mechanisms are car versus pedestrian accidents and motor vehicle crashes.
- Most cases result from blunt force to the trunk.
  » Intrusion of the flexible rib cage results in pulmonary contusions, the most common thoracic injury type seen in this population.
- The more cartilaginous nature of the pediatric chest wall protects it from bony fractures from most blunt forces.
  » Diagnosis of rib fractures implies significant kinetic energy transfer and thus the risk of multiple injuries (usually truncal and head).
- Risk of aortic and other major vascular injuries is secondary to shearing from rapid deceleration mechanisms and is far less common than in the adult population.
  » Lack of atherosclerosis fibrosis and calcification at

Table 18.4.1. INJURY RISKS BASED ON MECHANISM

Injury type	Example	Suspected injuries
Mild to moderate blunt forces to the trunk	• Motor vehicle collision; restraints used • Fall from minor height • Low-speed car versus pedestrian	• Pulmonary contusion (without rib fracture) • Simple pneumothorax
Major thoracic blunt force, crushing mechanism	• High-speed motor vehicle collision • High-speed car versus pedestrian • Fall from a significant height	• Rib fractures • Pulmonary contusion • Simple hemopneumothorax • Tension hemo- and/or pneumothorax • Other mediastinal structure contusion, crush, or direct disruption (tracheobronchial tree, myocardium, aorta, superior vena cava, esophagus)
Penetrating injuries		• Hemo- and/or pneumothorax with or without tension • Cardiac tamponade

the ligamentum arteriosum in younger children partially accounts for this.

» Major vascular injuries in children, when they do occur, are frequently fatal at the scene, with only 7% to 20% of such cases actually reaching hospital alive.

Physical Exam

- Initial assessment is concurrent with initial management.
- Follow the principles of Advanced Trauma Life Support (ATLS) for the primary survey.
- Depending on the mechanism and suspicion of thoracic or other injuries, secure the airway, ensure adequate oxygenation, and obtain adequate vascular access.
- Perform emergent chest decompression in cases consistent with tension pneumothorax, presenting with:
  » Increased work of breathing
  » Tracheal deviation
  » Reduced or absent breath sounds
  » Hyperresonance to chest percussion
  » Profound hemodynamic instability with hypotension unresponsive to IV fluids (assume potential of tension hemo/pneumothorax)
- Decompress with 14G to 16G angiocatheter (anterior chest, 2nd intercostal space) followed by placement of chest tube.
- If hemo/pneumothorax is suspected based on more "subtle findings" (e.g., reduced breath sounds), but there are no signs of tension and the patient is hemodynamically stable, obtain an emergent chest X-ray (CXR) while preparing for the potential need for a chest tube.
- If there is profound hemodynamic instability, place bilateral chest tubes.
- Elevated jugular venous pressure is suggestive of an obstructive phenomenon such as tension pneumothorax or cardiac tamponade.
  » Palpation of the chest wall may further demonstrate rib fractures and subcutaneous emphysema in this setting.

Investigations

Chest X-ray

- A chest X-ray (CXR) (anteroposterior [AP] view) should be obtained if the patient is hemodynamically stable and the injury mechanism was blunt force without direction to a specific body part.
  » If the CXR is normal, no further imaging is required.
  » Rib fracture(s) alone, without any other signs of thoracic injury on CXR, do not require further investigation.
  » If CXR is suggestive of pulmonary contusion but there is no hemo/pneumothorax and mediastinal

contour is normal, no further imaging is required beyond a repeat CXR (dependent on the clinical progression of the patient).

- A CT scan may be more sensitive in identifying pulmonary contusions at an earlier stage; however, studies suggest that visualization on CXR is a more reliable indicator of the need for ventilator support than what is visualized on a CT scan.

CT Scan

- Indications for a CT scan include the following:
  » Patient **must** be hemodynamically stable
  » Patient has a widened mediastinum
    › If the mediastinal silhouette is abnormal, consider the risk of mediastinal vascular injury and obtain a CT scan with IV contrast.
- The intrathoracic presence of stomach or bowel contents is diagnostic of traumatic diaphragmatic hernia, however an elevated, indistinct, or irregular diaphragmatic border is suggestive of diaphragmatic hernia and requires a CT scan (or operation if patient is hemodynamically unstable) for definitive diagnosis.
  » In both instances, surgical consultation is required.

Management

- Indications for a chest tube are:
  » Symptomatic hemo/pneumothorax
  » Postdecompression of a tension pneumothorax
  » Pneumothorax in a patient on positive pressure ventilation
- Consider a chest tube in patients who have a pneumothorax and are to be transported to another facility.
- A chest tube may not be required for small hemo/pneumothoraces visible on CXR but without clinical symptoms.
- A chest tube is not required for incidental pneumothoraces discovered on CT scan only.
- The need for a second tube is dependent on the efficacy of the initial tube to control air leakage.
  » If pneumothorax persists despite full suction (-20 cm H_2O), insert a second tube.
- The need for a second tube and/or suspicion of a massive hemothorax should trigger an emergent surgical consultation.
- Size guidelines for chest tubes:
  » Toddlers — 20 Fr
  » School-age children — 24 Fr
  » Teenagers/adolescents — 28 Fr to 32 Fr
- A smaller tube size can be used if there is only a simple pneumothorax and the goal is simply to evacuate the air.
- If the patient has a diagnosed or suspected hemothorax, use a minimum chest tube size of 20 Fr to avoid clotting within the tube.

TRAUMA

SPECIFIC INJURIES

RIB FRACTURES

- The pediatric chest wall is pliable, so blunt forces are transmitted to the internal organs, most commonly resulting in pulmonary contusions.
- The presence of a rib fracture should raise concern that the injury was caused by a significant force or child abuse (see Chapter 1.7).
  - » Fractures of the first rib especially should be investigated further for esophageal or great vessel injuries.
- Due to the low incidence of rib fractures in pediatric patients, flail chest is not common.

Management

- Manage rib fractures with:
  - » Analgesia
  - » Chest tube if pneumothorax is present
  - » Physiotherapy

PULMONARY CONTUSION

- No specific intervention other than supportive care is required.
- Use IV fluids judiciously to reduce the risk of pulmonary edema.

HEMO/PNEUMOTHORAX

- If a small hemo/pneumothorax (< 15%) is visible and there are no cardiorespiratory symptoms and no plan for positive pressure ventilation, observation may be sufficient.
  - » Need for a repeat CXR depends on the time proximity to the actual injury (e.g., if 12 hours have passed since the injury, it is unlikely to require any intervention; if the first CXR was done within 1 hour of the injury, consider a repeat CXR in 1 to 2 hours, depending on the patient's clinical status).
- If there is significant hemo/pneumothorax, especially if it is symptomatic, place a chest tube and repeat the CXR to ensure adequate lung expansion.
- There are no clear criteria for the diagnosis of a "massive hemothorax" in children.
  - » Consider the need for surgical intervention (thoracotomy) if there is rapid evacuation of ≥ 20% of blood volume upon initial chest tube placement.

PNEUMOMEDIASTINUM

- Pneumomediastinum may be related to an acute lung injury or to the disruption of major air-containing mediastinal viscus: larynx, tracheobronchial tree, or esophagus.
  - » Clinical findings and other findings on CXR should guide further investigation and management.
- The absence of significant clinical symptoms and other injuries visualized on CXR suggests minor disruption contained by the mediastinal tissue, and conservative observation is all that is required.
- If the condition is associated with clinical symptoms (e.g., respiratory distress, hoarseness, dyspnea, chest pain) or another major thoracic injury is visualized on CXR (e.g., large pneumothorax), then consider the following:
  - » Esophagoscopy
  - » Laryngoscopy/tracheobronchoscopy

MYOCARDIAL INJURY

- In Canada, the vast majority of cases of myocardial injury are due to blunt-force mechanisms.
- Three-quarters of cases will have associated injuries:
  - » Head injury, including intracerebral bleeding
  - » Rib fractures
  - » Lung injury
  - » Abdominal organ (spleen and kidney) injury
- Presentation can vary from asymptomatic to the presence of a new murmur to dysrhythmias.
- Elevated creatine kinase and/or troponins may or may not be present.
- If myocardial injury is suspected, confirm with an echocardiogram.
- Massive cardiac rupture may occur but is rarely survivable beyond the scene of injury.
- Maintain a high degree of suspicion if there are signs of cardiac tamponade (see "Tamponade," below).
- Visualize through the cardiac window with point-of-care ultrasound.

TAMPONADE

- Tamponade occurs when a myocardial injury results in blood accumulating in the pericardial sac.
  - » When the amount of fluid is significant, cardiac output is compromised.
- CXR may show an enlarged heart, but this is difficult to interpret with an AP view.
- ECG findings include:
  - » Low voltage
  - » Electrical alternans
- Clinical findings of tamponade are Beck's triad:
  - » Elevated neck veins
  - » Muffled heart sounds
  - » Hypotension

Management

- If the patient is unstable and has compromised cardiac contractility, consider bedside pericardiocentesis.
- Obtain an emergent surgical consultation for a pericardial window in the operating room.

ESOPHAGEAL INJURIES

- See "Pneumomediastinum," above.

REFERENCES

Allen CJ, Straker RJ, Tashiro J, et al. Pediatric vascular injury: experience of a level 1 trauma center. *J Surg Res*. 2015;196(1):1–7. https://doi.org/10.1016/j.jss.2015.02.023. Medline:25796108

Kaptein YE, Talving P, Konstantinidis A, et al. Epidemiology of pediatric cardiac injuries: a National Trauma Data Bank analysis. *J Pediatr Surg*. 2011;46(8):1564–1571. https://doi.org/10.1016/j.jpedsurg.2011.02.041. Medline:21843725

Kuniyoshi Y, Kamura A, Yasuda S, Tashiro M, Toriyabe Y. Laryngeal injury and pneumomediastinum due to minor blunt neck trauma: case report. *J Emerg Med*. 2017; 52(4):e145–e148. Medline:27818032

Pryor SD, Lee LK. Clinical outcomes and diagnostic imaging of pediatric patients with pneumomediastinum secondary to blunt trauma to the chest. *J Trauma*. 2011;71(4):904–908. https://doi.org/10.1097/TA.0b013e31820edfbe. Medline:21460747

Rosenberg G, Bryant AK, Davis KA, Schuster KM. No breakpoint for mortality in pediatric rib fractures. *J Trauma Acute Care Surg*. 2016;80(3):427–432. https://doi.org/10.1097/TA.0000000000000955. Medline:26713973

Wylie J, Morrison GC, Nalk K, et al. Lung contusion in children: early computed tomography versus radiography. *Pediatr Crit Care Med*. 2009;10(6):643–647. https://doi.org/10.1097/PCC.0b013e3181a63f58. Medline:19455072

18.5

Abdominal Trauma

Rahim Valani

- Trauma is the leading cause of death in children > 1 year of age.
  - » Abdominal trauma is the third leading cause of death in this group.
- The incidence of blunt abdominal injury is 9 per 100 000 children.
  - » Blunt injuries make up 85% of abdominal trauma cases.
  - » Intraabdominal injuries occur in 5% to 10% of pediatric patients with blunt abdominal trauma.
- The most common organs injured are:
  - » Liver and spleen — median grade 3 injury for both
  - » Kidneys
  - » Pancreas
  - » Hollow viscera
- Common causes of blunt abdominal trauma are:
  - » Traffic/car accident
  - » Fall from height
  - » Handlebar injuries
  - » Contact and noncontact sport injuries
  - » Nonaccidental trauma (NAT)
- Mortality in children with abdominal injuries is predominantly due to associated head injury (see Chapter 18.1).

Diagnosis

- The sensitivity of diagnosing significant intraabdominal injuries by pain on physical exam in a patient with a Glasgow Coma Scale (GCS; see *Table 18.1.1*) score of 15 is 79% with a specificity of 8%.
  - » Sensitivity decreases to 51% with GCS 14, and 32% with GCS 13.
- Concerning signs include:
  - » Abdominal tenderness or bruising
  - » Lacerations over the torso
  - » Seatbelt sign
  - » Abdominal tenderness or rigidity
  - » Abdominal distension
  - » Referred shoulder pain
  - » Vomiting

Investigations

- Commence investigations only once initial management has been completed (see "Initial Management," below).

CT Scan

- CT scan is the imaging of choice in hemodynamically stable patients.
  - » There is no increased benefit to using oral contrast.
  - » The split bolus method allows arterial and venous enhancement with a single scan.
    - › The first slow bolus provides solid organ, portal, and venous enhancement.
    - › The second faster bolus provides angiographic enhancement.
- For isolated abdominal injuries, the rate of intraabdominal injuries after a negative CT scan is 0.19% with a negative predictive score (NPV) of 99.8%.
- There is a concern regarding radiation dose in patients having CT scans; the use of the Pediatric Emergency

Care Applied Research Network (PECARN) criteria for reducing the need for abdominal CT scans may be helpful.

- CT scan may be omitted if patient:
  › Is GCS ≥ 14
  › Has no complaints of abdominal pain
  › Has no history of vomiting after the injury
  › Has no abdominal tenderness
  › Has no thoracic wall trauma
  › Has no abdominal bruising or seatbelt sign
  › Has no absent or decreased breath sounds
» CT scan has a sensitivity of 97%, a specificity of 42.5% and an NPV of 99.9% with the PECARN head injury decision rule.

Ultrasound

- See Chapter 1.8 on point-of-care ultrasound (POCUS).
- FAST scans have not been shown to reduce the number of CT scans.
  » The overall sensitivity of FAST scans ranges from 30% to 90%.
- There are issues regarding the presence of free fluid that can be present in the absence of injury.
  » Physiologic free fluid in pediatric patients is estimated to occur in 6% to 22% of cases.
- FAST scan can be modified or used in combination with clinical exam and laboratory studies to help increase sensitivity and specificity.
  » Positive FAST scan combined with aspartate transaminase (AST) or alanine transaminase (ALT) > 100 IU/L increases the sensitivity to 88% and specificity to 98%.
  » The use of contrast-enhanced ultrasound improves the sensitivity of abdominal scans to detect hemoperitoneum from 91% to 96%.

Management

Initial Management

- Follow the protocols of advanced trauma life support (ATLS) with ABCDE:
  » **A**irway
  » **B**reathing
  » **C**irculation
  » **D**isability
  » **E**xposure
- Complete primary and secondary surveys and attend to life-threatening injuries.
- Obtain trauma panel bloodwork that includes liver enzymes and amylase/lipase.

- An unstable patient or a patient with peritonitis may require an urgent laparotomy.

Further Management

- Involve the pediatric surgeon early in the management of intraabdominal injuries.
- Hospital admission should ideally be at a center that manages pediatric trauma patients.
- 90% to 96% of solid organ injuries can be managed conservatively.
  » Management of blunt liver and spleen injury is dependent on the hemodynamic stability of the patient and not the grade of the injury.
- Regular hemoglobin checks are no longer required once the patient is hemodynamically stable.
  » Repeat testing of hemoglobin in a stable patient has limited utility; instead, rely more on the vital signs and clinical assessment to guide repeat testing.
  » A transfusion threshold of 70 has been shown to be safe.
- For hemodynamically unstable patients, a laparotomy should be considered.
- The following are indications for surgical exploration of the injury:
  » 40 mL/kg blood transfusion in 24 hours
  » Biliary and urine leaks
  » Vascular complications
- Consider angioembolization for vascular assessment and management.
  » The most common sites of bleeding where angioembolization is used are the pelvic area, spleen, and liver.
- Consider endoscopic retrograde cholangiopancreatogram (ERCP) for liver trauma patients with major bile leak injuries.
  » Consider sphincterotomy and stenting to decrease biliary tract pressures
- Manage pain (see Chapter 1.4).

Disposition

- For isolated abdominal injuries and in cases where there is no evidence of intraabdominal injury, patients can be safely discharged home from the emergency department (ED) or after a short observation unit stay.
- The following are criteria for being discharged home safely:
  » Normal CT scan (NPV of 96% to 100%)
  » Asymptomatic
  » No other indication for admission
  » Appropriate follow-up / reliable caregiver

SPECIFIC INJURY PATTERNS

HANDLEBAR INJURIES

- Handlebar injuries are most commonly from bicycle handlebars, but may be from other sources including motorcycles, scooters, quad bikes, and jet skis.
- Handlebar injuries are most common in children 6 to 14 years of age.
- Handlebars can injure other regions as well, but the most common injury site is the abdomen (see Table 18.5.1).

Table 18.5.1. LOCATION OF HANDLEBAR INJURIES IN PEDIATRIC PATIENTS

Site	Incidence of injury
Abdomen	64%
Face	13%
Chest	12%
Thigh	11%

SEATBELT SYNDROME

- Seatbelts syndrome is a triad of abdominal wall bruising, internal abdominal injury, and spinal fractures.
- The prevalence of seatbelt syndrome is difficult to estimate.
  - » Reports vary from 1.3% to 16%.
  - » The highest risk is in children 4 to 9 years of age.
- Abdominal wall bruising where the lap belt was in contact with the abdomen at the time of the injury is a characteristic finding.
- The injury occurs because of improper placement of the lap belt.
  - » In a child, the lap belt rests high on the abdomen when:
    - › The appropriate booster seat is not used
    - › The belt slips from the pelvis to the abdomen
- Injuries result from rapid deceleration force with hyperflexion of the torso, leading to:
  - » Bowel/gastrointestinal (GI) injuries
    - › There is a 9% to 21% risk of solid organ injury.
    - › There is an 11% to 25% risk of bowel injury, most commonly in the small bowel.
      - · In order of most to least likely, the injury may occur in the jejunum, the duodenum, or the ileum.
    - › A CT scan can detect 76% to 98% of bowel injuries.
  - » Spine injuries
    - › Chance fracture may occur from compression of the anterior vertebral body and transverse fracture that extends to the posterior elements.

REFERENCES

Adelgais KM, Kuppermann N, Kooistra J, et al; Intra-Abdominal Injury Study Group of the Pediatric Emergency Care Applied Research Network (PECARN). Accuracy of the abdominal examination for identifying children with blunt intra-abdominal injuries. *J Pediatr.* 2014;165*(6)*:1230–1235.e5. https://doi.org/10.1016/j.jpeds.2014.08.014. Medline:25266346

Berona K, Kang T, Rose E. Pelvic free fluid in asymptomatic blunt abdominal trauma patients: a case series and review of the literature. *J Emerg Med.* 2016;50*(5)*:753–758. https://doi.org/10.1016/j.jemermed.2016.01.003. Medline:26884127

Braungart S, Beattie T, Midgley P, Powis M. Implications of a negative abdominal CT in the management of pediatric blunt abdominal trauma. *J Pediatr Surg.* 2017;52*(2)*:293–298. https://doi.org/10.1016/j.jpedsurg.2016.11.028. Medline:27912976

Bregstein JS, Lubell TR, Ruscica AM, Roskind CG. Nuking the radiation: minimizing radiation exposure in the evaluation of pediatric blunt trauma. *Curr Opin Pediatr.* 2014;26*(3)*:272–278.

Djordjevic I, Slavkovic A, Marjanovic Z, Zivanovic D. Blunt trauma in pediatric patients: experience from a small centre. *West Indian Med J.* 2015;64*(2)*:126–130. Medline:26360685

Ellison AM, Quayle KS, Bonsu B, et al; Pediatric Emergency Care Applied Research Network (PECARN). Use of oral contrast for abdominal computed tomography in children with blunt torso trauma. *Ann Emerg Med.* 2015;66*(2)*:107–114.e4. https://doi.org/10.1016/j.annemergmed.2015.01.014. Medline:25794610

Haasz M, Simone LA, Wales PW, et al. Which pediatric blunt trauma patients do not require pelvic imaging? *J Trauma Acute Care Surg.* 2015;79*(5)*:828–832. https://doi.org/10.1097/TA.0000000000000848. Medline:26496109

Koyama T, Skattum J, Engelsen P, Eken T, Gaarder C, Naess PA. Surgical intervention for paediatric liver injuries is almost history: a 12-year cohort from a major Scandinavian trauma centre. *Scand J Trauma Resusc Emerg Med.* 2016;24*(1)*:139. https://doi.org/10.1186/s13049-016-0329-x. Medline:27899118

Leung VJ, Grima M, Khan N, Jones HR. Early experience with a split-bolus single-pass CT protocol in paediatric trauma. *Clin Radiol.* 2017;72*(6)*:497–501. https://doi.org/10.1016/j.crad.2017.01.004. Medline:28190515

Mahajan P, Kuppermann N, Tunik M, et al; Intra-abdominal Injury Study Group of the Pediatric Emergency Care Applied Research Network (PECARN). Comparison of clinical suspicion versus a clinical prediction rule in identifying children at risk for intra-abdominal injuries after blunt torso trauma. *Acad Emerg Med.* 2015;2*(9)*:1034–1041. https://doi.org/10.1111/acem.12739

Menaker J, Blumberg S, Wisner DH, et al; Intra-abdominal Injury Study Group of the Pediatric Emergency Care Applied Research Network (PECARN). Use of the focused assessment with sonography for trauma (FAST) examination and its impact on abdominal computed tomography use in hemodynamically stable children with blunt torso trauma. *J Trauma Acute Care Surg.* 2014;77*(3)*:427–432. https://doi.org/10.1097/TA.0000000000000296. Medline:25159246

Miele V, Piccolo CL, Galluzzo M, Ianniello S, Sessa B, Trinci M. Contrast-enhanced ultrasound (CEUS) in blunt abdominal trauma. *Br J Radiol.* 2016;89*(1061)*:20150823. https://doi.org/10.1259/bjr.20150823. Medline:26607647

Nataraja RM, Palmer CS, Arul GS, Bevan C, Crameri J. The full spectrum of handlebar injuries in children: a decade of experience. *Injury.* 2014;45*(4)*:684–689. https://doi.org/10.1016/j.injury.2013.07.022. Medline:24321415

Notrica DM. Pediatric blunt abdominal trauma: current management. *Curr Opin Crit Care.* 2015;21*(6)*:531–537. https://doi.org/10.1097/MCC.0000000000000249. Medline:26418761

Sellars ME, Deganello A, Sidhu PS. Paediatric contrast-enhanced ultrasound (CEUS): a technique that requires co-operation for rapid implementation into clinical practice. *Ultraschall Med.* 2014;35*(3)*:203–206. https://doi.org/10.1055/s-0034-1366567. Medline:24871612

Szadkowski MA, Bolte RG. Seatbelt syndrome in children. *Pediatr Emerg Care.* 2017;33*(2)*:120–125. Medline:28141769

TRAUMA

Tummers W, van Schuppen J, Langeveld H, Wilde J, Banderker E, van As A. Role of focused assessment with sonography for trauma as a screening tool for blunt abdominal trauma in young children after high energy trauma. *S Afr J Surg.* 2016;54(2):28–34. Medline:28240501

van As AB. Paediatric trauma care. *Afr J Paediatr Surg.* 2010;7(3):129–133. https://doi.org/10.4103/0189-6725.70409. Medline:20859013

Westgarth-Taylor C, Loveland J. Paediatric pancreatic trauma: a review of the literature and results of a multicentre survey on patient management. *S Afr Med J.* 2014;104(11 Pt 2):803–807. https://doi.org/10.7196/SAMJ.8920. Medline:26038793

Wisner DH, Kuppermann N, Cooper A, et al. Management of children with solid organ injuries after blunt torso trauma. *J Trauma Acute Care Surg.* 2015;79(2):206–214, quiz 332. https://doi.org/10.1097/TA.0000000000000731. Medline:26218687

18.6

Musculoskeletal Trauma I: Introduction and Upper Limbs

Joe Nemeth

GENERAL INTRODUCTION

- Musculoskeletal (MSK) trauma is common in pediatric patients.
  » MSK system is involved in 20% of injuries that require a visit to the ED.
  » Rates of incidence have a bimodal distribution.
    › The first peak occurs in children < 1 year of age.
    › The second peak occurs in teenage children.

- The most common causes of MSK trauma are:
  » Falls
  » Motor vehicle accidents
- Pediatric MSK injuries have unique characteristics.
  » Bones are more porous and vascular than those of adults because of their lower mineral content.
  » The periosteum is flexible.

Table 18.6.1. SALTER-HARRIS CLASSIFICATION SYSTEM
Adapted from Salter and Harris (1963).

Type	Incidence	Radiological findings	Comments	Management
I	6%	• Can be subtle or absent (may only be seen in certain views such as oblique) • Transverse fracture through the epiphysis • Epiphysis separates/displaces from metaphysis • No associated fragments of bone / cortical disruption	None	• Immobilize the fracture (using appropriate splint), apply cold compress, and elevate. • Orthopedic follow-up is not usually necessary unless a reduction is needed. • Distal fibula fractures (most common) can be followed up by the patient's GP as the risk of growth disturbance is extremely low.
II	75%	• Fracture through the physis and proximally through the metaphyseal bone • Triangular-shaped fragment of metaphysis not associated with epiphysis	None	• Carry out a closed reduction and immobilization of the fraction in a splint or cast, apply ice, provide analgesia, and request orthopedic follow-up.
III	7% to 10%	• Fracture line starting at physis, through the epiphysis, and then distally into the articular joint.	• Diagnosis is based on the appearance of the epiphyseal fragment not associated with the metaphyseal fracture. • CT or MRI may be required for appropriate evaluation of full injury.	• Early reduction of the fracture in the ED is important; consult orthopedics for possible open reduction or ORIF.
IV	10%	• Fracture line originates at the articular surface and goes distally into the epiphysis and physis to the metaphysis.	• There is a high risk of growth disturbance (growth retardation).	• Early reduction of the fracture in the ED is important; consult orthopedics, as reduction is usually ORIF.
V	< 1%	• Usually involves the knee or ankle • Fracture due to significant compressive/axial load forces crushing the physis and displacing the epiphysis	• Poor outcomes are common, especially since this type is often misdiagnosed as type I. • History is very important and should point toward type V; a high index of suspicion is needed.	• Immobilize the fracture and request orthopedic consultation with early follow-up to monitor bone growth.

ED emergency department. **ORIF** open reduction and internal fixation.

» Healing occurs more rapidly due to highly vascularized periosteum that is thickened and osteogenic.
» There are unique fracture patterns based on mechanism of injury.
  › Bones bow rather than fracture completely (ulna and fibula).
  › Torus/buckle fractures occur with compression forces (distal radius).
» Epiphyseal plates are weaker than ligaments and tendons.
  › Growth plate injuries are more common (use Salter-Harris classification — see *Table 18.6.1*, above).
  › Dislocations and ligamentous injuries are uncommon.
• Certain mechanisms of injury are more common based on age.
» In patients < 12 months of age, fractures often occur from injury caused by someone else (nonaccidental trauma [NAT], delivery).
» In patients >18 months of age, injuries often occur from activities such as walking and running.
» In teenagers, injuries often occur from sports or high-risk activities.
• Patient's size plays a role in the type of injury.
» The area of injury depends on where the force and impact occurred.

Physical Exam

• Fractures may not be obvious on X-ray, but if the patient is functionally impaired or there is obvious edema of the limb or a fat pad on the X-ray, immobilize the affected area (with splint, not circumferential cast) and arrange for follow-up with a repeat X-ray.
• Always assess neurovascular status before and after splinting/casting a patient.
• Examine the joints above and below the injured area.

Diagnosis

Classification of Pediatric Fractures

• Pediatric fractures may be classified as:
» Plastic deformity
  › A plastic deformity usually occurs in the forearm (radius and/or ulna) and lower leg (tibia and/or fibula).
» Buckle fracture
  › This is a compression fracture that is usually seen at the junction of the metaphysis and diaphysis (could be very subtle on X-ray).
» Greenstick fracture
  › In a greenstick fracture, the bone is bent but the fracture does not traverse the width of the bone.

» Complete fractures:
  › Spiral
  › Oblique
  › Transverse
  › Physeal injuries

Salter-Harris Classification

• The Salter-Harris classification is used to describe physeal (growth plate) bone injuries.
• The classification is based on the extent of a fracture in relation to the metaphysis, physis, epiphysis, and joint.
• The growth plates are weak points in pediatric bones so are at risk of fractures.
• Physeal cartilage is less elastic and therefore less resistant to stress compared to adult bone.
• 21% to 30% of pediatric long bone fractures are physeal.
» The rate of incidence of physeal fractures steadily increases with age, reaching a peak between the ages of 9 and 16 years.
  › The peak in females is between 9 and 12 years of age.
  › The peak in males is between 12 and 15 years of age.
» Physeal injuries are most commonly due to sports (68%), falls (26%), and motor vehicle accidents (6%).
» The most common sites of injury are the distal growth plates of the radius and ulna (due to flexion and extension).
  › The least common site is the distal femur, but fractures to the distal femur can have the highest incidence of complications.
• Radiological films are required for appropriate classification of physeal injuries

Management

• See *Table 18.6.1*.

Complications

• Be aware of complications of fractures that may require further management:
» Physeal arrest
» Nonunion
  › Nonunion is extremely rare in pediatric patients and mainly occurs at the lateral condyle of the distal humerus.
» Delayed union
» Nerve and/or vascular injury
» Compartment syndrome
» Refracture
» Infection
» Myositis ossificans

UPPER LIMB INJURIES

CLAVICLE FRACTURES

- The clavicle has fibrocartilaginous articulation with the sternum (sternoclavicular joint) and the acromion (acromioclavicular joint).
- Fractures usually result from direct or indirect trauma to the shoulder region.
  » The most common cause is a fall on the shoulder.
  » Traffic accidents and sports injuries are commonly involved.
  » Clavicle fractures caused by direct blow to the clavicle and indirect fractures secondary to energy transmitted from a fall onto an outstretched hand (FOOSH) are less common.
- Incidence of clavicle fractures peaks between 13 and 20 years of age.
  » Clavicle fractures are usually displaced in children > 10 years old.
  » They are usually nondisplaced in children < 10 years old.
- Middle-third clavicle fractures have the highest rate of incidence compared to medial-third and lateral-third fractures.
  » Proximal-third fractures account for 5% of clavicular fractures.
    › They result from axial compression of the shoulder toward the midline.
  » Middle-third fractures account for 85% of clavicular fractures.
    › They are usually caused by a fall onto the shoulder.
    › In neonates, this type of fracture is usually from obstetrical causes.
  » Distal-third fractures account for 10% of clavicular fractures.
    › They are caused by force on the apex of the shoulder.

History

- On history, ask about:
  » Well-localized pain that worsens with arm movements
  » Snapping or cracking felt at the time of injury

Physical Examination

- Clavicle fractures are easy to miss in infants and young children if they are not specifically looked for.
- Clavicle fractures are classified according to Allman classification:
  » Group I fracture: middle-third (most common in children)
    › Group I fractures present with:
      · A visible bulge and hematoma.
      · Point tenderness
      · Crepitus and motion of the fragment that can be felt with direct palpation

  » Group II fracture: distal-third
    › Group II fractures can be mistaken for acromio-clavicular joint disruption.
    › They have a point of maximal tenderness that is usually more medial, on the bone and not the joint.
    › They present with pain and tenderness around the acromioclavicular joint that worsens with adduction of the arm.
  » Group III fracture: proximal-third (least common)
    › Group III fractures are usually associated with high-energy trauma (e.g., motor vehicle accident) and head, neck, and chest injuries.
    › They should be suspected in any young individual with medial clavicle or sternoclavicular injury.
    › They may occur with physeal injury (Salter-Harris type I or II).
- Patient should be examined for:
  » Open fractures
  » Tenting of the skin — this can lead to skin necrosis
  » Lung and/or neurovascular damage in the upper extremity
  » Associated injuries secondary to trauma, especially with proximal-third fractures
  » Scapular fracture with high-energy mechanisms

Investigations

- Imaging (X-ray) is the primary type of investigation.
  » Anteroposterior (AP) views are generally sufficient to assess middle-third fractures.
  » 45° cephalic-tilt view can be helpful to better assess the clavicle.
  » Posteroanterior (PA) views of the chest can help compare the fracture to the uninjured side, especially for shortening of the clavicle.
  » Oblique views should be obtained if a distal fracture is suspected.
- Proximal-third fractures are usually occult. A CT scan may be indicated to assess the extent of the fracture and associated injuries.
- Consider bedside ultrasound as a diagnostic tool.

Management

- Most nondisplaced fractures can be treated conservatively with immobilization of the arm in a sling.
- Obtain an orthopedic referral if the patient has:
  » An open fracture or severe tenting of the skin
  » A neurovascular injury
  » Complete fracture displacement (> 100%)
  » A comminuted fracture
  » A shortened clavicle
  » A group III fracture with posterior displacement
- If there is any displacement of the bone, especially in adolescents, consult an orthopedist regarding the possibility of ORIF.

Complications

- Complications of clavicle fractures include:
  » Malunion/nonunion
    › This affects up to one-third of nonoperatively-managed, completely displaced, angulated, or shortened fractures.
  » Subclavian vein or artery compression
  » Brachial plexus injury or thoracic outlet syndrome
  » Callus formation at the fracture site (cosmetic)

HUMERAL SHAFT FRACTURES

- Humeral shaft fractures account for less than 10% of fractures in children, but occurrence varies with age group.
  » The peak rates of incidence are in children < 3 years of age (from falls) and in children > 12 years of age (from sports injuries and trauma).
- These fractures are usually due to a FOOSH or direct trauma to the humerus.
  » A fracture that happens due to a minor trauma should raise suspicion of a pathological fracture (i.e., bone cyst, malignancy, osteopenia).
- Humeral shaft fractures can also be associated with high-energy polytrauma such as motor vehicle collisions.
- In children < 3 years of age, nonaccidental trauma (NAT) should be suspected, especially when the mechanism seems inconsistent with the fracture pattern (see Chapter 1.7).

History

- On history, ask about:
  » The history of the fall or direct trauma to the humerus
  » Midarm pain
- Note that swelling and/or deformity may not be evident.

Physical Examination

- Eliminate associated injuries when the mechanism of injury is significant.
- Conduct a neurovascular examination.
  » Vascular injuries are rare unless there is significant deformity.
  » Radial nerve injuries are more common with displaced fractures or following manipulation.
- Conduct a skin examination.
  » Any wound or puncture in the area should be considered an open fracture.
- If there is significant deformity, look for:
  » Radial nerve injury
  » Vascular injuries

- » "Occult" open fractures
  › Any wound or puncture wound along the arm should be considered a sign of open fracture and treated accordingly.

Investigations

- AP and lateral view X-rays of the humerus are generally sufficient for diagnosis.

Management

- Ensure that the patient has adequate analgesia.
- Immobilize the fracture to prevent further displacement of the bone and for the patient's comfort.
- Obtain an immediate orthopedic consultation for:
  » Open fractures
  » Displacement > 100%
  » Neurovascular injury
  » Grossly displaced fractures or angulation of:
    › More than 20° of varus/valgus
    › More than 20° in sagittal plane
    › More than 15° of rotation
    › More than 2 cm shortening
- Provide orthopedic follow-up in 7 to 10 days for an incomplete or moderately displaced closed fracture.
- Immobilization with a sling and swathe or shoulder immobilizer may be sufficient for minimally displaced or incomplete fractures.
- Completely or moderately displaced fractures can be managed with a sugar-tong splint or hanging cast in older children.

SUPRACONDYLAR FRACTURES

- In children, the supracondylar region of the distal humerus is made of thin, weak bone compared to the elbow joint capsule and collateral ligament.
- Supracondylar fractures account for 3% to 16% of all pediatric fractures, and 60% of elbow fractures.
  » The peak rate of incidence occurs between 5 and 10 years of age.
- This type of fracture is caused by a forced extension mechanism with axial loading (FOOSH in 70% of cases).
  » The older the child is, the higher the energy required to produce a facture.
  » 5% of supracondylar fractures are flexion-type injuries.
    › These are caused by direct posterior-anterior force on a flexed elbow (i.e., fall onto a flexed elbow).

History

- On history, ask about:
  » History of a fall
  » Elbow pain and refusal to move the joint

TRAUMA

Physical Examination

- Assess the patient for:
  - » Swelling and hematoma around the elbow joint
  - » Antalgic positioning (i.e., flexed elbow, no movement)
- Do not passively move the arm.
- Immobilize the arm before imaging if there is gross bone displacement.
- Perform a neurovascular examination.
  - » Assess the patient's pulse, capillary refill, coloration, and temperature.
  - » Conduct a motor exam: "1-2-3 finger counting" (thumb extension "1," spreading the fingers against resistance "2," pincer grasp/OK sign "3").
  - » Conduct a sensory exam: palmar surface of D1 to D3, dorsal webspace between D1 and D2, and ulnar side of D5.
- Examine skin for open fracture.

Investigations

- Imaging (X-ray) is the primary type of investigation.
- A true lateral X-ray view of the humerus and elbow is generally sufficient to make the diagnosis.
- On a normal X-ray, the anterior humeral line (traced along the anterior side of the humeral shaft) should cross the middle third of the capitulum and the radio-capitular line (line drawn parallel to the radius shaft, in its center), then pass through the center of the radial head and the capitulum.
- On lateral X-rays, the fracture line is usually seen at the distal humerus.
  - » Follow the anterior humeral line, which should cross the middle third of the capitulum.
  - » Assess the radiocapitellar line.
    - › Any disruption in that line may indicate a fracture-dislocation.
- On AP X-rays, the fracture line is typically transverse and seen on the distal humerus, through the olecranon fossa.
- Indirect signs of fracture include:
  - » Any posterior fat pad
  - » Sail sign (enlarged anterior fat pad)
  - » Anterior humeral line anterior to the capitulum or passing through its anterior third
  - » Misalignment of the radial head, neck, and capitulum (radiocapitular line disrupted) indicates a fracture-dislocation
- Assess the ossification centers of the elbow.
  - » Knowing the ossification centers helps to distinguish fractures from growth centers on X-rays.
  - » Order of ossification (CRITOE):
    - › **Capitulum** (ossification occurs at approximately age 1)

- › **Radial head** (age 3)
- › **Internal epicondyle** (age 5)
- › **Trochlea** (age 7)
- › **Olecranon** (age 9)
- › **External epicondyle** (age 11)
  - » Make sure no ossification center is "missing" and that no new one has been "created."
  - » Always obtain AP and lateral views of the forearm (common site for associated injuries).
- Look for the following items:
  - » Brachial artery injury
    - › This artery can be cut during initial injury or during manipulation of bony fragments.
    - › An intimal tear can cause vascular insufficiency and thrombosis.
    - › This is more common with posterolateral displacement.
      - · Median nerve injury (including anterior interosseous branch) is frequently associated.
  - » Compartment syndrome (see Chapter 6.1)
  - » Elbow dislocation
  - » Forearm and wrist fractures
    - › Fracture of the forearm, especially the distal radius, coexists in up to 5% of supracondylar fractures.
  - » Median nerve injury
    - › This is more common with posterolateral displacement.
    - › It is characterized by weakness of flexion in the hand, weak pincer grasp.
    - › Patients experience loss of sensation on the palmar surface of D1-D2-D3.
  - » Radial nerve injury
    - › This is more common with posteromedial displacement.
    - › It is characterized by weakness of wrist extension and thumb extension ("thumbs-up" sign).
    - › Patients experience loss of sensation over webspace between D1 and D2.
  - » Ulnar nerve injury
    - › This is more common with flexion-type injuries.
    - › It is characterized by weakness of wrist flexion and finger spreading ("high-five" sign)
    - › Patients experience altered sensation on ulnar side of D4 to D5.
- Supracondylar fractures are classified according to Gartland classification:
  - » Gartland type I — minimal displacement, usually greenstick or torus fracture
    - › Type I fractures can be occult with only indirect signs of effusion on imaging.
    - › The anterior and posterior humeral lines are intact.
  - » Gartland type II — displacement, posterior cortex intact

> › A component of rotation is possible.
> › The anterior humeral line crosses the capitulum anteriorly.
> » Gartland type III — disrupted anterior and posterior cortex
>> › The fracture is displaced posterolaterally (most common), posteromedially, or anterolaterally (usually flexion-type injury).

Management

- Provide appropriate analgesia and possible splinting before imaging.
- Do not manipulate the bony fragments.
- Obtain an urgent orthopedic referral for:
  - » Open fracture
  - » Neurovascular compromise
  - » Gartland type II or III supracondylar fracture
  - » Evidence or suspicion of compartment syndrome
- Specific management is based on the type of fracture:
  - » Gartland type I — Immobilize the fracture with posterior splint and sling.
    - › Avoid circumferential casts due to risk of compartment syndrome.
    - › Obtain an orthopedic consult within 7 days.
  - » Gartland type II — Perform a closed reduction with cast.
    - › Surgery is required if the fracture is irreducible.
  - » Gartland type III — Consult orthopedics for ORIF.
  - » Flexion-type injury — Because they are more unstable, they are more likely to require fixation.

FOREARM FRACTURES

- The radius and ulna are joined together by the proximal radioulnar joint, distal radioulnar joint, interosseous membrane, and annular ligament around the radial head.
- Imaging (X-ray) is the primary type of investigation.
  - » All identified forearm fractures should have AP and true lateral wrist and elbow X-rays.

MONTEGGIA FRACTURES

- The peak rate of incidence of Monteggia fractures occurs between 4 and 10 years of age, although Monteggia fractures are rare in children (< 1% of forearm fractures).
- A Monteggia fracture is defined as:
  - » Fracture of the proximal third of the ulna or plastic deformation of the ulna
  — and —
  - » Dislocation of the radial head
- Suspect this type of fracture if the patient has a history of FOOSH or has sustained a direct blow to the ulna.

- Monteggia fractures are classified according to Bado classification:
  - » Bado type I (most common type in children) — proximal ulnar shaft fracture with apex displaced anteriorly with anterior radial head dislocation
    - › A type I–equivalent injury consists of a radial head fracture rather than dislocation.
  - » Bado type II — ulnar shaft fracture apex and radial head dislocation are directed posteriorly
    - › Occasionally, the elbow can dislocate posteriorly, a type II–equivalent injury.
  - » Bado type III — fractured ulnar metaphysis with radial head dislocated laterally
  - » Bado type IV — fractured ulnar and radial shafts with radial head dislocated anteriorly

Physical Exam

- Patient has a decreased range of motion at the elbow.
- Patient has pain with mobilization and palpation of the forearm and elbow joint.

Investigations

- Imaging should include AP and true lateral forearm X-rays.
  - » Look for:
    - › Posterior interosseous nerve neurapraxia in up to 10% of cases
    - › Weakness of fingers in extension
    - › Sensory deficit on the dorsal aspect of the wrist

Management

- Request urgent consultation with a pediatric orthopedist.
- Perform a closed reduction of the ulna and radial head dislocation with long-arm casting for Bado fracture types I, II, and III.
  - » Immobilize the fracture in flexion-supination.
- For Bado type IV fractures, unstable fractures, or delay in diagnosis, operative management is warranted.

Complications

- Neurapraxia is a complication in 10% of cases (posterior interosseous nerve).
  - » It usually resolves spontaneously.
- Delay in diagnosis or misdiagnosis can lead to chronic instability or decreased range of motion of the elbow.

GALEAZZI FRACTURES

- The peak rate of incidence of Galeazzi fractures occurs between 9 and 13 years of age — less frequent than in the adult population.
- This type of fracture usually results from axial loading of the forearm with extreme supination or pronation; FOOSH is the most common mechanism.

- Galeazzi fractures are missed in more than one-third of cases.
- This type of fracture is defined as:
  » Distal radius fracture
  — and —
  » Concomitant disruption of the distal radioulnar joint (DRUJ)
    › DRUJ injury in the pediatric population can present as a displaced ulnar physeal injury or a dislocation of the distal ulna; the ulnar shaft is intact.
- Galeazzi fractures are classified as:
  » Type I: dorsal displacement of the distal radius (usually results from pronation)
  » Type II: volar displacement of the distal radius (usually results from supination)

Physical Exam

- Assess patient for:
  » Radial deformity
    › Sometimes a deformity or prominence of the ulnar head can be seen.
  » Limitation of wrist motion and pain with mobilization
  » Pain upon palpation of the wrist
  » Neurovascular symptoms
- Conduct a DRUJ instability test.
  » Anterior-posterior shearing force is applied to the distal ulna and radius.
  » A positive test, pain, or more instability compared to the contralateral side indicates disruption of the DRUJ.

Investigations

- Imaging (X-ray) is the primary type of investigation.
  » AP and true lateral X-rays of the wrist and proximal forearm are essential to diagnosis.
  » Contralateral side views are often helpful for comparison.
  » Findings include:
    › Displaced distal radial shaft fracture
    › DRUJ disruption signs (subtle)
    › Widened DRUJ on AP view
    › Ulnar styloid fracture
    › Shortening of the radius by 5 mm or more

Management

- Request urgent consultation with an orthopedic surgeon.
- Closed reduction and casting in young children is recommended; internal fixation is recommended for adolescents.

BUCKLE FRACTURES

- The peak rate of incidence for this type of fractures occurs at around 5 to 10 years of age, before the pubertal growth spurt.
- Torus fractures occur most commonly at the distal radius.
  » The typical mechanism is FOOSH.
  » Buckle factures can also occur at the distal tibia, fibula, and femur.

Physical Exam

- Assess patient for:
  » Soft tissue swelling
  » Point tenderness over bony injury
- A mass over the fracture area may be palpable.

Investigations

- Radiological findings may be subtle, as distinct fractures are not seen.
  » Inspect the metaphyseal contour for any deformities in the cortex, such as:
    › Asymmetry
    › Bulging
    › Deviation from the cortical margin
  » Look for soft tissue swelling.
  » Oblique views may help with diagnosis.

Management

- Reduction is usually not required unless there is significant angulation.
- Immobilize the fracture in a splint and follow-up with GP or orthopedics.
  » Follow-up after 1 week if reduction was needed.
- Removable splints are associated with less pain and repeat visits due to problems with the cast.
- Simple torus fracture of distal radius does not require orthopedics follow-up.

ACKNOWLEDGEMENT

The author would like to acknowledge Dr. Caroline Hosatte-Ducassy and Dr. Anali Maneshi for their assistance with this chapter.

REFERENCES

Black KJ, Duffy C. Musculoskeletal disorders in children. In: Tintinalli JE, Stapczynski JS, Ma OJ, et al, editors. *Tintinalli's emergency medicine: a comprehensive study guide.* 8th ed.; 2016.

Caine D, DiFiori J, Maffulli N. Physeal injuries in children's and youth sports: reasons for concern? *Br J Sports Med.* 2006;40(9):749–760. https://doi.org/10.1136/bjsm.2005.017822. Medline:16807307

Carson S, Woolridge DP, Colletti J, Kilgore K. Pediatric upper extremity injuries. *Pediatr Clin North Am.* 2006;53(1):41–67, v. https://doi.org/10.1016/j.pcl.2005.10.003. Medline:16487784

Della-Giustina K, Della-Giustina DA. Emergency department evaluation and treatment of pediatric orthopedic injuries. *Emerg Med Clin North Am.* 1999;17(4):895–922, vii. https://doi.org/10.1016/S0733-8627(05)70103-6. Medline:10584108

Herring J. *Tachdjian's pediatric orthopaedics: from the Texas Scottish Rite Hospital for Children.* 4th ed. 3 vols. Philadelphia; 2007.

Khosla S, Melton LJ III, Dekutoski MB, Achenbach SJ, Oberg AL, Riggs BL. Incidence of childhood distal forearm fractures over 30 years: a population-based study. *JAMA.* 2003;290(11):1479–1485. https://doi.org/10.1001/jama.290.11.1479. Medline:13129988

Leary JT, Handling M, Talerico M, Yong L, Bowe JA. Physeal fractures of the distal tibia: predictive factors of premature physeal closure and growth arrest. *J Pediatr Orthop.* 2009;29(4):356–361. https://doi.org/10.1097/BPO.0b013e3181a6bfe8. Medline:19461377

Marx JA, Rosen P. *Rosen's emergency medicine: concepts and clinical practice.* 8th ed.; 2014.

Mencio GA, Swiontknowski MF. *Green's skeletal trauma in children.* 5th ed.; 2015.

Moore KL, Dalley AF, Agur AMR. *Clinically oriented anatomy.* 8th ed.; 2017.

Noonan KJ, Price CT. Forearm and distal radius fractures in children. *J Am Acad Orthop Surg.* 1998;6(3):146–156. https://doi.org/10.5435/00124635-199805000-00002. Medline:9689186

Salter R, Harris WR. Injuries involving the epiphyseal plate. *J Bone Joint Surg Am.* 1963;45(3):587-622.

Villarin LA Jr, Belk KE, Freid R. Emergency department evaluation and treatment of elbow and forearm injuries. *Emerg Med Clin North Am.* 1999;17(4):843–858, vi. https://doi.org/10.1016/S0733-8627(05)70100-0. Medline:10584105

Wu J, Perron AD, Miller MD, Powell SM, Brady WJ. Orthopedic pitfalls in the ED: pediatric supracondylar humerus fractures. *Am J Emerg Med.* 2002;20(6):544–550. https://doi.org/10.1053/ajem.2002.34850. Medline:12369030

18.7

Musculoskeletal Trauma II: Lower Limbs

Joe Nemeth

FEMORAL SHAFT FRACTURES

- The femoral shaft is divided into proximal-third (subtrochanteric), middle-third (midshaft), and distal-third (supracondylar, intercondylar, and condylar) sections.
- Femoral fractures are the most common reason for hospitalization for pediatric orthopedic trauma.
- These fractures are more common in males than in females (2:1).
- More than 60% of femoral fractures in children occur in the shaft.
- There is a bimodal rate of incidence, with an initial peak at 2 to 3 years of age followed by a peak at 17 to 18 years of age.
  - » In children, falls are the most common mechanism of injury.
    - › Relatively low-energy injuries can cause femoral shaft fracture (e.g., fall while running).
  - » In adolescents, higher-energy mechanisms are usually involved due to stronger cortical bone.
  - » In infants and toddlers, the most common causes are falls and child abuse.
    - › Maintain a high level of suspicion for nonaccidental trauma (NAT) in all nonambulating children, especially with an unclear history or trivial mechanism (see Chapter 1.7).
    - › The fracture is usually a distal femur fracture.

- Pathologic causes should be suspected for fractures that result from minor trauma.
  - » Consider the following:
    - › Bone cyst
    - › Fibrous dysplasia
    - › Osteogenesis imperfecta
    - › Malignancy

History

- Patients usually have a history of significant trauma.
- Determine:
  - » How the injury occurred
  - » What kind of energy or forces were involved
  - » What the mechanism was
    - › Consider Waddell's triad: femoral fracture, intrathoracic or intraabdominal injury, and head injury.
- The child may complain of thigh pain, inability to bear weight, and a feeling of instability.
- Younger children may be irritable and refuse to walk.

Physical Exam

- The child may refuse to weight bear on the affected leg.
- Examine the patient for:
  - » Shortening of the affected limb
  - » Gross deformity

» Swelling or hematoma of the thigh
» Pain and/or crepitus on palpation
- Always perform a neurovascular examination and a hip and knee exam.
- Look for associated injuries due to the high energy required to break the femur.

Investigations
- Diagnosis is usually made clinically.
  » Imaging is helpful to classify the fractures and rule out associated injuries.
- Anteroposterior (AP) and lateral X-rays of the femur are generally sufficient for diagnosis.
- Always obtain imaging for the ipsilateral hip and knee to rule out associated injuries.

Management
- In an isolated femoral shaft fracture, analgesia and immobilization are the first steps.
- Treat open fractures with antibiotics and tetanus pro-phylaxis if indicated.
- Consider informing the child protection team if there is suspicion of child abuse or NAT.
  » The American Academy of Orthopedic Surgeons recommends that all children < 3 years of age with a diaphyseal fracture should be evaluated for child abuse.
- Obtain an immediate consultation with a pediatric orthopedist.
- Treatment options depend on the age and size of the patient and the fracture pattern.
  » Children < 6 months of age can usually be treated with a Pavlik harness or spica cast.
  » Spica casting with or without traction is usually con-sidered in children < 5 years of age.
  » Surgical management is required for:
    › Children > 5 years of age
    › Limb shortening > 2 cm
    › Open fracture
    › Multiple fractures or polytrauma
    › Very proximal or distal fractures
    › Length-unstable fractures (spiral or comminuted)

DISTAL FEMORAL FRACTURES
- Leg growth continues until approximately 14 years of age (in female children) to 16 years of age (in male children).
  » Growth of the femur relies on the distal physis, which provides 70% of femoral length and 40% of lower limb growth.
- Metaphyseal fractures (supracondylar femoral frac-tures) are the most common type of distal femoral fracture.

» For distal physeal fractures, Salter-Harris type II is the most common (see *Table 18.6.1*).
- The popliteal fossa (posterior aspect of distal femur and knee joint) contains important neurovascular structures:
  » Popliteal artery and vein
  » Posterior tibial nerve and common peroneal nerve (which travel along the popliteal artery)

Risk Factors
- Distal femoral fractures usually result from high-energy mechanisms.
- Males are more at risk than females.
- The peak rates of incidence occur in older children and teenagers.
- The physis is weaker than the knee ligaments in chil-dren, and it fails under stress.
  » Varus or valgus stress on the knee causes disruption of the physis and a distal physeal fracture.

History
- On history, ask about:
  » High-energy trauma or sports-related injury
  » Inability to walk
  » Pain over the knee or thigh

Physical Exam
- Patient is unable to bear weight on the affected limb.
- Observe the patient for:
  » Pain and swelling of the distal femur and knee joint
  » Tenderness on palpation of the physis
- Look for varus or valgus instability of the knee during the exam.

Investigations
- Obtain AP and lateral X-rays of the knee and entire femur and hip, looking for:
  » Disruption of the bony cortex
  » Soft tissue swelling around the physis
- Oblique and tunnel views might be needed for occult fractures.
- Stress views are not needed as they may exacerbate the instability of the fracture.
- CT scan, MRI, or ultrasound might be warranted in certain clinical contexts, such as history and physical findings that are highly suspicious for distal femoral fracture, but no fracture is seen on the X-rays.
- Doppler ultrasound or CT angiography is warranted in children with signs of vascular injury.
- Review and document these specific items:
  » Popliteal artery injury, especially with displaced epiphysis

› Look for popliteal hematoma and signs of vascular damage.
› Assess pedal and tibialis posterior pulses and temperature, color, and capillary refill of the foot.
» Peroneal nerve injury
› Motor and sensory exam of foot.
› Assess ankle flexion/dorsiflexion and sensation on lateral and superior aspect of foot.
» Other injuries associated with trauma and the possibility of child abuse

Management

- Provide analgesia and immobilization.
- Obtain an immediate orthopedic consultation for:
  » Nondisplaced fractures
    › Nondisplaced fractures require long leg casting with close clinical follow-up.
  » Displaced metaphyseal or Salter-Harris type I or II fractures
    › These fractures require closed reduction and percutaneous pinning.
  » Salter-Harris type III and IV or irreducible fractures
    › These fractures require open reduction and internal fixation (ORIF).
- Consider serial physical examination, Doppler ultrasound, or the ankle-brachial index to evaluate the integrity of the vascularity.
  » Obtain an urgent consultation with vascular surgery if there is a high level of suspicion for vascular injury.
- If the mechanism of injury is suspicious and the patient has significant pain over the distal femur, a close orthopedic follow-up is warranted to assess the patient for a Salter-Harris type I fracture (potential for growth arrest).

TIBIA AND FIBULA FRACTURES

- Tibia and fibula fractures are the most common long bone fractures of the lower extremities.
- They constitute 15% of all pediatric fractures.
- These fractures are most common in males younger than 10 years of age.
- The type of fracture depends on the direction of the force of energy:
  » Direct force — transverse or segmental fracture
  » Indirect force — oblique/spiral fracture
- The most common causes by age include are:
  » < 4 years of age — fall from height, bicycling injury
  » > 4 years of age — motor vehicle accident, being struck by a motor vehicle as a pedestrian
  » Teenagers — sports-related injury
- Nerve or vascular damage with closed injuries is uncommon.

Investigations

- Obtain AP and lateral X-rays, including the ankle and knee views.
- Consider oblique views if the fracture is not visible on standard views and there is a high index of suspicion for injury.

Management

- For proximal tibial metaphysis:
  » Treat with closed reduction with correction of any valgus angulation of greenstick fractures
  » Fracture needs to be immobilized in a long leg cast with the knee in extension
    › This is usually done with adequate sedation or under general anesthesia.
- For tibia/fibula shaft fractures:
  » Treat with closed reduction with specific attention to maintaining tibial length, angulation, and no rotation
  » Immobilize with a long leg cast with the knee flexed 20° to 60°
- Indications for operative treatment include:
  » Segmental fractures
  » Unstable fracture
  » Neurovascular injury
  » Open fracture

TODDLER'S FRACTURE

- A toddler's fracture is an oblique fracture of the distal tibial shaft without a fibular fracture.
- It usually occurs in children 9 months to 6 years of age.
- This type of fracture can be caused by a trivial injury, so the history may not contribute much information.
  » The refusal to weight bear or the presence of a limp may be the only evidence of injury.

Physical Exam

- Exam is unremarkable.
  » Localized tenderness may be found.

Investigations

- Obtain standard AP and lateral X-rays.
- Consider oblique views if the fracture is not visible on standard views as the findings may be subtle.

Management

- If no fracture is identified on X-rays:
  » Immobilize the limb with a long leg cast
  » Redo X-rays in 7 to 10 days
    › Look for subperiosteal thickening suggestive of new bone formation.

ANKLE FRACTURES

- Younger children are more prone to epiphyseal injuries, whereas teenagers have more fractures that resemble adult injuries.
- Distal tibial epiphysis is the second most common epiphyseal injury site (second to the distal radius).
- Ankle fractures may be classified according to the Dias-Tachdjian modification of the Lauge-Hansen classification of pediatric ankle fractures:
  » Supination — inversion
  » Pronation — inversion, external rotation
  » Supination — plantar flexion
  » Supination — external rotation

Investigations

- Obtain the standard 3 views of the ankle on X-ray: AP, lateral, and mortise.
- The Ottawa ankle rules can be used in the pediatric population for children over 10 years of age.
  » These rules have a sensitivity of 98.5% to 100% and sensitivity of 24%.
- Look for pain in the malleolar zone and any of:
  » Bone tenderness at the posterior edge of the lateral malleolus
  — or —
  » Bone tenderness at the posterior edge of the medial malleolus
  — or —
  » Inability to weight bear both immediately and in the emergency department (ED)

Management

- Most ankle fractures can be treated with closed reduction with external immobilization.
- Operative management is indicated for:
  » Open fracture
  » Inability to maintain reduction
  » Displaced intraarticular or physeal fractures

TRIPLANAR FRACTURES

- Triplanar fractures of the distal tibia are caused by external rotation on a supinated foot.
- The average age of injury is 13 to 14 years of age.
- 50% of patients will have an associated fibula fracture.

Investigations

- Obtain standard AP, lateral, and mortise X-ray views of the ankle.
  » Salter-Harris type III is usually seen on AP view.
  » Salter-Harris type II is usually seen on lateral view.
  » AP view will show fracture through the epiphysis with a widened mortise.

Management

- Management is primarily surgical.
  » Nonoperative treatment may be considered if the fracture is minimally displaced (< 2 mm).
  » Immobilize the fracture in a long leg cast with the foot internally rotated.

TILLAUX FRACTURE

- A Tillaux fracture is a Salter-Harris type III fracture of the anterolateral portion of the distal tibia.
  » It is usually seen in patients 13 to 16 year of age due to asymmetrical closure of the distal tibial physis.
- It is caused by external rotation of the ankle.
  » It is often misdiagnosed as a sprain given the typical age of patients.

Management

- Management is closed reduction to reduce displacement of the fracture to < 2 mm.
  » Operative treatment is indicated if closed reduction is unsuccessful.

FOOT FRACTURES

- The most common fractures of the foot occur at the metatarsals (MTs).
  » Most foot fractures occur in MT 2 to MT 5.
  » About 10% of fractures occur at the base MT 5.
- Fractures are usually due to:
  » Crush injury
  » Axial loading
  » Fall/jump from a height
  » Repetitive stress (most common with MT 2)

MT 5 FRACTURES

- MT 5 fractures carry a risk of nonunion based on location of the injury (watershed area in Zone II, proximal to mid-MT area):
  » Zone I fracture — avulsion fracture from peroneus brevis
    › Treat Zone I fractures with a short leg cast or boot.
  » Zone II fracture (Jones fracture) — fracture of the proximal diaphysis in the watershed area
    › Immobilize Zone II fractures with a short leg case and advise the patient to not bear weight.
  » Zone III fracture — usually a stress fracture
    › Advise the patient to bear weight as tolerated; no immobilization is recommended.

LISFRANC FRACTURES

- The Lisfranc joint is the tarsometatarsal (TMT) joint.
- Mechanisms of injury include:
  » Impact load while standing on toes

- » Direct heel-toe compression
- » Fall backward while the foot is in a fixed position
- Lisfranc fractures may be classified as:
  - » Type A — total incongruity
    - › The entire TMT joint is shifted.
  - » Type B — partial incongruity
    - › This is the most common pattern in children.
  - » Type C — divergent
    - › MT 1 is displaced medially and the other 4 MTs are displaced laterally.

Investigations

- Obtain standard AP, lateral, and oblique X-rays.
  - » Weight bearing can help accentuate abnormalities.
- Look for the following specific X-ray findings:
  - » On oblique view:
    - › Alignment of lateral border of MT 1 with medial cuneiform
    — and —
    - › Medial aspect of MT 2 lined up with medial aspect of medial cuneiform
  - » Fracture at the base of MT 2
  - » Separation ≥ 2 mm between the base of MT 1 and MT 2

Management

- Management can be conservative if displacement is < 2 mm and the fracture can be reduced anatomically.
- Otherwise, operative management is necessary.

ACKNOWLEDGEMENT

The author would like to acknowledge Dr. Caroline Hosatte-Ducassy and Dr. Anali Maneshi for their assistance with this chapter.

REFERENCES

Clare MP. Lisfranc injuries. *Curr Rev Musculoskelet Med.* 2017;10(1):81–85. https://doi.org/10.1007/s12178-017-9387-6. Medline:28188544

Dowling S, Spooner CH, Liang Y, et al. Accuracy of Ottawa Ankle Rules to exclude fractures of the ankle and midfoot in children: a meta-analysis. *Acad Emerg Med.* 2009;16(4):277–287. https://doi.org/10.1111/j.1553-2712.2008.00333.x. Medline:19187397

Herring JA. *Tachdjian's pediatric orthopedics: from the Texas Scottish Rite Hospital for Children.* 5th ed. Philadelphia, PA: Elsevier/Saunders; 2014.

Lau S, Bozin M, Thillainadesan T. Lisfranc fracture dislocation: a review of a commonly missed injury of the midfoot. *Emerg Med J.* 2017;34(1):52–56. https://doi.org/10.1136/emermed-2015-205317. Medline:27013521

Llopis E, Carrascoso J, Iriarte I, Serrano MP, Cerezal L. Lisfranc injury imaging and surgical management. *Semin Musculoskelet Radiol.* 2016;20(2):139–153. https://doi.org/10.1055/s-0036-1581119. Medline:27336449

McTimoney M, Purcell L; Canadian Paediatric Society Paediatric Sports and Exercise Medicine Section. Ankle sprains in the paediatric athlete. *Paediatr Child Health.* 2007;12(2):133–135.

Mencio GA, Swiontkowski MF. *Green's skeletal trauma in children.* 5th ed. Philadelphia, PA: Elsevier/Saunders; 2015.

Ribbans WJ, Natarajan R, Alavala S. Pediatric foot fractures. *Clin Orthop Relat Res.* 2005;(432):107–115. https://doi.org/10.1097/01.blo.0000156451.40395.fc. Medline:15738810

18.8

Pediatric Burns

Haley F. M. Augustine, Matthew Choi

- The highest fatality rate from burns in the pediatric population occurs in patients between 0 and 5 years of age.
- Scalds and flame are the major causes of burns (accounting for 50% of burn-related admissions).
- Contact burns are common in the pediatric population (e.g., fireplace, heating elements).
- There is a trend of decreasing incidence of accidental burns.
- The rate of incidence of intentional burns is 1% to 4.2% of cases.

- Types of burns:
  - » Scald
  - » Flame
  - » Contact
  - » Chemical
  - » Electrical
  - » Inhalation
  - » Frostbite (see Chapter 20.1)

Physical Exam

- Burn severity is classified based on the depth of penetration:

» First-degree
  › First-degree burns are confined to the epidermis.
  › They are painful, erythematous, and they blanche to the touch.
» Second-degree (partial thickness):
  › Superficial second-degree (superficial partial thickness)
    · The superficial dermis is affected.
    · These burns are painful, blanche to the touch, and often blister.
    · They reepithelialize without skin-grafting surgery.
  › Deep second-degree (deep partial thickness)
    · The deep dermis is affected.
    · These burns are painful to pinprick.
    · Deep second-degree burns reepithelialize but involve a prolonged healing time and increased scar burden.
    · Treat deep second-degree burns with surgical debridement and skin grafting.

Note: It is difficult to differentiate superficial and deep second-degree burns on first assessment.

» **Third-degree (full thickness)**
  › Third-degree burns are hard, leathery, painless, and have no hair follicles.
  › They reepithelialize from wound edges but have an exceedingly long healing time and excessive scar burden.
  › Treat third-degree burns with surgical debridement and skin grafting.

Management

Initial Management

- Burns should be treated as a trauma activation — first evaluate and manage the patient's ABCs and intervene as needed.
- Remove all the patient's clothing, evaluate the extent of injuries, then cover the patient for warmth.
- Assess specific issues related to burns:
  » Inhalational injury
    › Assess patients for tachypnea, stridor, hoarseness, singed nasal hairs, and carbonaceous sputum.
    › Full-thickness circumferential burns to the chest may require an escharotomy to assist with ventilation.
    › Obtain bloodwork to assess for inhalation injury, including arterial blood gas (ABG) and carboxyhemoglobin.
    › Pulse oximetry may be falsely normal.
  » Fluids
    › Obtain immediate intravenous access for bloodwork and fluid resuscitation.
    › Insert a urinary catheter to monitor urine output as a measure of resuscitation.
  » Temperature
    › Keep the patient warm after burn assessment.
    › Do not place cooling objects on the burn as this causes hypothermia.
  » Burns
    › Estimate total body surface area (TBSA) and depth of burns (first-, second-, or third-degree).
      · Note that only second- and third-degree burns are included in the TBSA calculation.
      · See *Figure 18.8.1*.
    › The TBSA calculation guides resuscitation.
    › Circumferential burns may require urgent escharotomy.

Other Aspects of Management

- To manage pain:
  » Provide early and adequate analgesia -This is important for lasting psychological effects.
  » Administer nonsteroidal anti-inflammatory drugs (NSAIDs) and acetaminophen with or without morphine or another opioid analgesic
- Use appropriate dressings.
  » Use antimicrobial dressings to keep the burn moist and minimize the microbial burden.
    › Consider Bactigras and Polysporin.
    › Consider silver-based dressings: Acticoat, Aquacel Ag, Mepilex Ag, Flamazine.
  » Consult plastic surgery to determine their recommendations for dressing coverage and for evaluation for surgery.
- Antibiotics are not routinely given.
- Obtain a tetanus vaccine update.
- **Transfer patient to a burn center if**:
  » The TBSA of second-degree (partial thickness) burns is > 10% (see *Figure 18.8.1*)
  » The patient has third-degree (full thickness) burns
  » The burn is chemical or electrical
  » The burn is an inhalation injury
  » The burns involve the face, hands, feet, genitalia, perineum, major joints
  » There is concomitant trauma, with the burn posing the greatest risk to the patient
  » There are preexisting medical conditions affecting mortality
  » The current facility lacks qualified personnel or equipment for care of burned children
  » The patient requires special social, emotional, or rehabilitative support

The Lund and Browder Burn Chart

- Use the Lund and Browder burn chart (*Figure 18.8.1*) to determine TBSA.
  » Body surface area distribution varies with anthropomorphic differences through infancy and childhood.

» The Lund and Browder burn chart is the most accurate method of estimating TBSA.

» Only include second- and third-degree burns in the TBSA calculation.

Figure 18.8.1. LUND AND BROWDER BURN CHART

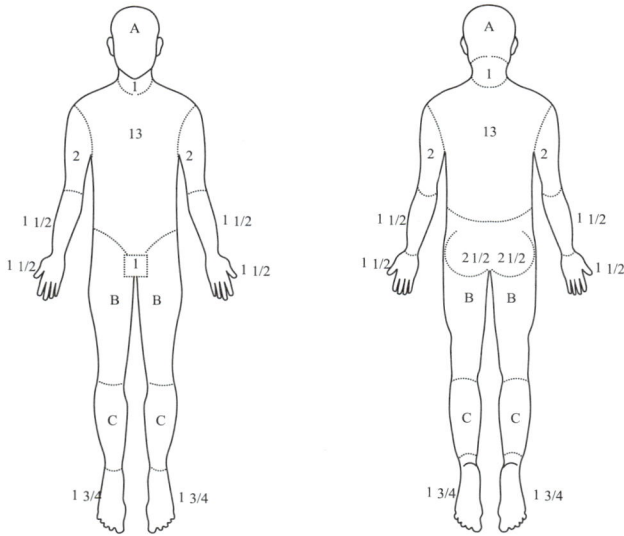

Area	Age					
	0	1	5	10	15	Adult
A = half of head	9 ½	8 ½	6 ½	5 ½	4 ½	3 ½
B = half of one thigh	2 ¾	3 ¼	4	4 ½	4 ½	4 ¾
C = half of one lower leg	2 ½	2 ½	2 ¾	3	3 ¼	3 ½

Region	Partial-thickness / second-degree burns (%)*	Full-thickness / third-degree burns (%)
Head		
Neck		
Anterior trunk		
Posterior trunk		
Right arm		
Left arm		
Buttocks		
Genitalia		
Right leg		
Left leg		
Total burn		

*Do not include erythema or first-degree burns

Investigations

- Obtain laboratory studies:
  » Complete blood count (CBC)
  » Electrolytes (monitor K+), extended electrolytes
  » Urea, creatinine
  » Arterial blood gas (ABG)
  » Carboxyhemoglobin
  » Lactate
  » Coagulation parameters
  » Creatine kinase
  » Liver function tests
- Obtain, as indicated:
  » Chest X-ray (CXR)
    › CXR is typically normal in the early stages of inhalation injury.
  » Electrocardiogram (ECG) and urine analysis (if burn is electrical)
    › Look for signs of hyperkalemia on ECG and rhabdomyolysis on urine analysis.
  » Compartment pressures (if compartment syndrome is suspected)
    › See Chapter 6.1 on compartment syndrome.

RESUSCITATION TREATMENT

BURN SHOCK

- Burn shock occurs in pediatric patients with TBSA > 10%.
- Note that children have a small circulating volume.
- Delays as short as 30 minutes may result in profound shock and worse outcomes.

Pathophysiology

- Burn shock is caused by shock-related systemic capillary leak in response to burn injury.
- It continues 18 to 24 hours after the injury.
- Resuscitation is required in addition to maintenance fluids.

Management

Fluid Management

- Ringer's lactate is the ideal fluid for fluid management.
- For children < 1 year of age, add dextrose solution (D5W ½ normal saline).
  » Sodium supplementation may be required.
- The Parkland formula is used to calculate 24-hour fluid requirement:
  » Fluid requirement = 4 mL × weight (kg) × % TBSA burned
    › Half the fluid volume is administered during the initial 8 hours of treatment from the time of injury.
    › The second half is given during the subsequent 16 hours.
    › Continue to monitor urine output as a marker of resuscitation.

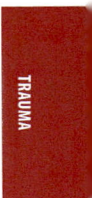

TRAUMA

Resuscitation Monitoring

- Evaluate pulse pressure, mental status, extremity color, and capillary refill.
- A urinary catheter is essential for burns > 20% TBSA.
  - » Titrate fluids to urine output of 1 mL/kg per hour (2 mL/kg per hour in infants).
- Late signs of hypovolemia are:
  - » Hypotension
  - » Decreased urine output
  - » Tachycardia
- Obtain bloodwork; ABG with pH base deficit or lactic acid reflects tissue perfusion.

SPECIFIC TYPES OF BURNS

INHALATION INJURY

- Inhalation injury is the primary contributor to burn mortality.

Physical Exam

- On physical exam, check patient for:
  - » Facial burns
  - » Singed nasal hair
  - » Carbonaceous sputum
  - » Altered mental status (agitation or stupor)
  - » Respiratory distress (dyspnea, stridor, hoarseness, wheezing)
  - » Elevated carboxyhemoglobin level (> 10%)
  - » Hoarseness
  - » Pharyngeal erythema and edema
  - » Smoke inhalation
    - › Smoke inhalation may result in carbon monoxide poisoning with hypoxia.
    - › Carboxyhemoglobin levels are > 10% in carbon monoxide poisoning.
      - · See Chapter 19.16 on carbon monoxide toxicity and management.
    - › Measure ABG and carboxyhemoglobin levels.

Management

- Place the patient on 100% oxygen.
- Secure the patient's airway immediately if signs of obstruction are present. Provide:
  - » Ventilator support
  - » Humidification of 100% oxygen
  - » Antibiotics for any signs of infection
- Consider early intubation in the following situations:
  - » Signs and symptoms of severe inhalation injury
  - » Large burns resulting in airway edema and requiring large volumes of fluid resuscitation
    - › Children are more prone to airway obstruction due to smaller trachea aperture.
  - » Anticipated long transfer time between hospitals

- Inhalation injuries have higher fluid resuscitation requirements.
- Consider bronchoscopy with pulmonary toilet.

FACIAL BURNS

- Burns to this vascular area of the body result in excessive edema.
- Elevate the head of the bed.
- Conduct a full eye exam, including fluorescein staining to evaluate the patient for corneal injury.
- Obtain an ophthalmology consult if there is ocular involvement.

COMPARTMENT SYNDROME

- See Chapter 6.1 for more information on compartment syndrome.
- Evaluate patients with circumferential burns for compartment syndrome.
- Signs and symptoms of compartment syndrome are:
  - » Pain on passive stretching
  - » Tense compartments on palpation
  - » Paresthesia
  - » Absent pulses
- The decision to intervene should be based on the clinical indications.
  - » If there are circumferential third-degree burns, escharotomy (incision through burn eschar) is advised in anticipation of massive fluid shifts with edema and compartment syndrome.
  - » A pressure testing of > 30 mmHg is an indication for fasciotomy (incision through fascia).

ELECTRICAL BURNS

- Electrical burns are typically high-voltage injuries (> 1000 volts) when all ages are considered.
- Pediatric electrical burns are often low-voltage household injuries (e.g., outlets, chewing on cords).
- Contact points have a higher risk of compartment syndrome.
- Monitor the patient's electrolytes, particularly potassium, and watch for acidosis.

ORGAN-SPECIFIC ELECTRICAL BURN INJURIES

- For cardiac injuries, initiate cardiac monitoring and workup (ECG, troponins, creatine kinase).
- For renal injuries, assess renal function.
  - » Obtain bloodwork: creatinine, urea.
  - » Assess patients for tea-colored urine (suggests myoglobinuria).
  - » Maintain adequate urine output to minimize myoglobin precipitation.
    - › This may require bicarbonate or mannitol.

NONACCIDENTAL INJURY

- See Chapter 1.7 for more information on nonaccidental injury.
- Maintain a high degree of suspicion in pediatric burn cases, including:
  - » Inconsistent history
  - » Delay in treatment
  - » Pattern of injury (e.g., cigarette burns, immersion burns, concomitant injuries)
- Maintain a low threshold for contacting children's aid services.

REFERENCES

Advanced Burn Life Support Advisory Committee. *Advanced burn life support course: provider manual.* Chicago, IL: American Burn Association; 2007.

American College of Surgeons Committee on Trauma. Guidelines for the operation of burn centers. In: American College of Surgeons Committee on Trauma, editor. *Resources for optimal care of the injured patient.* Chicago, IL: American College of Surgeons, 2006.

Feldman JJ. Facial burns. In: McCarthy JG, editor. *Plastic surgery.* vol. 3. Philadelphia, PA: WB Saunders; 1990.

Herndon D, et al. *Total burn care.* 4th ed. Philadelphia, PA: Saunders-Elsevier; 2012.

Hettiaratchy S, Papini R. Initial management of a major burn: II—assessment and resuscitation. *BMJ.* 2004;329*(7457)*:101–103. https://doi.org/10.1136/bmj.329.7457.101. Medline:15242917

Spinks A, Wasiak J, Cleland H, Beben N, Macpherson AK. Ten-year epidemiological study of pediatric burns in Canada. *J Burn Care Res.* 2008;29*(3)*:482–488. https://doi.org/10.1097/BCR.0b013e3181776ed9. Medline:18388560

18.9

Genitourinary Trauma

Kirstin Weerdenburg

- The majority of genitourinary (GU) injuries are the result of blunt trauma and can be associated with injury to other systems.
- The most frequent mechanisms of injury include:
  - » Motor vehicle and pedestrian collisions (most common)
  - » Falls
  - » Sports-related incidents (cycling, water sports)
- Initial management should follow the principles of acute trauma management and/or resuscitation.

Clinical Pitfalls

- Hematuria may be absent in patients with vascular pedicle or penetrating kidney injuries.
- A digital rectal exam is not useful for detecting a urethral injury.
- If urethral damage is suspected, do not insert a Foley catheter blindly (i.e., without obtaining imaging first).
- If suspected urethral damage occurs during Foley catheter placement, **do not** remove the catheter. Perform a retrograde urethrogram.
- Consider child abuse in the differential diagnosis for genital injury.
- Search for a hair tourniquet in unexplained penile or clitoral swelling.

- Vaginal exam is often forgotten on the secondary screen in trauma management.

KIDNEY INJURIES

- The kidneys are the most commonly injured structures in the GU tract.
- Injuries are typically minor and not life threatening, so conservative follow-up is the main management plan.
- Children are considered more susceptible to kidney injury than adults due to:
  - » The relatively larger size of the kidneys in proportion to the abdomen
  - » Inadequate protection of the organs due to weaker abdominal musculature
  - » A pliable rib cage that transmits forces rather than fracturing
  - » Less perinephric fat and fascia
- Kidneys with preexisting disease or conditions can be considered more susceptible to injury, even following relatively mild injury.

Physical Exam

- Kidney injuries can present with the any of the following signs and symptoms:
  - » Hematuria (microscopic or gross)

» Flank tenderness or pain
» Flank hematoma
» Palpable flank mass
» Abdominal tenderness, pain, or rigidity
» Paralytic ileus
» Hypovolemic shock

- Note that hematuria may be absent in patients with vascular pedicle or penetrating kidney injuries.

Classification

- Kidney injury severity is classified according to the injury severity scale devised by Moore, Cogbill, Malangoni, Jurkovich, and Champion (1996) and used by the American Association for the Surgery of Trauma (AAST); we refer the reader to these resources for more details.
- Injuries are graded between I and V, from least to most severe injury.

Investigations

- Urinalysis should be completed in all children with multisystem trauma or suspected isolated kidney injury.
- A CT scan is indicated in children with any of the following:
  » Gross hematuria
  » Microscopic hematuria > 50 red blood cells per high-power field (> 50 RBCs/HPF)
  » Major associated injuries
  » Mechanism of injury with significant deceleration forces
  » Hypotension
- Currently, a CT scan is preferred over conventional intravenous pyelogram.
  » Ultrasound may show disruption of renal parenchyma and free fluid in the abdomen but has poor sensitivity and specificity.

Management

- Use of conservative management is now increasingly accepted in children with blunt renal trauma.
  » Conservative management includes minimally invasive procedures such as percutaneous drainage, stent placement, and angioembolization, as well as observation.
  » Operative management includes laparotomy, renal exploration, and resection.
- Management can vary by center but is usually based on the grade of the injury and the hemodynamic stability of the patient (see *Table 18.9.1*).

Complications

- Possible early complications of kidney injury are:
  » Hemorrhage

» Urine extravasation
» Urinoma formation
» Ureteric obstruction
» Hydronephrosis

- Possible late complications of kidney injury are:
  » Hypertension
  » Arteriovenous fistula
  » Renoalimentary fistula

Table 18.9.1. MANAGEMENT OF KIDNEY INJURIES

Grade	Hemodynamically stable	Hemodynamically unstable
I	• Continued monitoring of urinalysis for hematuria, and if ongoing, consider repeat imaging study	• Evaluate for other causes of hemodynamic instability
II, III	• Admission for observation and continued monitoring of urinalysis for hematuria	• Evaluate for other causes of hemodynamic instability; consider repeat imaging study
IV, V	• Conservative management with admission for observation or use of minimally invasive procedures currently supported in the literature	• Early operative intervention

URETER INJURY

- Injury to the ureter is not common in children with trauma.
- Common sites of injury are:
  » Ureterorenal junction
  » Ureteropelvic junction
  » Ureterovesicular junction
- Injury to the ureter should be suspected in patients with the following injuries:
  » Fracture of the transverse process of the lumbar vertebrae
  » Pelvic fracture
  » Hip fracture
  » Lower rib fracture
  » Splenic laceration
  » Liver laceration
  » Diaphragmatic rupture

Physical Exam

- An enlarging flank mass in the absence of signs of retroperitoneal bleeding can be indicative of urinary extravasation.
- Physical examination may be unremarkable and urinalysis can be normal as the presence of hematuria is inconsistent and is an unreliable sign of this type of injury.

Investigations

- Request a CT scan or intravenous pyelogram.
- A retrograde pyelogram may be more reliable but is rarely performed as an initial evaluation.

Management

- Management depends on the level of injury, with placement of a ureteral stent indicated in most cases.

Complications

- Possible complications of ureter injury are:
  » Urinoma formation
  » Strictures
  » Hydronephrosis
  » Pyelonephritis

URINARY BLADDER INJURY

- Children are more susceptible to urinary bladder injuries due to:
  » Higher location of the bladder in the abdomen compared to adults (risk increases with improperly fastened seat or lap belts)
  » Bladder fullness (if present)
- Injuries can be classified as:
  » Contusion
  » Rupture
  » Extraperitoneal, intraperitoneal, or combined
    › Extraperitoneal injuries are typically associated with pelvic fractures of the anterior ring and are either related to laceration or penetration by the pelvic bone.
    › Intraperitoneal injuries are due to blunt trauma leading to a burst mechanism of a full, distended bladder.

Physical Exam

- Bladder injuries can present with the following signs and symptoms:
  » Abdominal or pelvic pain or tenderness
  » Hematuria (microscopic or gross)
  » Dysuria
  » Inability to void

Investigations

- The best method of evaluation is a retrograde cystogram, which is only done after a retrograde urethrogram to evaluate the patient for urethral injury.
- Cystography is indicated in children with:
  » Gross hematuria
  » Inability to void
  » Abnormal external GU examination
  » Multiple associated injuries
- Conventional cystography has been found to be more accurate than CT cystography at distinguishing intraperitoneal from extraperitoneal bladder injury.
  » CT cystography is often recommended when trauma patients are undergoing CT scanning for other associated injuries.

Management

- Management depends on the type of injury.
  » Contusions are managed conservatively with or without urethral catheterization.
  » Extraperitoneal injuries are typically managed non-operatively, with a urethral catheter or suprapubic drainage.
  » Intraperitoneal injuries are managed operatively.
- Bladder injuries may be missed on a CT scan if retrograde filling is not used to distend the bladder.

Complications

- Possible complications of urinary bladder injury are:
  » Infection
  » Persistent hematuria
  » Urinary incontinence
  » Bladder instability
  » Fistula

URETHRA INJURY

- The urethra is more frequently injured in males because it is longer and fixed to the urogenital diaphragm.
  » These injuries are classified based on the location (urogenital diaphragm discriminates anterior or posterior position).
- In addition to blunt trauma, injuries to the urethra can be associated with:
  » High-velocity falls onto the perineum
  » Straddle injuries
- Injury to the urethra can be associated with pelvic fractures.
- A digital rectal exam is not useful for detecting urethral injury and is especially limited in supine or obese patients.

Physical Exam

- Injuries to the urethra most commonly present with the following signs and symptoms:
  » Blood at the urethral meatus (considered the hallmark of urethral injuries)
  » Dysuria
  » Inability to void
  » Swelling of the penis as the patient voids
  » Perineal, periurethral, and/or scrotal or labial hematoma and/or edema
  » High-riding prostate in adolescent male patients

Investigations

- All male patients suspected of a urethral injury should have a retrograde urethrogram.
- Evaluation should be initiated in females with blood at the urethral meatus or with resistance upon catheterization.
- A CT scan can be used to evaluate the patient for other injuries as well.

Management

- Blind placement of a urethral catheter is discouraged until the urethra has been evaluated with imaging.
- Management remains controversial due to infrequency of this type of GU injury.
  - » Initial management should ensure drainage of the bladder either by suprapubic cystostomy or urethral realignment (if possible).
  - » Subsequent management in males is based on the location of the injury (anterior or posterior) and the severity, and includes catheter placement and/or immediate or delayed surgical repair.
  - » Subsequent management in females is directed at primary surgical repair of the defect without delay.

Complications

- Possible complications of urethra injury are:
  - » Strictures
  - » Urinary incontinence
  - » Impotence

GENITAL INJURIES

- In males, penile injuries most commonly occur due to blunt trauma, whereas scrotal injury occurs as a result of a straddle or sports injury.
- In females, trauma occurs most commonly due to straddle injury.
- Screen for incidental circulatory compromise (i.e. hair tourniquet).
- It is important to recognize sexual abuse as a possible cause of genital injury in both genders (see Chapter 1.7 on child abuse).

Physical Exam

- Males with injuries to the scrotum, testicle(s), or penis may present with the following signs or symptoms:
  - » Tenderness or pain
  - » Edema
  - » Hematoma
  - » Laceration
- Females may present with the following signs or symptoms:
  - » Vulvar hematoma
  - » Urinary retention
  - » Laceration of the perineum that is either superficial or deep and may involve the vagina, urethra, or rectum

Investigations

- In male patients, ultrasonography can help determine the extent of injury to the scrotum and its contents; however, it should not be relied on to exclude significant injury in a grossly abnormal testicle.
- Examination in females typically requires general anesthetic and may require urethroscopy, cystoscopy, vaginoscopy, and/or proctoscopy.

Management

- Scrotal injures can be observed if mild, but surgical exploration may be required to evacuate a hematoma, control bleeding, and/or repair a ruptured or dislocated testicle.
- Superficial penile shaft lacerations can be repaired with absorbable sutures under local anesthesia or a penile block, whereas more extensive lacerations require surgical consultation.
- Superficial female perineal lacerations can be treated conservatively with sitz baths until healed, whereas deep lacerations may be more extensive and require surgical consultation.

Complications

- Possible complications of genital injury are:
  - » Infection
  - » Tissue loss/scarring
  - » Infertility
  - » Fistula
  - » Dyspareunia

REFERENCES

Delaney KM, Reddy SH, Dayama A, Stone ME Jr, Meltzer JA. Risk factors associated with bladder and urethral injuries in female children with pelvic fractures: an analysis of the National Trauma Data Bank. *J Trauma Acute Care Surg.* 2016;80(3):472–476. https://doi.org/10.1097/TA.0000000000000947. Medline:26713981

Fleisher GR, Ludwig S. *Textbook of pediatric emergency medicine.* 6th ed. Philadelphia, PA: Lippincott Williams & Wilkins; 2010. Chapter 112, Genitourinary trauma; p. 1316–1327.

Henderson CG, Sedberry-Ross S, Pickard R, et al. Management of high grade renal trauma: 20-year experience at a pediatric level I trauma center. *J Urol.* 2007;178(1):246–250, discussion 250. https://doi.org/10.1016/j.juro.2007.03.048. Medline:17499798

LeeVan E, Zmora O, Cazzulino F, Burke RV, Zagory J, Upperman JS. Management of pediatric blunt renal trauma: a systematic review. *J Trauma Acute Care Surg.* 2016;80(3):519–528. https://doi.org/10.1097/TA.0000000000000950. Medline:26713980

Moore EE, Cogbill TH, Malangoni, MA, Jurkovich, GJ, Champion, HR. Scaling system for organ specific injuries. *Curr Op Crit Care.* 1996;2(6):450–462.

Pichler R, Fritsch H, Skradski V, et al. Diagnosis and management of pediatric urethral injuries. *Urol Int.* 2012;89(2):136–142. https://doi.org/10.1159/000336291. Medline:22433843

Toxicology

19.1

General Approach to Poisoning

Qamar Amin

- Most poisonings in younger children are usually accidental and are rarely fatal (i.e., they are unintentional and involve small doses).
- Poisonings in older children are similar to those in adults (i.e., they are intentional and involve larger doses).
- The number of poison-related deaths is small (about 2.5% of annual childhood deaths from unintentional injury).
- The American Association of Poison Control Centers (AAPCC) reports 1.5 million potentially toxic exposures per year for children and adolescents.
- Children < 6 years of age represent 79% of these exposures.
  - » Usually only 1 xenobiotic (poison) is involved.
- Unlike poisoning cases in adults, in pediatric poisoning:
  - » Cases usually do not involve intent to do self-harm or commit suicide
  - » Ingestion is usually nonlethal
  - » The ingested dose is usually small, but careful evaluation is necessary as a single pill can kill
  - » Patients usually present for evaluation within 1 hour or as soon as ingestion is discovered

History

- A thorough history is critical in the evaluation of a poisoned pediatric patient and should be taken from the patient or caregiver and/or prehospital personnel.
  - » Identify empty pill bottles, containers, or packaging of the poison as soon as possible to determine the poison so care can be optimized.
  - » Immediately give special thought to drugs that can kill in small doses (commonly referred to as "one kill pills") such as:
    - › Antihistamines
    - › Clonidine
    - › Toxic alcohols — methanol, ethylene glycol
    - › Methadone
    - › Sulfonylureas
    - › Sustained-release beta-blockers and calcium channel blockers
    - › Tricyclic antidepressants
- Take special care to look for other signs and symptoms of abuse; if abuse is suspected, contact the local Children's Aid Society (see Chapter 1.7).

Management

- The priority of care in a patient with poisoning is to rapidly assess ABCs.
- Consider gastric decontamination and administration of specific antidotes as next steps.
  - » Depending on the presentation, decontamination may be a required first step to prevent spread to healthcare providers.
  - » Most poisons require only supportive therapy; however, specific antidotes exist for some poisons, and should be administered as soon as one has been identified (see *Table 19.1.1*, below).
- Consultation with a toxicologist or poison control center should be undertaken as soon as possible in all ingestions presenting to the ED.

Decontamination

OROGASTRIC LAVAGE

- Orogastric lavage is rarely recommended in the pediatric population.
- It is sometimes used for serious ingestions (e.g., calcium channel blockers, tricyclic antidepressants) in patients who present within the first hour.
- Absolute contraindications include:
  - » Ingestion of caustic substances (risk of perforation)
  - » Non–life-threatening ingestions
  - » Decreased level of consciousness without a secured airway

- Patients should be positioned in a left-lateral decubitus position
- 24F tubes are recommended for toddlers; 20F tubes are recommended for adolescents.

Table 19.1.1. KNOWN ANTIDOTES FOR COMMON SUBSTANCES

Substance	Antidote
ASA	• Urinary alkalinization
Acetaminophen	• N-acetylcysteine (Mucomyst)
Anticholinergics	• Physostigmine (only with severe agitation or delirium and peripheral toxicity)
Anticoagulants	• Vitamin K • Fresh frozen plasma • Octaplex
Beta-blockers and calcium channel blockers	• Calcium chloride / gluconate • Glucagon • Insulin • Intralipid
Carbon monoxide	• Oxygen
Cholinergics	• Atropine • Pralidoxime (2-PAM)
Cyanide	• Hydroxocobalamin • Sodium nitrate
Digoxin	• Digoxin Fab (Digibind)
Heavy metals (arsenic, copper, lead, mercury)	• Dimercaprol • Calcium EDTA • Penicillamine • Succimer
Iron	• Deferoxamine
INH	• Pyridoxine
Opioids	• Naloxone
SSRIs	• Cyproheptadine
Toxic alcohols (methanol, ethylene glycol)	• Fomepizole, ethanol

ASA acetylsalicylic acid. **EDTA** ethylenediaminetetraacetate. **INH** isoniazid. **SSRIs** selective serotonin reuptake inhibitors.

NASOGASTRIC LAVAGE

- Nasogastric (NG) lavage has a better safety margin compared to orogastric lavage; it is proven to be beneficial in reducing the amount of toxin adsorbed in an adult population but is unstudied in the pediatric population.
- It is recommended for use only in patients with serious ingestions who present within the first hour or who have ingested a toxin that has a delayed adsorption.
- 24F tubes are recommended for toddlers; 20F tubes are recommended for adolescents.

ACTIVATED CHARCOAL

- Activated charcoal (AC) is the most popular technique for gastrointestinal (GI) decontamination.
- AC decreases systemic toxicity by adsorbing toxins present in the gastrointestinal tract.
- AC is best used for substances that:
  » Undergo enterohepatic circulation
  » Have a low volume of distribution
  » Have a lower fraction of plasma protein binding
- AC is recommended for use in patients who present within the first hour after ingestion.
  » AC may be considered up to 2 hours post-exposure; consult your local poison control center for advice.
- Calculate the dose as 1 g/kg of body weight.
  » Mixing the charcoal with ice or in a flavored drink may make it more palatable for pediatric patients.
- Major complications may include aspiration, pneumonitis, and vomiting.
  » Antiemetics such as ondansetron or dimenhydrinate are often needed to mitigate and reduce the symptoms of nausea and vomiting.

MULTIPLE-DOSE ACTIVATED CHARCOAL

- Multiple-dose activated charcoal (MDAC) is given every 4 hours for 4 doses.
- It is most commonly indicated for:
  » Theophylline
  » Phenobarbital
  » Dapsone
  » Carbamazepine
  » Quinine
- MDAC carries the additional risk of bowel obstruction.

WHOLE BOWEL IRRIGATION

- Whole bowel irrigation irrigates and propels the toxin through the GI tract for elimination before it can be absorbed systemically.
- It is recommended for use in cases of body packing/stuffing, ingestions of enteric coated substances, and substances that will not bind to AC:
  » Lithium
  » Iron and other heavy metals
  » Sustained-release medications
- To perform whole bowl irrigation, administer polyethylene glycol orally or via an NG tube until rectal effluents are clear.
- Recommended dosing, based on age, is:
  » 9 months to 6 years of age: 25 mL/kg per hour up to 500 mL/hour
  » 6 to 12 years of age: 1000 mL/hour
  » Adolescents: 1500 to 2000 mL/hour

URINARY ALKALINIZATION

- Urinary alkalization with intravenous sodium bicarbonate enhances the elimination of some toxins, most notably salicylates.
- It works on weak acids by increasing ionization; weak acids are trapped in the renal tubules and eventually excreted in the urine.

SALICYLATE POISONING

- In cases of salicylate poisoning, after assessing the pH, potassium, and creatinine:
  » Administer a bolus of sodium bicarbonate — 25 to 50 mL IV of an 8.4% solution over 1 hour
    › Use additional boluses of sodium bicarbonate as needed.
  » Check urine pH every 15 to 30 minutes until the desired pH is achieved, then check hourly to avoid systemic alkalemia
    › The target is to achieve a urinary pH of 7.5 to 8.5.
- Urine output should not exceed 200 mL/hour.
- Urinary alkalinization is discontinued when the salicylate level falls below 1.8 mmol/L.
- See Chapter 19.3 for more on salicylate toxicity.

Specific Antidotes

- Most toxic ingestions require only supportive management; however, there are several substances for which antidotes are available (see *Table 19.1.1*).

Investigations

- Test blood glucose by finger-stick method.
- Consider the following laboratory studies:
  » Serum electrolytes and osmolarity
  » Venous blood gas
  » Lactate
  » Anion gap and osmolar gap calculations
  » Specific toxin levels — acetaminophen, ASA, ethanol
  » Other serum drug levels as needed
- Consider drug screens.
  » Drug screens have no utility in medical management but may be warranted in cases of nonvolitional exposure.
- Consider imaging studies:
  » Electrocardiogram (ECG)
  » Radiography

  › Consider radiography on a case-by-case basis as most toxins are radiolucent
  › The following may be seen on plain film radiography:
    · Chloral hydrate
    · Calcium
    · Drug packets
    · Iron and other metals
    · Neuroleptic agents
    · Sustained-release medications
    · Enteric coated preparations

Disposition

- Typically, a 6-hour observation period is sufficient for observation postingestion in an asymptomatic patient, with reassessments 2 and 4 hours postexposure.
- Some asymptomatic patients may require longer observation periods depending on the particular agent's pharmacological properties (e.g., sustained-release products).
- Poison control centers and hospital pharmacy services should be consulted for advice on the posttreatment management of a patient with poisoning.

Note: Anticipation of instability in stable-presenting patients is of utmost importance in poisoned children as they can decline rapidly (e.g., in cases of a "one kill pill" ingestion).

REFERENCES

Grierson R, Green R, Sitar DS, Tenenbein M. Gastric lavage for liquid poisons. *Ann Emerg Med.* 2000;35(5):435–439. https://doi.org/10.1016/S0196-0644(00)70004-7. Medline:10783405

Höjer J, Troutman WG, Hoppu K, et al; American Academy of Clinical Toxicology; European Association of Poison Centres and Clinical Toxicologists. Position paper update: ipecac syrup for gastrointestinal decontamination. *Clin Toxicol (Phila).* 2013;51(3):134–139. https://doi.org/10.3109/15563650.2013.770153. Medline:23406298

Hollander JE, McCracken G, Johnson S, Valentine SM, Shih RD. Emergency department observation of poisoned patients: how long is necessary? *Acad Emerg Med.* 1999;6(9):887–894. https://doi.org/10.1111/j.1553-2712.1999.tb01235.x. Medline:10490249

Horton DK, Berkowitz Z, Kaye WE. Secondary contamination of ED personnel from hazardous materials events, 1995-2001. *Am J Emerg Med.* 2003;21(3):199–204. https://doi.org/10.1016/S0735-6757(02)42245-0. Medline:12811712

Hostelage C, Meekins P. Decontamination of the poisoned patient. In: Roberts JR, Hedges JR, editors. *Clinical procedures in emergency medicine.* 4th ed., Saunders; 2004. p. 824–40.

Osterhoudt K. The toxic toddler: drugs that can kill in small doses. *Contemp Pediatr.* 2000;17:73–89.

Proudfoot AT, Krenzelok EP, Vale JA. Position paper on urine alkalinization. *J Toxicol Clin Toxicol.* 2004;42(1):1–26. https://doi.org/10.1081/CLT-120028740. Medline:15083932

19.2

Acetaminophen Toxicity

Bandar Baw, Emily Austin

- Acetaminophen (APAP; also called paracetamol) is an over-the-counter medication used to treat mild pain and fever in both pediatric and adult populations; it has minimal anti-inflammatory effects.
- The therapeutic dose is 10 to 15 mg/kg to a maximum dose of 75 mg/kg per day; patients exceeding this amount are at risk of developing either acute (within 8 hours) or multiple supratherapeutic (within 24 hours) toxicity that could lead to hepatotoxicity.
- There are variable strengths and combinations of APAP formulas on the market, some of which are controlled because of opioid components such as codeine, oxycodone, or hydrocodone.
- Most APAP toxicity in children is unintentional; deliberate overdoses are more commonly seen in teenagers and adults.
  - » Accidental APAP overdose in pediatric population often results from miscalculation of therapeutic dose by a caregiver.
  - » APAP-containing combination products (widely available over-the-counter and in prescription formulations) carry an increased risk of leading to APAP toxicity, and an accompanying risk of opioid or other agent toxicity.
- APAP is the leading cause of acute liver failure in North America.
  - » In the United States, 4.7% of isolated APAP overdoses result in death.
  - » Pediatric exposure to APAP as single drug overdose was found in more than 22 000 cases in 2015.

Pharmacology

- Immediate-release APAP is rapidly absorbed by the GI tract; peak serum levels are attained within 30 to 60 minutes after a therapeutic dose.
  - » Sustained-release APAP formulations act more slowly; peak absorption levels are attained about 2 hours after a therapeutic dose.
- In an acute overdose setting, peak plasma concentrations of immediate-release acetaminophen formulas occur at 4 hours.

Toxicology

- At therapeutic doses, approximately 95% of acetaminophen is metabolized through sulfation and glucuronidation pathways into nontoxic metabolites that are then excreted in the urine.
  - » In the pediatric population, the sulfation route is utilized much more than in adults, who rely vastly on the glucuronidation pathway.
  - » The remaining 5% of acetaminophen is metabolized through a different pathway, mainly CYP2E1 (a cytochrome P-450 enzyme found largely in the liver), to produce the toxic metabolite N-acetyl-p-benzoquinone imine (NAPQI).
  - » A much smaller amount (< 1%) is excreted unchanged in the urine.

APAP Metabolism

APAP Metabolism Pathways

- Sulfation 40% to 50%
- Glucuronidation 45% to 50%
- P-450 5% (produces toxic NAPQI)
- Excreted unchanged in the urine (< 1%)

- At therapeutic doses of acetaminophen, only a small amount of NAPQI is made, and the liver has adequate stores of glutathione to bind and detoxify the NAPQI.
- In an overdose, the nontoxic metabolic pathways (sulfation and glucuronidation) become saturated, and more APAP is metabolized through the CYP450 system, producing greater amounts of the toxic byproduct NAPQI.
  - » The increased amount of NAPQI overwhelms the glutathione stores and cannot be adequately detoxified.
  - » Glutathione depletion leads to an increase in reactive oxygen free radicals.
  - » NAPQI goes on to covalently bind proteins, leading to inflammation and the necrosis of hepatocytes.
- In a massive overdose, the parent compound (i.e. APAP, and not the toxic metabolite NAPQI) can lead to toxicity.
  - » APAP acts as an oxidative stressor, inhibiting mitochondrial aerobic metabolism and preventing normal adenosine triphosphatase (ATP) production.

Risk Factors

- Pediatric groups with higher susceptibility to APAP toxicity include:
  - » Children < 2 years of age

> › Children in this age group tend to metabolize more NAPQI through P-450 isoenzymes.
- » Infants and younger patients with acute illness that might leave them acutely malnourished and lacking adequate glutathione replacement
- » Patients with chronic liver disease
- » Patients with induced CYP450 isoenzymes, whether drug-induced (isoniazid, rifampin, phenobarbital, carbamazepine) or due to genetic polymorphism

Physical Exam

- The clinical presentation for acetaminophen toxicity is has 3 stages:
  - » Stage 1
    - › Patients may be clinically asymptomatic at this stage, or present with nausea and vomiting but no abnormalities in liver function.
  - » Stage 2
    - › Stage 2 occurs 8 to 24 hours after ingestion.
    - › Patients appear clinically stable.
    - › Laboratory tests show biochemical evidence of liver injury: aspartate transaminase (AST) and alanine transaminase (ALT) levels of 1000 IU/L.
  - » Stage 3
    - › Stage 3 occurs about 48 hours after ingestion.
    - › Patients develop acute liver failure as a result of liver necrosis and are unable to maintain homeostatic functions.
    - › AST and ALT levels are higher than 10 000 IU/L; evidence of end-organ dysfunction may be apparent (e.g., encephalopathy).
- Massive APAP overdose (1 g/kg) may result in rapid loss of consciousness and severe metabolic acidosis. This is likely because of both inhibiting mitochondrial respiration and pyroglutamic acid (5-oxoproline) additive effects.

Investigations

- Laboratory investigations for patients with suspected APAP poisoning to assess toxicity include:
  - » Serum acetaminophen concentration
    - › In patients presenting with an acute overdose, serum acetaminophen concentration should be measured 4 hours after exposure.
  - » AST or ALT
  - » International normalized ratio (INR)
  - » Creatinine
  - » Lactate
  - » Venous blood gas (VBG) or arterial blood gas (ABG)
- Conduct other investigations as appropriate:
  - » Complete blood count (CBC)
  - » Electrolytes
  - » Blood urea nitrogen (BUN) and creatinine
  - » Glucose
  - » ASA and ethanol levels
  - » Serum osmolality

- » Electrocardiogram (ECG)
- » Chest X-ray as needed

Management

- Because of the effectiveness of N-acetylcysteine (NAC) as an antidote for acetaminophen toxicity, decontamination has much smaller role in an isolated acetaminophen overdose.
  - » Activated charcoal is not indicated unless a patient presents within 1 hour and has a potential multidrug ingestion

N-Acetylcysteine

- NAC has multiple mechanisms of actions for treating acetaminophen-induced hepatotoxicity.
  - » It serves as a precursor to glutathione synthesis.
  - » It donates a sulfur group, enhancing the sulfation pathway.
  - » It is a direct free radical scavenger and nonspecific antioxidant.
  - » It works to improve oxygen supply to hepatocytes.
- Using the Rumack-Matthew nomogram, the acetaminophen level should be plotted to determine the need to start treatment with NAC.
  - » If administered within 6 to 8 hours of an acute acetaminophen overdose, NAC appears to be almost entirely effective at preventing acute liver injury.
  - » Ensure that administration of NAC is started within this time period without delay even before the APAP level or the presence of liver damage has been assessed.
  - » NAC can be helpful even if administered after evidence of hepatotoxicity is present.
- Indications for NAC include:
  - » Acute APAP overdose with APAP level above the treatment line on the Rumack-Matthew nomogram
  - » Supratherapeutic APAP ingestion with elevated AST or ALT
  - » Chronic APAP overdose with elevated AST or ALT, or evidence or liver failure (e.g., elevated INR)
  - » Unknown type or time of APAP ingestion with evidence of liver injury (elevated AST or ALT) and elevated APAP level
- When administering NAC:
  - » Give a loading dose of 150 mg/kg over 1 hour
    - › Follow this with a maintenance dose of 50 mg/kg over 4 hours.
      - · Follow this with 100 mg/kg over 16 hours.
  - » Diluent volume is based on the patient's weight
- Complications associated with IV NAC include:
  - » Nausea and vomiting (associated with PO, not IV)
  - » Nonimmune anaphylactic reaction (anaphylactoid reaction)
  - » Bronchospasm
  - » Hypotension

Liver Transplant

- Acute liver failure due to APAP-induced hepatotoxicity is known to have a mortality of about 30% without liver transplantation.
- Predicting which patients are likely to survive without transplantation is challenging. The most validated and clinically useful set of criteria is the King's College criteria.
  - » King's College criteria are not validated in the pediatric population.
  - » Mortality is known to be 80% to 90% in patients who do not undergo liver transplant and who meet King's College criteria.

King's College criteria for APAP-induced liver failure — Indications for liver transplant

Based on O'Grady, Alexander, Hayllar, Williams (1989).

1. Arterial pH < 7.3 or blood lactate > 3 mmol/L after adequate volume resuscitation, irrespective of the grade

— **or** —

2. Blood lactate > 3.5 mmol/L after volume resuscitation

— **or** —

3. All 3 of:
   - Grade III or IV encephalopathy
   - INR > 6.5
   - Serum creatinine > 300 μmol/L

REFERENCES

Alhelail MA, Hoppe JA, Rhyee SH, Heard KJ. Clinical course of repeated supratherapeutic ingestion of acetaminophen. *Clin Toxicol (Phila)*. 2011;49(2):108–112. https://doi.org/10.3109/15563650.2011.554839. Medline:21370947

Blieden M, Paramore LC, Shah D, Ben-Joseph R. A perspective on the epidemiology of acetaminophen exposure and toxicity in the United States. *Expert Rev Clin Pharmacol*. 2014;7(3):341–348. https://doi.org/10.1586/17512433.2014.904744. Medline:24678654

Bunchorntavakul C, Reddy KR. Acetaminophen-related hepatotoxicity. *Clin Liver Dis*. 2013;17(4):587–607, viii. https://doi.org/10.1016/j.cld.2013.07.005. Medline:24099020

Emmett M. Acetaminophen toxicity and 5-oxoproline (pyroglutamic acid): a tale of two cycles, one an ATP-depleting futile cycle and the other a useful cycle. *Clin J Am Soc Nephrol*. 2014;9(1):191–200. https://doi.org/10.2215/CJN.07730713. Medline:24235282

Fenves AZ, Kirkpatrick HM III, Patel VV, Sweetman L, Emmett M. Increased anion gap metabolic acidosis as a result of 5-oxoproline (pyroglutamic acid): a role for acetaminophen. *Clin J Am Soc Nephrol*. 2006;1(3):441–447. https://doi.org/10.2215/CJN.01411005. Medline:17699243

Green JL, Heard KJ, Reynolds KM, Albert D. Oral and intravenous acetylcysteine for treatment of acetaminophen toxicity: a systematic review and meta-analysis. *West J Emerg Med*. 2013;14(3):218–226. https://doi.org/10.5811/westjem.2012.4.6885. Medline:23687539

Hanly LN, Chen N, Aleksa K, et al. N-acetylcysteine as a novel prophylactic treatment for ifosfamide-induced nephrotoxicity in children: translational pharmacokinetics. *J Clin Pharmacol*. 2012;52(1):55–64. https://doi.org/10.1177/0091270010391790. Medline:21263015

Heard KJ. Acetylcysteine for acetaminophen poisoning. *N Engl J Med*. 2008;359(3):285–292. https://doi.org/10.1056/NEJMct0708278. Medline:18635433

Hinson JA, Roberts DW, James LP. *Adverse drug reactions*. Berlin, Heidelberg: Springer; c2010. Mechanisms of acetaminophen-induced liver necrosis; p. 369–405. https://doi.org/10.1007/978-3-642-00663-0_12.

Lancaster EM, Hiatt JR, Zarrinpar A. Acetaminophen hepatotoxicity: an updated review. *Arch Toxicol*. 2015;89(2):193–199. https://doi.org/10.1007/s00204-014-1432-2. Medline:25537186

Losek JD. Acetaminophen dose accuracy and pediatric emergency care. *Pediatr Emerg Care*. 2004;20(5):285–288. https://doi.org/10.1097/01.pec.0000125655.20443.7a. Medline:15123898

Mowry JB, Spyker DA, Brooks DE, Zimmerman A, Schauben JL. 2015 Annual Report of the American Association of Poison Control Centers' National Poison Data System (NPDS): 33rd Annual Report. *Clin Toxicol (Phila)*. 2016;54(10):924–1109. https://doi.org/10.1080/15563650.2016.1245421. Medline:28004588

O'Grady J, Alexander G, Hayllar K, Williams R. Early indicators of prognosis in fulminant hepatic failure. *Gastroenterol*. 1989;97(2):439–45.

19.3

Salicylates

Patrick Weldon

- Historically, salicylates are a leading cause of fatal poisoning in children. However, rates of poisoning are decreasing due to safety initiatives and increased use of alternative anti-inflammatory/antipyretic medications in the pediatric age group.
- Despite this, significant potential for morbidity/mortality due to salicylate toxicity still exists.
- Epidemiological data from the American Association of Poison Control Centers' (AAPCC) National Poison Data System (2014) shows that:
  - » Of approximately 24 700 reported exposures to salicylates (all forms), there were 15 fatalities
  - » Over 50% of cases were in children < 19 years of age, and of these there were 2 fatalities
  - » There were approximately 5000 cases of intentional ingestion

Pharmacology

- Common forms of salicylates are:
  - » Acetylsalicylic acid (ASA, Aspirin)
    - › There are many over-the-counter preparations of ASA, including enteric-coated and combination formulations.
  - » Methyl salicylate
    - › This is an ingredient in a number of topical preparations / liniments.
    - › Oil of wintergreen is concentrated methyl salicylate.
      - · 1 mL contains salicylate equivalent to 1.4 g ASA.
  - » Salicylic acid (topical keratolytic)
- Toxicity can result from both ingestion and, rarely, excessive topical exposure.

Pharmacokinetics

- Single therapeutic doses are rapidly absorbed.
  - » The peak serum level typically occurs about 1 hour postingestion.
  - » Enteric-coated formulations have delayed absorption, with peak concentrations at about 4 to 6 hours.
- Salicylate is a weak acid, existing in ionized and non-ionized forms as in the equilibrium expression:

$$HSal \leftrightarrow H+ + Sal-.$$

  - » At physiologic pH, salicylate exists mainly in ionized form.
  - » The equilibrium is shifted to the left (unionized) by acidic pH.
  - » Unionized forms can easily diffuse across cell membranes into tissues (e.g., across the blood-brain barrier), where toxic effects are exerted.
- The half-life of salicylate in therapeutic doses is approximately 2 to 4 hours.
- Salicylate is largely (approximately 90%) protein bound, metabolized in the liver, and eliminated in urine.

Toxicity

- There is no absolute correlation between the salicylate dose and clinical symptoms. In general, a single acute ingestion of:
  - » 150 to 300 mg/kg results in mild toxicity
  - » 300 to 500 mg/kg results in moderate toxicity
  - » > 500 mg/kg results in severe toxicity / death
- Toxicity is more severe at lower doses when ingestion is chronic.
- In cases of salicylate overdose, absorption can be delayed due to salicylate-induced pylorospasm and bezoar formation.
  - » Peak serum levels occur up to 24 hours postingestion.
  - » Normal metabolic pathways become saturated, resulting in delayed, dose-dependent elimination with half-lives up to 20 to 30 hours.

Toxic effects

RESPIRATORY EFFECTS

- Stimulation of the medullary respiratory center results in hyperventilation and respiratory alkalosis.
- With severe toxicity, patients can develop acute respiratory distress syndrome (ARDS).

GASTROINTESTINAL EFFECTS

- Nausea and vomiting result directly from gastric irritation and are centrally mediated via stimulation of the chemoreceptor trigger zone.
- Hemorrhagic gastritis can occur from direct mucosal irritation.

METABOLIC EFFECTS

- Uncoupling of oxidative phosphorylation and interference with the tricarboxylic acid cycle lead to increased glucose utilization with eventual hypoglycemia, production of organic acids, hyperthermia, and diaphoresis.
- This results in increased anion gap metabolic acidosis.

CENTRAL NERVOUS SYSTEM EFFECTS

- Tinnitus is typically the earliest central nervous system (CNS) symptom and can occur with therapeutic doses.
- Neuronal cell damage occurs from impaired energy metabolism (as above) and cytotoxic effects of salicylates.
- Symptoms include irritability/agitation, lethargy, and stupor, and can progress to seizures, coma, and cerebral edema in severe cases.

HEMATOLOGIC EFFECTS

- Toxicity may cause platelet dysfunction and coagulopathy.

CIRCULATORY EFFECTS

- Hypovolemia secondary to fluid losses from hyperthermia, vomiting, and hyperventilation may occur.

Diagnosis

- A high index of suspicion is required as the initial symptoms of salicylate intoxication can be subtle and nonspecific.
- Early symptoms include:
  - » Tinnitus
  - » Gastrointestinal symptoms (nausea and vomiting)
  - » Tachycardia
  - » Hyperventilation with both increased rate and depth of respiration and concomitant respiratory alkalosis on blood gas tests

- As the toxicity progresses, metabolic acidosis develops, with more pronounced CNS symptoms.
  » Mixed metabolic acidosis with respiratory alkalosis on blood gas tests is often seen.
  » In younger children, the period of respiratory alkalosis can be shorter due to the smaller functional reserve.
    › Patients can present early with only metabolic acidosis.
- With progressive toxicity, patients develop respiratory acidosis from CNS depression with or without ARDS in addition to metabolic acidosis.
  » This results in worsening acidemia, further exacerbating toxicity.
- Later findings include seizures, coma, and cerebral edema.
  » Mortality is generally due to severe CNS toxicity.

History
- History should include:
  » Time/chronicity of ingestion
  » Calculated mg/kg dose
  » Possible coingestions
  » Whether the overdose was intentional or accidental
  » Clinical symptoms, including tinnitus

Investigations
- Initiate initial bloodwork:
  » Blood gas with lactate
  » Electrolytes
  » Calcium
  » Glucose
  » Creatinine
  » Blood urea nitrogen (BUN)
  » Liver function tests
  » International normalized ratio (INR) / partial thromboplastin time (PTT)
  » Salicylate levels
  » Acetaminophen levels (based on suspicion of coingestion)
- Based on clinical presentation, initiate other investigations, such as:
  » Electrocardiogram (ECG)
  » Chest X-ray (CXR)

Interpretation of Salicylate Levels
- Higher salicylate levels generally correlate with toxicity but **must be taken in the context of clinical findings and blood pH**.
- Lower/falling salicylate levels in the context of acidosis or progression of clinical symptoms can reflect wider distribution into tissues and more severe toxicity.
- There is higher risk of toxicity at lower serum levels in the context of chronic ingestions.

- Levels should be monitored every 2 hours (with serum pH) until they consistently decline and clinical symptomatology / acid-base status shows improvement.
- The Done nomogram was developed to correlate the degree of toxicity with salicylate levels at 6 to 60 hours following a single acute ingestion.
  » This has been found to have limited clinical utility and is no longer recommended for use in guiding management.

Management
- All suspected significant salicylate ingestions should be managed in conjunction with a local poison control center or toxicologist.
- Therapy relies on prompt supportive care, limiting salicylate entry into the CNS, and enhancing its elimination.
  » No antidote for salicylate toxicity exists.

Supportive Care
- Supportive care for salicylate toxicity involves:
  » Respiratory management
    › The decision to intubate should be taken with caution, as there is a risk of significant clinical deterioration both during intubation and postintubation.
    › Hypoventilation during rapid sequence intubation produces respiratory acidosis, and maintenance of respiratory alkalosis is challenging with mechanical ventilation.
      · These effects result in acute worsening of systemic acidosis, leading to increased salicylate diffusion into the CNS and worsening toxicity.
  » Circulatory management
    › Hypovolemia can exacerbate toxicity and should be treated with IV crystalloids as needed.
  » Glucose management
    › Toxicity can result in CNS hypoglycemia despite normal serum glucose levels.
    › Patients with suspected salicylate toxicity and altered mental status should be treated with a dextrose bolus (0.5 to 1 g/kg) and continuous infusion regardless of serum level.

Limiting Absorption
- Activated charcoal binds salicylate effectively (see Chapter 19.1 for more on activated charcoal).
  » Give a single dose for acute ingestion within 2 hours of presentation.
  » Consider multiple doses if prolonged absorption is suspected (i.e., ingestion of enteric-coated preparations, bezoars).
- Whole bowel irrigation (WBI) is not typically recommended but can be considered in large ingestions of enteric-coated ASA.

Enhancing Elimination

- Serum/urine alkalinization is the mainstay of therapy.
  - » Alkalinization of serum drives the reaction to the right, increasing the amount of salicylate in ionized form.
  - » "Traps" ionize alicylate in blood, which prevents diffusion into the CNS, limiting toxicity.
  - » Concomitant alkalinization of the urine keeps the ionized form of salicylate in the urine, enhancing elimination.
  - » Increasing urine pH from 6 to 8 can result in a ten-fold increase in salicylate elimination.
- Serum/urine alkalinization:
  - » Is indicated in patients with suspected salicylate ingestion with clinical symptoms and/or metabolic acidosis regardless of availability of salicylate level
  - » Should be consider treatment in asymptomatic patients with significantly elevated salicylate level (> 2.9 to 3.6 mmol/L).

DOSING

- Give an IV bolus of 1 to 2 mEq/kg followed by infusion of 3 ampules of sodium bicarbonate mixed in 1 L of 5% dextrose solution and run at 1.5 to 2 times the maintenance rate.

MONITORING

- While patients are on alkalinization therapy, monitor blood gas, electrolytes, glucose (every 1 to 2 hours), and urine pH (hourly).
  - » Aim for blood pH 7.4 to 7.55 and urine pH 7.5 to 8.
- Close monitoring and potassium supplementation (20 to 40 mEq/L potassium chloride) is required to maintain effective alkalinization.
  - » Hypokalemia promotes acidification of urine through potassium reabsorption from the tubules in exchange for hydrogen.

Hemodialysis

- Salicylates are readily removed by intermittent hemodialysis.
- Hemodialysis allows for the correction of acid-base / electrolyte abnormalities.
- Hemodialysis is indicated if:
  - » Salicylate > 7.2 mmol/L regardless of clinical symptoms
    - › The threshold is lower with renal failure / chronic ingestion.
  - » Severe (pH < 7.2) or refractory acidosis
  - » Altered mental status or signs of cerebral edema
  - » ARDS/hypoxia requiring supplemental oxygen

Disposition

- All patients requiring alkalinization should be admitted to hospital.
- Obtain a PICU consultation for any patient for whom hemodialysis or intubation is being considered.

REFERENCES

American College of Medical Toxicology. Guidance document: management priorities in salicylate toxicity. *J Med Toxicol*. 2015;11(1):149–152. https://doi.org/10.1007/s13181-013-0362-3. Medline:25715929

Done AK. Salicylate intoxication. Significance of measurements of salicylate in blood in cases of acute ingestion. *Pediatrics*. 1960;26:800–807. Medline:13723722

Dugandzic RM, Tierney MG, Dickinson GE, Dolan MC, McKnight DR. Evaluation of the validity of the Done nomogram in the management of acute salicylate intoxication. *Ann Emerg Med*. 1989;18(11):1186–1190. https://doi.org/10.1016/S0196-0644(89)80057-5. Medline:2817562

Gaudreault P, Temple AR, Lovejoy FH Jr. The relative severity of acute versus chronic salicylate poisoning in children: a clinical comparison. *Pediatrics*. 1982;70(4):566–569. Medline:7122154

Greenberg MI, Hendrickson RG, Hofman M. Deleterious effects of endotracheal intubation in salicylate poisoning. *Ann Emerg Med*. 2003;41(4):583–584. https://doi.org/10.1067/mem.2003.128. Medline:12705252

Juurlink DN, Gosselin S, Kielstein JT, et al; EXTRIP Workgroup. Extracorporeal treatment for salicylate poisoning: systematic review and recommendations from the EXTRIP Workgroup. *Ann Emerg Med*. 2015;66(2):165–181. https://doi.org/10.1016/j.annemergmed.2015.03.031. Medline:25986310

Kuzak N, Brubacher JR, Kennedy JR. Reversal of salicylate-induced euglycemic delirium with dextrose. *Clin Toxicol (Phila)*. 2007;45(5):526–529. https://doi.org/10.1080/15563650701365800. Medline:17503260

Lugassy DM. Salicylates. In: Hoffman RS, Howland M, Lewin NA, Nelson LS, Goldfrank LR, eds. *Goldfrank's Toxicologic Emergencies, 10e*. New York, NY: McGraw-Hill; 2015.

Madan RK, Levitt J. A review of toxicity from topical salicylic acid preparations. *J Am Acad Dermatol*. 2014;70(4):788–792. https://doi.org/10.1016/j.jaad.2013.12.005. Medline:24472429

Mowry JB, Spyker DA, Brooks DE, McMillan N, Schauben JL. 2014 Annual Report of the American Association of Poison Control Centers' National Poison Data System (NPDS): 32nd Annual Report. *Clin Toxicol (Phila)*. 2015;53(10):962–1147. https://doi.org/10.3109/15563650.2015.1102927. Medline:26624241

O'Malley GF. Emergency department management of the salicylate-poisoned patient. *Emerg Med Clin North Am*. 2007;25(2):333–346, abstract viii. https://doi.org/10.1016/j.emc.2007.02.012. Medline:17482023

Proudfoot AT, Krenzelok EP, Vale JA. Position paper on urine alkalinization. *J Toxicol Clin Toxicol*. 2004;42(1):1–26. https://doi.org/10.1081/CLT-120028740. Medline:15083932

Stolbach AI, Hoffman RS, Nelson LS. Mechanical ventilation was associated with acidemia in a case series of salicylate-poisoned patients. *Acad Emerg Med*. 2008;15(9):866–869. https://doi.org/10.1111/j.1553-2712.2008.00205.x. Medline:18821862

TOXICOLOGY

19.4

Toxic Alcohols

Emily Austin, Bandar Baw

- Alcohols are found in many products, including spirits, solvents, and additives to some dietary and pharmaceutical products.
- Although any alcohol may cause toxicity if consumed in a high enough quantity, not every alcohol is a toxic alcohol.
  » Toxic alcohols are defined as those with metabolic byproducts that cause toxicity; it is not the parent compound itself that causes toxicity.
  » The most common toxic alcohols seen clinically are methanol and ethylene glycol.
  » Isopropanol ingestion is a common presentation but does not have a toxic byproduct and is not considered a toxic alcohol.
  » Other less common ingestions are glycol ethers, propylene glycol, and polyethylene glycol.
- The American Association of Poison Control Centers (AAPCC, 2015) data shows:
  » Methanol exposure in 2117 cases (17% of which were children < 12 years of age)
  » Ethylene glycol exposure in 6892 cases (> 10% were children < 12 years of age), the vast majority of which were the result of automotive product exposures such as antifreeze
- Other possible toxic alcohol exposures are:
  » Isopropyl alcohol
  » Less common toxic alcohol exposures:
    › Glycol ethers — usually found in automotive fluids such as brake and hydraulic products, as well as paints and other industrial products
    › Propylene glycol — found as a preservative in IV medications
      · Propylene glycol can cause severe anion gap metabolic acidosis and renal failure.
    › Polyethylene glycol — an alcohol polymer of ethylene glycol
- Polyethylene glycol does not cause toxicity because it is not absorbed by human intestines.
  » It is used medically as an osmotic laxative.

Pharmacology

- Alcohols in general (including toxic alcohols) have rapid absorption rates, and peak plasma concentrations occur within the hour.
- Alcohols follow zero-order kinetic metabolism.

- Alcohol dehydrogenase is the enzyme responsible for the metabolism of parent compounds including ethanol.
  » Ethanol has a much higher affinity to alcohol dehydrogenase than do methanol (× 16) and ethylene glycol (× 60).

Toxicology

- See below for specific alcohol toxicologies.
- Higher-concentration toxic alcohols can be fatal at very low doses (as low as 0.2 mL/kg), which means only a few milliliters can kill a younger pediatric patient.
- The parent compounds of methanol, ethylene glycol, and isopropanol are not themselves toxic.
  » These act as alcohols and can lead to inebriation, gastritis, or pancreatitis.

Investigations

- A patient with suspected toxic alcohol ingestion should have the following bloodwork to assess the extent and severity of toxicity:
  » Complete blood count (CBC)
  » Electrolytes and extended electrolytes
  » Blood urea nitrogen (BUN) and creatinine
  » Glucose
  » Venous blood gas
  » Serum osmolality
  » International normalized ratio (INR)
  » Lactate
  » Acetylsalicylic acid (ASA), acetaminophen (APAP), and ethanol serum concentrations
  » Toxic alcohol levels — methanol, ethylene glycol and/or isopropanol serum concentrations
- Consider an electrocardiogram (ECG).
- Other causes of altered level of consciousness should be sought; the treating physician should arrange for imaging such as a CT scan of the head if necessary.

Physical Exam

- In the early postexposure period, bloodwork may show only an elevated osmolar gap but no anion gap metabolic acidosis.
  » The initial stage consists of "alcohol effects," which may include altered mental state due to inebriation with risk of aspiration and respiratory depression.

» Abdominal pain, vomiting, and upper gastrointestinal upset may occur.

» There is a possibility of hematemesis and pancreatitis.

- The effects of toxic byproducts start to appear after a few hours; these include:
  » Worsening level of consciousness
  » Anion gap metabolic acidosis
  » Pulmonary or cerebral edema
  » Hypotension
  » Myoglobinuria
  » Acute renal injury
  » Evidence of end organ dysfunction

- It should be noted that the absence of an osmolar gap does not rule out toxic alcohol poisoning for the following reasons:
  » Blood sample may have been drawn after most of the parent compound had been metabolized
  » The dose of toxic alcohol ingested may not be high enough to elevate the osmolar gap, though it may still cause toxicity (see *Figure 19.4.1*).
    › Some patients have a baseline osmolar gap in the negative spectrum (e.g., –2). In such patients, the presence of active osmotic compounds would cause the osmolar gap to become slightly positive (e.g., + 2), but not above the classic abnormal osmolar gap of 10.

Figure 19.4.1. RELATIONSHIP BETWEEN OSMOLAR GAP AND ANION GAP IN TOXIC ALCOHOL POISONING

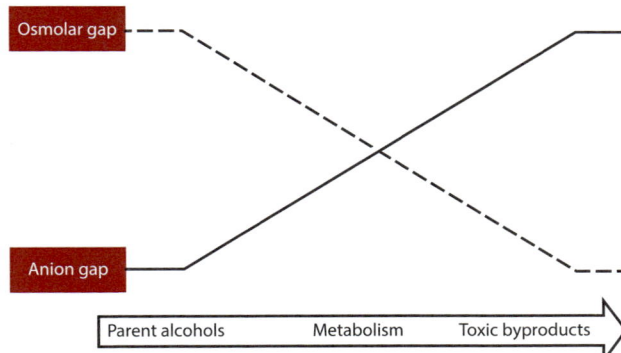

- See below for clinical presentations of specific alcohol toxicities.

Management

- Decontamination is limited in toxic alcohol ingestion due to the rapid absorption rate.
  » A nasogastric (NG) tube and suction may prevent further absorption of large doses or early presentation of toxicity.
  » There is no role for activated charcoal in isolated toxic alcohol ingestion.

- Management of toxic alcohol toxicity can be divided into 3 categories:
  » Category 1 — Supportive treatment
  » Category 2 — Blocking the conversion of the parent compound to the toxic byproduct
  » Category 3 — Enhancing the elimination of both parent alcohols and their toxic byproducts with hemodialysis

Category 1 Management

- Secure the airway and administer fluid and pressors for hypotension.
- Correct severe acidemia with sodium bicarbonate.
  » Administer a loading dose of 1 to 2 mEq/kg IV.
    › Loading dose may be repeated until pH 7.45 is reached.
  » Administer an IV infusion of 150 mEq/L in D5W at 1 to 2 times the maintenance dose.
  » Check pH frequently to prevent undertreatment or overshooting alkalosis.

Category 2 Management

- Indications for enzyme blocking are:
  » Presence of symptoms with clinical suspicion
  » Osmolar gap with the right clinical suspicion
  » Plasma ethylene glycol concentration > 3.22 mmol/L
  » Plasma methanol concentration > 6.24 mmol/L

- Use either fomepizole or ethanol, both of which are competitive inhibitors of the alcohol dehydrogenase enzyme.
  » Fomepizole
    › Administer a loading dose of 15 mg/kg.
    › Follow with a maintenance dose of 10 mg/kg every 12 hours.
    › Fomepizole is safer and more cost-effective than ethanol treatment.
      · It is less prone to medication errors compared to ethanol treatment.
  » Ethanol
    › Ethanol is not expensive but requires strict and intensive monitoring.
      · Risks and complications outweigh its lower cost.
    › The treating physician must keep ethanol at 22 mmol/L for optimum inhibition of alcohol dehydrogenase.
    › Downsides include:
      · Risk of undertreatment may lead to toxic alcohol poisoning
      · Risk of overdosing can lead to aspiration, airway obstruction, respiratory depression, or hypotension
      · Risk of developing hyponatremia or hypoglycemia
      · Need for frequent blood sampling
      · Need for intensive cardiac and nursing monitoring

TOXICOLOGY

Category 3 Management

- Indications for dialysis are:
  - » Plasma ethylene glycol concentration > 4 mmol/L
  - » Plasma methanol concentration > 15.9 mmol/L
  - » High clinical suspicion with osmolar gap of > 10 mOsm/L or double gap (presence of both osmolar gap and anion gap)
  - » Severe acidosis
  - » Evidence of end organ dysfunction (e.g., acute renal injury, blindness, pulmonary edema)

METHANOL

- Methanol is commonly found in:
  - » Illegal (homemade) spirits
  - » Windshield-wiper fluid (up to 60% of methanol ingestion toxicity)
  - » Airplane fuel
  - » Paint removers
  - » Some solvents
- At toxic levels and untreated, methanol exposure has a death rate of 28%; blindness occurs in about one-third of survivors.

Toxicology

- Methanol is metabolized into the toxic byproducts formaldehyde and formic acid.
  - » Formic acid damages optic nerve/disc and basal ganglia and can lead to a variety of visual complaints and findings in addition to necrosis of the putamen and caudate nuclei, which may contribute to Parkinson disease–like features.
    - › Folate (folinic acid) facilitates the conversion of formic acid into water and carbon dioxide in the minor pathway (see Figure 19.4.2).

Figure 19.4.2. METHANOL METABOLISM

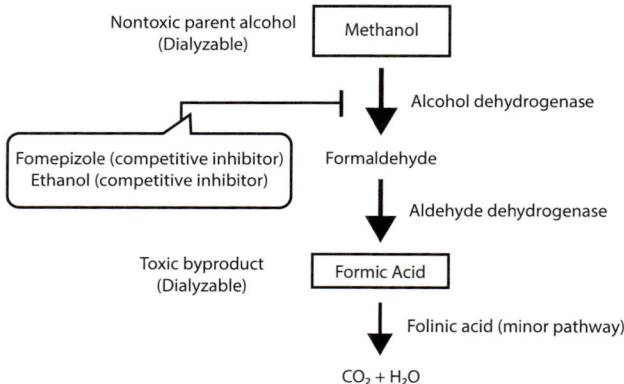

Physical Exam

- Patients exposed to methanol may present with visual complaints such as blurred, hazy, or "snow-field" vision; in severe cases, they present with complete blindness.

- Survivors may sustain basal ganglia necrosis and may develop Parkinson's disease–like symptoms later in life.

Management

- Manage as for general toxic alcohol exposure.
- As an adjunctive therapy, administer folinic acid (leucovorin), which assists in minor pathways of methanol metabolism.
  - » Folinic acid is the activated form of folic acid.
  - » It is used in methanol overdose to facilitate minor nontoxic pathway.
  - » Administer 1 mg/kg IV may repeated once in 4 hours.

ETHYLENE GLYCOL

- Ethylene glycol has a sweet taste, which could contribute to its frequent ingestion by children and pets.
- It is found in automobile antifreeze.

Toxicology

- Ethylene glycol is metabolized into oxalic acid and glycolic acid.
  - » These acids cause direct renal injury, hypocalcemia, and oxalate crystals in the urine.
    - › Thiamine and pyridoxine assist in converting byproducts into nontoxic compounds in minor quantities, which are in turn excreted (see Figure 19.4.3).

Figure 19.4.3. ETHYLENE GLYCOL METABOLISM

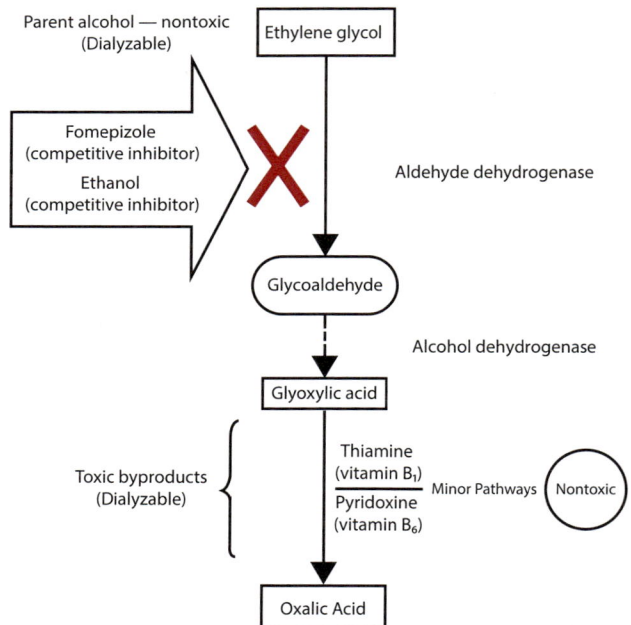

Physical Exam

- Patients with ethylene glycol toxicity may present with acute renal injury with elevated creatinine, urinary calcium oxalate crystals, and hypocalcemia.

- Severe hypocalcemia may lead to QTc prolongation and ventricular dysrhythmias.
- If antifreeze containing fluorescein dye (used by mechanics to identify leaks) was ingested, then the patient's urine may illuminate under UV lights, however this is not sufficient for detecting ethylene glycol exposure.

Management

- Manage as for general toxic alcohol exposure.
- As an adjunctive therapy, administer vitamins that assist in minor pathways of ethylene glycol metabolism:
  » Pyridoxine (vitamin B6)
    › Administer 50 mg IV/IM every 6 hours.
  » Thiamine (vitamin B1)
    › Thiamine is used in ethylene glycol toxicity along with pyridoxine as adjunct therapy to enhance minor pathway of ethylene glycol detoxification.
    › Administer 50 mg IV every 8 hours.

ISOPROPYL ALCOHOL (ISOPROPANOL)

- Isopropyl alcohol is mostly found as rubbing alcohol (up to 70%) and in other solvents and disinfectants.
- It may be used as a cheap ethanol substitute by some alcohol abusers.

Toxicology

- Isopropanol is metabolized into the nontoxic compound acetone.
  » Acetone is a ketone; there is no anion gap metabolic acidosis.

REFERENCES

Barceloux DG, Bond GR, Krenzelok EP, Cooper H, Vale JA; American Academy of Clinical Toxicology Ad Hoc Committee on the Treatment Guidelines for Methanol Poisoning. American Academy of Clinical Toxicology practice guidelines on the treatment of methanol poisoning. *J Toxicol Clin Toxicol.* 2002;40(4):415–446. https://doi.org/10.1081/CLT-120006745. Medline:12216995

Brent J. Fomepizole for ethylene glycol and methanol poisoning. *N Engl J Med.* 2009;360(21):2216–2223. https://doi.org/10.1056/NEJMct0806112. Medline:19458366

Davis LE, Hudson D, Benson BE, Jones Easom LA, Coleman JK. Methanol poisoning exposures in the United States: 1993-1998. *J Toxicol Clin Toxicol.* 2002;40(4):499–505. https://doi.org/10.1081/CLT-120006753. Medline:12217003

Flomenbaum N. *Goldfrank's toxicologic emergencies* [ed. by] Neal E. Flomenbaum…[et al.]. New York, NY: McGraw-Hill, 2006.

Lachenmeier DW, Rehm J, Gmel G. Surrogate alcohol: what do we know and where do we go? *Alcohol Clin Exp Res.* 2007;31(10):1613–1624. https://doi.org/10.1111/j.1530-0277.2007.00474.x. Medline:17681034

Lepik KJ, Sobolev BG, Levy AR, et al. Medication errors associated with the use of ethanol and fomepizole as antidotes for methanol and ethylene glycol poisoning. *Clin Toxicol (Phila).* 2011;49(5):391–401. https://doi.org/10.3109/15563650.2011.580754. Medline:21740138

Miller H, Barceloux DG, Krenzelok EP, Olson K, Watson W. American Academy of Clinical Toxicology practice guidelines on the treatment of ethylene glycol poisoning. *J Toxicol Clin Toxicol.* 1999;37(5):537–560. https://doi.org/10.1081/CLT-100102445. Medline:10497633

Mowry JB, Spyker DA, Brooks DE, Zimmerman A, Schauben JL. 2015 Annual Report of the American Association of Poison Control Centers' National Poison Data System (NPDS): 33rd Annual Report. *Clin Toxicol (Phila).* 2016;54(10):924–1109. https://doi.org/10.1080/15563650.2016.1245421. Medline:28004588

Mycyk MB, Aks SE. A visual schematic for clarifying the temporal relationship between the anion and osmol gaps in toxic alcohol poisoning. *Am J Emerg Med.* 2003;21(4):333–335. https://doi.org/10.1016/S0735-6757(03)00079-2. Medline:12898493

Roberts DM, Yates C, Megarbane B, et al, *and the EXTRIP Work Group.* Recommendations for the role of extracorporeal treatments in the management of acute methanol poisoning: a systematic review and consensus statement. *Crit Care Med.* 2015;43(2):461–472. https://doi.org/10.1097/CCM.0000000000000708. Medline:25493973

Roy M, Bailey B, Chalut D, Senécal PE, Gaudreault P. What are the adverse effects of ethanol used as an antidote in the treatment of suspected methanol poisoning in children? *J Toxicol Clin Toxicol.* 2003;41(2):155–161. https://doi.org/10.1081/CLT-120019131. Medline:12733853

Zakharov S, Pelclova D, Navratil T, et al. Fomepizole versus ethanol in the treatment of acute methanol poisoning: Comparison of clinical effectiveness in a mass poisoning outbreak. *Clin Toxicol (Phila).* 2015;53(8):797–806. https://doi.org/10.3109/15563650.2015.1059946. Medline:26109326

Zakharov S, Pelclova D, Navratil T, et al. Efficiency of acidemia correction on intermittent versus continuous hemodialysis in acute methanol poisoning. *Clin Toxicol (Phila).* 2017; 55(2):123–132.

19.5

Caustics

K. A. Sutherland, Wesley Palatnick

- Caustics are corrosive, acidic, or alkaline agents that cause tissue injury on direct contact.
- Common products that can cause injuries include:
  » Liquids
    › Drain cleaners — 30% potassium hydroxide / lye (NaOH or KOH) or 93% sulfuric acid (H_2SO_4)
    › Household or industrial bleach — sodium hypochlorite (NaClO)
    › Toilet bowl cleaners — hydrogen chloride (HCl)
    › Swimming pool chemicals — e.g., 70% sodium hypochlorite (NaHClO), 70% calcium hypochlorite (Ca[ClO]$_2$)
  » Airbag deployment chemicals (alkali powder)
  » Cement — contains lime (CaO), which can be corrosive
  » Methamphetamine-manufacturing chemicals — hydrogen chloride (HCl), sulfuric acid (H_2SO_4), sodium hydroxide (NaOH), ammonium hydroxide (NH_4OH), anhydrous ammonia (NH_3), metallic lithium
  » Pills that can induce esophageal erosion — doxycycline, tetracycline, potassium chloride, ASA
- Factors influencing the extent of injury include:
  » Type of agent (acid vs alkali)
  » Concentration of solution
  » Volume
  » Viscosity
  » Duration of contact
  » pH — injury increases with pH > 11 or < 3
  » Titratable acid/alkaline reserve
  » Presence or absence of food in the stomach
  » Form — crystals/solids can have prolonged tissue adherence resulting in more severe burns
  » Superimposed thermal injury from acid-base reactions

Toxicology

- Phases of injury include:
  » Necrosis
  » Bacterial/polymorphonuclear leukocyte invasion
  » Vascular thrombosis
  » Superficial tissue sloughing
  » Granulation tissue formation
  » Collagen deposition, reepithelialization (after > 1 week to several months)
  » When ingested, esophageal stricture formation (after weeks to years)

Alkaline Agents

- Alkaline agents (e.g., lye [NaOH or KOH], ammonia [NH_3]) are proton acceptors, and dissociate into conjugate acids and free hydroxide ions.
- Local effects include liquefaction necrosis, fat saponification, and protein disruption, allowing deep penetration of alkaline agent into tissue

Acidic Agents

- Acidic agents (e.g., hydrochloric acid [HCl], sulfuric acid [H_2SO_4]) are proton donors, and dissociate into conjugate bases and free hydrogen ions.
- The local effects include desiccation of epithelial cells and coagulation necrosis with eschar formation limiting further penetration.
- Perforation of the stomach may lead to damage to spleen, liver, pancreas, and kidneys.
- Systemic absorption may lead to metabolic acidosis, hemolysis, renal failure, and disseminated intravascular coagulation.

ORAL INGESTION

Physical Exam

- Initial presenting complaints include:
  » Oral, chest, or abdominal pain
  » Vomiting, drooling
  » Wheezing, coughing, stridor, dysphonia for injuries to the oropharynx and tracheobronchial tree
  » Burns to the face, lips, or oral cavity from spillage or secondary contamination after vomiting
- Ominous findings include:
  » Systemic toxicity
  » Acidosis
  » Hemodynamic instability with hypotension
  » Tachycardia
  » Fever

- Alkali injury is more likely to affect the esophagus.
- Acid injury is more likely to affect the stomach.
- Perform repeated assessments and watch for emergent issues such as:
  » Airway edema — consider early intubation
  » Esophageal or gastric perforation — requires an urgent surgery referral
- Intentional ingestions may have a greater degree of oropharyngeal sparing but a higher likelihood of serious injury.
- The correlation of clinical symptoms to the severity of esophageal burns is controversial.
  » Oropharyngeal burns are not predictive of distal injury.
  » Drooling and dysphagia have 100% sensitivity and 90% specificity.
  » Lack of oral burns is not predictive of lack of distal injury.
- Possible findings 2 to 8 weeks postinjury include:
  » Dysphagia
  » Food impaction secondary to esophageal strictures
  » Pyloric stenosis
  » Gastric outlet obstruction
- Possible findings 40 to 50 years postinjury include:
  » Increased risk of esophageal cancer

Investigations

- Consider coingestants and document the time of ingestion, the amount and type of product ingested, and if there was suicidal intent.
- Order an electrocardiogram (ECG).
  » Dissociated fluoride from hydrofluoric acid ingestions may result in severe hypocalcemia which may cause QTc prolongation, torsades de pointes, or other ventricular dysrhythmias.
- Order appropriate diagnostic imaging, such as:
  » Screening chest or abdominal X-ray to look for peritoneal/mediastinal air.
  » Considering CT scan if the pretest probability of a significant caustic ingestion is high.
- Contrast esophageal studies are *not* useful as they do not gauge the depth of injury.
  » If done, use water-soluble contrast due to the risk of perforation.
- Order an endoscopic exam within 12 to 24 hours.
  » This provides prognostic and diagnostic information.
    › Patients with minimal injury may be discharged.
  » An endoscopic exam enables the safe insertion of a nasogastric (NG) tube for nutrition.
  » Indications for endoscopic exam include:
    › Intentional ingestions
    › Unintentional ingestions with stridor, pain, vomiting, and/or drooling

  » Contraindications for endoscopic exam include:
    › Ingestion of household-strength bleach — endoscopy is not required in this context
    › Asymptomatic patients — endoscopy is controversial in this context
    › 24 hours or more of elapsed time since ingestion — after 24 hours, wound softening causes higher risk of perforation

Injury Grade

- Determine the injury grade (based on findings at endoscopy):
  » Grade 1 — edema, hyperemia
  » Grade 2 — superficial ulcers, whitish membranes, exudates, friability, hemorrhage
    › Grade 2a — noncircumferential
    › Grade 2b — circumferential
  » Grade 3 — transmural involvement with deep tissue injury, necrotic mucosa, frank perforation of stomach or esophagus
- Initial depth of injury correlates with the risk of esophageal stricture formation.
  » Grade 1 injuries do not progress to stricture.
  » 15% to 30% of all Grade 2 burns progress to stricture, with up to 75% of circumferential Grade 2 burns developing strictures.
  » Up to 90% of Grade 3 burns result in stricture.

Management

- Perform early intubation if the patient presents with signs or symptoms of upper airway injury:
  » Hoarse or muffled voice
  » Odynophagia
  » Drooling
  » Tongue or pharyngeal edema
- Surgical management is indicated in the following contexts:
  » Peritonitis
  » Severe chest and abdominal pain
  » Evidence of perforation on endoscopy or diagnostic imaging
  » Refractory hypotension
- Stricture prevention is crucial.
- Controversial treatments include:
  » Antacids, and H2 blockers
  » Fluid dilution with milk or water
    › Given the risk of perforation, this should never be forced upon individuals who do not want to swallow.
    › Fluid dilution can cause thermal reaction and subsequent burn.
    › It has limited efficacy after 30 minutes postingestion.

» Careful NG aspiration immediately after acid ingestion
  › Blind NG tube placement is contraindicated if the probability of perforation is high.
  › **Do not use** with alkali ingestion given the high risk of esophageal perforation.
» Prophylactic antibiotics and corticosteroids
  › In Grade 2 and 3 burns, steroid therapy increases the risk of severe complications such as brain abscess, gastrointestinal hemorrhage, pneumonia, esophagogastric necrosis, osteoporosis, and prepyloric ulcer formation; therefore, steroids are now not routinely recommended.
  › Prophylactic antibiotic use is only recommended if steroids are administered.

- Contraindicated treatments include:
  » Neutralization of ingested corrosive with a weak acid or alkali
    › This may cause thermal reactions and worsen the injury.
  » Ipecac induction of emesis
    › This causes reexposure of the esophageal mucosa to the caustic material.
  » Activated charcoal
    › This interferes with tissue evaluation.
    › Most caustics are not adsorbed by charcoal.
  » Gastric lavage
    › Gastric lavage raises concerns regarding perforation of friable tissue.

DERMAL EXPOSURE

Management

- Remove all the patient's clothing.
- Brush away dry chemical agents.
- Use copious irrigation.
  » Prolonged gentle irrigation is recommended over high-pressure irrigation.
  » Irrigation is especially recommended with strong alkalis, as they combine with protein and fat to form soluble protein complexes that permit the passage of hydroxyl ions deep into tissue.
- There is a theoretical risk of exothermic reaction when water comes into contact with elemental metals.
  » Apply mineral oil to the skin prior to irrigation.
- Avoid neutralizing acid and alkali burns with weak alkali or acid solutions, respectively, as they may also cause exothermic reactions and resultant thermal burns.

OCULAR INJURY

- Alkali burns are more common than acid burns.
- Unilateral involvement is more common than bilateral injury.

- Mechanisms of injury:
  » Splash injury from chemical handling
  » Exploding batteries
  » Airbag deployment
  » Intentional assault

Pathophysiology

- Pathophysiology of alkali burns:
  » Interaction with lipids in the corneal epithelium, causing liquefactive necrosis with deep penetration through the stroma
  » Rapid injury may cause complete blindness in < 1 minute

Injury Grade

- Injury Grades 1 and 2 present with hyperemia, conjunctival ecchymosis, and/or defects in the corneal epithelium.
  » In Grade 1 injuries, the cornea appears hazy.
- Injury Grades 3 and 4 present with mydriasis, gray iris discoloration, early cataract formation, and/or blood vessel thrombosis.
  » In Grade 3 injuries, ischemia in less than half of the limbus.
  » In Grade 4 injuries, there is necrosis of bulbar and tarsal conjunctiva.

Management

- Irrigate the eye immediately and copiously, starting with tap water at the scene.
  » A Morgan lens will facilitate irrigation.
    › Using a Morgan lens has the risk of trapping the burn between the lens and the conjunctiva, worsening the injury.
    › Replace the lens between liter bags of normal saline.
  » Continue irrigation until pH = 7.4 (near–physiologic level)
    › More irrigation may be required even after normal pH has been reached.
- Apply topical anesthetics repeatedly to reduce pain.
- Evert the upper eyelid and inspect the area for particulate matter.
- Perform slit-lamp examination with fluorescein staining to assess for corneal abrasion.
- Consider the use of ocular antibiotics if abrasion is present.
- Obtain an immediate ophthalmologic consultation and follow-up.
- Consider cycloplegics to decrease the potential for papillary constriction (with the guidance of the consultant ophthalmologist).

SPECIAL CASES

HYDROFLUORIC ACID

- Hydrofluoric acid is commonly used in glass etching, rust removal, cement and brick cleaning, the manufacturing of high-octane gasoline, and the production of microelectronics.
- The dissociated fluoride anion is extremely electronegative, scavenging cations such as calcium and magnesium, and inhibiting Na-K ATPase pump.
- Hydrofluoric acid acts like an alkali despite being an acid.
  » It causes liquefactive necrosis of the skin and eyes, worsening the burn.
- Systemic toxicity is life threatening if exposure covers > 2% total body surface area (TBSA).
- Dermal exposure may cause necrosis with eschar and vesicle formation.
- Emergency department (ED) presentation is often delayed, as the onset of severe symptoms such as pain is often delayed.
- Systemic toxicity includes:
  » Profound hypocalcemia and hypokalemia
  » Dysrhythmias (QT prolongation, ventricular arrhythmias)

Management

- Irrigate immediately and copiously with water.
- Remove formed blisters.
- Local infiltration and intravenous or intraarterial infusion of calcium has been used to treat severe extremity exposures.
- Apply 3.5 g of calcium gluconate powder in a water-soluble lubricant to affected areas and cover with an occlusive dressing.
  » Commercial preparations of calcium gluconate powder are available.
  » A latex surgical glove may be used as an occlusive for hand exposure with trephination of nails.
    › Administer intraarterial calcium gluconate for significant hand exposure in addition to the above therapy.
- Provide local infiltration of 10% calcium gluconate (0.5 mL/cm^2).

BUTTON BATTERIES, CONVENTIONAL ALKALINE CYLINDRICAL BATTERIES

- Batteries present both obstructive and chemical hazards (see also Chapter 14.6, "Foreign Body Aspiration and Ingestion").
- Button batteries contain metallic salts (lithium, mercury, nickel, zinc, cadmium, and silver bathed in NaOH or KOH).
- Obstruction caused by batteries may cause pressure necrosis or caustic injury after leakage of the alkaline medium.
- Ulceration, perforation, or fistula formation may occur if not treated quickly.

Investigations

- Use radiographic evaluation to see:
  » Batteries in airway or esophagus
    › Immediate removal is required.
  » Gastric or intestinal batteries
    › Watchful waiting is recommended.
    › Perform follow-up radiographs to document the passage of the batteries.

CEMENT

- Cement is a special case as many do not appreciate its caustic nature and potential to cause injury.
- Cement is composed of salicylates and calcium aluminates.
- When dry cement is combined with water, hydrolysis occurs resulting in a solution of basic lime hydrate with a pH of 10 to 14.
- Brush away dry material and rinse with copious water.
- Manage as you would any other dermal alkali exposure.

PHENOL (CARBOLIC ACID)

- Phenol is a starting material for organic polymer and plastic production, and is used in the agricultural, cosmetic, and medical fields.
- It causes protein denaturation and coagulation necrosis.
- Systemic toxicity presents with dysrhythmias, hypotension, seizures, and coma.
- Treat with supportive therapy.

REFERENCES

Appelqvist P, Salmo M. Lye corrosion carcinoma of the esophagus: a review of 63 cases. *Cancer*. 1980;45(10):2655–2658. https://doi.org/10.1002/1097-0142(19800515)45:10<2655::AID-CNCR2820451028>3.0.CO;2-P. Medline:7378999

Homan CS, Maitra SR, Lane BP, Thode HC Jr, Davidson L. Histopathologic evaluation of the therapeutic efficacy of water and milk dilution for esophageal acid injury. *Acad Emerg Med*. 1995;2(7):587–591. https://doi.org/10.1111/j.1553-2712.1995.tb03594.x. Medline:8521203

Homan CS, Maitra SR, Lane BP, Thode HC, Sable M. Therapeutic effects of water and milk for acute alkali injury of the esophagus. *Ann Emerg Med*. 1994;24(1):14–20. https://doi.org/10.1016/S0196-0644(94)70155-5. Medline:8010543

Howell JM, Dalsey WC, Hartsell FW, Butzin CA. Steroids for the treatment of corrosive esophageal injury: a statistical analysis of past studies. *Am J Emerg Med*. 1992;10(5):421–425. https://doi.org/10.1016/0735-6757(92)90067-8. Medline:1642705

Mamede RC, de Mello Filho FV. Ingestion of caustic substances and its complications. *Sao Paulo Med J*. 2001;119(1):10–15. https://doi.org/10.1590/S1516-31802001000100004. Medline:11175619

TOXICOLOGY

Nuutinen M, Uhari M, Karvali T, Kouvalainen K. Consequences of caustic ingestions in children. *Acta Paediatr.* 1994;83(*11*):1200–1205. https://doi.org/10.1111/j.1651-2227.1994.tb18281.x. Medline:7841737

Pelclová D, Navrátil T. Do corticosteroids prevent oesophageal stricture after corrosive ingestion? *Toxicol Rev.* 2005;24(*2*):125–129. https://doi.org/10.2165/00139709-200524020-00006. Medline:16180932

Rosenberg N, Kunderman PJ, Vroman L, Moolten SE. Prevention of experimental esophageal stricture by cortisone. II. Control of suppurative complications by penicillin. *AMA*

Arch Surg. 1953;66(*5*):593–598. https://doi.org/10.1001/archsurg.1953.01260030610007. Medline:13039730

Rumack BH, Burrington JD. Caustic ingestions: a rational look at diluents. *Clin Toxicol.* 1977;11(*1*):27–34. https://doi.org/10.3109/15563657708989816. Medline:577479

Salzman M, O'Malley RN. Updates on the evaluation and management of caustic exposures. *Emerg Med Clin North Am.* 2007;25(*2*):459–476. https://doi.org/10.1016/j.emc.2007.02.007. Medline:17482028

19.6

Opioid Overdose

Eric Flynn, Wesley Palatnick

- Opioids are commonly prescribed medications for both acute and chronic pain.
- Illicit opioids such as heroin are a common cause of overdose and emergency department (ED) visits.
  - » Prescription opioid overdose and misuse of prescription opioids has surpassed heroin overdose as a cause of fatalities in the ED, in correlation with the dramatic increase in the use of prescription opioids in the past 10 years.

Pharmacology

- An opioid is defined as any compound that interacts with an opioid receptor. They may be derived from opium (opiates) or may be synthetic or semisynthetic.
- Opioids act on 3 major receptor types:
  1. Mu
  2. Kappa
  3. Delta
     › These receptors are widely distributed throughout the central and peripheral nervous system.
     › Different opioids may have both agonist and antagonist effects at different receptors, which explains the multiple effects of opioid medications.

Physical Exam

- Opioid overdose is a clinical diagnosis.
- The opioid toxidrome consists of:
  - » Miosis
    › Note that pupil findings may not be present.
  - » Respiratory depression
  - » Central nervous system (CNS) depression
- A respiratory rate of < 12 breaths per minute is the best indicator for reversal with naloxone.

Table 19.6.1. TOXIC EFFECTS OF OPIOIDS

Organ system	Toxic effects of opioids
Respiratory system	• Decreased respiratory drive • Hypoventilation • Bronchoconstriction • Acute lung injury
Central nervous system	• Analgesia • Antitussive • Sedation/Coma
Ophthalmic	• Miosis
Dermatologic	• Flushing • Pruritus
Cardiovascular	• Bradycardia • Vasodilation
Gastrointestinal	• Hypomotility

Investigations

- Test for common coingestions by testing:
  - » Serum ethanol level
  - » Serum acetaminophen level
    › Acetaminophen is combined with opioids in a number of pharmaceutical preparations.
- Use bedside glucose determination to rule out hypoglycemia.
- Perform additional investigations as needed.

Management

- Initial treatment focuses on management of ABCs and good supportive care.
- Activated charcoal has no proven benefit more than 1 hour postingestion.
  - » Activated charcoal should not be given routinely in opioid overdose.

Naloxone

- Naloxone is a competitive opioid receptor antagonist that reverses opioid effects.
- It can be administered IV, IM, IN, IO, or via an endotracheal tube (ETT).
- The time of onset for naloxone is as follows:
  » IV/IO: 1 to 2 minutes
  » IM: 2 to 5 minutes
  » IN: 8 to 13 minutes
- Naloxone's duration of effect is 30 to 120 minutes depending on route of administration.

Note: Most opioids have a longer duration of effect than naloxone, so repeated doses or continuous infusion may be required.

- Naloxone should be dosed in pediatric patients as follows:
  » For full reversal in resuscitation setting (American Heart Association guidelines for special circumstances of resuscitation):
    › < 5 years of age or < 20 kg: 0.1 mg/kg IV/IO/ETT
    › > 5 years of age or > 20 kg: 2 mg IV/IO/ETT
  » For reversal of respiratory depression:
    › 0.01 mg/kg IV/IM and titrate to effect
      · Administer a subsequent dose of 0.1 mg/kg, repeated every 2 to 3 minutes as required.
- Naloxone should be dosed in adolescent and adult patients as follows:
  » Apneic dosing: 0.4 to 2 mg IV
  » Respiratory depression: 0.04 to 0.4 mg IV
    · Repeat every 2 to 3 minutes and titrate to effect.
- If multiple doses of naloxone are required to reverse the opioid effect, the initial dose may be delivered via continuous infusion at two-thirds the strength of the effective bolus dose per hour.
  » A smaller initial dose in continuous infusion minimizes adverse effects of naloxone.
  » The dose per hour can be increased as necessary via continuous infusion.
- Tracheal intubation may be required if naloxone administration is ineffective.

Disposition

- Patients can be safely discharged 2 to 4 hours after the last dose of naloxone if there is no ongoing evidence of opioid intoxication.

REFERENCES

American Heart Association. Special circumstances of resuscitation file [Internet]. Dallas, TX: American Heart Association; 2015 Available from: https://eccguidelines.heart.org/wp-content/themes/eccstaging/dompdf-master/pdffiles/part-10-special-circumstances-of-resuscitation.pdf

Boyer EW. Management of opioid analgesic overdose. *N Engl J Med.* 2012;367(2):146–155. https://doi.org/10.1056/NEJMra1202561. Medline:22784117

Chyka PA, Seger D. Position statement: single-dose activated charcoal. American Academy of Clinical Toxicology; European Association of Poisons Centres and Clinical Toxicologists. *J Toxicol Clin Toxicol.* 1997;35(7):721–741. https://doi.org/10.3109/15563659709162569. Medline:9482427

Clarke SF, Dargan PI, Jones AL. Naloxone in opioid poisoning: walking the tightrope. *Emerg Med J.* 2005;22(9):612–616. https://doi.org/10.1136/emj.2003.009613. Medline:16113176

Dart RC, Surratt HL, Cicero TJ, et al. Trends in opioid analgesic abuse and mortality in the United States. *N Engl J Med.* 2015;372(3):241–248. https://doi.org/10.1056/NEJMsa1406143. Medline:25587948

Goldfrank L, Weisman RS, Errick JK, Lo MW. A dosing nomogram for continuous infusion intravenous naloxone. *Ann Emerg Med.* 1986;15(5):566–570. https://doi.org/10.1016/S0196-0644(86)80994-5. Medline:3963538

Hoffman JR, Schriger DL, Luo JS. The empiric use of naloxone in patients with altered mental status: a reappraisal. *Ann Emerg Med.* 1991;20(3):246–252. https://doi.org/10.1016/S0196-0644(05)80933-3. Medline:1996818

Holstege CP, Borek HA. Toxidromes. *Crit Care Clin.* 2012;28(4):479–498. https://doi.org/10.1016/j.ccc.2012.07.008. Medline:22998986

Kelly AM, Kerr D, Dietze P, Patrick I, Walker T, Koutsogiannis Z. Randomised trial of intranasal versus intramuscular naloxone in prehospital treatment for suspected opioid overdose. *Med J Aust.* 2005;182(1):24–27. Medline:15651944

Kleinman ME, Chameides L, Schexnayder SM, et al. Part 14: pediatric advanced life support: 2010 American Heart Association guidelines for cardiopulmonary resuscitation and emergency cardiovascular care. *Circulation.* 2010;122(18 Suppl 3):S876–S908. https://doi.org/10.1161/CIRCULATIONAHA.110.971101. Medline:20956230

Martin WR. Naloxone. *Ann Intern Med.* 1976;85(6):765–768. https://doi.org/10.7326/0003-4819-85-6-765. Medline:187095

Marx JA, Hockberger RS, Walls RM, et al. *Rosen's emergency medicine concepts and clinical practice.* 8th ed. Philadelphia, PA: Elsevier Saunders; 2014.

National Vital Statistics System. Multiple cause of death file [Internet]. Atlanta, GA: Centers for Disease Control and Prevention; 2012. Available from: http://www.cdc.gov/nchs/data/dvs/Record_Layout_2012.pdf

Nelson LS, Lewin NA, Howland MA, et al. *Goldfrank's toxicologic emergencies.* 9th ed., McGraw-Hill; 2011.

Robertson TM, Hendey GW, Stroh G, Shalit M. Intranasal naloxone is a viable alternative to intravenous naloxone for prehospital narcotic overdose. *Prehosp Emerg Care.* 2009;13(4):512–515. https://doi.org/10.1080/10903120903144866. Medline:19731165

Substance Abuse and Mental Health Services Administration. Results from the 2011 National Survey on Drug Use and Health: summary of national findings, NSDUH series H-44, HHS publication no. (SMA) 12–4713 [Internet]. Rockville, MD: Substance Abuse and Mental Health Services Administration; 2012. Available from: https://www.samhsa.gov/data/sites/default/files/Revised2k11NSDUHSummNatFindings/Revised2k11NSDUHSummNatFindings/NSDUHresults2011.htm

Waldhoer M, Bartlett SE, Whistler JL. Opioid receptors. *Annu Rev Biochem.* 2004;73(1):953–990. https://doi.org/10.1146/annurev.biochem.73.011303.073940. Medline:15189164

TOXICOLOGY

19.7

Street Drugs I: Cocaine, GHB, and Cannabis

Erik Hildahl, Wesley Palatnick

COCAINE

- Cocaine is primarily a recreational drug in adolescents and teens 12 to 18 years of age.
  - » Ingestion is almost entirely accidental in individuals < 12 years of age.
  - » There are a number of reported cases of children < 12 years of age being exposed.
  - » There are reports of children < 4 months of age manifesting toxicity from second-hand crack cocaine smoke.
- In 2011, in the United States, there were 5904 cocaine-related emergency department (ED) visits by children aged 12 to 18 years of age.
  - » Cocaine is second only to marijuana for illicit drug–related ED visits.
- Patients or caregivers may withhold history of cocaine use from ED care providers, making diagnosis difficult.
- Cocaine is one of the most common causes of cardiac arrest in pediatric patients < 18 years of age.
  - » Myocardial infarction has been reported in patients as young as 17 years of age after cocaine use.

Pharmacology

- Cocaine is derived from the leaves of *Erythroxylum coca*.
  - » Leaves are processed into cocaine hydrochloride, a white powder.
  - » Cocaine powder can be nasally insufflated, applied to mucous membranes, orally ingested, or dissolved in water and injected.
  - » It can also be converted to free-base ("crack") cocaine and smoked.
- Cocaine blocks the reuptake of the catecholamines norepinephrine and dopamine at the presynaptic adrenergic terminals.
  - » These catecholamines accumulate at postsynaptic receptors.
    - › This results in sympathomimetic effects that are dose dependent.
  - » Significant vasoconstriction occurs due to alpha-adrenergic receptor stimulation.
    - › This also causes increased endothelin-1 (vasoconstrictor) and decreased nitric oxide (vasodilator) concentrations.

- Absorption of the drug is rapid from all sites (mucous membranes, lung tissue, GI tract).
- Cocaine is 90% bound to proteins and has a volume of distribution of 2.7 L/kg in healthy individuals.
- Cocaine is a weak base and a small molecule.
  - » It diffuses freely across the placenta and blood-brain barrier.

Onset of Action

- Smoking or IV injection results in onset of action within seconds.
  - » Peak plasma concentration is reached in 2 to 5 minutes.
  - » The maximum "high" after injection occurs in approximately 1 to 5 minutes.
- Nasal insufflation results in onset of action in 1 to 5 minutes.
  - » Peak plasma concentration is reached in 30 to 60 minutes.
- Oral ingestion results in onset of action in 30 to 60 minutes.
  - » Peak plasma concentration is reached in 60 to 90 minutes.

Metabolism and Elimination

- Metabolism is primarily hepatic.
- Cocaine is rapidly metabolized by the liver into its major metabolites benzoylecgonine and ecgonine methyl ester (EME).
- Benzoylecgonine and EME are eliminated in the urine.
- About 1% to 9% of cocaine is excreted unchanged in the urine.

Physical Exam

- The symptoms of sympathomimetic toxidrome include:
  - » Central nervous system (CNS) excitation
  - » Mydriasis
  - » Tachycardia
  - » Hypertension
  - » Diaphoresis
  - » Hyperthermia
- Chest pain is the most frequent symptom in cocaine users presenting to the ED.

- Young children may present differently from adolescents.
  - » Presenting complaint may be:
    - › Seizure
    - › Myoclonus
    - › Dystonia
    - › Lethargy
    - › Coma
- Cocaine exposure should be considered in a patient with the first onset of unexplained seizures.

Toxicity

Neurologic Effects

- Neurologic effects of cocaine include:
  - » Stroke
    - › Both ischemic and hemorrhagic strokes have been reported.
    - › Stroke is usually due to preexisting disease such as arteriovenous malformation (AVM) or aneurysm.
  - » Seizures
    - › Seizures may also occur, especially in children.

Cardiovascular Effects

- Cocaine increases myocardial oxygen demand and reduces coronary artery blood flow (through coronary artery vasoconstriction or spasm).
- Cocaine users have a higher incidence of myocardial infarction than nonusers.
- Takotsubo cardiomyopathy (reversible left ventricular apical ballooning) due to catecholamine excess has also been described.
  - » Dilated cardiomyopathy can develop in chronic users.
- Patient may present with tachydysrhythmias.
  - » Sinus tachycardia is the most common abnormal rhythm.
- Brugada pattern on electrocardiogram (ECG) has been associated with cocaine use.
  - » It is caused by blockage of cardiac sodium channels.
- Torsades de pointes has also been described.
  - » It is caused by blockage of cardiac potassium channels resulting in prolonged QT.

Respiratory Effects

- Patients may experience spontaneous pneumothorax/ pneumomediastinum.
  - » This occurs predominantly after smoking crack cocaine.
  - » Prolonged Valsalva maneuver, done to increase the high, may lead to over-distension and rupture of alveoli.
- Patients may develop "crack lung" — an acute pulmonary syndrome with hypoxia, hemoptysis, respiratory failure, and diffuse alveolar infiltrates.

- Smoking cocaine can induce bronchospasm and significantly exacerbate underlying respiratory issues (e.g., asthma).

Dermatologic Effects

- Skin rash or infection at injection sites may be present.
  - » They are usually secondary to "skin popping" (injecting the drug subcutaneously).
- Patients may have vasculitic rash that is not explained by more common causes such as rheumatologic diseases.
  - » Vasculitic rash is caused mainly by levamisole-contaminated cocaine (see "Levamisole," below).

Otorhinolaryngologic (ENT) Effects

- Chronic nasal insufflation can lead to nasal septum perforation.

Musculoskeletal Effects

- Rhabdomyolysis is common in the setting of agitated delirium or hyperthermia related to cocaine use.

Hematologic Effects

- Patients may have increased thrombogenicity.
  - » Cocaine enhances platelet aggregation and decreases fibrinolysis (which increases endogenous tissue plasminogen activator inhibitor).

Investigations

- Cocaine use is primarily a clinical diagnosis.
- Consider the following investigations:
  - » Toxicology screening
    - › Toxicology screening is not routinely recommended.
      - · It does not distinguish recent from remote cocaine use.
      - · False negatives occur in very dilute urine.
    - › Screening should be performed if unintentional poisoning or child abuse or neglect is suspected.
    - › Cocaine metabolites can be detected for up to 72 hours in urine.
    - › Metabolites can also be detected in blood, urine, saliva, and hair.
  - » ECG
    - › The most common finding on ECG is sinus tachycardia.
    - › Cocaine can prolong PR, QRS, and QT intervals.
      - · A variety of dysrhythmias are possible, including wide complex tachycardias.
    - › ST may be elevated in setting of myocardial infarction or Takotsubo cardiomyopathy.
  - » Bloodwork
    - › Routine bloodwork is recommended in moderate or severe presentations.
      - · Include creatine kinase (CK) and myoglobin to rule out rhabdomyolysis.

» Imaging
› Order a chest X-ray (CXR) if patient has chest pain or respiratory symptoms.

Management

- Any suspected cocaine exposure in a child should raise suspicion of child neglect or abuse (see Chapter 1.7).
- Initial treatment should focus on management of ABCs and good supportive care.
  » Manage airway.
    › If intubation is required, avoid succinylcholine.
    › There is a possible risk of hyperkalemia due to rhabdomyolysis.
    › Acetylcholinesterase metabolizes both cocaine and succinylcholine.
      · Using succinylcholine can theoretically prolong cocaine effects.
  » Check the patient's temperature and glucose.
- Benzodiazepines are first-line therapy.
  » CNS depressive effects counteract the stimulatory effects of cocaine.
  » Treat agitation, tremulousness, hypertension, and tachycardia.

Decontamination

- Gastric lavage is not recommended.
- Whole bowel irrigation (WBI) may be useful in the management of a body packer (an individual who ingests multiple drug packets to smuggle the drug across an international border).
- It is recommended that activated charcoal be given prior to polyethylene glycol (PEG) bowel irrigation if both are to be used.
  » However, patients requiring emergent surgery for a ruptured drug packet may be at risk for significant intraperitoneal contamination if charcoal is administered.
- Activated charcoal is generally not recommended for routine presentations; however, one can consider giving activated charcoal to body stuffers (individual who ingest his cocaine when faced with possible arrest by law enforcement) to prevent toxicity.

Specific Management Issues

CHEST PAIN

- Benzodiazepines are first-line treatment for chest pain.

MYOCARDIAL INFARCTION

- The American Heart Association (AHA) recommends:
  » Initial treatment with ASA/benzodiazepines
  » Consideration of nitroglycerin/nitroprusside if patient is still symptomatic after benzodiazepines
  » Using phentolamine if the previous medications are not effective in managing blood pressure

- Controversy remains over the use of beta-blockers.
  » In patients exposed to cocaine there is a risk of unopposed alpha stimulation, so beta-blockers should be avoided.
- Otherwise, follow the usual treatment for myocardial infarction.
  » Consider angiogram / percutaneous coronary intervention (PCI) and the usual antithrombotic/antiplatelet agents.
  » The vast majority of myocardial infarctions in children will likely be due to vasospasm and are unlikely to benefit from thrombolytic therapy or PCI.

DYSRHYTHMIAS

- Benzodiazepines are the mainstay of therapy for dysrhythmias due to their sympatholytic effect.
- Consider intravenous magnesium for significant ventricular dysrhythmias.
- Amiodarone is not recommended as it has beta-adrenergic antagonist effects.
- Tachydysrhythmias may not improve with cardioversion until underlying toxicity improves.

HYPERTHERMIA

- Aggressive external cooling may be required.

Other Considerations

LEVAMISOLE

- Levamisole is a common adulterant added to cocaine to add bulk or volume and boost the effects of the cocaine.
- It is primarily used today as an anthelminthic in veterinary medicine.
  » It was previously used to treat pediatric arthritis and nephrotic syndrome.
  » It was taken off the market due to significant side effects.
  » The most common complications include agranulocytosis (in 10% of patients) and vasculitis, which often affects the cheeks, ears, and lower extremities.
    › These complications usually improve with cessation of cocaine use.

BODY STUFFERS

- Body stuffers are individuals who intentionally consume the drug, either in whole form or within a wrapping or package in order to avoid arrest by law enforcement.
- Body stuffing carries a risk of significant toxicity.
- Activated charcoal can be considered if the patient presents within 1 hour of ingestion and significant ingestion is likely.
- These patients should be observed for a period of time in the ED.

BODY PACKERS

- Body packers are individuals who intentionally consume multiple well-wrapped packets of drugs with the intention of smuggling them over an international border.
- Body packing has been reported in children as young as 6 years old.
- Diagnosis is based mostly on history and plain abdominal X-rays.
  - » If suspicion is high, consider a CT scan to identify packages.
- WBI with PEG can be considered to increase the transit time of packets in the bowel.
- Activated charcoal should not be used.
- There is a risk of perforation, so patients may require emergent surgery if the packets leak.
- There is a high risk of intraperitoneal contamination.
- Known body packers with small bowel obstruction or signs of acute toxicity should have an emergent laparotomy for removal.

GAMMA-HYDROXYBUTYRIC ACID OR GAMMA-HYDROXYBUTYRATE

- Gamma-hydroxybutyric acid (GHB) is primarily a drug of abuse, with the highest incidence of use in individuals aged 18 to 25.
- The drug is available from a number of sites online.
- As a pharmaceutical (trade name Xyrem), it is approved for use to treat narcolepsy.
- Many cases of accidental intoxication in children have been described, involving:
  - » Accidental ingestion of GHB-related solvents
  - » Ingestion of toy beads coated in a GHB analog (gamma butyrolactone [GBL])
  - » Ingestion of GHB-laced soft drinks by children and adolescents
- In low doses, GHB produces euphoria.
- In higher doses, it produces an altered level of consciousness, coma, respiratory depression, and possibly death.
- GHB is abused in multiple ways, including:
  - » As a cheaper "high" than other drugs or alcohol (and without the hangover)
  - » In combination with ecstasy (MDMA or 3,4-methylenedioxymethamphetamine) to extend its effects (especially at raves)
  - » As a "downer" after stimulant use
  - » By bodybuilders as a workout supplement as it is purported to enhance growth hormone release
  - » To facilitate sexual assault

Pharmacology

- GHB exists endogenously at low levels in the human body.
- It is both a precursor and a metabolite of the inhibitory neurotransmitter gamma-aminobutyric acid (GABA).
- Endogenous GHB is thought to act primarily on GHB receptors in the brain, modulating dopamine, acetylcholine, endogenous opioids, and glutamate release.
- Exogenous GHB is thought to act at the GABA-B receptor.
  - » It decreases dopamine and acetylcholine concentrations.
- Peak absorption time is from 23 to 45 minutes post exposure depending on the dose.
  - » Peak blood concentrations occur 25 to 60 minutes postingestion.
  - » Onset of clinical effects typically occurs 15 to 20 minutes after exposure, with peak effects 30 to 60 minutes postexposure.
  - » GHB has a prolonged half-life in patients with cirrhosis.
- GHB is lipid soluble and can easily cross the blood–brain barrier.
  - » It does not bind significantly to plasma proteins.
- GHB is subject to first-pass metabolism by the cytochrome P450 system in the liver.
  - » It is converted to succinic semialdehyde by GHB dehydrogenase.
  - » After metabolism, the byproducts are eliminated rapidly.
- 1,4-butanediol is metabolized by alcohol dehydrogenase to gamma-hydroxybutyraldehyde, then by aldehyde dehydrogenase to form GHB.
  - » Ethanol coingestion can prolong metabolism due to competition for the enzyme alcohol dehydrogenase.

Physical Exam

- Low doses of GHB result in:
  - » Short-term anterograde amnesia
  - » Hypotonia
  - » Euphoria
  - » Drowsiness
- High doses of GHB result in:
  - » Respiratory depression
  - » Bradycardia
  - » Hypotension
  - » Coma
  - » Death
- The most common presentation involves:
  - » Vital signs:
    - › Bradycardia
      - · Bradycardia is usually asymptomatic.
    - › Hypotension

› Bradypnea/apnea
› Hypothermia
» CNS signs and symptoms:
› Labile level of consciousness
› Drowsiness leading to coma
› Myoclonus
› Usually miotic pupils that are poorly reactive to light
» Seizures — extremely rare
» Other
› Agitation or bizarre behavior (especially when emerging from coma)
› Emesis
› Urinary or bowel incontinence
» Possible hypokalemia, hypernatremia, and elevated creatine kinase (CK)
- Death may occur due to respiratory failure.
» Almost all reported deaths have occurred in the prehospital setting.
- Complete recovery can be expected in 4 to 8 hours.

Investigations

- Diagnosis is primarily clinical.
- ECG usually shows sinus bradycardia and possibly U waves.
- Laboratory workups are generally unremarkable.
» Blood and urine testing is not routinely recommended.
- If sexual assault is suspected, urine and serum GHB levels should be sent to the toxicology laboratory as soon as possible.
» The window for detection of GHB is very small — in urine, it can be detected for < 12 hours, and in blood < 6 hours.
» Blood and urine values are difficult to interpret due to naturally occurring endogenous GHB.
› Suggested cutoff is 4 mg/L in serum and 6 mg/L in urine.
- An accurate diagnosis can be difficult due to cointoxicants, especially other sedative-hypnotics.
- Quantitative GHB levels are not clinically relevant in the acute setting.
» There is no correlation between serum levels and degree of coma / time to awakening.

Management

- Initial treatment should focus on the management of ABCs and good supportive care.
» Focus on respiratory and cardiac support.
» Patients should be in a monitored setting (continuous blood pressure, cardiac, and pulse oximetry).
» Consider intubation in patients unable to protect their own airway.
› Vomiting is common in GHB toxicity.

› Respiratory arrest is the most common cause of death.
- Consider atropine for symptomatic bradycardia (rarely needed).
- Administer intravenous crystalloids for hypotension.

Antidotes and Decontamination

- The following are not recommended as antidotes as they have not shown any benefit and may possibly be harmful:
» Physostigmine
» Naloxone
» Flumazenil
- Dialysis (hemoperfusion, hemofiltration) is not recommended due to rapid GHB clearance and short duration of clinical symptoms.
» However, dialysis could theoretically be used because GHB has a low molecular weight, minimal protein binding, and a relatively small volume of distribution, making it amenable to elimination through dialysis.
- Activated charcoal is not recommended due to risk of aspiration.
» Mortality from GHB is very low with good supportive care, so risks likely outweigh benefits.
» Activated charcoal is of minimal benefit as GHB is rapidly absorbed.

CANNABIS (MARIJUANA)

- Cannabis is the most commonly used illicit drug in the United States among all age groups.
» In 2013, in the United States, 2.4 million people 12 years of age or older used marijuana for the first time.
» Almost 50% of youth in the United States 12 to 17 years of age believed it was "fairly easy" or "very easy" for them to obtain marijuana.
- In Canada, 21% of students in grades 7 to 12 have used cannabis in the last 12 months.
- Children are the most vulnerable population for unintentional and preventable poisonings.
» Cannabis ingestion has the potential to be fatal in young children.
- With changing laws in certain states in the United States, presentations to emergency departments have been increasing.
» One study demonstrated increased pediatric presentations after marijuana was legalized in Colorado.
» With the pending legalization of marijuana in Canada, a similar trend may occur.

Pharmacology

- Cannabinoids are compounds that bind to cannabinoid receptors.

- *Cannabis sativa* is the plant commonly referred to as "marijuana" or "hemp."
  - » It contains 2 major active biochemicals: tetrahydro-cannabinol (THC) and cannabidiol.
    - › THC is the main psychoactive constituent.
    - › Cannabidiol is thought to be responsible for other medical-related effects (e.g., anticonvulsant).
- Cannabis is available in several forms.
  - » Marijuana is made from the dried leaves and flowers of the plant.
  - » Hashish is made from the viscous resin of the plant.
  - » Nabilone is a synthetic pharmaceutical that mimics THC and is approved for use in Canada and the United States to treat nausea and as an adjunct analgesic for neuropathic pain.
- Absorption amounts vary based on the route of exposure:
  - » Inhalation
    - › Approximately 10% to 35% of available THC is absorbed.
    - › Peak plasma concentrations occur in 8 minutes.
  - » Ingestion
    - › Approximately 5% to 20% of available THC is absorbed.
    - › Effects are noted in 1 to 3 hours, with peak serum concentrations in 2 to 6 hours.
- Metabolism/elimination is primarily hepatic, with metabolites excreted in the urine.
  - » Elimination half-life varies greatly among individuals.
  - » Metabolites can be detected in urine for several weeks in chronic users.
- The chemicals found in cannabis are lipid soluble and accumulate in fatty tissues.

Clinical Uses

- Cannabis has been used for a wide variety of medical conditions:
  - » Nausea
  - » Chronic pain — most common medical use of cannabis
  - » Glaucoma
  - » Anorexia
  - » Asthma
  - » Depression
  - » Anxiety
  - » Seizures
  - » Muscle spasticity
- It has recently been used to treat refractory seizures in pediatric patients.
  - » Evidence for this use is anecdotal.
  - » The American Epilepsy Society concluded that the ratio of risk to benefit does not support use for seizures at this time.

History

- Gather information about:
  - » Recreational use
    - › Psychologic effects are variable — most report relaxation, feelings of well-being, and increased appetite.
    - › Physiologic effects include mild increase in heart rate, decreased vascular resistance, and conjunctival injection.
  - » Signs of acute toxicity:
    - › Lethargy
    - › Sedation
    - › Postural hypotension
    - › Slurred speech
    - › Slow reaction time
    - › Decreased coordination / muscle strength
  - » Accidental consumption by children
    - › Consumption can be life threatening due to respiratory depression / coma.
    - › Ingestion is almost exclusively through the oral route.
      - · Onset is slow (1 to 3 hours) and duration of effects is prolonged.
    - › The effects noted are mostly neurologic.
      - · Agitation, psychosis, diaphoresis, lethargy, apnea, and coma have been reported.
    - › Patients may also present with hypotonia, hyporeflexia, tremor, and emesis.

Toxicity

Acute Use

- Patients may experience dysphoria, fear, panic attacks, and/or psychosis.
- There is some evidence that marijuana can increase risk of stroke as well as myocardial infarction.

Chronic Use

RESPIRATORY EFFECTS

- Chronic use can lead to clinical findings of chronic obstructive pulmonary disease (COPD).
- Marijuana also contains carcinogens that can theoretically increase the risk of cancer.

NEUROLOGIC EFFECTS

- Marijuana use at a young age is associated with poor school performance and high dropout rates.
- Chronic heavy cannabis use is also possibly linked to lower IQ in young adults and adolescents.

PSYCHOSIS/SCHIZOPHRENIA

- Cannabis use may precipitate psychotic reactions in those who are vulnerable or predisposed.
- It is unclear from longitudinal studies whether cannabis use increases the risk of developing schizophrenia.

TOXICOLOGY

REPRODUCTIVE EFFECTS

- Chronic marijuana users have been reported to have reduced fertility.

Cannabis Hyperemesis Syndrome (CHS)

- Cannabis hyperemesis syndrome (CHS) is similar to cyclic vomiting syndrome.
- It is characterized by recurrent episodes of nausea, vomiting, and abdominal pain in the setting of chronic, heavy cannabis use.
  » Episodes are separated by symptom-free periods.
- Suspect CHS when no other organic cause can be identified.
- Uniquely, symptoms almost immediately resolve when bathing or showering in hot water.
  » This is part of the diagnostic criteria.
- Conventional antiemetics may be tried but are often ineffective.
- CHS can be treated with benzodiazepines.
- There is anecdotal evidence that haloperidol or topical capsaicin cream may be an effective treatment.

Investigations

- Diagnostic testing is generally not clinically relevant.
- THC metabolites can be detected in plasma or urine.
  » In urine drug screens, THC is generally present for about 8 days in casual users and up to several weeks in heavy users.

Management

- Initial treatment focuses on the management of ABCs and good supportive care.
- Benzodiazepines are useful for agitation, psychosis, and CHS.
- Gastrointestinal (GI) decontamination is not recommended unless other coingestions warrant its use.
  » Clinical effects are rarely serious, and the risks outweigh the benefits.
- Patients with accidental ingestions should be observed in the ED.
  » If a patient is symptomatic, observation is recommended for up to 24 hours or until symptoms resolve.
  » If a patient is asymptomatic, observation is recommended for at least 6 hours (the upper limit of time to peak plasma levels).
- Although most poisonings in young children are accidental, abuse or neglect as a cause of poisoning must be considered, with referral to the appropriate child protection agency.

SYNTHETIC CANNABINOIDS

- Synthetic cannabinoids are compounds that bind to cannabinoid receptors.
  » They act like antagonists at the cannabinoid receptors and have different clinical effects than naturally-occurring cannabis.
- The most common of these illicit synthetic compounds are known as "K2" or "spice."
  » Others include "Aroma," "Mr. Smiley," "Zohai," "Eclipse," "Black Mamba," "Blaze," and "Dream."
- They were originally sold as incense or herbs to avoid legal ramifications.
- Synthetic cannabinoids are now listed as Schedule 1 controlled substances in the United States.
- There were over 4500 calls to the American Association of Poison Control Centers from 2010 to 2011 for synthetic cannabinoids.

Diagnosis

- Patient may present with sympathomimetic symptoms:
  » Diaphoresis
  » Agitation
  » Restlessness
- Other symptoms can include:
  » Psychosis
  » Dystonia
  » Tachycardia
  » GI disturbances
  » Seizures
  » Coma

Investigations

- Synthetic cannabinoids generally do not show up on routine urine toxicology screens.
- Specific assays are available but are not clinically relevant due to the long processing time required.
- Consider routine blood testing, including CK, as there is a risk of rhabdomyolysis with significant agitation.

Management

- Initial treatment focuses on the management of ABCs and good supportive care.
- Benzodiazepines are useful for agitation or psychosis.
- If rhabdomyolysis is suspected, ensure adequate urine output with the infusion of crystalloid.

REFERENCES

Abanades S, Farré M, Segura M, et al. Disposition of gamma-hydroxybutyric acid in conventional and nonconventional biologic fluids after single drug administration: issues in methodology and drug monitoring. *Ther Drug Monit.* 2007;29(1):64–70. https://doi.org/10.1097/FTD.0b013e3180307e5e. Medline:17304152

Allain F, Minogianis EA, Roberts DC, Samaha AN. How fast and how often: the pharmacokinetics of drug use are decisive in addiction. *Neurosci Biobehav Rev.* 2015;56:166–179. https://doi.org/10.1016/j.neubiorev.2015.06.012. Medline:26116543

Andresen H, Sprys N, Schmoldt A, Mueller A, Iwersen-Bergmann S. Gamma-hydroxybutyrate in urine and serum: additional data supporting current cut-off recommendations. *Forensic Sci Int.* 2010;200(1-3):93–99. https://doi.org/10.1016/j.forsciint.2010.03.035. Medline:20418032

Bania TC, Chu J. Physostigmine does not affect arousal but produces toxicity in an animal model of severe γ-hydroxybutyrate intoxication. *Acad Emerg Med.* 2005;12(3):185–189. https://doi.org/10.1197/j.aem.2004.09.020. Medline:15741579

Barrueto F Jr, Gattu R, Mazer-Amirshahi M. Updates in the general approach to the pediatric poisoned patient. *Pediatr Clin North Am.* 2013;60(5):1203–1220. https://doi.org/10.1016/j.pcl.2013.06.002. Medline:24093904

Beno S, Calello D, Baluffi A, Henretig FM. Pediatric body packing: drug smuggling reaches a new low. *Pediatr Emerg Care.* 2005;21(11):744–746. https://doi.org/10.1097/01.pec.0000186428.07636.18. Medline:16280948

Brenneisen R, Elsohly MA, Murphy TP, et al. Pharmacokinetics and excretion of gamma-hydroxybutyrate (GHB) in healthy subjects. *J Anal Toxicol.* 2004;28(8):625–630. https://doi.org/10.1093/jat/28.8.625. Medline:15538955

Broséus J, Gentile N, Esseiva P. The cutting of cocaine and heroin: a critical review. *Forensic Sci Int.* 2016;262:73–83. https://doi.org/10.1016/j.forsciint.2016.02.033. Medline:26974713

Carstairs SD, Fujinaka MK, Keeney GE, Ly BT. Prolonged coma in a child due to hashish ingestion with quantitation of THC metabolites in urine. *J Emerg Med.* 2011;41(3):e69–e71. Medline:20634020

Chyka PA, Seger D, Krenzelok EP, Vale JA; American Academy of Clinical Toxicology; European Association of Poisons Centres and Clinical Toxicologists. Position paper: single-dose activated charcoal. *Clin Toxicol (Phila).* 2005;43(2):61–87. https://doi.org/10.1081/CLT-51867. Medline:15822758

Cipriani F, Mancino A, Pulitanò SM, Piastra M, Conti G. A cannabinoid-intoxicated child treated with dexmedetomidine: a case report. *J Med Case Reports.* 2015;9(1):152. https://doi.org/10.1186/s13256-015-0636-2. Medline:26138711

Cohen J, Morrison S, Greenberg J, Saidinejad M. Clinical presentation of intoxication due to synthetic cannabinoids. *Pediatrics.* 2012;129(4):e1064–e1067. https://doi.org/10.1542/peds.2011-1797. Medline:22430444

De Knegt VK, Breindahl T, Harboe KM, et al. Gamma-hydroxybutyrate and cocaine intoxication in a Danish child. *Clin Case Rep.* 2016 Mar;4(3):228–231. https://doi.org/10.1002/ccr3.492.

Detyniecki K, Hirsch L. Marijuana use in epilepsy: the myth and the reality. *Curr Neurol Neurosci Rep.* 2015;15(10):65. https://doi.org/10.1007/s11910-015-0586-5. Medline:26299273

Dinis-Oliveira RJ. Metabolomics of cocaine: implications in toxicity. *Toxicol Mech Methods.* 2015;25(6):494–500. Medline:26249365

Driedger GE, Dong KA, Newton AS, Rosychuk RJ, Ali S. What are kids getting into these days? A retrospective chart review of substance use presentations to a Canadian pediatric emergency department. *CJEM.* 2015;17(4):345–352. https://doi.org/10.1017/cem.2015.13. Medline:25993915

Filloux FM. Cannabinoids for pediatric epilepsy? Up in smoke or real science? *Transl Pediatr.* 2015;4(4):271–282. Medline:26835389

Haller C, Thai D, Jacob P III, Dyer JE. GHB urine concentrations after single-dose administration in humans. *J Anal Toxicol.* 2006;30(6):360–364. https://doi.org/10.1093/jat/30.6.360. Medline:16872565

Heard K, Cleveland NR, Krier S. Benzodiazepines and antipsychotic medications for treatment of acute cocaine toxicity in animal models--a systematic review and meta-analysis. *Hum Exp Toxicol.* 2011;30(11):1849–1854. https://doi.org/10.1177/0960327111401435. Medline:21382911

Larocque A, Hoffman RS. Levamisole in cocaine: unexpected news from an old acquaintance. *Clin Toxicol (Phila).* 2012;50(4):231–241. https://doi.org/10.3109/15563650.2012.665455. Medline:22455354

Lee MO, Vivier PM, Diercks DB. Is the self-report of recent cocaine or methamphetamine use reliable in illicit stimulant drug users who present to the Emergency Department with chest pain? *J Emerg Med.* 2009;37(2):237–241. https://doi.org/10.1016/j.jemermed.2008.05.024. Medline:19081702

McCord J, Jneid H, Hollander JE, et al; American Heart Association Acute Cardiac Care Committee of the Council on Clinical Cardiology. Management of cocaine-associated chest pain and myocardial infarction: a scientific statement from the American Heart Association Acute Cardiac Care Committee of the Council on Clinical Cardiology. *Circulation.* 2008;117(14):1897–1907. https://doi.org/10.1161/CIRCULATIONAHA.107.188950. Medline:18347214

Michaud K, Grabherr S, Shiferaw K, Doenz F, Augsburger M, Mangin P. Acute coronary syndrome after levamisole-adultered cocaine abuse. *J Forensic Leg Med.* 2014;21:48–52. https://doi.org/10.1016/j.jflm.2013.10.015. Medline:24365689

Neijzen R, van Ardenne P, Sikma M, Egas A, Ververs T, van Maarseveen E. Activated charcoal for GHB intoxication: an in vitro study. *Eur J Pharm Sci.* 2012;47(5):801–803. https://doi.org/10.1016/j.ejps.2012.09.004. Medline:23017433

Pélissier F, Claudet I, Pélissier-Alicot AL, Franchitto N. Parental cannabis abuse and accidental intoxications in children: prevention by detecting neglectful situations and at-risk families. *Pediatr Emerg Care.* 2014;30(12):862–866. https://doi.org/10.1097/PEC.0000000000000288. Medline:25407034

Pinto JM, Babu K, Jenny C. Cocaine-induced dystonic reaction: an unlikely presentation of child neglect. *Pediatr Emerg Care.* 2013;29(9):1006–1008. https://doi.org/10.1097/PEC.0b013e3182a3204d. Medline:24201982

Schep LJ, Knudsen K, Slaughter RJ, Vale JA, Mégarbane B. The clinical toxicology of γ-hydroxybutyrate, γ-butyrolactone and 1,4-butanediol. *Clin Toxicol (Phila).* 2012;50(6):458–470. https://doi.org/10.3109/15563650.2012.702218. Medline:22746383

Schrot RJ, Hubbard JR. Cannabinoids: medical implications. *Ann Med.* 2016;48(3):128–141. https://doi.org/10.3109/07853890.2016.1145794. Medline:26912385

Schwartz BG, Rezkalla S, Kloner RA. Cardiovascular effects of cocaine. *Circulation.* 2010;122(24):2558–2569. https://doi.org/10.1161/CIRCULATIONAHA.110.940569. Medline:21156654

Silverberg D, Menes T, Kim U. Surgery for "body packers"—a 15-year experience. *World J Surg.* 2006;30(4):541–546. https://doi.org/10.1007/s00268-005-0429-7. Medline:16568225

Substance Abuse and Mental Health Services Administration. Results from the 2011 National Survey on Drug Use and Health: Summary of National Findings, NSDUH Series H-44, HHS Publication No. (SMA) 12–4713 [Internet]. Rockville, MD: Substance Abuse and Mental Health Services Administration; 2012. Available from: https://www.samhsa.gov/data/sites/default/files/Revised2k11NSDUHSummNatFindings/Revised2k11NSDUHSummNatFindings/NSDUHresults2011.htm

Substance Abuse and Mental Health Services Administration. Results from the 2013 National Survey on Drug Use and Health: Summary of National Findings, NSDUH Series H-48, HHS Publication No. (SMA) 14–4863 [Internet]. Rockville, MD: Substance Abuse and Mental Health Services Administration; 2014. Available from: https://www.samhsa.gov/data/sites/default/files/NSDUHresultsPDFWHTML2013/Web/NSDUHresults2013.pdf

Thai D, Dyer JE, Jacob P, Haller CA. Clinical pharmacology of 1,4-butanediol and gamma-hydroxybutyrate after oral 1,4-butanediol administration to healthy volunteers. *Clin Pharmacol Ther.* 2007;81(2):178–184. https://doi.org/10.1038/sj.clpt.6100037. Medline:17192771

van Amsterdam JG, van Laar M, Brunt TM, van den Brink W. Risk assessment of gamma-hydroxybutyric acid (GHB) in the Netherlands. *Regul Toxicol Pharmacol.* 2012;63(1):55–63. https://doi.org/10.1016/j.yrtph.2012.03.005. Medline:22440552

Volkow ND, Baler RD, Compton WM, Weiss SR. Adverse health effects of marijuana use. *N Engl J Med.* 2014;370(23):2219–2227. https://doi.org/10.1056/NEJMra1402309. Medline:24897085

Wallace EA, Andrews SE, Garmany CL, Jelley MJ. Cannabinoid hyperemesis syndrome: literature review and proposed diagnosis and treatment algorithm. *South Med J.* 2011;104(9):659–664. https://doi.org/10.1097/SMJ.0b013e3182297d57. Medline:21886087

TOXICOLOGY

Wang GS, Roosevelt G, Heard K. Pediatric marijuana exposures in a medical marijuana state. *JAMA Pediatr.* 2013;167(7):630–633. https://doi.org/10.1001/jamapediatrics.2013.140. Medline:23712626

Wang GS, Roosevelt G, Le Lait MC, et al. Association of unintentional pediatric exposures with decriminalization of marijuana in the United States. *Ann Emerg Med.* 2014;63(6):684–689. https://doi.org/10.1016/j.annemergmed.2014.01.017. Medline:24507243

Wehrman J. Fake marijuana spurs more than 4,500 calls to US poison centers [Internet]. AAPCC; 2011. Available from: http://www.aapcc.org/dnn/Portals/0/prrel

Wolff V, Armspach JP, Lauer V, et al. Cannabis-related stroke: myth or reality? *Stroke.* 2013;44(2):558–563. https://doi.org/10.1161/STROKEAHA.112.671347. Medline:23271508. *Erratum in: Stroke.* 2013;44:e15. https://doi.org/10.1161/STR.0b013e318286ba9d

Zvosec DL, Smith SW. Agitation is common in γ-hydroxybutyrate toxicity. *Am J Emerg Med.* 2005;23(3):316–320. https://doi.org/10.1016/j.ajem.2005.02.003. Medline:15915404

Zvosec DL, Smith SW, Litonjua R, Westfal RE. Physostigmine for gamma-hydroxybutyrate coma: inefficacy, adverse events, and review. *Clin Toxicol (Phila).* 2007;45(3):261–265. https://doi.org/10.1080/15563650601072159. Medline:17453877

19.8

Street Drugs II: Amphetamine Derivatives and Hallucinogens

Emily Austin, Bandar Baw

Role for Diagnostic Drug Testing

- Serum and urine testing is often available for some, but not all, "street" drugs.
- Toxicology screening is estimated to influence the management of < 15% of cases of poisoning or drug overdose.
- Urine immunoassay tests are the most widely available and are commonly referred to as "tox screens."
  » They are not useful in the acute management of a patient.
  » They are notorious for giving a false positive due to cross-reactivity to another substance.
  » The specific false positive / false negative profile is assay dependent (i.e., varies by assay manufacturer).
  » True positives do not mean that a person is necessarily intoxicated by that drug, but rather that the individual could have been recently exposed to it.
- Many drugs are not detected by common urine immunoassay screens at all.

AMPHETAMINE DERIVATIVES: METHAMPHETAMINE, MDMA, SYNTHETIC CATHINONES

Pharmacology

- Amphetamine derivatives are a group of compounds that share a similar chemical structure (phenylethylamine backbone).
- The addition of different side chains or a substitution on the phenylethylamine ring results in a different profile of catecholamine and serotonin simulation.

- As a general mechanism of action, amphetamine-derived drugs activate the sympathetic nervous system through:
  » Releasing biogenic amines (dopamine [DA], norepinephrine [NE], and serotonin [5-HT]) from presynaptic nerve terminals
  » Inhibiting the neuronal reuptake of these neurotransmitters
  » Blocking the breakdown of biogenic amines through inhibition of the monoamine oxidase enzyme

Physical Exam

- The desired effects from the use of amphetamine-derived drugs include:
  » Hyperarousal
  » Increased sensation of pleasure
  » Hallucinogenic effects
- Acute toxicity from these drugs is characterized by a hyperadrenergic state with:
  » Hyperthermia
  » Tachycardia
  » Hypertension
  » Central nervous system (CNS) stimulation that presents as seizures or agitation
- Several complications are reported, including:
  » Rhabdomyolysis
  » Hepatic and renal failure
  » Disseminated intravascular coagulopathy
  » Dysrhythmias
  » Vascular catastrophes (dissection, intracranial hemorrhage)
  » Cardiovascular collapse
  » Death

- Patients may display symptoms of both sympathomimetic toxicity and serotonin toxicity.

Investigations

- The diagnosis of amphetamine-derived compound exposure is most often based on clinical history and presentation.
- There is no role for toxicology testing.
- Useful laboratory studies include:
  » Electrolytes
  » Glucose
  » Blood urea nitrogen (BUN)
  » Creatine kinase (CK)
  » Urinalysis and urine dipstick (for rhabdomyolysis)
- An electrocardiogram (ECG) should be done.
- A CT scan of the brain is indicated if intracerebral hemorrhage is suspected.

Management

- Acute management is focused on emergency and supportive measures, with consideration of a patient's ABCs and temperature.
- Patients can be very agitated, and chemical sedation is often necessary.
  » First-line and main pharmacologic agents for sedation are the benzodiazepines. These should be delivered in rapidly escalating doses.
  » Antipsychotics may be effective, but have several associated risks including lowering the seizure threshold, altering temperature regulation (through anticholinergic effects), and precipitating cardiac dysrhythmias.
- Hyperthermia should be aggressively treated with sedation, external cooling measures, and, in certain patients, paralysis.
- Seizures are treated with benzodiazepines and barbiturates.
- Hypertension should be treated by first addressing any agitation.
  » Alpha-adrenergic antagonists (phentolamine) and vasodilators (nitroprusside and nitroglycerin) are indicated if severe hypertension persists.
- Patients are often hypovolemic and should be given fluid hydration, usually in the form of intravenous fluids, to maintain urine output at approximately 1 to 2 mL/kg per hour.

METHAMPHETAMINE

- Methamphetamine is known by many different names, including "speed," "meth," "yaba," "crystal," and "ice."
- It is most often consumed by snorting, injection, or ingestion.

- A crystalline form of methamphetamine ("ice") has a lower melting point and can be smoked.
- Methamphetamine can be easily synthesized at a low cost in clandestine laboratories by amateur chemists; this illicit manufacturing has contributed to increased use of methamphetamine globally.
- Methamphetamine shares the basic amphetamine structure, and also shares the mechanism of action of amphetamine-derived drugs (see "Pharmacology," above).
  » Methamphetamine is a more lipophilic compound and has more rapid and more pronounced CNS stimulatory effects.

MDMA

- MDMA is an abbreviation of the compound's chemical name: 3,4-methylenedioxymethamphetamine.
- It is a derivative of methamphetamine and is known by the names "ecstasy," "molly," "X," or "E," among others.
- MDMA is typically available in tablet form and consumed by ingestion.
- Significant variability in the amount of MDMA in tablets has been reported, with quantities ranging from 1 to 270 mg per tablet.
- "Molly" is marketed as "pure" MDMA, without any of the adulterants that might be found in a tablet.
  » It usually comes in powder form that can be snorted or ingested.
  » Despite claims of users to the contrary, contamination of "molly" is also reported.
- MDMA is has approximately one-tenth the CNS stimulant effects of the basic amphetamine compound but is a much more potent stimulus for serotonin release.
  » This preference for enhanced serotonin signaling distinguishes MDMA from amphetamine and methamphetamine.
- Acutely, MDMA use produces increased wakefulness and arousal (similar to amphetamine-derived drugs in general).
  » Users also describe a sense of euphoria, well-being, enhanced sexual arousal, and greater sociability.
- The sympathetic effect of MDMA can lead to similar presentation in overdose as other amphetamine-derived drugs.
- Severe hyponatremia is reported with MDMA use.
  » MDMA and its metabolites lead to vasopressin secretion, which, in combination with overhydration, can lead to significant hyponatremia.
  » Treatment of these patients involves free water restriction and, in certain situations, hypertonic saline.

SYNTHETIC CATHINONES

- Cathinone is a naturally-occurring beta-ketone amphetamine analogue found in the leaves of the khat plant (*Catha edulis*).
- In several countries in the Middle East and East Africa, it is popular to chew the fresh leaves of the khat plant to experience stimulant and psychoactive effects.
  - » Only the fresh leaves of the khat plant contain the cathinone compounds, so leaves must be chewed within a few days of harvest.
- Chewing khat has been associated with an increased risk of myocardial infarction, cardiomyopathy, peptic ulcer disease, and oral cancers.
- Synthetic cathinone derivatives are some of the newer sympathomimetic drugs to become popular on the drug scene.
  - » Common synthetic cathinones include methcathinone, mephedrone, methylone, and butlyone, though over 30 molecules are known to exist.
  - » On the street, these chemicals have many names, including "bath salts," "meow meow," and "bubbles."
- The term "bath salts" came about from the initial packaging and distribution of these drugs into small sachets labeled "Bath Salts" and "Not for Human Consumption."
  - » This was an attempt by illicit manufacturers to circumvent drug laws by using slightly altered chemical structures.
- Synthetic cathinones are most commonly consumed by snorting or ingesting a powder.
  - » A technique called "bombing" is also reported, whereby the powder is wrapped in cigarette paper and ingested.
- Synthetic cathinones act similarly to amphetamines and MDMA, leading to increased sympathetic nervous system activity and increased serotonin signaling.
- Cardiac, psychiatric, and neurologic signs and symptoms are the most common adverse effects reported in the literature related to synthetic cathinones, though patients are known to present with hyperthermia, rhabdomyolysis, and other manifestations of sympathetic nervous system toxicity.
- The most common symptoms of patients presenting with synthetic cathinone toxicity is agitation, ranging from mild agitation to severe psychosis.
- There are a few case reports of hyponatremia and cerebral edema associated with synthetic cathinone use.
- In general, there is no specific treatment for patients presenting with a synthetic cathinone exposure beyond the aggressive supportive measures discussed above.

HALLUCINOGENS

- Hallucinogens are a diverse group of compounds that alter and distort perception, thought, and mood.
- The lysergamide-, tryptamine-, and phenylethylamine-derived hallucinogens share a common site of action: the central serotonin receptors.
  - » 5-HT2A receptors seem to have the highest density in the cerebral cortex and are the known target of the above-mentioned hallucinogens.
- The clinical effects associated with hallucinogen use include psychologic effects.
  - » Patients are often fully oriented, alert, and aware.
- Hallucinogens rarely produce life-threatening toxicity in and of themselves.
  - » There are many reports of patients experiencing significant trauma as a result of the decisions made while under the influence of these drugs.
  - » Users experiencing panic reactions or dysphoric reactions are the most common presentation to the ED from hallucinogen use.
  - » Psychosis and depression have also been reported.

LYSERGAMIDES

- Lysergamides are hallucinogenic compounds that occur both naturally and synthetically.
- Natural lysergamide compounds are found in several species of morning glory (*Rivea corymbosa, Ipomoea violacea*) and Hawaiian baby woodrose (*Argyreia nervosa*), though in different concentrations.
- To experience hallucinogenic effects, a user would need to ingest 200 to 300 seeds of a morning glory plant, compared to approximately 5 to 10 seeds of a Hawaiian baby woodrose plant.
- Lysergic acid diethylamide, or LSD, is a water-soluble compound that is impregnated into blotter paper or formulated into a powder.
  - » The desired effects users seek include heightened awareness of visual and auditory stimuli with perceptual distortions and hallucinations.
  - » A "bad trip" occurs when LSD produces anxiety, bizarre behavior, and aggression.
  - » The effects of LSD generally last approximately 10 to 12 hours.

TRYPTAMINES

- Tryptamines, like the lysergamide compounds, are found in both natural and synthetic forms.
- Tryptamine molecules are defined by their shared chemical structure. Two endogenous tryptamine molecules exist in humans: serotonin and melatonin.
  - » Naturally-occurring tryptamine molecules include psilocybin, bufotenine (found in the skin of some toad species), and *N,N*-dimethyltryptamine (DMT).

- Psilocybin is a naturally-occurring psychoactive compound found in certain mushroom species and ingested as "magic mushrooms."
  - » Psilocybin-containing mushrooms are known to grow in natural environments but have also been grown by consumers at home using purchased kits online.

SALVIA DIVINORUM

- *Salvia divinorum* is a plant that grows naturally in Oaxaca, Mexico.
- It has been used for centuries in religious ceremonies and is available for purchase online.
- Salvinorin A is the active compound in *Salvia divinorum* and one of the most potent natural hallucinogens.
- Salvinorin A binds to the kappa opioid receptor, which is distinct from the mu opioid receptor.
- Users experience hallucinations, typically lasting 1 to 2 hours.

KRATOM

- Kratom comes from the leaves of the *Mitragyna speciosa* tree, which is native to Asia and Africa.
- The active compounds in kratom are mitragynine and 7-hydromitragynine.
  - » They activate opioid receptors as well as norepinephrine and serotonin receptors.
  - » This receptor activity has led people who are seeking relief from opioid dependence to use kratom.
- Hallucinations are reported with heavy use.

PHENCYCLIDINE AND KETAMINE

- Phencyclidine and ketamine are related drugs that act as "dissociative anesthetics."
- Phencyclidine was introduced as a general anesthetic in the 1950s but was found to be associated with a significant rate of postoperative psychosis, so its use was quickly limited to veterinary medicine.
- Ketamine is an analogue of phencyclidine.
  - » Ketamine has < 10% of the potency of phencyclidine and a significantly shorter duration of action.
- Both ketamine and phencyclidine are available in powder, tablet, capsule, and liquid form.
- These drugs are abused through injection, ingestion, or nasal insufflation.
  - » Phencyclidine has been sprayed onto a leaf material and smoked.
  - » Phencyclidine is referred to by many names, including "angel dust," "PeaCe Pill," and "elephant tranquilizer."
  - » Ketamine has been called "Special K" and "Vitamin K," among other names.

Mechanism of Action

- Phencyclidine and ketamine block signaling at the NMDA-receptor in the brain, leading to a dissociative state.
- Both drugs also weakly inhibit the reuptake of norepinephrine, dopamine, and serotonin.

Toxicity

- Ketamine and phencyclidine produce similar clinical presentations of acute toxicity, though the effects of ketamine are significantly shorter in duration.
- Both drugs lead to dissociation between the somatosensory cortex and the higher brain centers.
  - » Patients often present in a catatonic state.
- Rarely, patients may present with hyperthermia.
- Patients are often tachycardic and mildly hypertensive.
- Neurologic symptoms include ataxia and nystagmus.
- Patients often experience amnesia.
- Patients can display symptoms and signs of psychosis in a way that is often indistinguishable from schizophrenia.
- Recovery from ketamine is associated with an emergence phenomenon, consisting of agitation and delirium.
- A unique adverse effect associated with chronic ketamine abuse is evidence of urinary symptoms, including ulcerative cystitis.

Investigations

- The phencyclidine immunoassay in many commercial urine toxicology screens shows significant cross-reactivity for dextromethorphan, as well as other drugs (see *Table 19.8.1*).

Table 19.8.1. COMMON INTERFERENCES IN TOXICOLOGIC BLOOD OR URINE TESTS
Adapted from Olson (2011).

Substance	Common interferences
Amphetamines (urine immunoassay)	• Selegiline (MAO-B for Parkinson's treatment; metabolizes to amphetamine) • Pseudoephedrine, bupropion, labetalol, ranitidine, sertraline, trazodone
Benzodiazepines	• Test results in **false negative** if the drug does not metabolize to oxazepam or nordiazepam (e.g., Ativan)
Morphine, codeine	• Some opioids cross-react (hydromorphone, heroin) but others do not (oxycodone, methadone) • **Common false positives:** Rifampin, ofloxacin, and other quinolones
Phencyclidine	• **Common false positives:** Chlorpromazine, dextromethorphan, diphenhydramine, ibuprofen, imipramine, ketamine, meperidine
Tetrahydrocannabinol	• **Common false positives:** Pantoprazole, NSAIDs, riboflavin, efavirenz, promethazine

Management

- Toxicity from phencyclidine and ketamine is managed through aggressive supportive care.
- Airway, breathing, and circulatory issues must be addressed with all the usual modalities.
- Patients may be hyperthermic.
  - » Measure core temperature and initiate cooling if required.
- Patients with phencyclidine and ketamine toxicity are often agitated.
  - » Nonpharmacologic modalities are important, including a quiet room with as few disruptive sounds and stimuli as possible.
  - » Benzodiazepines are the best and safest pharmacologic agents for managing the agitation.
  - » Benzodiazepines are also effective for emergent reactions (emergence phenomenon).

REFERENCES

Al-Motarreb A, Al-Habori M, Broadley KJ. Khat chewing, cardiovascular diseases and other internal medical problems: the current situation and directions for future research. *J Ethnopharmacol.* 2010;132(3):540–548. https://doi.org/10.1016/j.jep.2010.07.001. Medline:20621179

Andrabi S, Greene S, Moukaddam N, Li B. New drugs of abuse and withdrawal syndromes. *Emerg Med Clin North Am.* 2015;33(4):779–795. https://doi.org/10.1016/j.emc.2015.07.006. Medline:26493523 *Erratum in: Emerg Med Clin North Am.* 2016;34(1):xv.

Banks ML, Worst TJ, Rusyniak DE, Sprague JE. Synthetic cathinones ("bath salts"). *J Emerg Med.* 2014;46(5):632–642. https://doi.org/10.1016/j.jemermed.2013.11.104. Medline:24565885

Berger KJ, Guss DA. Mycotoxins revisited: part II. *J Emerg Med.* 2005;28(2):175–183. https://doi.org/10.1016/j.jemermed.2004.08.019. Medline:15707814

Boulanger-Gobeil C, St-Onge M, Laliberté M, Auger PL. Seizures and hyponatremia related to ethcathinone and methylone poisoning. *J Med Toxicol.* 2012;8(1):59–61. https://doi.org/10.1007/s13181-011-0159-1. Medline:21755421

Carey JL, Babu KM. Hallucinogens. In: Hoffman RS, Howland M, Lewin NA, Nelson LS, Goldfrank LR, eds. *Goldfrank's toxicologic emergencies.* 10th ed. New York, NY: McGraw-Hill; 2015.

Coppola M, Mondola R. Synthetic cathinones: chemistry, pharmacology and toxicology of a new class of designer drugs of abuse marketed as "bath salts" or "plant food". *Toxicol Lett.* 2012;211(2):144–149. https://doi.org/10.1016/j.toxlet.2012.03.009. Medline:22459606

Jang DH. Amphetamines. In: Hoffman RS, Howland M, Lewin NA, Nelson LS, Goldfrank LR, eds. *Goldfrank's toxicologic emergencies.* 10th ed. New York, NY: McGraw-Hill; 2015.

Kalant H. The pharmacology and toxicology of "ecstasy" (MDMA) and related drugs. *CMAJ.* 2001;165(7):917–928. Medline:11599334

Morgan CJA, Curran HV; Independent Scientific Committee on Drugs. Ketamine use: a review. *Addiction.* 2012;107(1):27–38. https://doi.org/10.1111/j.1360-0443.2011.03576.x. Medline:21777321

National Institute on Drug Abuse. Commonly abused drugs charts [Internet]. Bethesda, MD: National Institute on Drug Abuse; 2017. Available from: https://www.drugabuse.gov/drugs-abuse/commonly-abused-drugs-charts.

Nichols DE. Hallucinogens. *Pharmacol Ther.* 2004;101(2):131–181. https://doi.org/10.1016/j.pharmthera.2003.11.002. Medline:14761703

Olmedo RE. Phencyclidine and ketamine. In: Hoffman RS, Howland M, Lewin NA, Nelson LS, Goldfrank LR, editors. *Goldfrank's Toxicologic Emergencies.* 10th ed. New York, NY: McGraw-Hill; 2015.

Olsen KR. *Poison & drug overdose.* 6th ed. USA: McGraw Hill; 2011.

Prosser JM, Nelson LS. The toxicology of bath salts: a review of synthetic cathinones. *J Med Toxicol.* 2012;8(1):33–42. https://doi.org/10.1007/s13181-011-0193-z. Medline:22108839

Schep LJ, Slaughter RJ, Beasley DM. The clinical toxicology of metamfetamine. *Clin Toxicol (Phila).* 2010;48(7):675–694. https://doi.org/10.3109/15563650.2010.516752. Medline:20849327

Tournebize J, Gibaja V, Kahn JP. Acute effects of synthetic cannabinoids: Update 2015. *Subst Abus.* 2017;38(3):344–366. https://doi.org/10.1080/08897077.2016.1219438. Medline:27715709

19.9

Methemoglobinemia

Katrina F. Hurley

- Iron associated with hemoglobin is in the ferrous state (Fe^{2+}); when it oxidizes to the ferric (Fe^{3+}) state, it is known as methemoglobin.
- The body's normal *in vivo* methemoglobin level is 1% to 2%.
- Ferric iron is returned to a ferrous state by:
  - » NADH methemoglobin reductase
    - › This is the main pathway that utilizes NADH from the Meyerhof glycolytic pathway.
    - › Low activity of NADH methemoglobin reductase in infants results in higher baseline levels.
  - » NADPH methemoglobin reductase
    - › NADPH methemoglobin reductase uses NADPH from the hexose monophosphate shunt pathway.

Pathophysiology

- Methemoglobin has a high affinity for oxygen.
  - » It compromises the release of oxygen to tissues (functional anemia), causing a leftward shift of the oxygen dissociation curve.
- Symptoms generally appear with methemoglobin levels > 10%.

- Symptoms include a saturation gap that may lead to clinical cyanosis and oxygen saturation of < 90% despite a normal PO_2 on an arterial blood gas test.
  - » The saturation gap refers to the difference between the measured oxygen saturation (pulse oximetry) and the calculated oxygen saturation on the arterial blood gas test.

Etiology

- Methemoglobinemia can be congenital or acquired.
  - » Congenital cases are rare and may be caused by hemoglobin M or NADH methemoglobin reductase deficiency.
  - » Acquired cases are usually caused by the oxidizing effects of nitrates and nitrites stemming from:
    - › Gastrointestinal overgrowth of nitrite-producing bacteria
    - › Antibiotics, including dapsone, quinolones, and sulfonamides
    - › Industrial compounds, including aniline dyes, naphthalene, and phenols
    - › Local anesthetics, including lidocaine, benzocaine, and prilocaine
    - › Dietary nitrates (e.g., nitrate-contaminated well water)
    - › Amyl nitrite from a "Lilly kit" for cyanide poisoning
    - › Cardiovascular medications, including nitroglycerin and nitroprusside

Diagnosis

- Suspect methemoglobinemia in patients with cyanosis that is not helped by the administration of oxygen.
  - » In patients with underlying cardiopulmonary or hematologic disease, symptoms may occur at lower methemoglobin levels.
  - » In cases of methemoglobinemia, blood is chocolate-colored or dark.
- Confirm diagnosis with cooximetry:
  - » Absorption at 570 mm and 670 mm
  - » Carboxyhemoglobin may also be detected

Management

- For initial management, focus on management of ABCs, including 100% supplemental oxygen.
- Identify and remove the oxidant stress when possible.
  - » Topical sources should be cleaned off.
- Individuals with normal red blood cell metabolism will correct methemoglobinemia over a period of hours.
- Persistently symptomatic methemoglobinemia may be treated with hyperbaric oxygen to ensure the reoxygenation of tissues and accelerated reduction of methemoglobin.
- Admit the patient to hospital to investigate underlying causes.

Table 19.9.1. CORRELATION OF METHEMOGLOBIN AND SYMPTOMATOLOGY FOR PREVIOUSLY HEALTHY INDIVIDUALS

Methemoglobin level	Possible presenting symptoms*
< 10%	• Usually asymptomatic
10% to 20%	• Cyanosis • Usually mild (e.g., fatigue)
20% to 50%	• Dyspnea • Exertion intolerance • Headache • Irritability • Tachypnea • Tachycardia
> 50%	• End-organ hypoxia (more evident) • Metabolic acidosis • CNS symptoms: lethargy, coma, and seizures • Cardiac symptoms: dysrhythmias
> 70%	• Life threatening symptoms • Death

CNS central nervous system.

*Note that presenting symptoms are also affected by the patient's hemoglobin levels. An underlying anemia would lead to symptoms at lower levels of methemoglobin.

Methylene Blue

- When symptoms are significant, administer the antidote: methylene blue.
- The mechanism of action for methylene blue action is as follows:
  - » Methylene blue is reduced to leukomethylene blue, accepting electrons from NADPH.
  - » Leukomethylene blue then reduces methemoglobin ($Fe3+$) to the ferrous state ($Fe2+$) and converts back to methylene blue.
- Indications for methylene blue are:
  - » Signs of organ hypoxia (seizures, altered mental status, dysrhythmias)
  - » Significant change in vital signs secondary to tissue hypoxia
  - » Methemoglobin levels > 20% regardless of symptoms
- Give methylene blue 1 to 2 mg/kg as a 1% solution IV over 5 min.
  - » If symptoms are still severe after 1 hour, consider administering a second dose.
- Use caution when administering methylene blue in patients with glucose-6-phosphate dehydrogenase (G6PD) deficiency as it may cause hemolysis.

REFERENCES

Furuta K, Ikeo S, Takaiwa T. et al. Identifying the cause of the "saturation gap": two cases of Dapsone-induced methemoglobinemia. *Intern Med.* 2015;54(13):1639–1641. https://doi.org/10.2169/internalmedicine.54.3496. Medline:26134197

Greer FR, Shannon M American Academy of Pediatrics Committee on Nutrition; American Academy of Pediatrics Committee on Environmental Health. Infant methemoglobinemia: the role of dietary nitrate in food and water. *Pediatrics.* 2005;116(3):784–786. https://doi.org/10.1542/peds.2005-1497. Medline:16140723

Guay J. Methemoglobinemia related to local anesthetics: a summary of 242 episodes. *Anesth Analg.* 2009;108(3):837–845. https://doi.org/10.1213/ane.0b013e318187c4b1. Medline:19224791

Khanal R, Karmacharya P, Pathak R, Poudel DR, Ghimire S, Alweis R. Do all patients with acquired methemoglobinemia need treatment? A lesson learnt. *J Community Hosp Intern Med Perspect.* 2015;5(5):29079. https://doi.org/10.3402/jchimp.v5.29079. Medline:26486118

Lindenmann J, Fink-Neuboeck N, Schilcher G, Smolle-Juettner FM. Severe methaemoglobinaemia treated with adjunctive hyperbaric oxygenation. *Diving Hyperb Med.* 2015;45(2):132–134. Medline:26165539

McDonagh EM, Bautista JM, Youngster I, Altman RB, Klein TE. PharmGKB summary: methylene blue pathway. *Pharmacogenet Genomics.* 2013;23(9):498–508. https://doi.org/10.1097/FPC.0b013e32836498f4.

Nelson KA, Hosteller MA. An infant with methemoglobinemia. *Hosp Physician.* 2003;39(2):31–38, 62.

19.10

Cyanide Toxicity

Bandar Baw

- The total number of cyanide exposures mentioned in a 2015 report by the American Association of Poison Control Centers (AAPCC) was 9646 cases (0.4% of total human exposures).
- Cyanide can be found in both natural substances and artificial chemicals.
  - » Natural cyanogenic sources include cassava roots and amygdalin, which is found in the kernels of apricots, peaches, bitter almonds, cherry pits, and apple seeds.
  - » Some alternative and herbal medicines contain naturally occurring cyanide compounds, which are used for their medicinal properties, such as antitumor activity, and have been reported to cause cyanide toxicity in the pediatric population.
  - » Artificial cyanide is found in potassium cyanide (used in mining and other chemical syntheses) and acetonitrile (used in some cosmetics and in nail polish remover).
  - » Iatrogenic cyanide poisoning has been reported after prolonged infusion of antihypertensive nitroprusside.
  - » Hydrogen cyanide gas can result from the combustion of plastic, wool, and other materials found in household furniture.
- In pediatric patients, death from smoke injuries is mostly due to toxic inhalation rather than from the burns themselves.
  - » Most fatalities are from smoke inhalation.
    - › Pediatric fire victims have been confirmed postmortem to have high cyanide levels in their blood, occasionally higher than carbon monoxide.
  - » Carbon monoxide toxicity is discussed in Chapter 19.16.
- The pediatric population is more susceptible to developing cyanide toxicity from cyanogenic plant ingestion and smoke inhalation compared to their adult counterparts.
- Cyanide is one of the most toxic substances and has the potential to be used in chemical warfare or terrorist activities.

Toxicity

- If not immediately detoxified, the cyanide molecule acts as rapid cellular asphyxiant, binding to cytochrome oxidase and blocking the electron transport chain in mitochondria.
  - » The action of these substances is similar to carbon monoxide, hydrogen sulfide, salicylic acid, and iron: all are cellular asphyxiants.
- This cellular toxicity forces cells to switch to anaerobic metabolism and, therefore, leads to the accumulation of severe lactic acid.
- Cell damage also occurs from free radicals and reactive oxygen production.

Diagnosis

- Both the rate at which toxicity takes effect and the severity of cyanide toxicity depend on the type and route of exposure.
  - » Toxicity occurs in seconds with hydrogen cyanide gas inhalation.
  - » Toxicity occurs in minutes with cyanide salt ingestion.
  - » Toxicity occurs in hours from ingestion of cyanogenic natural products or the initiation of IV nitroprusside.

- Severe, fast-occurring cyanide toxicity may result in sudden loss of consciousness.
  - » Toxicity affects the brain quickly, accompanied by aggressive cardiovascular collapse and severe metabolic acidosis.
- A subtler onset of exposure may result in a nonspecific clinical picture such as:
  - » Headache
  - » Abdominal pain
  - » Nausea and vomiting
  - » Altered level of consciousness — confusion
  - » Ataxia
  - » Seizure
- Cherry-red skin might occur due to underutilization of oxygen by affected tissues, which leads to increase oxygen contents in venous blood.
- Chronic exposure or survivors of severe cyanide toxicity may show evidence of:
  - » Neurologic manifestations such as:
    - › Extrapyramidal and movement disorders
    - › Vertigo
    - › Ataxia
  - » Cardiac complications such as dysrhythmia and conduction disorders

Investigations

- The key to the diagnosis of cyanide toxicity is having a high clinical suspicion supported by the correct clinical scenario that matches initial bloodwork.
  - » Key features of this clinical scenario are abrupt loss of consciousness, severe anion gap metabolic acidosis, and high lactate level.
- Venous blood gas analysis may reveal severe anion gap metabolic acidosis.
  - » This is caused by lack of oxygen utilization by cells in the presence of cellular asphyxia.
  - » Venous oxygen saturation may be higher than normal.
- Lactate level > 10 mmol/L (> 8 mmol/L in some literature) has positive predictive value for cyanide toxicity when it is difficult to diagnose in smoke inhalation injury.
- The carboxyhemoglobin level should also be obtained in all smoke inhalation patients to determine the extent of concomitant CO toxicity.
- The cyanide level can be obtained (in some laboratories) but has very limited use in treatment in the emergency department (ED) in patients with potential cyanide toxicity.
- Begin treatment if clinical suspicion of cyanide toxicity is high rather than waiting for confirmation of the cyanide level.

Management

- Treating patients with cyanide toxicity may carry risks to healthcare providers.
  - » Extreme caution should be taken to prevent cross-contamination.
  - » Personal protective equipment should be used appropriately.
  - » Decontaminate as necessary based on time and route of exposure (e.g., dermal, oral, or inhalation).
- General supportive treatment measures include:
  - » Airway management
  - » Aggressive intravenous fluid resuscitation
  - » Use of inotropes/vasopressors
  - » Treatment of seizure
- Severe metabolic acidosis can be treated with sodium bicarbonate (1 to 2 mEq/kg IV bolus followed by 150 mEq/L in 5% dextrose solution at 1.5 times the maintenance dose).
- Cyanide can be detoxified through one of the following 2 major pathways:
  1. Reaction with sodium thiosulfate to form less toxic thiocyanate, which is excreted by the kidneys
  2. Reaction with hydroxocobalamin to form cyanocobalamin (vitamin B_{12}), which is also excreted by the kidneys

Antidotes

- There are 2 main classic treatments for cyanide toxicity using the following antidotes:
  1. Cyanide antidote kit, which includes 3 compounds: amyl nitrite (inhaled, when IV access is lacking), sodium nitrite, and sodium thiosulfate
     - › Mechanism:
       - · Nitrites oxidize hemoglobin to produce methemoglobin.
       - · Methemoglobin binds to cyanide, taking it away from cytochrome oxidase in the mitochondria and restoring cellular respiration.
       - · Sodium thiosulfate enhances the conversion of cyanide to form thiocyanate (less toxic, excreted by kidneys).
     - › Sodium nitrite 0.2 mL/kg of 3% solution (6 mg/kg) is infused at 2.5 to 5 mL/min (to a maximum dose of 10 mL of 3% solution or 300 mg IV) followed immediately by sodium thiosulfate.
       - · Use sodium nitrite with caution in patients with preexisting low hemoglobin levels or methemoglobinemia.
       - · There is a possible risk of decreased oxygen-carrying capacity from nitrite-induced methemoglobinemia, especially with concomitant CO toxicity in fire victims.
       - · Administer sodium thiosulfate 1 mL/kg of 25% solution (250 mg/kg; maximum dose 12.5 g IV over 10 minutes) **or** 412 mg/kg infusion at 0.625 to 1.25 g/min.

› Amyl nitrite is mainly used when intravenous access is not readily available or to bridge time until venous access is available.
  · The capsule is crushed and inhaled.

2. Hydroxocobalamin (vitamin B_{12} precursor)
  › Hydroxocobalamin comes with a possible risk of nitrite-induced methemoglobinemia in children (hypotension, increased risk of overshooting methemoglobinemia, and decreased oxygen-carrying capacity).
  › It has been used with fewer side effects and better results for detoxification after cyanide exposure.
  › Hydroxocobalamin combines with cyanide to form cyanocobalamin (vitamin B_{12}).
    · Cyanocobalamin is excreted by the kidneys.
  › Dose at 70 mg/kg (to a maximum dose of 5 g) IV; this can be repeated at half the dose if necessary within 30 minutes.
  › Side effects include hypertension and reddish discoloration of urine and sweat.

• Due to the higher risks of (mainly) hypotension and decreased oxygen-carrying capacity in all populations, suggestions have been made to limit cyanide antidote use to only 2 compounds: hydroxocobalamin and sodium thiosulfate.
  » This eliminates the nitrite components of cyanide antidotes in pediatric patients

Table 19.10.1. CYANIDE ANTIDOTE DOSES

Drug	Initial dose	Maximum dose	Notes
Hydroxocobalamin	70 mg/kg IV	5 g	
Sodium thiosulfate	1 mL/kg of 25% solution (250 mg/kg)	12.5 g (50 mL)	
Amyl nitrite	Inhalation for 30 seconds	May repeat every 30 seconds × 4	Should be used only if IV access is lacking
Sodium nitrite	0.2 mL/kg of 3% solution (6 mg/kg) infused at 2.5 to 5 mL/min	300 mg (10 mL)	Followed immediately by sodium thiosulfate

REFERENCES

Abraham K, Buhrke T, Lampen A. Bioavailability of cyanide after consumption of a single meal of foods containing high levels of cyanogenic glycosides: a crossover study in humans. *Arch Toxicol.* 2016;90(3):559–574. https://doi.org/10.1007/s00204-015-1479-8. Medline:25708890

Anseeuw K, Delvau N, Burillo-Putze G, et al. Cyanide poisoning by fire smoke inhalation: a European expert consensus. *Eur J Emerg Med.* 2013;20(1):2–9. https://doi.org/10.1097/MEJ.0b013e328357170b. Medline:22828651

Ariffin WA, Choo KE, Karnaneedi S. Cassava (ubi kayu) poisoning in children. *Med J Malaysia.* 1992;47(3):231–234. Medline:1491651

Barillo DJ. Diagnosis and treatment of cyanide toxicity. *J Burn Care Res.* 2009;30(1):148–152. https://doi.org/10.1097/BCR.0b013e3181923b91. Medline:19060738

Baud FJ, Barriot P, Toffis V, et al. Elevated blood cyanide concentrations in victims of smoke inhalation. *N Engl J Med.* 1991;325(25):1761–1766. https://doi.org/10.1056/NEJM199112193252502. Medline:1944484

Baud FJ, Borron SW, Bavoux E, Astier A, Hoffman JR. Relation between plasma lactate and blood cyanide concentrations in acute cyanide poisoning. *BMJ.* 1996;312(7022):26–27. https://doi.org/10.1136/bmj.312.7022.26. Medline:8555853

Bebarta VS, Tanen DA, Lairet J, Dixon PS, Valtier S, Bush A. Hydroxocobalamin and sodium thiosulfate versus sodium nitrite and sodium thiosulfate in the treatment of acute cyanide toxicity in a swine (Sus scrofa) model. *Ann Emerg Med.* 2010;55(4):345–351. https://doi.org/10.1016/j.annemergmed.2009.09.020. Medline:19944487

Caravati EM, Litovitz TL. Pediatric cyanide intoxication and death from an acetonitrile-containing cosmetic. *JAMA.* 1988;260(23):3470–3473. https://doi.org/10.1001/jama.1988.03410230088034. Medline:3062198

Cescon DW, Juurlink DN. Discoloration of skin and urine after treatment with hydroxocobalamin for cyanide poisoning. *CMAJ.* 2009;180(2):251. https://doi.org/10.1503/cmaj.080727. Medline:19153403

Dart RC. Hydroxocobalamin for acute cyanide poisoning: new data from preclinical and clinical studies; new results from the prehospital emergency setting. *Clin Toxicol (Phila).* 2006;44(Suppl 1):1–3. https://doi.org/10.1080/15563650600811607. Medline:16990188

Dart RC, Bogdan GM. Acute cyanide poisoning: causes, consequences, recognition and management. *Frontline First Responder.* 2004;2:19–22.

Geller RJ, Barthold C, Saiers JA, Hall AH. Pediatric cyanide poisoning: causes, manifestations, management, and unmet needs. *Pediatrics.* 2006;118(5):2146–2158. https://doi.org/10.1542/peds.2006-1251. Medline:17079589

Hamel J. A review of acute cyanide poisoning with a treatment update. *Crit Care Nurse.* 2011;31(1):72–81, quiz 82. https://doi.org/10.4037/ccn2011799. Medline:21285466

Hammer GB, Lewandowski A, Drover DR, et al. Safety and efficacy of sodium nitroprusside during prolonged infusion in pediatric patients. *Pediatr Crit Care Med.* 2015;16(5):397–403. https://doi.org/10.1097/PCC.0000000000000383. Medline:25715047

Huzar TF, George T, Cross JM. Carbon monoxide and cyanide toxicity: etiology, pathophysiology and treatment in inhalation injury. *Expert Rev Respir Med.* 2013;7(2):159–170. https://doi.org/10.1586/ers.13.9. Medline:23547992

Meyer S, Gortner L, Larsen A, et al. Complementary and alternative medicine in paediatrics: a systematic overview/synthesis of Cochrane Collaboration reviews. *Swiss Med Wkly.* 2013;143:w13794. Medline:23740212

Mowry JB, Spyker DA, Brooks DE, McMillan N, Schauben JL. 2014 annual report of the American Association of Poison Control Centers' National Poison Data System (NPDS): 32nd annual report. *Clin Toxicol (Phila).* 2015;53(10):962–1147. https://doi.org/10.3109/15563650.2015.1102927. Medline:26624241 *Erratum in: Clin Toxicol (Phila).* 2016;54(7):607. https://doi.org/10.1080/15563650.2016.1190547

O'Brien DJ, Walsh DW, Terriff CM, Hall AH. Empiric management of cyanide toxicity associated with smoke inhalation. *Prehosp Disaster Med.* 2011;26(5):374–382. https://doi.org/10.1017/S1049023X11006625. Medline:22336184

Sauer H, Wollny C, Oster I, et al. Severe cyanide poisoning from an alternative medicine treatment with amygdalin and apricot kernels in a 4-year-old child. *Wien Med Wochenschr.* 2015;165(9-10):185–188. https://doi.org/10.1007/s10354-014-0340-7. Medline:25605411

Thompson JP, Marrs TC. Hydroxocobalamin in cyanide poisoning. *Clin Toxicol (Phila).* 2012;50(10):875–885. https://doi.org/10.3109/15563650.2012.742197. Medline:23163594

19.11

Digoxin Toxicity

Vincent Lim, Zoë Piggott

- Digoxin falls into a broad group of medications known as cardioactive steroids.
- Cardioactive steroids are used therapeutically for congestive heart failure as well as for rate control in atrial tachydysrhythmias.
- Preparations are administered PO — one of the only PO inotropes available — or IV.
- Another cardioactive steroid that is available but less commonly used is digitoxin (available in Europe).
  - » The important differences between digitoxin and digoxin are pharmacokinetic.
    - › Digitoxin has nearly 100% bioavailability, undergoes predominantly hepatic rather than renal metabolism, and has a longer half-life (6 to 7 days) than digoxin.
- There are also a number of plants with cardioactive steroid properties that have been implicated in cardioactive steroid toxicity:
  - » Foxglove (plants belonging to the *Digitalis* genus; e.g., *D. purpurea*)
  - » Oleander (*Nerium oleander* and *Thevetia peruviana*)
  - » Lily-of-the-valley (*Convallaria majalis*)
  - » Dogbane (*Apocynum cannabinum*)
  - » Red squill (*Urginea maritima*)

Pharmacology

- Digoxin causes physiologic changes to the heart by:
  - » Inhibiting the Na-K ATPase pump
    - › This increases cytosolic calcium, resulting in increased inotropy.
    - › In excess, the increase in intracellular calcium causes an elevation in the resting membrane potential, which increases cardiac myocyte irritability and results in tachydysrhythmias.
      - · This is further exacerbated by hypokalemia.
  - » Decreasing the rate of depolarization at the sinoatrial (SA) node and decreasing the rate of conduction through the atrioventricular (AV) node by the combination of indirect vagal stimulation and direct effects on the myocardium
    - › In excess, this can result in bradydysrhythmias and heart blocks.
  - » Increasing automaticity and decreasing repolarization times of the atria and ventricles
    - › In excess, this can result in tachydysrhythmias.

- Onset of action is:
  - » PO — 1 to 6 hours
  - » IV — 5 to 60 minutes

Table 19.11.1. AGE DEPENDENCE OF HALF-LIFE AND VOLUME OF DISTRIBUTION OF DIGOXIN*

Volume of distribution	Half-life
	Premature = 61 to 170 hours
Neonates = 7.5 to 10 L/kg	Neonates = 35 to 45 hours
Infants/Children = up to 16 L/kg	Infants = 18 to 25 hours
	Children = 18 to 36 hours
Adults = 5 to 7 L/kg	Adults = 36 to 48 hours
Adults (with renal failure) = 4 to 5 L/kg	Adults (with end-stage renal disease) = 3.5 to 5 days

*Therapeutic concentration: ACCF/AHA 2013 guidelines recommend 0.5 to 0.9 ng/mL

Clinical Presentation

- Digoxin toxicity may be either acute or chronic.
- Toxicity most commonly occurs in extremes of age (i.e., either in young children or the elderly) and in those with impaired renal function.
  - » Toxicity in children is most commonly the result of a dosing or administration error rather than accidental overdose.
- Digoxin toxicity can result in almost any type of cardiac dysrhythmia (tachycardia or bradycardia).
  - » The most common electrocardiogram (ECG) findings are:
    - › Frequent premature ventricular contractions
    - › Bradycardia with varying AV blocks
    - › Selected atrial dysrhythmias
  - » ECG rhythms most suggestive of digoxin toxicity (higher *specificity*) include:
    - › Bidirectional ventricular tachycardia
    - › Atrial fibrillation with slow ventricular rate
    - › Junctional tachycardia
    - › New bigeminy
  - » Acute poisoning more commonly results in bradydysrhythmias or AV blocks.
  - » Chronic poisoning more commonly results in tachydysrhythmias or ventricular dysrhythmias.

- » In pediatric patients, bradydysrhythmias and AV blocks are more common.
- 80% of patients have central nervous system (CNS), gastrointestinal (GI), and/or visual symptoms.
  - » Onset of symptoms is more gradual in chronic toxicity.
  - » The wide range of possible signs and/or symptoms includes:
    - › CNS — fatigue, weakness, confusion, decreased level of consciousness, seizures, paresthesia, headaches
    - › GI — nausea, vomiting, anorexia, diarrhea, abdominal pain
    - › Visual disturbances — blurry vision, halo, changes in color perception

Diagnosis

- Digoxin toxicity requires a high index of suspicion, particularly in children.
- It should be considered in any patient who is taking digoxin and has vague or nonspecific symptoms or dysrhythmias.
- Diagnosis relies on the measurement of the digoxin level.
  - » Steady state level (obtained 6 to 8 hours after ingestion) is more important than peak concentration.
  - » Measurement may be impractical in an acute overdose and may result in an inappropriately long delay to treatment.
- The half-life of digoxin may be shortened to 13 to 15 hours after the ingestion of a large quantity.

Investigations

- Investigations should include ECG, electrolyte levels, and digoxin level.

Management

- Initial treatment should focus on the management of ABCs and good supportive care.
- Consider activated charcoal if the patient presents within 1 hour of an acute ingestion (25 to 50 g; see Chapter 19.1).
- Avoid insertion of a nasogastric (NG) or orogastric (OG) tube due to vagal stimulation.

DigiFab

- Significant toxicity is treated with DigiFab, a digoxin-specific antibody.
  - » Treatment can be empirical.
    - › For acute ingestion of an unknown quantity with clinical toxicity or cardiac arrest give 10 to 20 vials for larger (adult-sized) children or adults, 5 to 10 vials for children.
    - › For chronic toxicity give 1 to 2 vials for children,

3 to 6 vials for larger (adult-sized) children or adults.
  - » Treatment can also be based on a calculation if the ingested quantity is known or if the digoxin level is at a steady state.
    - › **For acute ingestion of known quantity**:

$$\text{Number of vials} = \frac{\text{Total ingestion}\,(\text{mg})}{0.5\,(\text{mg}\,/\,\text{vial})} \times 80\ \text{Bioavailability}$$

    - › **For chronic toxicity with known steady state level**:

$$\text{Number of vials} = \frac{\text{Serum digoxin concentration}\,(\text{ng}\,/\,\text{mL}) \times \text{Patient weight}\,(\text{kg})}{100}$$

- Indications for DigiFab administration are:
  - » Acute ingestion > 0.3 mg/kg or > 4 mg
  - » Steady state concentration > 5 ng/mL
  - » Serum potassium > 5 to 5.5 mmol/L
  - » Hemodynamically significant tachydysrhythmias or cardiac arrest
  - » Bradycardias and heart blocks not responsive to atropine
  - » Coingestion of other cardiotoxic medications
  - » Serum digoxin level > 15 ng/mL at any time or > 10 ng/mL 6 hours postingestion, regardless of symptoms
- Administration of DigiFab may falsely elevate serum digoxin levels.
  - » Monitor patients' responses to therapy clinically as serum concentrations will be unreliable once DigiFab is administered.

Complications

- Electrolyte abnormalities often associated with digoxin toxicity include:
  - » Hypokalemia
    - › Hypokalemia is more common in chronic toxicity.
    - › It can potentiate the effects of digoxin toxicity.
    - › Treat with slow potassium replacement and monitor closely.
  - » Hyperkalemia
    - › Hyperkalemia is more common in acute toxicity.
    - › Consider treating with calcium gluconate or calcium chloride.
      - · Use of these substances for hyperkalemia remains controversial.
      - · There is a theoretical risk of developing "stone heart."
    - › Treat hyperkalemia with other usual hyperkalemia therapies in addition to DigiFab:
      - · Inhaled beta agonist (salbutamol)
      - · Insulin/glucose
  - » Hypomagnesemia
    - › Initiate replacement therapy with magnesium sulfate 25 to 50 mg/kg IV to a maximum of 2 g over 20 minutes.

- For bradycardia and bradydysrhythmias:
  » Administer atropine (0.02 mg/kg per dose up to 1 mg)
  » Consider pacing
    › Pacing is generally not recommended because of risk of increased dysrhythmias due to irritated myocardium.
    › If pacing is unavoidable, transcutaneous is preferred over transvenous.
    › It may be necessary for bradycardia or bradydysrhythmia that is unresponsive to atropine if DigiFab is unavailable or delayed.
- For tachycardia and tachydysrhythmias:
  » Use cardioversion for unstable tachydysrhythmias, defibrillation for pulseless ventricular tachycardia/ventricular fibrillation.
  » Do not perform any vagal maneuvers due to the risk of precipitating bradydysrhythmias/asystole.
  » Consider lidocaine, which suppresses ventricular automaticity in the setting of digoxin toxicity, if DigiFab is unavailable or delayed.
    › Give lidocaine 1 to 1.5 mg/kg IV bolus, then 30 to 50 mcg/kg per minute.
    › **Avoid** other antiarrhythmics, especially Class Ia sodium channel blockers, as they may worsen AV blocks, hypotension, and arrhythmias.
- There is no role for hemodialysis due to the high degree of protein binding and the large volume of distribution.

Disposition

- Patients exhibiting any signs or symptoms of digoxin toxicity require hospital admission.
  » Patients who are symptomatic and/or require DigiFab should be admitted to the intensive care unit for close monitoring.
  » Patients with only mild signs and symptoms of digoxin toxicity should be admitted for continuous cardiac monitoring, as well as serial ECGs and measurement of electrolytes and digoxin level.
- Asymptomatic patients who have ingested a large quantity of digoxin require cardiac monitoring for a minimum of 12 hours with or without admission to the ICU, with serial ECGs and measurement of electrolytes and digoxin level to determine the need for DigiFab.

- Asymptomatic patients with suspected digoxin toxicity should be placed on cardiac monitors for at least 6 hours with serial measurement of electrolytes and digoxin level and can be discharged if electrolytes remain unchanged and digoxin level is not rising (based on expert opinion).

REFERENCES

Bayer MJ. Recognition and management of digitalis intoxication: implications for emergency medicine. *Am J Emerg Med.* 1991;9(2 Suppl 1):29–32, discussion 33–34. https://doi.org/10.1016/0735-6757(91)90165-G. Medline:1997019

Cole JB. Cardiovascular drugs. In: Hockberger RS, Walls RM, Gausche-Hill M, eds. *Rosen's emergency medicine: concepts and clinical practice.* 9th ed. Philadelphia, PA: Elsevier; 2017.

Eichhorn EJ, Gheorghiade M. Digoxin. *Prog Cardiovasc Dis.* 2002;44(4):251–266. https://doi.org/10.1053/pcad.2002.31591. Medline:12007081

Gittelman MA, Stephan M, Perry H. Acute pediatric digoxin ingestion. *Pediatr Emerg Care.* 1999;15(5):359–362. https://doi.org/10.1097/00006565-199910000-00017. Medline:10532672

Hack JB. Cardioactive steroids. In: Hoffman RS, Howland M, Lewin NA, Nelson LS, Goldfrank LR, eds. *Goldfrank's toxicologic emergencies.* 10th ed. New York, NY: McGraw-Hill; 2015.

Hickey AR, Wenger TL, Carpenter VP, et al. Digoxin immune fab therapy in the management of digitalis intoxication: safety and efficacy results of an observational surveillance study. *J Am Coll Cardiol.* 1991;17(3):590–598. https://doi.org/10.1016/S0735-1097(10)80170-6. Medline:1993775

Levine M, Nikkanen H, Pallin DJ. The effects of intravenous calcium in patients with digoxin toxicity. *J Emerg Med.* 2011;40(1):41–46. https://doi.org/10.1016/j.jemermed.2008.09.027. Medline:19201134

Levine M, O'Connor A. Digitalis (cardiac glycoside) poisoning. In: *UpToDate,* Post TW, ed. Waltham, MA: UpToDate. [cited 2016 Jan 29]. Available from: https://www.uptodate.com/contents/digitalis-cardiac-glycoside-poisoning

Lip GY, Metcalfe MJ, Dunn FG. Diagnosis and treatment of digoxin toxicity. *Postgrad Med J.* 1993;69(811):337–339. https://doi.org/10.1136/pgmj.69.811.337. Medline:8346128

Ma G, Brady WJ, Pollack M, Chan TC. Electrocardiographic manifestations: digitalis toxicity. *J Emerg Med.* 2001;20(2):145–152. https://doi.org/10.1016/S0736-4679(00)00312-7. Medline:11207409

Rahimtoola SH. Digitalis therapy for patients in clinical heart failure. *Circulation.* 2004;109(24):2942–2946. https://doi.org/10.1161/01.CIR.0000132477.32438.03. Medline:15210610

Thacker D, Sharma J. Digoxin toxicity. *Clin Pediatr (Phila).* 2007;46(3):276–279. https://doi.org/10.1177/0009922806294805. Medline:17416888

Yancy CW, Jessup M, Bozkurt B, et al; American College of Cardiology Foundation; American Heart Association Task Force on Practice Guidelines. 2013 ACCF/AHA guideline for the management of heart failure: a report of the American College of Cardiology Foundation/American Heart Association Task Force on Practice Guidelines. *J Am Coll Cardiol.* 2013;62(16):e147–e239. https://doi.org/10.1016/j.jacc.2013.05.019. Medline:23747642

TOXICOLOGY

19.12

Iron Overdose

David Lussier, Wesley Palatnick

Epidemiology

- Iron overdose used to be a leading poisoning cause of morbidity and mortality in children, but recently there has been a decreased incidence of unintentional iron ingestions and reduced iron-related mortality in children < 6 years of age.
  - » This is thought to be due in part to public health initiatives beginning in the late 1990s.
- The most recent epidemiological data from the American Association of Poison Control Centers' (AAPCC, 2013) National Poison Data System are as follows:
  - » Overdose cases of involving iron salts: 3910
  - » Overdose cases of involving vitamins: 12 221
  - » Most common age group: < 5 years old
  - » Most common reason for ingestion: unintentional
- Due to the common use of prenatal vitamins by pregnant mothers, there is a greater risk of children suffering from iron poisoning during the mother's pregnancy, and especially in the first 6 months postpartum.

Pharmacology

- Iron is incorporated into hemoglobin and myoglobin, and is also needed for enzyme and cytochrome activity.
- Iron is primarily absorbed in the proximal small bowel.
- Once absorbed, iron is stored intracellularly as ferritin or is bound to transferrin in the serum.
- Iron stores are regulated by altering iron absorption, since humans are unable to directly excrete iron.
  - » Most iron is lost through the sloughing of gastrointestinal (GI) mucosal cells or via menstruation.
- Iron preparations vary in their elemental iron content; iron salts include:
  - » Ferrous gluconate (12% elemental iron)
  - » Ferrous sulfate (20% elemental iron)
  - » Ferrous fumarate (33% elemental iron)
- Nonionic forms (carbonyl iron and iron polysaccharide) have higher elemental iron but lower toxicity due to slower absorption.
- Common sources of ingested iron include prenatal vitamins, multivitamins, and the "placebo row" of oral contraceptive pills.
- Overdoses involving iron-containing adult preparations are much more likely to cause serious toxicity than iron-containing children's vitamins.

- Enteric coated preparations have much lower bioavailability, take longer to reach peak serum iron concentration, and generally result in lower peak serum iron concentrations.

Toxicity

- Iron can participate in redox reactions, shifting from the ferrous (Fe^{2+}) to the ferric (Fe^{3+}) oxidation state.
- Ferric iron is toxic to many cellular processes through free radical production and lipid peroxidation.
- The causes of iron toxicity are multifactorial. Effects include:
  - » GI effects:
    - › Direct mucosa erosion
    - › Hepatic injury
      - · Hepatic injury is caused by iron accumulation in the liver through the portal circulation.
  - » Metabolic acidosis
    - › Metabolic acidosis is cause by hydration of ferric ions in plasma, which generates 3 hydrogen ions (H^+), leading to the disruption of the Krebs cycle and the electron transport chain.
  - » Hypovolemia
    - › Hypovolemia is caused by capillary leaking and third spacing.
    - › It exacerbates acidotic state.
  - » Cardiovascular effects:
    - › Hypotension
      - · Hypotension is caused by the direct negative inotropic effect iron may have on the heart.
  - » Possible postarteriolar dilation and venous pooling
  - » Coagulopathy
    - › Coagulopathy may result from direct thrombin inhibition.
- Peak serum iron concentrations occur 2 to 3 hours after therapeutic dosing and up to 4 to 6 hours after an acute overdose.
  - » Peak serum iron concentrations may be delayed if an enteric coated product is ingested.
- Toxic and lethal doses are not firmly established; commonly accepted values are:
  - » 20 to 60 mg/kg of elemental iron — may cause clinical toxicity
    - › Serious outcomes are unlikely but have been reported at these doses.

» 200 to 250 mg/kg of elemental iron — estimated lethal doses

› **Note that fatalities have been reported at levels as low as 70 mg/kg.**

Physical Exam

- Iron toxicity is divided into 5 stages that may progress quickly or overlap, so it is important to determine the phase by clinical and laboratory assessment and not solely by time after ingestion.
  » Stage 1: GI toxicity (onset within a few hours)
    › Stage 1 symptoms include abdominal pain, nausea, vomiting, diarrhea, GI bleeding.
  » Stage 2: relative stability (onset within 6 to 24 hours)
    › A patient in stage 2 must not be mistaken for a patient with only mild poisoning who may only experience stage 1.
    › Stage 2 symptoms are subtle and include hypovolemia, hypoperfusion, and acidosis.
  » Stage 3: shock and acidosis (onset after 4 hours and up to 4 days)
    › Shock that occurs soon after toxic ingestion is most likely hypovolemic and is potentially exacerbated in cases of GI bleeding.
    › After 24 to 48 hours, patients may show signs of distributive shock and eventually cardiogenic shock.
    › Circulatory shock is the most common cause of death in iron overdose.
    › Further stage 3 symptoms include poor peripheral perfusion, lethargy, altered level of consciousness, possible multisystem organ failure, and coagulopathy.
  » Stage 4: hepatotoxicity (onset after 12 hours and up to several days)
    › Fulminant hepatic failure may develop from the liver's exposure to high concentrations of iron from the portal circulation and its ability to passively absorb large amounts of iron.
    › Fulminant hepatic failure is the second most common cause of death in iron overdose.
  » Stage 5: Bowel obstruction (onset after 2 to 8 weeks)
    › Bowel obstruction is due to the initial bowel injury and subsequent scarring and stricture formation.
    › It typically affects the stomach or proximal small bowel, though cases of distal small bowel involvement with ingestion of enteric-coated products have been reported.

History

- History should include the time of ingestion, type of iron preparation, calculated mg/kg dose, other coingestions, and whether the overdose was intentional or accidental.

Investigations

Bloodwork

- Laboratory workups are suggested for patients who present with systemic toxicity and who have ingested an unknown quantity of elemental iron or a known quantity of more than 30 to 40 mg/kg.
- Appropriate laboratory tests include the following:
  » Complete blood count (CBC), electrolytes, creatinine, urea, glucose, coagulation profile, liver enzymes, lactate, blood gas, and type and screen.
  » Serum iron concentration
    › Peak serum iron concentration occurs 4 to 6 hours postingestion with a non–enteric-coated product and up to 8 hours with an extended-release preparation.
    › Serum iron concentration > 54 μmol/L is usually associated with GI toxicity and has been associated with systemic toxicity.
    › Serum iron concentration > 90 μmol/L is associated with serious systemic toxicity.
    › Low serum iron concentration cannot be used to rule out serious toxicity, as levels do not always correlate with the severity of the ingestion and a single serum iron concentration measurement may not represent the peak serum iron concentration
    › Serial serum iron concentrations may be required
    › Serum iron concentrations are inaccurate after the administration of deferoxamine (unless determined by atomic absorption spectroscopy).
    › Total serum iron-binding capacity (TIBC) levels are not accurate in iron overdose and should not be used.

Imaging

- Abdominal X-rays are recommended with ingestions > 30 to 40 mg/kg of elemental iron.
- Visualization of radiopaque pills in the stomach can help confirm ingestion and guide management.
- Adult tablets with a higher elemental iron content are more likely to be radiopaque than chewable vitamins or liquid preparations.
- Negative radiographs cannot be used to exclude the ingestion of iron-containing substances, especially if the radiographs are delayed for several hours after ingestion or if multivitamins or a liquid iron preparation is ingested.

Management

- Focus initial treatment on management of ABCs and good supportive care.
- Contact the local poison control center and/or a toxicologist.

- Place patients under observation.
  » Observation is recommended for asymptomatic patients who have ingested < 20 mg/kg of elemental iron or patients with a serum iron concentration < 54 μmol/L.
  » If no symptoms develop in 6 hours, it is unlikely that any systemic symptoms will develop.
    › Patients may be discharged with appropriate follow-up.
  » Patients who have ingested enteric coated preparations may have delayed toxicity and should be placed under longer observation or admitted to hospital.
- Commence therapeutic treatments (active management).
  » Therapeutic treatments should be considered in cases of ingestion of > 20 mg/kg of elemental iron, serum iron concentration > 54 μmol/L, or severe GI symptoms.
  » Therapeutic treatments are indicated in cases of ingestion > 60 mg/kg of elemental iron, serum iron concentration > 90 μmol/L, or evidence of systemic toxicity.
- Limit iron absorption.
  » The efficacy of gastric lavage is controversial and therefore is not routinely recommended; if performed:
    › Use a large-bore nasogastric (NG) or orogastric (OG) tube since many tablets are too large to be removed using a small tube, and the iron tablets may have formed a bezoar.
    › Perform a repeat abdominal X-ray after lavage to assess the need for further decontamination.
    › Use normal saline solution for lavage.
  » Whole bowel irrigation (WBI) (see Chapter 19.1) is the preferred gastric decontamination procedure and is indicated for serious ingestions with a significant number of tablets visible on abdominal X-ray, especially if they are still evident after gastric lavage.
  » Serial abdominal X-rays can be used to monitor treatment.
- Consider chelation therapy using deferoxamine.
  » Indications for chelation therapy include serum iron concentration > 90 μmol/L and severe GI symptoms or evidence of systemic symptoms when an iron level is not readily available.
  » In chelation therapy, deferoxamine binds free ferric (Fe^{3+}) iron in the blood forming ferrioxamine, which is excreted via the kidneys as orange-colored urine known as "vin rose."
  » The standard dose of deferoxamine is 15 mg/kg per hour.
    › The maximum recommended dose is 6 g in 24 hours.
    › Recommendations for the duration of therapy are variable and controversial.
      · Common endpoints include the resolution of systemic symptoms such as shock and/or acidosis, or change in urine color from vin rose back to normal.
  » Adverse effects of deferoxamine include:
    › Hypotension
      · Hypotension is the most common adverse effect.
      · It is dose-related.
    › Acute respiratory distress syndrome due to free radical damage to the lungs
    › Decrease in renal function (ensure adequate hydration)
    › Anaphylactoid reactions
    › *Yersinia enterocolitica* sepsis

REFERENCES

Abhilash KP, Arul JJ, Bala D. Fatal overdose of iron tablets in adults. *Indian J Crit Care Med.* 2013;17(5):311–313. https://doi.org/10.4103/0972-5229.120326. Medline:24339645

Anderson BD, Turchen SG, Manoguerra AS, Clark RF. Retrospective analysis of ingestions of iron containing products in the united states: are there differences between chewable vitamins and adult preparations? *J Emerg Med.* 2000;19(3):255–258. https://doi.org/10.1016/S0736-4679(00)00234-1. Medline:11033271

Burkhart KK, Kulig KW, Hammond KB, Pearson JR, Ambruso D, Rumack B. The rise in the total iron-binding capacity after iron overdose. *Ann Emerg Med.* 1991;20(5):532–535. https://doi.org/10.1016/S0196-0644(05)81609-9. Medline:2024794

Chyka PA, Butler AY. Assessment of acute iron poisoning by laboratory and clinical observations. *Am J Emerg Med.* 1993;11(2):99–103. https://doi.org/10.1016/0735-6757(93)90099-W. Medline:8476468

Chyka PA, Butler AY, Holley JE. Serum iron concentrations and symptoms of acute iron poisoning in children. *Pharmacotherapy.* 1996;16(6):1053–1058. Medline:8947978

Gumber MR, Kute VB, Shah PR, et al. Successful treatment of severe iron intoxication with gastrointestinal decontamination, deferoxamine, and hemodialysis. *Ren Fail.* 2013;35(5):729–731. https://doi.org/10.3109/0886022X.2013.790299. Medline:23635030

Howland MA. Risks of parenteral deferoxamine for acute iron poisoning. *J Toxicol Clin Toxicol.* 1996;34(5):491–497. https://doi.org/10.3109/15563659609028006. Medline:8800186

Juurlink DN, Tenenbein M, Koren G, Redelmeier DA. Iron poisoning in young children: association with the birth of a sibling. *CMAJ.* 2003;168(12):1539–1542. Medline:12796332

Kaczorowski JM, Wax PM. Five days of whole-bowel irrigation in a case of pediatric iron ingestion. *Ann Emerg Med.* 1996;27(2):258–263. https://doi.org/10.1016/S0196-0644(96)70334-7. Medline:8629765

Klein-Schwartz W. Toxicity of polysaccharide--iron complex exposures reported to poison control centers. *Ann Pharmacother.* 2000;34(2):165–169. https://doi.org/10.1345/aph.19225. Medline:10676823

Klein-Schwartz W, Oderda GM, Gorman RL, Favin F, Rutherfoord Rose S. Assessment of management guidelines. Acute iron ingestion. *Clin Pediatr (Phila).* 1990;29(6):316–321. https://doi.org/10.1177/000992289002900604. Medline:2361339

Mowry JB, Spyker DA, Cantilena LR Jr, McMillan N, Ford M. 2013 Annual report of the American Association of Poison Control Centers' national poison data system (NPDS): 31st annual report. *Clin Toxicol (Phila).* 2014;52(10):1032–1283. https://doi.org/10.3109/15563650.2014.987397. Medline:25559822

Perrone J. Iron. In: Hoffman RS, Howland M, Lewin NA, Nelson LS, Goldfrank LR, eds. *Goldfrank's toxicologic emergencies.* 10th ed. New York, NY: McGraw-Hill; 2015.

Tenenbein M. Benefits of parenteral deferoxamine for acute iron poisoning. *J Toxicol Clin Toxicol.* 1996;34(5):485–489. https://doi.org/10.3109/15563659609028005. Medline:8800185

Tenenbein M. Toxicokinetics and toxicodynamics of iron poisoning. *Toxicol Lett.* 1998;102-103:653–656. https://doi.org/10.1016/S0378-4274(98)00279-3. Medline:10022330

19.13

Lead Poisoning

Helen Yaworski, Wesley Palatnick

- Lead is a naturally occurring element found in soil and water.
- The incidence of lead poisoning (plumbism) is significantly lower since lead was removed from household paint and gasoline, but:
  - » Up to 1 million children in the United States still have lead levels > 0.48 µmol/L
  - » Preschoolers living in older, urban housing areas and those born outside Canada and the United States are most at risk of plumbism
- Lead levels in soil are higher in urban centers, especially in and around firing ranges, old buildings, and smelters.
- Lead may be found in:
  - » Paint and pigments (as a stabilizer)
  - » Gasoline (as an antiknock additive)
  - » Acid batteries
  - » Lead pipes
  - » Ceramics
  - » Glass
  - » Solder
- The major sources that result in toxic levels of lead include:
  - » Lead-based paint in homes built before 1970
  - » Contaminated soil
  - » "Take-home exposure" from parents' work or hobbies, such as:
    - › Radiator repair, battery reclamation, ammunition manufacturing, ceramics, stained glass, furniture refinishing
  - » Toys, especially imported ones
  - » Water contaminated by lead pipes
  - » Leaded gasoline (phased out in Canada in 1990)
  - » Alternative medicines

Pharmacology

Absorption

- Absorption rate is highest through inhalation of fumes or contaminated dust.
- Gastrointestinal (GI) absorption is higher in children than in adults (50% vs 15%).
- If lead remains in the stomach, the acidic environment increases the rate and amount absorbed.

- Greater GI absorption occurs when the diet is deficient in iron, calcium, and trace minerals.
- Absorption may occur from retained bullet fragments, especially if the fragment is in a joint.

Distribution

- Lead is rapidly distributed via the bloodstream.
- It crosses the blood-brain barrier, particularly in infants and children.
- It crosses the placenta and accumulates in the fetus.
- It concentrates in bone, where it can stay partitioned for decades, to be released during times of high bone turnover.

Elimination

- Lead is primarily excreted by the kidneys.
- Small amounts of lead are eliminated in bile, shed skin, hair, and nails.

Toxicity

- The toxic effects of lead are mediated by three major mechanisms:
  - » Lead acts as an electron acceptor, binding with sulfhydryl ligands and affecting structural proteins and enzymes.
  - » Because lead is similar to calcium, it interferes with calcium-dependent reactions, including second-messenger systems, mitochondrial energy-production systems, and neurotransmitters.
  - » Lead may cause mutagenesis, at least in nonhuman animals.
- Children are at higher risk of lead toxicity due to a number of factors:
  - » They are closer to the source (contaminated soil, dust)
  - » They explore using hand-to-mouth behavior -Developmentally delayed children are at increased risk due to prolonged period of hand-to-mouth activity.
  - » They absorb more lead from a given source than adults
  - » Their bodies sequester less lead into bone
  - » Their renal excretion is less efficient
  - » Their body systems (including the central nervous system [CNS]) are still developing

Diagnosis

- Toxicity is usually a result of chronic accumulation.
- Lead poisoning can be subtle and insidious. Often cognitive symptoms, including hyperactivity and inability to listen to instructions, bring affected children to the attention of a physician.
- Although no blood lead level is considered safe, the degree of toxicity depends on the level in the blood.
  » Children are often more symptomatic than adults at any given blood level.
- Subclinical effects can occur at levels < 0.5 µmol/L.

Investigations

- Order tests as appropriate.
  » Microcytic anemia may be a clue to the diagnosis.
- Routine screening is no longer recommended.
- In the United States, screening of high-risk populations (urban, low income, areas with known high lead levels, children born outside North America) is recommended at 12 months of age.
- Health Canada recommends screening children in areas of known elevated lead levels or those with known soil contamination from smelters and other sources.

- There is concern of lead toxicity if:
  » Blood lead level > 0.48 µmol/L
  » Free erythrocyte protoporphyrin (FEP) level > 0.62 µmol/L
  » X-ray findings show recent lead ingestion

Management

- If the patient is asymptomatic, the initial treatment focuses on the management of ABCs and good supportive care.
- Contact the local poison control center and/or a toxicologist for management advice.
- In symptomatic, severe cases, supportive care may include:
  » Ventilator support
  » Benzodiazepines for seizure control
  » Titration of IV fluids to urine output of 1 to 2 mL/kg per hour
  » Measures to control intracranial pressure (ICP) — elevate head of bed, maintain normal carbon dioxide levels, consider dexamethasone and mannitol.
- In cases of acute ingestion, consider:
  » Whole bowel irrigation if lead is seen on abdominal X-ray
  » Endoscopic removal of lead chips within the GI tract seen on the abdominal X-ray

Table 19.13.1. EFFECT OF LEAD ON BODY SYSTEMS

System	Pathophysiology	Clinical effects
Neurologic	• Decreased dopamine, acetylcholine, and GABA release • Reduced "synaptic pruning," especially in the hippocampus • Structural changes similar to those seen in Alzheimer's disease • Microvascular changes • Peripheral neuropathy	• Cognitive impairment, poor memory; long-term effects may include decreased IQ, ADHD, anti-social behavior • Lethargy, fatigue, insomnia, decreased libido, headache, myalgias • Wrist or foot drop • Severe: cerebral edema, increased ICP,* ataxia, seizures, coma
Hematologic	• Inhibited pathways in heme synthesis • Altered energy metabolism, leading to fragile RBC membranes • Decreased erythropoiesis because of effects on the kidney	• Microcytic or normocytic anemia • Basophilic stippling • Hemolysis
Cardiovascular	• Calcium-activated increase in vascular tone	• Hypertension
Gastrointestinal	• Impaired GI motility, altered ion transport, spasmodic contractions	• "Lead colic" (crampy abdominal pain) • Constipation
Renal	• Decreased energy-dependent transport • Competitive decrease in excretion of uric acid	• Aminoaciduria, glucosuria, phosphaturia • Interstitial fibrosis (chronic) • Saturnine gout
Endocrine		• Adults: Decreased thyroid and adrenopituitary function • Children: Decreased growth hormone and insulin-like growth factor
Reproductive		• Decreased sperm count, increased rates of spontaneous abortion and pre-term delivery
Skeletal	• Decreased response to vitamin D_3 and osteoblast/osteoclast coupling • Premature calcification of growth plates	• Lead lines on X-ray • Short stature

GABA gamma-aminobutyric acid. **ICP** intracranial pressure. **RBC** red blood cell.

*Studies have shown a decrease in encephalopathy-linked deaths in children; however, these studies were completed at the same time that improved ICP treatments came into use. This suggests that the major reason for the decrease in deaths was not a decrease in cases of lead toxicity, but the better management of ICP.

Chelation Therapy

- Chelation therapy may be instituted if the patient presents with significant clinical toxicity or elevated lead levels (see *Table 19.13.2*, below).

Table 19.13.2. CHELATION INDICATIONS AND AGENTS

	Lead level	Treatment
Children	• Severe: 3.4 to 4.8 μmol/L or encephalopathy	• BAL **and** calcium disodium EDTA
	• Mild to moderate: 2.4 to 3.4 μmol/L	• BAL **and** calcium disodium EDTA
	• Asymptomatic: > 2.4 μmol/L	• Succimer
Adult	• Encephalopathy	• BAL **and** calcium disodium EDTA
	• > 4.8 μmol/L or symptoms suggesting encephalopathy	• BAL **and** calcium disodium EDTA
	• 3.4 to 4.8 μmol/L or mild symptoms	• Succimer
	• < 3.4 μmol/L	• Usually no chelation

BAL British anti-Lewisite.

- » Chelation therapy is usually indicated for lead levels > 2.17 μmol/L.
- » Chelating agents — agents that bind with lead to form a complex that is excreted renally — include:
  - › British anti-Lewisite (dimercaprol or BAL)
    - · Administer IM.
  - › Calcium disodium EDTA
    - · Administer IV.
  - › Succimer (dimercaptosuccinic acid [DMSA])
    - · Administer PO.
  - › D-penicillamine
    - · Administer PO.
    - · D-penicillamine has limited use due to side effects.

Further Management

- Considered third-line therapy.
- In all cases, other aspects of care and prevention include:
  - » Controlling the contaminated environment
    - › Refer the case to public health so they can investigate the potential source(s) of the lead and mitigate exposure.

- » Identifying of the source of lead
- » Removing lead-based paint
  - › Preferably, this is done by professionals while the family is out of the home.
- » Avoiding play in contaminated soil
- » Mopping floors to control contaminated dust
- » Avoiding the use of ceramics for food storage or preparation as the glaze may contain lead
- » Drinking cold water and allow the tap to run for a few minutes to flush water that has been standing in the pipes
- » Preventing contamination at or from work
  - › Use ventilation, masks, ensure work clothes are not worn at home, do not eat or smoke in work area.
- » Decreasing hand-to-mouth activity, cleaning toys and pacifiers frequently, washing hands before meals
- » Ensuring adequate iron, calcium, and zinc intake

REFERENCES

Dapul H, Laraque D. Lead poisoning in children. *Adv Pediatr.* 2014;61(1):313–333. https://doi.org/10.1016/j.yapd.2014.04.004. Medline:25037135

Harvey B, ed. *Managing elevated blood lead levels among young children: recommendations from the Advisory Committee on Childhood Lead Poisoning Prevention.* Atlanta, GA: Centre for Disease Control; 2002.

Health Canada. Lead information package – some commonly asked questions about lead and human health [Internet]. Ottawa (ON): Government of Canada; 2009 [cited 2016 Feb 14]. Available from: https://www.canada.ca/en/health-canada/services/environmental-workplace-health/environmental-contaminants/lead/lead-information-package-some-commonly-asked-questions-about-lead-human-health.html

Health Canada. Final human health state of the science report on lead [Internet]. Ottawa (ON): Government of Canada; 2013 [cited 2016 Feb 14]. Available from: https://www.canada.ca/en/health-canada/services/environmental-workplace-health/reports-publications/environmental-contaminants/final-human-health-state-science-report-lead.html

Markowitz M. Lead poisoning: a disease for the next millennium. *Current Prob Pediatrics.* 2000;30(3):62–70.

Warniment C, Tsang K, Galazka SS. Lead poisoning in children. *Am Fam Physician.* 2010;81(6):751–757.

Woolf AD, Goldman R, Bellinger DC. Update on the clinical management of childhood lead poisoning. *Pediatr Clin N Am.* 2007;54(2):271–294.

19.14

Organophosphate Toxicity

Aaron Guinn, Wesley Palatnick

- Organophosphates are a diverse group of chemicals characterized by a core phosphate group with a number of different organic side chains.
- They were originally developed and used as pesticides.
- Common examples of organophosphates include fenthion, malathion, parathion, chlorpyrifos, diazinon, dichlorvos, phosmet, and dimethoate.
  - » Nerve agents are also organophosphates but are generally considered separately due to differences in use (i.e., chemical warfare), as well as differences in the clinical management of toxicity.
- Clinically, organophosphates all share the characteristic of binding to and inhibiting acetylcholinesterase (AChE), the enzyme responsible for breaking down acetylcholine (ACh).
- Worldwide (and especially in developing countries) organophosphates are the most common cause of death due to toxic ingestion.

Toxicity

- Organophosphates are rapidly absorbed via inhalation, ingestion, or skin contact; toxicity can occur with exposure via any of these routes.
- Binding of the organophosphate molecule to AChE inhibits the activity of this enzyme, leading to elevated levels of ACh.
  - » Clinical effects of elevated ACh levels vary depending on the location of the affected ACh receptors (AChRs) in the body.
  - » Elevated ACh levels at muscarinic ACh receptors (mAChR) in the peripheral parasympathetic nervous system lead to bradycardia, bronchoconstriction, hypersecretion, miosis, and smooth muscle contraction in the gut.
  - » Elevated ACh levels at nicotinic acetylcholine receptors (nAChR) in the preganglionic receptors in the sympathetic nervous system and neuromuscular junction result in tachycardia, diaphoresis, muscle weakness and fasciculations, and mydriasis.
  - » Elevated ACh levels in the central nervous system (CNS) — both nAChR and mAChR — lead to agitation, confusion, lethargy, seizures, and coma.
  - » Binding of the organophosphate molecule to AChE becomes irreversible after a period of time (24 to 48 hours), a process known as "aging."
- The summation of all the effects listed above is cholinergic toxidrome.

- The mnemonic SLUDGE describes the clinical effects of toxicity:
  - » **S**alivation
  - » **L**acrimation
  - » **U**rination
  - » **D**iarrhea
  - » **G**astrointestinal (GI) distress
  - » **E**mesis
- The "Killer Bs" — bradycardia, bronchorrhea, and bronchospasm — are so named because they represent the leading causes of death from this type of poisoning.
- Organophosphates also bind to and inhibit a number of other enzymes in the body, such as butyrylcholinesterase (pseudocholinesterase) and neuropathy target esterase.

Physical Exam

- The onset of symptoms can be extremely rapid, sometimes within minutes.
  - » Muscarinic symptoms are usually the predominant clinical effects.
- Patients may initially be anxious or agitated; however, level of consciousness can rapidly decrease, and patients may become comatose and lose protective airway reflexes.
- Seizures may occur, although it is unclear if these are independent of hypoxia.
- Respiratory failure can occur rapidly. Its etiology is multifactorial and related to a depressed level of consciousness, bronchorrhea and bronchospasm, and potentially early neuromuscular weakness.
- After the resolution of the acute cholinergic crisis, certain patients are at risk of developing the intermediate syndrome: a delayed onset of muscle weakness due to effects of organophosphates at nAChR at the neuromuscular junction.
  - » Cranial nerve involvement may occur.
  - » If respiratory muscles are significantly weakened, hypercarbic respiratory failure may occur.
  - » An early symptom is the inability to raise the head off the bed while lying supine.
- The duration of symptoms depends on the severity of poisoning.
  - » Organophosphates with increased lipophilicity have a longer duration of toxicity.

Agent-Specific Differences

- Certain organophosphates (e.g., dimethoate) are associated with much more severe hypotension and cardiovascular effects than others.
- The time it takes for aging to occur is strongly influenced by the organic side chains of the organophosphate molecule; for instance:
  » Diethyl organophosphates take hours to age
  » Dimethyl organophosphates age much more rapidly
- Risk of intermediate syndrome is much higher with certain organophosphates (e.g., fenthion and malathion).
- Inhibition of neuropathy target esterase leads to organophosphate-induced delayed neuropathy.
  » Organophosphate-induced delayed neuropathy is a syndrome of axonal degradation and demyelination that:
    › Can occur after chronic exposure or several days to weeks after acute exposure
    › Generally presents with pain and distal muscle weakness
    › Can resemble Guillain-Barré syndrome (see Chapter 4.8)
  » The risk of organophosphate-induced delayed neuropathy varies significantly among organophosphates.

Diagnosis

- The diagnosis of organophosphate toxicity is a clinical one and should be suspected in any patient presenting with the signs and symptoms of a cholinergic toxidrome.
- In practice, the combination of the triad of pinpoint pupils, diaphoresis, and increased work of breathing should raise concern for significant organophosphate toxicity.
- If the diagnosis is in doubt, an atropine challenge may be performed.
  » In patients who do not have organophosphate toxicity and have normal AChE activity, administration of atropine 0.05 mg/kg in children will cause an increase in heart rate, dilated pupils, and drying of mucous membranes.
  » Absence of this response to a test dose of atropine is highly suggestive of organophosphate toxicity, unless the patient only had very mild symptoms to begin with.
- Decreased pseudocholinesterase and red cell acetylcholinesterase levels have also been used in the diagnosis of organophosphate toxicity.
  » Practically, the turnaround time on these tests is too long for them to be clinically useful.
  » Note also that there is a wide range of "normal" red cell acetylcholinesterase levels, so there may be a significant poisoning with an acetylcholinesterase level within the normal range.

- » Conditions that can decrease pseudocholinesterase levels include:
  - Liver disease
  - Pregnancy
  - Renal disease
  - Malnutrition
  - Hereditary pseudocholinesterase deficiency

Management

- Management begins with removal of the patient from the source of contamination, followed by external decontamination.
  » Healthcare workers should use universal precautions and ensure that they avoid becoming contaminated.
  » Contaminated clothing should be removed and placed in sealed bags.
  » Contaminated skin should be washed with soap and water.
- GI decontamination is not routinely recommended because:
  » Organophosphates are not bound to activated charcoal
  » There is a significant risk of pulmonary aspiration, as organophosphates are commonly dissolved in a hydrocarbon solvent.
- Initial airway management is critical as most deaths are related to respiratory failure.
  » Administer supplemental oxygen for hypoxia.
- Clinical deterioration can be rapid, so close monitoring and frequent reassessment is necessary.
- If indicated, intubation should ideally be performed via rapid sequence intubation to minimize the risk of hydrocarbon aspiration and hypoxia.
  » Succinylcholine should be avoided, as its effects may last significantly longer than usual due to organophosphate inhibition of pseudocholinesterase.
  » Benzodiazepines are useful as an induction agent, as they may be protective against organophosphate toxicity and decrease mortality.
  » Ketamine is also a reasonable choice for an induction agent due to its bronchodilatory effects and neutral hemodynamic profile.
- Seizures should be rapidly treated with benzodiazepines.
  » There is no role for phenytoin in cases of organophosphate toxicity.

Atropine

- Atropine is the antidote of choice in organophosphate toxicity.
- The usual initial dose of atropine in children is 0.015 to 0.05 mg/kg, doubling the previous dose every 5 minutes until the reversal of cholinergic symptoms occurs (atropinization).

- » Ideally, atropine is given IV, but can also be given via IO method or endotracheal tube (ETT).
  - › ETT dose is 2 to 3 times the IV dose, diluted in 5 mL of normal saline, followed by 5 positive-pressure breaths.
- Hypoxia should not delay administration of atropine.
- The goal of atropine administration is reversal of cholinergic symptoms.
  - » The usual suggested endpoint of atropine administration is the "drying of secretions."
  - » Extremely high doses of atropine may be required.
- Atropine reverses most features of the cholinergic toxidrome and the effects of excess ACh at mAChRs but has no effect at nicotinic receptors.
  - » It will not treat or prevent intermediate syndrome.
- Once the initial total therapeutic dose of atropine has been administered, a maintenance infusion of atropine may be started if required.
  - » The usual starting dose is 10% to 20% of the total dose of atropine required to manage the symptoms, delivered per hour.
- Excessive atropine administration will result in symptoms of anticholinergic toxicity.
- Glycopyrrolate may be used instead of atropine, but it does not cross the blood–brain barrier and so has no effect on CNS symptoms.

Oximes

- Oximes such as pralidoxime are administered to reverse the bond between the organophosphate and the ACHr, and must be given early before aging at both the nACHr and mAChR occurs.
  - » Oximes are the only treatment with an antinicotinic effect, though they have limited CNS penetration.
- The usual pediatric dose is a 30 mg/kg (to a maximum of 2 g) bolus over 20 minutes followed by a 10 to 20 mg/kg per hour (to a maximum of 0.65 g/hr) IV infusion rate.
- Side effects are generally mild and include dizziness, vomiting, tachycardia, and hypertension.

Disposition

- Symptomatic patients should be admitted to a monitored setting.
- Asymptomatic patients may be discharged from hospital once they have not required atropine or an oxime for at least 24 hours and there are no symptoms of respiratory muscle weakness.

REFERENCES

Abedin MJ, Sayeed AA, Basher A, Maude RJ, Hoque G, Faiz MA. Open-label randomized clinical trial of atropine bolus injection versus incremental boluses plus infusion for organophosphate poisoning in Bangladesh. *J Med Toxicol.* 2012;8(2):108–117. https://doi.org/10.1007/s13181-012-0214-6. Medline:22351300

Balali-Mood M, Abdollahi M, eds. *Basic and clinical toxicology of organophosphorus compounds.* London: Springer; 2014. https://doi.org/10.1007/978-1-4471-5625-3.

Blain PG. Organophosphorus poisoning (acute). *BMJ Clin Evid.* 2011:2102.

Buckley N, Eddleston M, Li Y, Bevan M, Robertson J. Oximes for acute organophosphate pesticide poisoning. *Cochrane Database Syst Rev.* 2011;2:CD005085. https://doi.org/10.1002/14651858.CD005085.pub2.

Connors NJ, Harnett ZH, Hoffman RS. Comparison of current recommended regimens of atropinization in organophosphate poisoning. *J Med Toxicol.* 2014;10(2):143–147. Medline:23900961

Eddleston M, Buckley NA, Checketts H, et al. Speed of initial atropinisation in significant organophosphorus pesticide poisoning—a systematic comparison of recommended regimens. *J Toxicol Clin Toxicol.* 2004;42(6):865–875. https://doi.org/10.1081/CLT-200035223. Medline:15533026

Eddleston M, Buckley NA, Eyer P, Dawson AH. Management of acute organophosphorus pesticide poisoning. *Lancet.* 2008;371(9612):597–607. https://doi.org/10.1016/S0140-6736(07)61202-1. Medline:17706760

Eddleston M, Dawson A, Karalliedde L, et al. Early management after self-poisoning with an organophosphorus or carbamate pesticide - a treatment protocol for junior doctors. *Crit Care.* 2004;8(6):R391–R397. https://doi.org/10.1186/cc2953. Medline:15566582

Eddleston M, Eyer P, Worek F, et al. Differences between organophosphorus insecticides in human self-poisoning: a prospective cohort study. *Lancet.* 2005;366(9495):1452–1459. https://doi.org/10.1016/S0140-6736(05)67598-8. Medline:16243090

Eddleston M, Eyer P, Worek F, et al. Pralidoxime in acute organophosphorus insecticide poisoning—a randomised controlled trial. *PLoS Med.* 2009;6(6):e1000104. https://doi.org/10.1371/journal.pmed.1000104. Medline:19564902

Eddleston M, Haggalla S, Reginald K, et al. The hazards of gastric lavage for intentional self-poisoning in a resource poor location. *Clin Toxicol (Phila).* 2007;45(2):136–143. https://doi.org/10.1080/15563650601006009. Medline:17364630

Eddleston M, Juszczak E, Buckley NA, et al; Ox-Col Poisoning Study collaborators. Multiple-dose activated charcoal in acute self-poisoning: a randomised controlled trial. *Lancet.* 2008;371(9612):579–587. https://doi.org/10.1016/S0140-6736(08)60270-6. Medline:18280328

Eddleston M, Mohamed F, Davies JO, et al. Respiratory failure in acute organophosphorus pesticide self-poisoning. *QJM.* 2006;99(8):513–522. https://doi.org/10.1093/qjmed/hcl065. Medline:16861715

Eddleston M, Szinicz L, Eyer P, Buckley N. Oximes in acute organophosphorus pesticide poisoning: a systematic review of clinical trials. *QJM.* 2002;95(5):275–283. https://doi.org/10.1093/qjmed/95.5.275. Medline:11978898

Gunnell D, Eddleston M, Phillips MR, Konradsen F. The global distribution of fatal pesticide self-poisoning: systematic review. *BMC Public Health.* 2007;7:357. https://doi.org/10.1186/1471-2458-7-357. Medline:18154668

Indira M, Andrews MA, Rakesh TP. Incidence, predictors, and outcome of intermediate syndrome in cholinergic insecticide poisoning: a prospective observational cohort study. *Clin Toxicol (Phila).* 2013;51(9):838–845. https://doi.org/10.3109/15563650.2013.837915. Medline:24047461

Johnson S, Peter JV, Thomas K, Jeyaseelan L, Cherian AM. Evaluation of two treatment regimens of pralidoxime (1 gm single bolus dose vs 12 gm infusion) in the management of organophosphorus poisoning. *J Assoc Physicians India.* 1996;44(8):529–531. Medline:9251423

Koksal N, Buyukbese MA, Guven A, Cetinkaya A, Hasanoglu HC. Organophosphate intoxication as a consequence of mouth-to-mouth breathing from an affected case. *Chest.* 2002;122(2):740–741. https://doi.org/10.1378/chest.122.2.740. Medline:12171860

Li Y, Tse ML, Gawarammana I, Buckley N, Eddleston M. Systematic review of controlled clinical trials of gastric lavage in acute organophosphorus pesticide poisoning. *Clin Toxicol (Phila).* 2009;47(3):179–192. https://doi.org/10.1080/15563650701846262. Medline:18988062

Little M, Murray L; Poison Information Centres of New South Wales, Western Australia, Queensland, New Zealand, and the Australian Capital Territory. Consensus statement: risk of nosocomial organophosphate poisoning in emergency departments. *Emerg Med Australas.* 2004;16(5-6):456–458. https://doi.org/10.1111/j.1742-6723.2004.00649.x. Medline:15537409

Namba T, Hiraki K. PAM (pyridine-2-aldoxime methiodide) therapy for alkylphosphate poisoning. *JAMA.* 1958;166(15):1834–1839.

Nelson L, Lewin N, Howland M, Hoffman M, Golfrank L, Flomenbaun

N. Antidotes in depth (A34): atropine. In: *Goldfrank's toxicologic emergencies.* 9th ed. New York: McGraw-Hill; 2010.

Nelson L, Lewin N, Howland M, Hoffman R, Goldfrank L, Flomenbaum N. Chapter 113: organic phosphorus compounds and carbamates insecticides. In: *Goldfrank's toxicologic Emergencies.* 9th ed. New York: McGraw-Hill; 2010.

Selden BS, Curry SC. Prolonged succinylcholine-induced paralysis in organophosphate insecticide poisoning. *Ann Emerg Med.* 1987;16(2):215–217. https://doi.org/10.1016/S0196-0644(87)80018-5. Medline:2432808

19.15

Tricyclic Antidepressant Toxicity

Zoë Piggott

- Tricyclic antidepressants (TCAs) are a class of medications that have proven efficacious in the treatment of major depressive disorder and neuropathic pain.
- TCAs are not considered first-line therapy for depression in pediatric patients.
- Several other less-common indications for antidepressant use exist, including:
  » Pediatric patients — ADHD
  » Teenage and adult patients — cyclic vomiting, irritable bowel syndrome, obsessive compulsive disorder (OCD)
- TCAs are still regularly prescribed in Canada despite the introduction of newer antidepressants (i.e., SSRIs and dual-action antidepressants) with better safety profiles.
  » In 2000, TCAs represented approximately 24% of the Canadian antidepressant prescription market share.

Pharmacology

- TCAs work by potentiating the action of endogenous central nervous system (CNS) neurotransmitters.
  » They inhibit the reuptake of both serotonin (5-HT) and norepinephrine (NE).
- TCAs are also antagonists/blockers of the following receptors:
  » Alpha-adrenergic receptors
  » Sodium channels, with particular effects seen with myocardial sodium channel blockade
  » Anticholinergic (largely antimuscarinic) activity
  » Histamine (H_1) receptors
  » Potassium channels

- The toxicity of TCAs is a direct extension of the following actions:
  » Lowered seizure threshold — increased availability of 5-HT and NE in the CNS
  » Hypotension (vasodilation) — alpha-adrenergic blockade (in vascular smooth muscle)
  » Antimuscarinic toxidrome (dry mouth, dilated pupils, ileus, flushed skin) — muscarinic ACh receptor blockade
  » Sedation or altered level of consciousness — histamine (H_1) receptor blockade
  » Dysrhythmias — sodium (Na) channel blockade, potassium (K) channel blockade
- TCAs have a high first-pass metabolism along with a large volume of distribution and extensive protein binding.
  » Removal through dialysis or forced diuresis is therefore not effective.
- Metabolism/clearance is predominantly via the hepatic cytochrome P450 enzyme system.
  » This can be affected by genetics and induction or inhibition by other medications or substances.
  » Many have active metabolites that are cleared renally.
- Half-life elimination takes approximately 1 day and may take up to 3 days.

Toxicity

- TCA toxicity should be included in the differential diagnosis of several commonly encountered clinical scenarios:
  » Fever and altered mental status
  » Attempted suicide by self-poisoning
  » Status epilepticus or new seizure-like episodes

- Toxicity may result from exploratory pill ingestion by toddlers.
- TCAs are more frequently lethal in overdose than the newer SSRIs and dual-action antidepressants.
  » They have a very narrow therapeutic window.
  » Older TCAs (e.g., dothiepin, amitriptyline) have much higher fatal toxicity indexes than newer TCAs (e.g., nortriptyline, imipramine), which in turn have higher fatal toxicity indexes than all SSRIs.

$$\text{Fatal toxicity index} = \frac{\text{number of associated deaths}}{\text{number of prescriptions}}$$

- TCA overdose may result in clinically significant toxicity after the ingestion of as little as 3 or 4 times the daily dose.
- In young children, > 5 mg/kg of most TCAs should be considered potentially toxic and may equate to only 1 or 2 pills.
  » Toxic doses may be even lower for select TCAs:
    › > 2.5 mg/kg for nortriptyline, desipramine, trimipramine
    › > 1 mg/kg for protriptyline

Diagnosis

- A helpful mnemonic for clinical manifestations of TCA toxicity is "TCAA":
  » **T**onic–clonic seizures
  » **C**ardiac toxicity
  » **A**nticholinergic toxidrome
  » **A**cidosis with elevated lactate
- System-specific toxic effects that may be observed include:
  » Central nervous system (CNS) effects (symptoms of NE and 5-HT excess):
    › Focal seizures
    › Agitation, altered mental status
    › Hypertonia and hyperreflexia
    › Coma
  » Cardiotoxic effects (sodium channel blockade) resulting in slowed myocyte depolarization:
    › Characteristic electrocardiogram (ECG) abnormalities (see below)
    › Ventricular dysrhythmias
  » Anticholinergic effects:
    › Dry mouth
    › Mydriasis
    › Flushing
    › Tachycardia
    › Fever
    › Ileus
    › Urinary retention
  » Peripheral vascular effects:
    › Vasodilation results in hypotension and poor end-organ perfusion

  » Acid-base homeostasis:
    › Lactic acidosis due to decreased peripheral vascular resistance and/or poor cardiac output
- Look for ECG abnormalities:
  » Sinus tachycardia (most common finding) resulting from:
    › Antimuscarinic effects
    › NE excess (i.e., sympathetic activation)
  » Prolonged PR interval
  » Wide QRS complex
  » Prolonged QT interval
  » Terminal 40-millisecond right axis deviation, manifested as tall R-wave in lead aVR (> 3 mm) or R:S ratio in lead aVR > 0.7.
    › This predicts a higher risk of seizures and cardiac dysrhythmias / cardiac instability, though sensitivity and specificity are only moderate.

Management

- Initial treatment should focus on management of ABCs and good supportive care.
- The following clinical priorities must be addressed immediately:
  » Airway maintenance and protection
    › Consider tracheal intubation in patients with severely depressed or deteriorating level of consciousness, as clinically appropriate.
  » Adequate oxygenation and ventilation
    › Supplemental oxygen as required.
    › It is important to consider preintubation respiratory rate and volume when choosing initial mechanical ventilation settings.
      · Respiratory compensation for metabolic acidosis may be required.
  » Circulatory support
    › Administer intravenous crystalloid boluses of 10 to 20 mL/kg as required for initial resuscitation.
    › Sodium bicarbonate therapy aids in improving myocardial function.
    › The vasopressor of choice is NE.
- Obtain an ECG.
- Contact the local poison center and/or a toxicologist.

Decontamination

- Gastric lavage is not the standard of care as it has never been shown to decrease drug absorption or improve patient outcomes.
- Activated charcoal is appropriate only in carefully selected patients with life-threatening ingestions presenting within 1 hour of ingestion (see Chapter 19.1).
  » Risk of aspiration and airway compromise should be carefully considered.
  » No good evidence exists to support multidose charcoal.

- Studies examining the effect of gastric decontamination on drug absorption have produced conflicting results.

Sodium Bicarbonate

- Sodium bicarbonate is the treatment of choice for TCA poisoning with dysrhythmia, seizures, or QRS > 100 milliseconds on ECG, as it:
  - » Narrows the QRS on ECG
  - » Prevents and terminates cardiac dysrhythmias
  - » Corrects hypotension
- Appropriate bicarbonate dosing:
  - » 1 to 2 mEq/kg IV bolus, followed by continuous IV infusion at 2 times the hourly maintenance rate
    - › Mix 150 mEq of sodium bicarbonate in 1 L of 5% dextrose solution.
- The postulated mechanisms of action of sodium bicarbonate are the following:
  - » Increase in serum pH decreases the proportion of available unbound (i.e., active) drug
  - » Correction of metabolic acidosis increases myocardial contractility
  - » Delivery of sodium ions to cardiac myocytes may overcome drug-induced sodium channel blockade
- Specific treatment goals include:
  - » Serum pH 7.45 to 7.55
  - » QRS < 100 milliseconds

Other Specific Treatments

- IV benzodiazepines are the treatment of choice for both agitation and seizure activity.
  - » Avoid phenytoin for seizure control as this medication also blocks sodium channels.
- Avoid Class Ia/Ic/III antiarrhythmic drugs.
  - » Like tricyclics, these medications delay myocyte depolarization.
  - » They may worsen QRS widening, QT prolongation, and dysrhythmias.
- Anticholinergic symptoms should be treated with supportive care and sodium bicarbonate (see above).
  - » Note that physostigmine remains contraindicated in TCA poisoning as it has been associated with precipitation of asystole and seizures.
- Adjuncts for refractory cardiotoxicity or hypotension are:
  - » Hypertonic (3%) saline 1 to 2 mL/kg IV bolus — increases extracellular sodium concentration.
  - » 20% lipid emulsion 1 to 1.5 mL/kg IV bolus — inactivates lipophilic drug molecules.
  - » Magnesium and/or lidocaine — controls arrhythmia.

Disposition

- Asymptomatic children who have ingested > 5 mg/kg (or an unknown amount) of TCA should be observed in the ED for 6 hours after the ingestion.

REFERENCES

Banks CJ, Furyk JS. Review article: hypertonic saline use in the emergency department. *Emerg Med Australas.* 2008;20(4):294–305. https://doi.org/10.1111/j.1742-6723.2008.01086.x. Medline:18462408

Barbey JT, Roose SP. SSRI safety in overdose. *J Clin Psychiatry.* 1998;59(15 Suppl 15):42–48. Medline:9786310

Blackman K, Brown SG, Wilkes GJ. Plasma alkalinization for tricyclic antidepressant toxicity: a systematic review. *Emerg Med (Fremantle).* 2001;13(2):204–210. https://doi.org/10.1046/j.1442-2026.2001.00213.x. Medline:11482860

Bosse GM, Barefoot JA, Pfeifer MP, Rodgers GC. Comparison of three methods of gut decontamination in tricyclic antidepressant overdose. *J Emerg Med.* 1995;13(2):203–209. https://doi.org/10.1016/0736-4679(94)00153-7. Medline:7775792

Brown TC. Sodium bicarbonate and tricyclic-antidepressant poisoning. *Lancet.* 1977;309(8007):375. https://doi.org/10.1016/S0140-6736(77)91189-8. Medline:64906

Cao D, Heard K, Foran M, Koyfman A. Intravenous lipid emulsion in the emergency department: a systematic review of recent literature. *J Emerg Med.* 2015;48(3):387–397. https://doi.org/10.1016/j.jemermed.2014.10.009. Medline:25534900

Crome P, Dawling S, Braithwaite RA, Masters J, Walkey R. Effect of activated charcoal on absorption of nortriptyline. *Lancet.* 1977;310(8050):1203–1205. https://doi.org/10.1016/S0140-6736(77)90440-8. Medline:73903

Dargan PI, Colbridge MG, Jones AL. The management of tricyclic antidepressant poisoning: the role of gut decontamination, extracorporeal procedures and fab antibody fragments. *Toxicol Rev.* 2005;24(3):187–194. https://doi.org/10.2165/00139709-200524030-00011. Medline:16390220

Everett AV. Pharmacologic treatment of adolescent depression. *Curr Opin Pediatr.* 2002;14(2):213–218. https://doi.org/10.1097/00008480-200204000-00012. Medline:11981293

Feighner JP. Mechanism of action of antidepressant medications. *J Clin Psychiatry.* 1999;60(4 Suppl 4):4–11, discussion 12–13. Medline:10086478

Fineberg NA, Reghunandanan S, Simpson HB, et al; Accreditation Task Force of The Canadian Institute for Obsessive Compulsive Disorders. Obsessive-compulsive disorder (OCD): Practical strategies for pharmacological and somatic treatment in adults. *Psychiatry Res.* 2015;227(1):114–125. https://doi.org/10.1016/j.psychres.2014.12.003. Medline:25681005

Flanagan RJ. Fatal toxicity of drugs used in psychiatry. *Hum Psychopharmacol.* 2008;23(S1 Suppl 1):S43–S51. https://doi.org/10.1002/hup.916. Medline:18098225

Gilron I, Baron R, Jensen T. Neuropathic pain: principles of diagnosis and treatment. *Mayo Clin Proc.* 2015;90(4):532–545. https://doi.org/10.1016/j.mayocp.2015.01.018. Medline:25841257

Glauser J. Tricyclic antidepressant poisoning. *Cleve Clin J Med.* 2000;67(10):704–706, 709–713, 717–719. https://doi.org/10.3949/ccjm.67.10.704. Medline:11060957

Hazell P, Mirzaie M. Tricyclic drugs for depression in children and adolescents. *Cochrane Database Syst Rev.* 2013;6(6):CD002317. Medline:23780719

Hejazi RA, McCallum RW. Cyclic vomiting syndrome: treatment options. *Exp Brain Res.* 2014;232(8):2549–2552. https://doi.org/10.1007/s00221-014-3989-7. Medline:24862509

Hemels ME, Koren G, Einarson TR. Increased use of antidepressants in Canada: 1981-2000. *Ann Pharmacother.* 2002;36(9):1375–1379. https://doi.org/10.1345/aph.1A331. Medline:12196054

Henry JA. Epidemiology and relative toxicity of antidepressant drugs in overdose. *Drug Saf.* 1997;16(6):374–390. https://doi.org/10.2165/00002018-199716060-00004. Medline:9241492

Henry K, Harris CR. Deadly ingestions. *Pediatr Clin North Am.* 2006;53(2):293–315. https://doi.org/10.1016/j.pcl.2005.09.007. Medline:16574527

Hoffman JR, Votey SR, Bayer M, Silver L. Effect of hypertonic sodium bicarbonate in the treatment of moderate-to-severe cyclic antidepressant overdose. *Am J Emerg Med.* 1993;11(4):336–341. https://doi.org/10.1016/0735-6757(93)90163-6. Medline:8216512

Hookway C, Buckner S, Crosland P, Longson D. Irritable bowel syndrome in adults in primary care: summary of updated NICE guidance. *BMJ*. 2015;350(Feb25 10):h701. https://doi.org/10.1136/bmj.h701. Medline:25716701

Jamaty C, Bailey B, Larocque A, Notebaert E, Sanogo K, Chauny JM. Lipid emulsions in the treatment of acute poisoning: a systematic review of human and animal studies. *Clin Toxicol (Phila)*. 2010;48(1):1–27. https://doi.org/10.3109/15563650903544124. Medline:20095812

Kerr GW, McGuffie AC, Wilkie S. Tricyclic antidepressant overdose: a review. *Emerg Med J*. 2001;18(4):236–241. https://doi.org/10.1136/emj.18.4.236. Medline:11435353

Knudsen K, Abrahamsson J. Magnesium sulphate in the treatment of ventricular fibrillation in amitriptyline poisoning. *Eur Heart J*. 1997;18(5):881–882. https://doi.org/10.1093/oxfordjournals.eurheartj.a015356. Medline:9152662

Kulig K, Bar-Or D, Cantrill SV, Rosen P, Rumack BH. Management of acutely poisoned patients without gastric emptying. *Ann Emerg Med*. 1985;14(6):562–567. https://doi.org/10.1016/S0196-0644(85)80780-0. Medline:2859819

Kupfer DJ, Frank E, Phillips ML. Major depressive disorder: new clinical, neurobiological, and treatment perspectives. *Lancet*. 2012;379(9820):1045–1055. https://doi.org/10.1016/S0140-6736(11)60602-8. Medline:22189047

Levitt MA, Sullivan JB Jr, Owens SM, Burnham L, Finley PR. Amitriptyline plasma protein binding: effect of plasma pH and relevance to clinical overdose. *Am J Emerg Med*. 1986;4(2):121–125. https://doi.org/10.1016/0735-6757(86)90155-5. Medline:3004528

Liebelt EL, Francis PD, Woolf AD. ECG lead aVR versus QRS interval in predicting seizures and arrhythmias in acute tricyclic antidepressant toxicity. *Ann Emerg Med*. 1995;26(2):195–201. https://doi.org/10.1016/S0196-0644(95)70151-6. Medline:7618783

McKinney PE, Rasmussen R. Reversal of severe tricyclic antidepressant-induced cardiotoxicity with intravenous hypertonic saline solution. *Ann Emerg Med*. 2003;42(1):20–24. https://doi.org/10.1067/mem.2003.233. Medline:12827118

Michael JB, Sztajnkrycer MD. Deadly pediatric poisons: nine common agents that kill at low doses. *Emerg Med Clin North Am*. 2004;22(4):1019–1050. https://doi.org/10.1016/j.emc.2004.05.004. Medline:15474780

Otasowie J, Castells X, Ehimare UP, Smith CH. Tricyclic antidepressants for attention deficit hyperactivity disorder (ADHD) in children and adolescents. *Cochrane Database Syst Rev*. 2014;9(9):CD006997. Medline:25238582

Pentel PR, Benowitz NL. Tricyclic antidepressant poisoning. Management of arrhythmias. *Med Toxicol*. 1986;1(2):101–121. https://doi.org/10.1007/BF03259831. Medline:3784839

Pentel PR, Peterson CD. Asystole complicating physostigmine treatment of tricyclic antidepressant overdose. *Ann Emerg Med*. 1980;9(11):588–590. https://doi.org/10.1016/S0196-0644(80)80232-0. Medline:7001962

Qin B, Zhang Y, Zhou X, et al. Selective serotonin reuptake inhibitors versus tricyclic antidepressants in young patients: a meta-analysis of efficacy and acceptability. *Clin Ther*. 2014;36(7):1087–1095.e4. https://doi.org/10.1016/j.clinthera.2014.06.001. Medline:24998011

Rosenbaum TG, Kou M. Are one or two dangerous? Tricyclic antidepressant exposure in toddlers. *J Emerg Med*. 2005;28(2):169–174. https://doi.org/10.1016/j.jemermed.2004.08.018. Medline:15707813

Rudorfer MV, Potter WZ. Metabolism of tricyclic antidepressants. *Cell Mol Neurobiol*. 1999;19(3):373–409. https://doi.org/10.1023/A:1006949816036. Medline:10319193

Schneir AB, Offerman SR, Ly BT, et al. Complications of diagnostic physostigmine administration to emergency department patients. *Ann Emerg Med*. 2003;42(1):14–19. https://doi.org/10.1067/mem.2003.232. Medline:12827117

Suchard JR. Assessing physostigmine's contraindication in cyclic antidepressant ingestions. *J Emerg Med*. 2003;25(2):185–191. https://doi.org/10.1016/S0736-4679(03)00169-0. Medline:12902007

Swartz CM, Sherman A. The treatment of tricyclic antidepressant overdose with repeated charcoal. *J Clin Psychopharmacol*. 1984;4(6):336–340. https://doi.org/10.1097/00004714-198412000-00008. Medline:6512002

Teece S, Hogg K. Gastric lavage in tricyclic antidepressant overdose. *Emerg Med J*. 2003;20(1):64. https://doi.org/10.1136/emj.20.1.64. Medline:12533375

Thanacoody HK, Thomas SH. Antidepressant poisoning. *Clin Med (Lond)*. 2003;3(2):114–118. https://doi.org/10.7861/clinmedicine.3-2-114. Medline:12737365

Thanacoody HK, Thomas SH. Tricyclic antidepressant poisoning: cardiovascular toxicity. *Toxicol Rev*. 2005;24(3):205–214. https://doi.org/10.2165/00139709-200524030-00013. Medline:16390222

von Wolff A, Hölzel LP, Westphal A, Härter M, Kriston L. Selective serotonin reuptake inhibitors and tricyclic antidepressants in the acute treatment of chronic depression and dysthymia: a systematic review and meta-analysis. *J Affect Disord*. 2013;144(1-2):7–15. https://doi.org/10.1016/j.jad.2012.06.007. Medline:22963896

Wille SM, Cooreman SG, Neels HM, Lambert WE. Relevant issues in the monitoring and the toxicology of antidepressants. *Crit Rev Clin Lab Sci*. 2008;45(1):25–89. https://doi.org/10.1080/10408360701713112. Medline:18293180

Woolf AD, Erdman AR, Nelson LS, et al. Tricyclic antidepressant poisoning: an evidence-based consensus guideline for out-of-hospital management. *Clin Toxicol (Phila)*. 2007;45(3):203–233. https://doi.org/10.1080/15563650701226192. Medline:17453872

Yates C, Galvao T, Sowinski KM, et al, *and the* EXTRIP workgroup. Extracorporeal treatment for tricyclic antidepressant poisoning: recommendations from the EXTRIP Workgroup. *Semin Dial*. 2014;27(4):381–389. https://doi.org/10.1111/sdi.12227. Medline:24712820

19.16

Carbon Monoxide Toxicity

Bandar Baw

Note: Exposure to combustion or fire can:

- Endanger the patient's ability to breathe
  » Swelling of the upper and lower airways mechanically impairs either airway movement or essential gas exchange.
    › Airway management for victims of burns and smoke inhalation is discussed in Chapter 1.2.
- Cause cellular asphyxiation
  » Inhaled toxins such as carbon monoxide and cyanide cause cellular asphyxiation.
    › Cyanide toxicity is discussed in Chapter 19.10.

- Carbon monoxide is a colorless, odorless, and tasteless gas resulting from incomplete combustion of carbon-containing materials.
- In North America, it accounts for more than 50 000 emergency department (ED) visits per year, which is equal to approximately 53 of every 100 000 ED visits.
  » Pediatric cases (< 15 years of age in one study) account for about 3% of total exposures.
  » > 50% of deaths occur at home.
- Public health measures encouraging the use of carbon monoxide detectors to prevent carbon monoxide–related deaths.
- Environmental conditions such as winter storms or electricity disruption may contribute to carbon monoxide toxicity outbreaks.
- Sources of carbon monoxide toxicity can be exposure to:
  » Fire
  » Automotive exhaust
  » Burning coal
  » Natural gas–powered equipment such as water heaters, furnaces, and stoves
  » Methylene chloride
- Carbon monoxide is produced naturally in the human body from various metabolic activities in minute quantities.
  » Smokers may have higher carbon monoxide levels, reaching up to 10% at any one time.

Pathophysiology

- Carbon monoxide is rapidly absorbed after inhalation.

- Once absorbed, carbon monoxide follows one of the following routes:
  » It binds to hemoglobin to form carboxyhemoglobin (COHb)
    › Hemoglobin has 200 times the affinity to bind with carbon monoxide compared to oxygen
    › Fetal (newborn) hemoglobin has a higher affinity to carbon monoxide than adult hemoglobin, which puts infants at greater risk of toxicity.
  » It binds to myoglobin
  » It dissolves in blood and can be diffused into tissue compartments, including the heart and brain, exerting direct cellular toxicity
- The half-life of carbon monoxide is:
  » 6 hours in room air (21% oxygen)
  » 90 minutes with 100% oxygen (positive pressure ventilation mask or endotracheal intubation)
  » 20 minutes after 2.5 atmosphere absolute (ATA) hyperbaric oxygen therapy

Toxicity

- Mechanisms of toxicity can be classified into the following effects:
  » Transportation hypoxia by:
    › Decreasing the ability of hemoglobin to carry and transport oxygen from lungs to tissues by mechanically binding to hemoglobin instead of oxygen molecules, resulting in the formation of carboxyhemoglobin (COHb) instead of normal oxyhemoglobin
    › Shifting the oxygen–hemoglobin dissociation curve to the left, making it harder for hemoglobin to release already-attached oxygen to the tissues
  » Cellular hypoxia (asphyxiation) through inhibition of mitochondrial respiratory function
  » Direct and indirect effects causing oxidative stress cascade
  » Direct myocardial dysfunction partially caused by carbon monoxide binding to myoglobin

Diagnosis

- Children are at higher risk of developing symptoms of toxicity at lower levels of carbon monoxide (< 10%) compared to adults.

- Carbon monoxide toxicity presents with a spectrum of symptoms depending on the acuity and severity of the exposure; the clinical picture correlates directly to the amount of carbon monoxide inhaled.
  » Mild exposure may result in nonspecific findings such as headache, dizziness, fatigue, and a feeling of generally unwellness.
    › Younger patients may present with irritability and uneasiness.
  » Moderate exposure may lead to nausea and vomiting, mild confusion, fussiness, poor feeding, or ataxia.
  » Severe exposure may result in end-organ dysfunction:
    › Seizures, altered level of consciousness, syncope, coma, ischemic stroke, myocardial infarction, dysrhythmia, hypotension, or death
- Late neuropsychiatric sequelae may occur in patients with chronic exposure or in survivors of severe toxicity (up to 10% of children exposed), likely from various ischemic or oxidative stress effects:
  » Personality changes
  » Mood swings
  » Memory deficit
  » Impaired concentration
  » Difficulty learning
  » Gross motor or sensory deficits
  » Gait disturbance
  » Peripheral neuropathy
  » Hearing loss
  » Visual loss
  » Psychosis
- Clinical hints of carbon monoxide toxicity include:
  » Family members presenting with nonspecific complaints at the same time
  » Pets with the same signs
  » Symptoms that resolve or improve once the person leaves the affected area (e.g., the home)
  » In winter, camping or being located in a poorly ventilated area
  » Lack of functioning carbon monoxide detector at home
- A high level of clinical suspicion is needed.

Investigations

- A regular pulse oximeter cannot be used to diagnose carbon monoxide toxicity as it cannot distinguish between oxyhemoglobin and COHb.
  » Cooximetry is the mainstay of diagnosis that gives [CO] level in venous blood (which is as accurate as an arterial blood sample).
    › Carbon monoxide concentration > 5% is abnormal in children.
  » Noninvasive pulse cooximetry has been used to detect carbon monoxide exposure with some accuracy as a screening tool in the emergency department (ED).
- The absolute carbon monoxide level does not reliably reflect the severity of carbon monoxide toxicity for many reasons, including:
  » Delayed presentation
  » Chronicity of exposure
  » Treatment with oxygen en route to the ED, affinity of different hemoglobin to carbon monoxide (fetal vs adult), and the presence of underlying coexisting medical conditions such as coronary artery disease.
- Blood gas testing may reveal:
  » Normal PaO_2
  » Metabolic acidosis
- An MRI or CT brain scan can show changes in white matter as well as basal ganglia that mainly reflects ischemic events.
- Initiate investigations to exclude exposure to other substances and concomitant end-organ dysfunction as appropriate.

Management

- Management starts by preventing exposure through public education and enforcing the use of functioning carbon monoxide detectors.
- Removing the patient from the affected site is the first decontamination method.
  » Use caution to prevent further exposure to first responders or other individuals near the scene.

Oxygen

- Oxygen supplementation decreases the half-life of carbon monoxide.
- For mild exposures, use of nonrebreather face mask oxygen may be sufficient.
- Intubation and 100% oxygen should be considered for airway concerns associated with moderate to severe exposure.
- Benefit of hyperbaric oxygen therapy is controversial.
  » Some randomized studies showed benefits.
  » A recent Cochrane Review failed to prove the effect of hyperbaric oxygen therapy on carbon monoxide–toxic patients.
  » Indications for hyperbaric oxygen therapy are:
    › Altered level of consciousness
    › Neurologic deficits
    › Cardiovascular dysfunction
    › Severe acidosis
    › Carbon monoxide > 25% (> 15% for pregnant patients)
  » Hyperbaric oxygen therapy is also used to prevent neuropsychological sequelae.
- Treatment should continue until carbon monoxide is < 5%.

REFERENCES

Buckley NA, Juurlink DN, Isbister G, Bennett MH, Lavonas EJ. Hyperbaric oxygen for carbon monoxide poisoning. *Cochrane Database Syst Rev.* 2011;*(4)*:CD002041. Medline:21491385

Centers for Disease Control and Prevention (CDC). Use of carbon monoxide alarms to prevent poisonings during a power outage--North Carolina, December 2002. *MMWR Morb Mortal Wkly Rep.* 2004;*53(9)*:189–192. Medline:15017373

Chung WS, Lin CL, Kao CH. Carbon monoxide poisoning and risk of deep vein thrombosis and pulmonary embolism: a nationwide retrospective cohort study. *J Epidemiol Community Health.* 2015;*69(6)*:557–562. https://doi.org/10.1136/jech-2014-205047. Medline:25614638

Hampson NB, Hauff NM. Carboxyhemoglobin levels in carbon monoxide poisoning: do they correlate with the clinical picture? *Am J Emerg Med.* 2008;*26(6)*:665–669. https://doi.org/10.1016/j.ajem.2007.10.005. Medline:18606318

Hampson NB, Weaver LK. Residential carbon monoxide alarm use: opportunities for poisoning prevention. *J Environ Health.* 2011;*73(6)*:30–33. Medline:21306092

Roth D, Herkner H, Schreiber W, et al. Accuracy of noninvasive multiwave pulse oximetry compared with carboxyhemoglobin from blood gas analysis in unselected emergency department patients. *Ann Emerg Med.* 2011;*58(1)*:74–79. https://doi.org/10.1016/j.annemergmed.2010.12.024. Medline:21459480

Roth D, Schreiber W, Herkner H, Havel C. Prevalence of carbon monoxide poisoning in patients presenting to a large emergency department. *Int J Clin Pract.* 2014;*68(10)*:1239–1245. https://doi.org/10.1111/ijcp.12432. Medline:24698635

Sircar K, Clower J, Shin MK, Bailey C, King M, Yip F. Carbon monoxide poisoning deaths in the United States, 1999 to 2012. *Am J Emerg Med.* 2015;*33(9)*:1140–1145. https://doi.org/10.1016/j.ajem.2015.05.002. Medline:26032660

Styles T, Przysiecki P, Archambault G, et al. Two storm-related carbon monoxide poisoning outbreaks—Connecticut, October 2011 and October 2012. *Arch Environ Occup Health.* 2015;*70(5)*:291–296. https://doi.org/10.1080/19338244.2014.904267. Medline:24971904

Suner S, Partridge R, Sucov A, et al. Non-invasive pulse CO-oximetry screening in the emergency department identifies occult carbon monoxide toxicity. *J Emerg Med.* 2008;*34(4)*:441–450. https://doi.org/10.1016/j.jemermed.2007.12.004. Medline:18226877

Thom SR. Carbon monoxide pathophysiology and treatment. In: Neuman TS, Thom SR, eds. *Physiology and Medicine of Hyperbaric Oxygen Therapy.* Milton, ON: Elsevier Canada; 2008.

Weaver LK. Clinical practice. Carbon monoxide poisoning. *N Engl J Med.* 2009;*360(12)*:1217–1225. https://doi.org/10.1056/NEJMcp0808891. Medline:19297574

Weaver LK, Hopkins RO, Chan KJ, et al. Hyperbaric oxygen for acute carbon monoxide poisoning. *N Engl J Med.* 2002;*347(14)*:1057–1067. https://doi.org/10.1056/NEJMoa013121. Medline:12362006

Wheeler-Martin K, Soghoian S, Prosser JM, et al. Impact of mandatory carbon monoxide alarms: an investigation of the effects on detection and poisoning rates in New York City. *Am J Public Health.* 2015;*105(8)*:1623–1629. https://doi.org/10.2105/AJPH.2015.302577. Medline:26066948

19.17

Adverse Drug Reactions

Michael Rieder

- Adverse drug reactions are common and are a major cause of mortality and morbidity.
- The minimum rate of adverse drug reaction for any given drug is 5%, with adverse drug reaction rates in some drugs being almost 100%.
- An adverse drug events occurs because of a combination of adverse drug reactions and drug errors, including:
  » Giving the wrong dose of a drug
  » Giving the wrong drug
  » Giving a drug via the wrong route
- Drug errors can be addressed by health care system changes, but adverse drug reactions often occur at usual therapeutic doses and with appropriately prescribed drugs.
- Suspected adverse drug reactions are common reasons for emergency department (ED) visits.

Classification

- Adverse drug reactions can be classified as either predictable or unpredictable.
  » Predictable adverse drug reactions are:
    › Side effects (e.g., fine hand tremor from salbutamol inhaler)
      · Side effects are usually self-limited.
      · They are often due to off-target effects.
      · They often improve over time (i.e., "treating through" is an option).
    › Secondary effects (e.g., pseudomembranous colitis from lincosamides)
      · Secondary effects are predictable but not inevitable results of the drug's pharmacologic effects.
    › Interactions (e.g., renal injury when clarithromycin is given with cyclosporine)
      · Interactions occur when drug, food, or infection alters the clearance of a concurrently administered drug.

TOXICOLOGY

› Toxicity (e.g., renal injury from high-dose aminoglycosides)

· Too much of anything is harmful ("Everything is poisonous, nothing is poisonous, it is all a question of dose" – French physiologist Claude Bernard).

» Unpredictable adverse drug reactions are:

› Intolerance (e.g., tinnitus at standard doses of salicylates)

· Intolerance leads to disabling side effects that occur at usual doses and usual drug concentrations in blood in uniquely susceptible populations.

› Allergic or pseudoallergic reactions (e.g., anaphylaxis from penicillin)

· Although very much overdiagnosed, drug allergies are among the most serious — and most dreaded — types of adverse drug reactions.

› Idiosyncratic reactions (e.g., Stevens-Johnson syndrome from sulfonamides)

· Idiosyncratic reactions are uncommon but very serious adverse drug reactions and often occur with drugs that undergo complex metabolism.

› Psychogenic reactions (e.g., multiple drug hypersensitivity)

· Psychogenic reactions are poorly understood adverse drug reaction patterns that are disabling for the patients impacted.

Diagnosis

- Timing is crucial.
  » Immediate onset reactions typically occur within 1 to 2 hours of administration of the drug.
  » Delayed reactions may take 1 to 2 weeks to develop and 1 to 6 weeks to resolve.
  » The longer a drug has been taken, the less likely it is that an adverse event is related to therapy unless there has been a dramatic change in the patient's condition or a new therapeutic agent has been administered.
- An adverse drug reaction can present in a variety of manners, but the most common possible adverse drug reaction presentation in pediatric emergency medicine settings is cutaneous (rash).
  » Cutaneous adverse drug reactions can present in a number of forms, but some of the most common are:
    › Urticaria
    › Vascular rashes
    › Mucositis
- Note that many other diseases present as rashes.
  » A common, non–adverse drug reaction cause of urticaria in children is infection.
  » The most common cause of nonspecific maculopapular rashes is viral infection.
- There is a high rate of overdiagnosis of suspected drug allergy or suspected adverse drug reaction in the ED.

» It is appropriate to be cautious in an emergency department (ED) setting but follow-up is needed for accurate diagnosis.

» Adverse drug reactions are usually described to patients as a drug allergy; avoid this, as it is an unfortunate misuse of the term.

› Diagnosis as a suspected adverse drug reaction would be more accurate in most cases (except in the case of suspected true allergy, e.g., anaphylaxis) and less likely to lead to problems with future therapy.

Management

- Follow the 5 A's of adverse drug reaction management.
  » **A**ppreciation
  » **A**ssessment
  » **A**nalysis
  » **A**ssistance
  » **A**ftermath
    › An important and often overlooked part of the management of suspected adverse drug reactions in the ED is arranging appropriate follow-up.

Appreciation

- When an undesired event occurs in a patient receiving a medication, the possibility that the drug may be responsible must be considered.
- It is very difficult to diagnose a problem that you do not consider to be part of the differential diagnosis.
- When undesired events occur in the context of therapy, physicians often ascribe them to the disease under treatment, whereas patients and families often ascribe them to the drug; the truth is often somewhere in-between.

Assessment

- A careful assessment of the event in question is essential; this includes:
  » Taking a history of the initial clinical problem being treated
  » Understanding the temporal course of therapy, including concurrent therapy and other conditions that are present
  » Taking a family history
  » Conducting a careful physical examination
- The precise details about the timing of when the adverse drug reaction occurred in context of the temporal course of therapy — and the timing of doses — is essential for an accurate assessment.
- A reliable source of drug information is essential.
  » The number of therapeutic agents available is very large and growing, and most physicians are only comfortable prescribing the drugs they routinely use.
  » A number of electronic drug resources are available, and a clinical pharmacist or drug information service

may be essential, especially for new or uncommonly used drugs.

Analysis

- After careful assessment and development of a differential diagnosis, the decision must be made as to the working diagnosis, which, in this context, is essentially a decision between drug-related versus non–drug-related diagnoses.
- In the ED, the diagnosis is typically suspected adverse drug reaction.
  - » In many cases, the diagnosis is presented to the patient and family as suspected drug allergy, which, as noted above, is a usually inaccurate and unfortunate use of the word "allergy."

Assistance

- In the infrequent case of immediately life-threatening reactions such as anaphylaxis, management of the ABCs according to established protocols is urgently required.
- Most suspected adverse drug reactions are managed by symptomatic treatment (e.g., treatment of urticaria is done predominately with antihistamines).
  - » In this context, conventional antihistamines such as diphenhydramine (1 mg/kg every 6 to 8 hours) are more effective than selective antihistamines.
  - » The majority of patients with suspected adverse drug reactions can be managed in this way.
  - » Part of management is usually to stop the presumed offending drug.
    - › However, in the case of a side effect (such as fine hand tremor associated with salbutamol therapy), continuing therapy ("treating through") is an option, with the awareness that the side effect will likely diminish and resolve over time.
    - › In the context of stopping a drug, the original diagnosis for which the drug was prescribed must be revisited; in the event that the original diagnosis has not been adequately addressed, alternate therapy may be required.
- The symptoms of the majority of adverse drug reactions can be expected to resolve over the following several days.
  - » In the case of a delayed reaction, it may take weeks for full resolution of symptoms.
- In the event of a serious adverse drug reaction such as Stevens-Johnson syndrome, hospitalization and

intervention such as immunomodulatory therapy may be required.

- » Immunomodulatory therapy may be administered by pulse corticosteroid therapy (prednisone or methylprednisolone 1 to 2 mg/kg per day for 5 days) or intravenous immunoglobulin (1 to 2 mg/kg).
- » Urgent consultation with an expert in the management of these conditions is prudent given their considerable morbidity and known mortality.

Aftermath

- Patients with very serious adverse drug reactions such as anaphylaxis or Stevens-Johnson syndrome need to be followed very closely and frequently require admission to hospital.
- Patients with less-severe reactions may require symptomatic treatment for several days; urgent follow-up should be available should their condition deteriorate.
- Follow-up should be arranged for patients with suspected adverse drug reactions to ascertain whether they have in fact had an adverse drug reaction and how this may influence future therapy.
  - » Follow-up may include diagnostic evaluation or drug rechallenge; this is often overlooked and can lead to a misdiagnosis of drug allergy, which can limit therapy for patients for years.
- The fact of sustaining an adverse drug reaction is likely to influence drug compliance in the future, so a discussion as to what drugs the patient should avoid — and what drugs are likely to be safe — is an important part of the care of patients with suspected adverse drug reactions and should be part of discharge instructions.
  - » For example — except in the case of anaphylaxis — cross-reactions between penicillins and cephalosporins are very rare and cephalosporins can be used as therapeutic alternatives.
    - › In the case of anaphylactic reactions, therapeutic alternatives include clindamycin.

REFERENCES

Noguera-Morel L, Hernández-Martín Á, Torrelo A. Cutaneous drug reactions in the pediatric population. *Pediatr Clin North Am.* 2014;61(2):403–426. https://doi.org/10.1016/j.pcl.2013.12.001. Medline:24636653

Rieder M. New ways to detect adverse drug reactions in pediatrics. *Pediatr Clin North Am.* 2012;59(5):1071–1092. https://doi.org/10.1016/j.pcl.2012.07.010. Medline:23036245

Swanson L, Colven RM. Approach to the patient with a suspected cutaneous adverse drug reaction. *Med Clin North Am.* 2015;99(6):1337–1348. https://doi.org/10.1016/j.mcna.2015.06.003. Medline:26476256

TOXICOLOGY

20.1

Hypothermia and Cold-Induced Injuries

Patrick Weldon

HYPOTHERMIA

- Hypothermia is responsible for approximately 1000 to 1500 deaths annually in the United States.

Risk Factors

- Risk factors for hypothermia include:
  - » Age
    - › Children are at increased risk due to:
      - · Increased ratio of surface area to body mass
      - · Decreased ability to recognize and escape cold environments
      - · Lower energy stores
    - › Neonates are at particular risk as they have very limited ability to produce heat through shivering.
    - › The elderly are also at increased risk due to impaired thermogenesis.
  - » Intoxication / substance abuse
  - » Homelessness
  - » Participation in outdoor cold-weather sports
  - » Underlying medical conditions (see information on secondary etiologies under "Differential Diagnosis," below)
  - » Major trauma
    - › Direct effects of both trauma and resuscitation (unwarmed IV fluids / blood) can predispose an individual to hypothermia.
    - › Hypothermia in trauma increases mortality (rate approaches 100% with body temperature < 32°C).
      - · Hypothermia is part of the "lethal triad in trauma" — hypothermia, coagulopathy, and acidosis — and should be aggressively treated.

Classifications

- Hypothermia is defined by a core temperature < 35°C.
- The classification of hypothermia is based on core temperature:

  - » Mild — 32°C to 35°C
  - » Moderate — 28°C to 32°C
  - » Severe — < 28°C
  - » "Profound hypothermia" — some experts use this term to classify < 24°C
- Classification generally correlates with clinical symptoms and signs.

Pathophysiology

- Normal thermoregulation reflects the balance of heat production and loss in the human body.
- Mechanisms of heat loss include:
  - » Radiation — responsible for about 60% of heat loss in normal conditions
  - » Conduction — responsible for minimal to 15% heat loss in air; this increases 25 times in water (immersion/submersion injuries)
  - » Convection — responsible for 5% to 25% of heat loss in still air; this increases up to 10 times with significant environmental wind
  - » Evaporation — responsible for 7% to 20% of heat loss at rest
  - » Respiration — responsible for 15% of heat loss at rest; this increases with exertion, altitude, and cold air
- All organ systems can be affected.
- With moderate to severe hypothermia, cellular metabolic rate slows and oxygen consumption decreases 6% for each 1°C decrease in temperature.
  - » This may offer cerebral protection against anoxia if severe hypothermia develops prior to the onset of cardiac arrest.
  - » There are multiple case reports / case series of patients with neurologically intact survival in severe hypothermia and with cardiac arrest despite prolonged resuscitation time (up to 7 hours).

» With severe hypothermia, prolonged resuscitation is indicated.

› Termination of resuscitation should be deferred until core temperature is > 32°C to 34°C even with no signs of life unless obvious lethal injuries are present or if the arrest/asphyxia event occurred prior to cooling (e.g., warm water drowning).

Diagnosis

- Clinical signs and symptoms follow a typical sequence with progressive hypothermia, though there is individual variability in the core temperature at which each occurs and overlap is possible.

MILD HYPOTHERMIA (32°C TO 35°C)

- Mild hypothermia reflects the body's compensatory mechanisms for maintaining core temperature.
- Shivering is triggered to generate heat.
- Patients with mild hypothermia may present with:
  » Cardiovascular effects:
    › Sympathetic stimulation resulting in peripheral vasoconstriction and increased heart rate (HR) and blood pressure (BP)
  » Respiratory effects:
    › Tachypnea
    › Bronchorrhea and bronchospasm
  » Renal effects:
    › Cold-induced diuresis
      · This is initially generated by increased mean arterial pressure (MAP) detected at the kidneys from peripheral vasoconstriction, leading to increased urine output.
  » Central nervous system (CNS) effects:
    › Slurred speech
    › Ataxia
  » Hematologic effects:
    › Increased hematocrit from intravascular depletion
    › Platelet and leukocyte sequestration
    › Coagulopathy from platelet sequestration and enzymatic dysfunction of coagulation cascade
  » Gastrointestinal effects:
    › Ileus
    › Pancreatitis
    › Impaired hepatic metabolism of drugs/toxins
- Compensatory mechanisms initially result in increased metabolic rate and oxygen consumption as well as hyperglycemia, which can progress to hypoglycemia with worsening hypothermia as energy stores are depleted.

MODERATE HYPOTHERMIA (28°C TO 32°C)

- Moderate hypothermia reflects the transition period to failure of compensatory mechanisms and progressive organ dysfunction.

- Shivering ceases.
- Patients with moderate hypothermia may present with:
  » Cardiovascular effects:
    › Progressive decrease in HR and BP
    › Slowed conduction with prolongation of all intervals
    › Atrioventricular (AV) blocks
    › Atrial flutter/fibrillation with slow ventricular response
    › J waves (Osborne waves)
      · Positive deflection of the J point is seen most prominently in precordial leads.
      · The size of J waves generally correlates with the degree of hypothermia.
      · J waves are characteristic but not pathognomonic of hypothermia.

Figure 20.1.1. J-WAVE

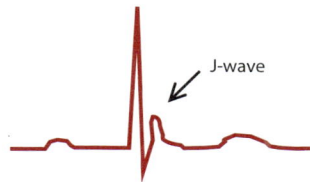

J-wave

  » Respiratory effects:
    › Progressively decreasing respiratory rate
    › Impaired airway reflexes with increased risk of aspiration
  » Renal effects:
    › Ongoing cold-induced diuresis due to tubular dysfunction, with decreased sodium and water reabsorption
  » CNS effects:
    › Increasingly altered level of consciousness
      · Patients can develop hallucinations and engage in paradoxical undressing.

SEVERE HYPOTHERMIA (< 28°C)

- Severe hypothermia reflects ongoing organ dysfunction with the absence of compensatory mechanisms; clinical findings in severe hypothermia can mimic death.
- Patients with severe hypothermia may present with:
  » Cardiovascular effects:
    › Progressive decrease in HR and BP
    › Vasodilation leading to flushing/erythema of skin
    › Increased risk of ventricular fibrillation due to myocardial irritability
    › Asystole
  » Respiratory effects:
    › Hypoventilation progressing to apnea
    › Pulmonary edema may develop
  » CNS effects:
    › Stupor progressing to coma
    › Pupillary response progressively more sluggish and eventually unreactive

> › Areflexia
> › Electroencephalogram (EEG) becomes isoelectric at about 24°C to 26°C
> » Musculoskeletal effects
> › Muscular rigidity due to actin-myosin dysfunction

Differential Diagnosis

- Consider a broad differential diagnosis when faced with a hypothermic patient.
  » Primary hypothermia is due to environmental exposure that increases heat losses via the mechanisms discussed above (see "Pathophysiology").
  » Secondary etiologies include:
    › Impaired thermoregulation due to CNS pathology, including:
      · Traumatic brain or spinal cord injury
      · Tumor
      · Congenital malformations
    › Impaired heat production due to:
      · Endocrine pathology (e.g., hypothyroidism, adrenal insufficiency)
      · Malnutrition or anorexia
      · Hypoglycemia
    › Increased heat loss due to:
      · Loss of skin barrier (e.g., burns, dermatitis)
      · Toxins that promote vasodilation or sedation (alcohol, benzodiazepines, opioids, clonidine)
    › Sepsis

Management

- Initial treatment should focus on supportive care, including assessment, management of ABCs, and rewarming the patient.

Airway/Breathing Management

- Intubate for apnea, respiratory failure, or cardiac arrest.
  » Give supplemental oxygen.
    › Oxygen should be warmed and humidified.

Circulation Management

- In severe hypothermia, assess patients for the presence of pulse/respiration for 30 to 60 seconds as physiologic changes (hypoventilation, severe bradycardia, muscle rigidity) can make detection challenging.
  » Arterial lines and point-of-care ultrasound can be useful adjuncts to determine the presence of a pulse.
  » If an organized cardiac rhythm is present, some experts recommend deferring compressions regardless of the degree of bradycardia to avoid precipitating ventricular fibrillation as cardiac output is likely sufficient to meet metabolic demands.
- Management of cardiac arrest should generally follow PALS/ACLS guidelines.
  » Use normal rate and depth for chest compressions.

> » Defibrillation may be attempted but it is unlikely to be successful when body temperature is < 30°C.
>   › Up to 3 initial shocks are recommended, then defer until the patient is rewarmed.
> » Epinephrine is associated with a higher rate of return of spontaneous circulation (ROSC) in animal models.
>   › Concerns exist for toxic accumulation with excessive doses due to decreased drug metabolism in hypothermia.
>   › American Heart Association (AHA) guidelines state that "it is reasonable to consider administration of a vasopressor concurrent with rewarming strategies."
>   › European guidelines suggest withholding medications until body temperature is 30°C, then doubling the administration interval until 34°C is reached.

ARRHYTHMIA MANAGEMENT

- Bradycardic and atrial arrhythmias typically resolve with rewarming and do not usually require pharmacologic treatment.
- Ventricular dysrhythmias are unlikely to respond to pharmacologic treatment (e.g., amiodarone) until the patient is sufficiently rewarmed.
  » Some evidence exists for the use of Bretylium but it is unavailable in North America.

FLUID RESUSCITATION

- Patients are typically significantly volume depleted due to diuresis and third-spacing; they require fluid resuscitation.
- IV crystalloids should be warmed to 40°C to 44°C to prevent further decrease in body temperature.

Temperature Monitoring

- Core temperature should be monitored using a low-reading thermometer or probe as conventional thermometers cannot read below 34°C.
  » Bladder or esophageal monitoring is more reliable as rectal probes can have significant time lag with regard to temperature changes.

Initial Investigations

- Order bloodwork:
  » Complete blood count (CBC), blood gas, glucose, electrolytes, blood urea nitrogen (BUN), creatinine, coagulation studies, lipase
    › Blood gas analyzers typically correct values to 37°C, which increases $PaCO_2$ and PaO_2 and decreases pH.
    › Management decisions and target values should be based on uncorrected values.
- Initiate ECG and continuous cardiac monitoring.
- Initiate other investigations/imaging as indicated based on the clinical picture and suspicion of secondary etiologies.

Rewarming

- Choice of initial rewarming strategy should be based on the degree of hypothermia and cardiovascular status, as well as institutional and provider capabilities.

PASSIVE EXTERNAL REWARMING

- Passive external rewarming prevents further heat loss by removing the patient from the cold environment and wet clothing.
- It allows for rewarming through the body's own heat-production mechanisms (e.g., shivering).
  » Adequate caloric intake must be ensured to meet energy needs.

ACTIVE EXTERNAL REWARMING

- Active external rewarming is the method of choice for mild to moderate hypothermia, combined with noninvasive internal methods (e.g., warm IV fluids, oxygen).
  » It can also be considered in severe hypothermia with stable cardiac status.
- Forced air (e.g., Bair Hugger) warming devices are preferred.
- Alternatives include electrical/chemical warming blankets and warm water immersion.
- Rewarming of the trunk versus periphery must be ensured to minimize risk of core afterdrop / rewarming shock (see below).
- Monitor the patient closely for burns.

ACTIVE INTERNAL REWARMING

- Noninvasive and invasive techniques of active internal rewarming exist.
  » Noninvasive techniques include administration of warmed, humidified oxygen and warmed IV fluids.
    › These techniques should be used for all patients.
  » Invasive techniques include:
    › Pleural lavage
      · Pleural lavage is the method of choice in severe hypothermia or cardiac arrest if extracorporeal membrane oxygenation (ECMO) / bypass is unavailable (see "Extracorporeal Techniques," below).
      · It involves 2 chest tubes (3rd IC space midclavicular and 6th IC space posterior axillary) with infusion/drainage of warmed normal saline.
      · The rewarming rate is about 3°C to 4°C per hour.
    › Bladder/peritoneal lavage
      · These alternatives have a lower rate of rewarming compared to pleural lavage.

EXTRACORPOREAL TECHNIQUES

- Extracorporeal techniques are the methods of choice in severe hypothermia or cardiac arrest.
- ECMO is the preferred modality.

- Alternatives include full cardiopulmonary bypass and hemodialysis.
- The rewarming rate is 6°C to 9°C per hour (hemodialysis is about 2°C to 4°C per hour).

Note: Failure of rewarming should prompt escalation of rewarming strategy and consideration of secondary etiologies.

Complications

- Complications during rewarming and post-rewarming include:
  » Afterdrop — continued core temperature decrease after removal of patient from the cold environment
    › Afterdrop is caused by return of cold blood to the core and ongoing core-to-periphery heat transfer.
    › Room temperature IV fluids may also contribute.
    › Afterdrop can precipitate arrhythmias.
  » Rewarming shock — worsening hypotension with initiation of rewarming
    › Contributing factors include peripheral vasodilation in the context of intravascular depletion and poor cardiac function with return of cold, acidic blood to the core.
    › Rewarming shock can progress to circulatory collapse.
    › Risk is increased with external rewarming without fluid resuscitation and core rewarming.
  » Other complications
    › Pulmonary edema
    › Rhabdomyolysis
    › Renal failure
    › Sepsis
    › Local cold injuries

Disposition

- Patients with mild hypothermia may be discharged home once rewarmed and stable.
- Patients with moderate to severe hypothermia require admission for monitoring and rewarming, preferably to a facility with pediatric critical care and ECMO capabilities.

LOCAL COLD-INDUCED INJURIES

FROSTBITE

Pathophysiology

- During freezing, tissue damage occurs both via the direct effects of ice crystal formation in the extracellular space and ischemic damage through vasoconstriction and microvascular thrombosis.
- With the rewarming of tissues, further damage occurs through reperfusion injury and ongoing microvascular damage.

ENVIRONMENTAL EMERGENCIES

- Multiple rewarming-refreezing cycles can exacerbate tissue damage and should be avoided.

Classification

FROSTNIP

- Frostnip is the mildest form of injury; it is reversible with no permanent tissue damage.
- The affected area develops pain followed by paresthesia, which resolves completely with rewarming.

FROSTBITE

- Frostbite is traditionally graded 1 to 4 but is now most often classified simply as superficial or deep.
  - » Superficial frostbite involves skin and subcutaneous tissues only.
    - › It is characterized by tissue pallor, edema, and subsequent formation of clear blisters.
    - › Damaged tissue typically heals with no permanent tissue loss.
  - » Deep frostbite can involve deeper structures, including muscles, bones, and joints.
    - › It often develops hemorrhagic blisters.
    - › Affected tissue evolves to varying degrees of necrosis and ulceration, with permanent tissue loss.

Management

- Identify and treat any concomitant, life-threatening conditions or injuries.
- Use minimal, gentle handling of affected areas to avoid further tissue damage.
- Rewarming is the primary treatment.
  - » Immerse affected tissue in circulating water at 40°C to 42°C for 20 to 45 minutes until tissue is supple and circulation is restored.
  - » The rewarming process is highly painful, and often requires narcotic analgesia.
- The debridement of affected areas should be delayed as the demarcation of viable from nonviable tissue can take several weeks.
  - » Early consultation with a plastic surgeon should occur with any significant tissue involvement.
  - » Management of blisters is controversial.
    - › Hemorrhagic blisters (signifying deep tissue involvement) should initially be left intact in most cases.
- Sterile, nonadherent, noncompressive, padded dressings should be applied, along with splinting of the affected area.
- Tetanus prophylaxis should be initiated (see Chapter 10.4).
- Antibiotics are not indicated unless signs of infection develop.

- Consider additional therapies:
  - » Intraarterial/intravenous tissue plasminogen activator (tPA) injections
    - › Within 24 hours, tPA injections have been shown to improve rates of tissue salvage in small studies.
    - › This can be considered in consultation with plastic surgery in severe cases.
  - » Potential adjunctive therapies
    - › Consider ASA, topical aloe vera, and hyperbaric oxygen, though benefits have not been well established.

PERNIO (CHILBLAINS)

- Pernio is characterized by localized inflammatory skin lesions and is triggered by an abnormal vascular response to nonfreezing cold.
- The condition is most common in females 15 to 30 years of age.
- It can be associated with underlying medical conditions, including systemic lupus erythematosus (SLE), anorexia nervosa, and cold agglutinin disease.

Diagnosis

- Pernio presents with single or multiple erythematous or violaceous edematous lesions that are typically accompanied by pain and pruritus.
  - » Pernio occurs about 12 to 24 hours following cold exposure.
  - » It is most common on dorsal surfaces of fingers and toes, but can also affect cheeks, nose, pinnae, shins, and thighs.
  - » It may evolve to blisters or ulcers with risk of secondary infection.
- Pernio is typically self-limited, resolving over 1 to 3 weeks, though it can have a chronic or recurrent course.

Management

- Rewarm the affected areas.
- Skin lesions require gentle wound care to prevent ulceration or secondary infection.
- Oral nifedipine may be of benefit in severe or prolonged cases.
- Limiting cold exposure is key to preventing recurrence.

IMMERSION (TRENCH) FOOT

- Immersion foot is tissue injury caused by prolonged exposure to a wet, nonfreezing cold environment.
  - » Historically, immersion foot was commonly seen in sailors and soldiers, but now it more typically occurs in the homeless population.

- The condition's clinical presentation follows 3 stages:
  1. Initial stage (24 to 48 hours)
     › This stage is characterized by vasoconstriction.
     › The affected extremity is cold and pale with variable degree of anesthesia.
  2. Hyperemic stage (2 to 6 weeks)
     › This stage is characterized by vasodilatation.
     › The affected extremity is hyperemic and swollen, with a painful, burning sensation.
     › Tissue damage with edema, blistering, and ulceration is present.
  3. Post-hyperemic stage (weeks or months)
     › The affected extremity is cyanotic but can be warm, with increased cold sensitivity.
     › Tissue damage or loss is ongoing.

Management

- Remove the patient from the wet environment and provide exposure to warm, dry air.
- Elevate the extremity to prevent edema.
- Provide meticulous wound care and protect pressure points to prevent further tissue damage and infection.

Complications

- Complications of immersion foot include:
  » Tissue loss due to liquefaction gangrene
  » Cellulitis, lymphangitis
  » Nerve injury
  » Persistent cold sensitivity of the vasculature of the affected extremity

REFERENCES

Brown DJ, Brugger H, Boyd J, Paal P. Accidental hypothermia. *N Engl J Med.* 2012;367(20):1930–1938. https://doi.org/10.1056/NEJMra1114208. Medline:23150960

Corneli HM. Accidental hypothermia. *J Pediatr.* 1992;120(5):671–679. https://doi.org/10.1016/S0022-3476(05)80226-4. Medline:1578300

Danzl DF, Pozos RS. Accidental hypothermia. *N Engl J Med.* 1994;331(26):1756–1760. https://doi.org/10.1056/NEJM199412293312607. Medline:7984198

Fisher JD, Schaefer C, Reeves JJ. Successful resuscitation from cardiopulmonary arrest due to profound hypothermia using noninvasive techniques. *Pediatr Emerg Care.* 2011;27(3):215–217. https://doi.org/10.1097/PEC.0b013e31820d8e04. Medline:21378525

Jurkovich GJ. Environmental cold-induced injury. *Surg Clin North Am.* 2007;87(1):247–267, viii. https://doi.org/10.1016/j.suc.2006.10.003. Medline:17127131

Kleinman ME, Goldberger ZD, Rea T, et al. American Heart Association focused update on adult basic life support and cardiopulmonary resuscitation quality: an update to the American Heart Association guidelines for cardiopulmonary resuscitation and emergency cardiovascular care. *Circulation.* 2017;CIR.0000000000000539:e1-e7. https://doi.org/10.1161/CIR.0000000000000539.

Meiman J, Anderson H, Tomasallo C; Centers for Disease Control and Prevention (CDC). Hypothermia-related deaths—Wisconsin, 2014, and United States, 2003-2013. *MMWR Morb Mortal Wkly Rep.* 2015;64(6):141–143. Medline:25695318

Simon TD, Soep JB, Hollister JR. Pernio in pediatrics. *Pediatrics.* 2005;116(3):e472–e475. https://doi.org/10.1542/peds.2004-2681. Medline:16140694

Soar J, Perkins GD, Abbas G, et al. European Resuscitation Council guidelines for resuscitation 2010 section 8. Cardiac arrest in special circumstances: electrolyte abnormalities, poisoning, drowning, accidental hypothermia, hyperthermia, asthma, anaphylaxis, cardiac surgery, trauma, pregnancy, electrocution. *Resuscitation.* 2010;81(10):1400–1433. https://doi.org/10.1016/j.resuscitation.2010.08.015. Medline:20956045

Vanden Hoek TL, Morrison LJ, Shuster M, et al. Part 12: cardiac arrest in special situations: 2010 American Heart Association guidelines for cardiopulmonary resuscitation and emergency cardiovascular care. *Circulation.* 2010;122(18 Suppl 3):S829–S861. https://doi.org/10.1161/CIRCULATIONAHA.110.971069. Medline:20956228

20.2

Drowning

Qamar Amin

- Drowning is defined as the process of experiencing respiratory impairment from submersion or immersion in a liquid.
- Contrary to popular belief, drowning fatality rates in children are among the lowest of any age group.
- Drowning is the second leading cause of unintentional injury for children aged 1 to 19 years.
  » An average of 473 drowning deaths occur in Canada each year, with an annual average of 1.4 per 100 000 of the general population.
  » The highest water-related fatality rates are seen in a bimodal age distribution in adults aged 20 to 34 years (1.6 per 100 000) and seniors 65 years and older (1.8 per 100 000).

Risk Factors

- Risk factors include:
  » Males
  » Warmer summer months, especially on the weekends
    › Two-thirds of pediatric drowning deaths occur in the spring and summer months.

ENVIRONMENTAL EMERGENCIES

- Open bodies of water
  - About three-quarters of drownings occur in natural bodies of water.
  - A smaller portion of drownings occurs in bathtubs and swimming pools.
- Medical conditions that predispose individuals to drowning, such as:
  - Seizure disorders
  - Behavioral disorders (e.g., autism) and developmental delay
  - Conditions that predispose individuals to cardiac syncope (e.g., prolonged QT syndrome)
- Absence of appropriate supervision
- Ethanol consumption
- Severe neurologic deficits occur in 5% to 10% of cases. Contributing factors include:
  - Prolonged submersion time
  - Prolonged resuscitation time
  - Delayed bystander CPR
  - Open-water settings
- Immersion syndrome refers specifically to syncope resulting from cardiac dysrhythmias from contact with water that is at least 5°C lower than body temperature.

Pathophysiology

- Unexpected submersion triggers breath-holding panic and a struggle to surface.
- Air hunger and hypoxia develop, and the victim begins to swallow water.
- As breath holding is overcome, involuntary gasping results in the aspiration of water and subsequent drowning.
- Aspiration of 1 to 3 mL/kg of water can destroy pulmonary surfactant, leading to alveolar collapse, atelectasis, noncardiogenic pulmonary edema, intrapulmonary shunting, and ventilation-perfusion mismatch.
- Eventual hypoxia metabolic respiratory acidosis ensues, leading to cardiovascular collapse and eventually death.

History

- Drownings are often witnessed, so gathering a good history from witnesses is critical. Ask about:
  - Events prior to drowning
  - Duration of submersion
  - Bystander CPR
  - Past medical history
  - Episodes of coughing, choking, or vomiting close to a body of water

Physical Exam

- Examination usually reveals respiratory symptoms:
  - Any sign of respiratory distress (hypoxia, increased work of breathing, cyanosis)
  - Crackles and wheezes (may be present)

- If the patient has sustained any central nervous system (CNS) injury, then some degree of lethargy up to a full-blown coma can be seen.
- Cardiac dysrhythmias may be present; consider immersion syndrome.

Investigations

- Order chest radiography.
- Obtain bloodwork:
  - Complete blood count (CBC), electrolytes, creatinine, and blood glucose
  - Venous blood gas (VBG) and lactate — to assess degree of hypoxia
- Electrocardiogram (ECG) should be obtained as soon as possible to scrutinize for any dysrhythmias, QT prolongation, or ischemic changes.
- Consider toxicology workup as needed.
- Consider CT imaging of the brain if it is clinically indicated (trauma or neurological symptoms).

Management

- Initiate resuscitation as per the Advanced Cardiovascular Life Support (ACLS) guidelines, with attention to core temperature.
  - Drowning victims may be hypothermic on presentation and should be rewarmed.
- Initial treatment focuses on management of ABCs and good supportive care.
  - If oxygen saturation is < 90%, provide supplemental oxygen or even consider positive pressure ventilation.
  - Intubate if the patient's $PaCO_2$ is > 50 mmHg.
- Stable patients should be monitored for 6 hours in the emergency department (ED); if no respiratory, cardiac, or neurologic symptoms develop, they can be discharged home.
- Empiric antibiotics or steroids are not recommended.
  - Antibiotics can be considered in cases of infection

Prognosis

- Risk factors for a poor prognosis include:
  - Submersion time > 5 minutes
    - Submersion time is the most important factor and can be extrapolated from the presence or absence of hypoxia.
  - CPR for > 10 minutes
- Patient age, rectal temperature, and water temperature are **not** significant predictors of outcome.

REFERENCES

American Academy of Pediatrics Committee on Injury, Violence, and Poison Prevention. Prevention of drowning. *Pediatrics.* 2010;126(1):178–185. https://doi.org/10.1542/peds.2010-1264. Medline:20498166

Ballesteros MA, Gutiérrez-Cuadra M, Muñoz P, Miñambres E. Prognostic factors and outcome after drowning in an adult population. *Acta Anaesthesiol Scand.* 2009;53(7):935–940. https://doi.org/10.1111/j.1399-6576.2009.02020.x. Medline:19496759

Drowning Prevention Research Centre Canada. *Canadian drowning report.* 2015 ed. Toronto, ON: Lifesaving Society of Canada; 2015.

Drowning Prevention Research Centre Canada. *Canadian drowning report.* 2016 ed. Toronto, ON: Lifesaving Society of Canada; 2016.

Ibsen LM, Koch T. Submersion and asphyxial injury. *Crit Care Med.* 2002;30(11 Suppl):S402–S408. https://doi.org/10.1097/00003246-200211001-00004. Medline:12528781

Orlowski JP, Szpilman D. Drowning. Rescue, resuscitation, and reanimation. *Pediatr Clin North Am.* 2001;48(3):627–646. https://doi.org/10.1016/S0031-3955(05)70331-X. Medline:11411297

Suominen P, Baillie C, Korpela R, Rautanen S, Ranta S, Olkkola KT. Impact of age, submersion time and water temperature on outcome in near-drowning. *Resuscitation.* 2002;52(3):247–254. https://doi.org/10.1016/S0300-9572(01)00478-6. Medline:11886729

Suominen PK, Vähätalo R. Neurologic long term outcome after drowning in children. *Scand J Trauma Resusc Emerg Med.* 2012;20(1):55. https://doi.org/10.1186/1757-7241-20-55. Medline:22894549

van Beeck E, Branch C, Szpilman D, A new definition of drowning: towards documentation and prevention of a global health problem. *B World Health Organ.* 2005;83(11):853–856.

Weiss J; American Academy of Pediatrics Committee on Injury, Violence, and Poison Prevention. Prevention of drowning. *Pediatrics.* 2010;126(1):e253–e262. https://doi.org/10.1542/peds.2010-1265. Medline:20498167

20.3

Heat Illness

Rahim Valani

- The human body has a narrow functional range (35°C to 41°C), with the resting internal temperature tightly regulated between 36.5°C and 37.5°C.
- The regulation of body temperature is achieved through 2 main regulatory mechanisms:
  1. Behavioral regulation, which includes:
     › The type of clothing the individual wears
     › Moving to a more comfortable location, such as to a warmer room or into the shade
     › Altering activity
  2. Physiological regulation, which includes:
     › Thermogenic response (shivering) in cold environments
     › Thermolytic responses (sudomotor response [sweating], blood flow redistribution) in hot environments
     › Exercise and exertional activity generate heat.
- The body requires intact cardiovascular and integumentary systems for thermoregulation.
  » Blood is transferred from the core to the skin to help with thermoregulation.
- Heat stress may be compensated or uncompensated; uncompensated heat stress may lead to heat illness.
  » When heat stress is compensated:
     › Core body temperature increases during exertion / exercise
     › A new steady state is achieved to increase metabolic demands and dissipate heat
  » When heat stress is uncompensated:
     › The body's cooling capacity is exceeded and the body cannot maintain a steady temperature
     › Continued stress leads to increased heat retention and risk of severe heat illness

Mechanisms of Heat Dissipation

- There are 4 main mechanisms of heat dissipation:
  1. Evaporation
     › Water vaporizes from the skin and respiratory tract.
     › This accounts for 7% to 20% of heat loss under normal circumstances; it increases to 70% with evaporation of sweat.
        · Evaporation of 1 L of sweat results in the loss of 580 kcal of heat.
     › Evaporation is the most effective cooling mechanism.
     › If the humidity in the environment is > 75%, then evaporation is ineffective.
  2. Radiation
     › Radiation is energy transfer through electromagnetic heat.
     › It accounts for 60% of heat loss.
  3. Convection
     › Convection is the transfer of heat to moving air/liquid.
     › The rate of heat transfer depends on the temperature of the convection current, the speed of the air circulation, and the amount of body surface exposed.
     › Convection accounts for 5% to 25% of heat loss.

4. Conduction
   › Conduction is the direct transfer of thermal energy to an adjacent cooler object.
   › The rate of heat transfer depends on the temperature difference between the two objects.
   › Conduction accounts for minimal to 15% of heat loss.

Risk Factors

- Individual factors include:
  » Extremes of age
  » Low fitness level
  » Dehydration
    › Every 1% drop in hydration increases the body temperature by 0.22°C.
  » Acclimatization
    › Full acclimatization requires 10 to 14 days, and involves:
      · Plasma volume expansion (estimated 5% to 7% increase)
      · Improved cutaneous blood flow
      · Lower threshold to begin sweating
      · Increased sweat output
      · Lower salt concentration in sweat
      · Lower skin and core temperature without major exertion
  » History of heat-related illness
  » Clothing / equipment use
- Environmental risk factors are:
  » Hot ambient temperature (temperature > 28°C)
  » High relative humidity
- Other risk-factors include:
  » Activity lasting > 1 hour
  » Medications, drug use, and supplements
  » Chronic medical conditions such as:
    › Sickle cell disease or trait
    › Skin conditions (eczema, psoriasis, burns)

HEAT RASH

- Heat rash is also known as "prickly heat."
- It is characterized by a pruritic, maculopapular, erythematous rash.
- The rash occurs due to blockage of the sweat ducts.
- Manage with:
  » Antihistamines — for the pruritus
  » Loose-fitting clothes during exercise

HEAT CRAMPS

- Heat cramps are exertional or exercise-associated muscle spasms.
- They can occur during or after exercise.

- Cramps are usually restricted to the muscle groups involved in the activity.
- Heat cramps are most commonly experienced by less-fit individuals who are not used to exercising or have not trained for an athletic event in which they are participating.
- Manage heat cramps with:
  » Rest
  » Rehydration with an electrolyte solution

HEAT SYNCOPE

- Heat syncope is the transient loss of consciousness.
- It is caused by blood pooling in the extremities.
- The syncope usually occurs after stopping exercise suddenly, standing for a prolonged period of time, and/or inadequate hydration.
- Manage heat syncope by:
  » Removing the patient from the heat source
  » Putting the patient in a supine position
  » Checking blood glucose
  » Beginning hydration (oral if tolerated, otherwise IV)
  » Considering an electrocardiogram (ECG)

HEAT EXHAUSTION

- Heat exhaustion is the inability to continue an activity in the heat.
- It presents with lethargy and profuse sweating.
- The condition is caused by heat stress and low circulating blood volume that impairs heat dissipation.
- The patient is usually tachycardic, hypotensive, and has a core temperature < 40°C
- Manage heat exhaustion by:
  » Giving IV fluid hydration
  » Considering bloodwork — specifically electrolytes, renal function, creatine kinase (CK), and coagulation tests
  » Obtaining an ECG

HEAT STROKE

- Heat stroke is extreme hyperthermia (core body temperature > 40°C).
- It is due to thermoregulatory failure that presents with profound central nervous system (CNS) dysfunction.
- Younger individuals usually develop exertional heat stroke (diaphoretic skin).
  » Classic heat stroke is usually from exposure to high temperatures within confined spaces.
    › It is more commonly seen in the elderly, those affected by medications or alcohol, and those with psychiatric conditions.

- Other organ systems can be affected, including:
  - » Respiratory
  - » Cardiovascular
  - » Hepatic
  - » Renal
  - » Hematological — specifically coagulation

Investigations

- Obtain an ECG.
- Obtain bloodwork:
  - » Complete blood count (CBC), electrolytes, renal function, hepatic function, CK, coagulation tests
- Order a toxicology screen.

Management

- Manage ABCs.
- Measure core temperature (esophageal, bladder, or rectal).
- Administer IV fluids.
- Cool the patient via:
  - » Air-conditioned room
    - › Air-conditioned rooms have a cooling rate of 0.03°C to 0.06°C per minute.
  - » Ice water immersion
    - › Water at 2°C has a cooling rate of 0.35°C per minute.
    - › Water at 14°C to 20°C has a cooling rate of 0.15°C to 0.19°C per minute.
  - » Ice packs
    - › Apply to the axilla, neck, and groin.
  - » Evaporative and convective cooling
    - › Apply ice packs and use convection fans.
    - › This is a common method used in mass gathering events.
  - » Cold IV fluids
    - › 4°C saline over 30 minutes cools the body by 1°C.

- › Room temperature saline over 30 minutes cools the body by 0.5°C.
- Consult ICU for admission.

Disposition

- Educate parents/caregivers and patients to prevent the recurrence of heat illness. Instruct them to:
  - » Ensure adequate hydration during activities
  - » Wear appropriate clothing for physical activities
  - » Learn to recognize the early signs/symptoms of heat illness such as fatigue, cramps, nausea, and dizziness
- Before returning to exercise after heat stroke, the patient should:
  - » Avoid exercising for at least 7 days after discharge
  - » Have a follow-up physical exam after 1 week
  - » Restart exercising in a cool environment and gradually increase duration and intensity
  - » Increase exercise intensity gradually over a period of weeks

REFERENCES
Atha WF. Heat-related illness. *Emerg Med Clin North Am.* 2013;31(4):1097–1108. https://doi.org/10.1016/j.emc.2013.07.012. Medline:24176481

Gaudio FG, Grissom CK. Cooling methods in heat stroke. *J Emerg Med.* 2016;50(4):607–616. https://doi.org/10.1016/j.jemermed.2015.09.014. Medline:26525947

Gomez CR. Disorders of body temperature. In: Biller J, Ferro JM, eds. *Handbook of clinical neurology* Vol. 120 (3rd series). Elsevier; 2014.

Périard JD, Racinais S, Sawka MN. Adaptations and mechanisms of human heat acclimation: applications for competitive athletes and sports. *Scand J Med Sci Sports.* 2015;25(Suuppl 1 Suppl 1):20–38. https://doi.org/10.1111/sms.12408. Medline:25943654

Pryor RR, Bennett BL, O'Connor FG, Young JM, Asplund CA. Medical evaluation for exposure extremes: heat. *Clin J Sport Med.* 2015;25(5):437–442. https://doi.org/10.1097/JSM.0000000000000248. Medline:26340737

Pryor RR, Roth RN, Suyama J, Hostler D. Exertional heat illness: emerging concepts and advances in prehospital care. *Prehosp Disaster Med.* 2015;30(3):297–305. https://doi.org/10.1017/S1049023X15004628. Medline:25860637

20.4

Electrical Injuries

Rahim Valani

- 3% of pediatric burns are due to electrical injuries.
- Most injuries happen at home and occur in children < 5 years of age.
  - » 70% of injuries are low voltage.

- » Electrical injuries are more common in males than in females.
- » High-voltage injuries are most often seen in teenagers.

- Electrical injuries can be classified by type of voltage:
  » Low voltage — < 1000 volts (V)
  » High voltage — > 1000 V
  » Lightning
  » Thermal burns
  » Voltaic arc
- Severity of injury is dependent upon:
  » Amount of voltage
  » Amperage
  » Type of current (direct or alternating)
    › Alternating current is considered more destructive as it produces tetanic contractions, making the patient "freeze up" and causing more injury.
  » Duration of exposure
  » Tissue resistance
    › Tissues, in decreasing order of resistance, are: bone, fat, tendon, skin, muscle, blood vessels, nerves.
      · Because of their low resistance, nerves and vessels are the first tissues to be injured; they also help propagate the electrical impulse to the rest of the body.
- For arcing, the extent of tissue damage depends on:
  » Proximity to the source
  » Surrounding water vapor / humidity
  » Clothing type

Physical Exam

- Presentation varies depending on the severity of injury:
  » Mild:
    › Altered level of consciousness
    › Amnesia/confusion
    › Paresthesias
  » Moderate:
    › Seizure
    › Respiratory arrest
    › Burns
  » Severe:
    › Cardiac arrest
    › Major trauma

Injury Types

- The injury can be due to electrical, thermal, and mechanical forces.

BURNS

- The conversion of electrical energy to thermal energy results in burns.
  » Entry and exit wounds are usually visible.
    › Burns are usually evident at contact points.
    › Current can also jump over flexed joints.
    › The amount of burn seen externally is deceiving — more damage occurs to the underlying tissue than what is seen.

- Other types of electrical injury burns are:
  » Arc burns
    › In an arc burn, current passes to the body externally, which can generate very high temperatures (> 2 000°C).
  » Flash burns
    › Flash burns are flame burns from electrical ignition of surroundings (e.g., clothing).

MECHANICAL INJURY

- Electrical injuries can lead to mechanical injuries when the patient thrown by the force of the shock, falls from a height, or experiences severe muscle contractions.
  » Look for fractures, contusion, and soft tissue injuries.
  » The most common areas of injury in the upper limbs are the hand, the elbow, and the axilla.

CARDIAC INJURY

- Cardiac injuries may be caused by a combination of electrical injury mechanisms.
  » Any type of cardiac rhythm / arrhythmia may be seen.
  » Mortality from electrical injuries is due to cardiac or respiratory arrest.
    › Mortality occurs in an estimated 3% to 14% of electrical injuries.

NEUROLOGIC INJURY

- 50% of patients involved in high voltage injuries with have some neurological impairment.
- Symptoms can be delayed from days to weeks
- Patients can present with:
  » Confusion, altered mental status, and seizure activity
  » Paresthesias, hemiplegia
  » Autonomic dysfunction
  » Keraunoparalysis — temporary paralysis that is seen after a lightning strike
    › Keraunoparalysis is due to vascular spasm that results in a pulseless extremity.
    › The lower limbs are affected twice as much as the upper limbs.
    › Symptoms resolve in a few hours.

Management

- Stabilize ABCs.
- Provide fluid resuscitation — use the Parkland formula (see Chapter 18.8).
- Examine the patient for other associated injuries:
  » Laceration/contusions
  » Fractures
  » Head and C-spine injuries
  » Visceral damage
  » Vascular damage — thrombosis, vasospasm, ischemic necrosis
    › Presentation of vascular injuries may be delayed.
  » Inhalation injury

Investigations

- Specific investigations include:
  » Electrocardiogram (ECG) / cardiac monitoring
    › Criteria for ongoing cardiac monitoring are:
      · Abnormal ECG
      · Loss of consciousness
      · Voltage
      · Cardiac history (congenital heart disease, history of Kawasaki disease, etc.)
    › Studies have shown that if the initial ECG is normal, then patients may not be at risk for late arrhythmia.
  » Bloodwork:
    › Complete blood count (CBC), creatine kinase (CK), and renal function
  » Urinalysis — check for myoglobin
    › If there is evidence of myoglobinuria/rhabdomyolysis, treat aggressively with fluids to ensure adequate urine output.

Disposition

- The decision to admit the patient to hospital depends on:
  » Type and extent of injury
  » Associated injuries (burn, fractures, head injury, etc.)
  » Associated neurologic injury
  » Reliability of parents/caregivers
  » Loss of consciousness
  » Initial ECG

ORAL ELECTRICAL BURNS

- Oral electrical burns are estimated to be 0.001% of all pediatric injuries that present to the emergency department (ED).
- 50% of cases occur in children < 3 years of age.
  » Cases are more common in males than in females.
- Injury usually occurs from:
  » Biting or mouthing an electrical cord
  » Mouthing a battery

Management

- Manage oral burns as you would other electrical injuries.
- Consider discharging the patient home if:
  » Parents/caregivers are reliable and know how to control the bleeding
  » Patient experiences no loss of consciousness
  » Patient has no other injury requiring hospital admission
  » ECG is normal
  » Patient is able to tolerate fluids by mouth
  » Appropriate follow-up has been arranged

Complications

- The most feared complication is injury to the labial artery, which may not be initially apparent.
  » It is usually seen on day 5 when the eschar falls off (but may be delayed up to 2 weeks).

REFERENCES

Bailey B, Gaudreault P, Thivierge RL. Experience with guidelines for cardiac monitoring after electrical injury in children. *Am J Emerg Med.* 2000;18(6):671–675. https://doi.org/10.1053/ajem.2000.16307. Medline:11043619

Caglar A, Ayyaz A, Guzecicek A, et al. Predictive factors for clinical severity and cardiopulmonary arrest in pediatric electrical injuries in Southeastern Turkey. *Pediat Emer Care.* 2016:

Glatstein MM, Ayalon I, Miller E, Scolnik D. Pediatric electrical burn injuries: experience of a large tertiary care hospital and a review of electrical injury. *Pediatr Emerg Care.* 2013;29(6):737–740. https://doi.org/10.1097/PEC.0b013e318294dd64. Medline:23714758

Nguyen BH, MacKay M, Bailey B, Klassen TP. Epidemiology of electrical and lightning related deaths and injuries among Canadian children and youth. *Inj Prev.* 2004;10(2):122–124. https://doi.org/10.1136/ip.2003.004911. Medline:15066980

Ogilvie MP, Panthaki ZJ. Electrical burns of the upper extremity in the pediatric population. *J Craniofac Surg.* 2008;19(4):1040–1046. https://doi.org/10.1097/SCS.0b013e318175f523. Medline:18650729

Umstattd LA, Chang CWD. Pediatric oral burns: incidence of emergency department visits in the United States, 1997–2012. *Otolaryngol Head Neck Surg.* 2016;155(1):94–98. https://doi.org/10.1177/0194599816640477. Medline:27048673

Abbreviations

A

AAPCC	American Association of Poison Control
AAST	American Association for the Surgery of Trauma
ACA	anterior cerebral artery
ACCP	American College of Chest Physicians
AChE	acetylcholinesterase
AChR	acetylcholine receptor
ACL	anterior cruciate ligament
ACLS	Advanced Cardiac Life Support
ADEM	acute disseminated encephalomyelitis
AHA	American Heart Association
ALL	acute lymphoblastic leukemia
ALOC	altered level of consciousness
ALT	alanine transaminase
ALTE	apparent life-threatening event
AML	acute myelogenous leukemia
ANC	absolute neutrophil count
AOM	acute otitis media
AOP	apnea of prematurity
APAP	acetaminophen
ARDS	acute respiratory distress syndrome
ART	antiretroviral therapy
ASA	acetylsalicylic acid, Aspirin
ASA	American Society of Anesthesiologists
ASD	atrial septal defect
ASOT	antistreptolysin O titer
AST	aspartate transaminase
ATLS	Advanced Trauma Life Support
ATP	adenosine triphosphate
AUB	abnormal uterine bleeding
AV	atrioventricular
AVM	arteriovenous malformation
AVN	avascular necrosis
AVNRT	atrioventricular nodal reentry tachycardia
AVP	arginine vasopressin
AVRT	atrioventricular reentry tachycardia

B

B_6	pyridoxine
BAL	British anti-Lewisite (dimercaprol)
BAL	bronchial alveolar lavage
BCG	Bacillus Calmette–Guérin
BLS	basic life support
BUN	blood urea nitrogen
BV	bacterial vaginosis
BVM	bag valve mask

C

CAH	congenital adrenal hyperplasia
CAS	child aid services
CBC	complete blood count
CBF	cerebral blood flow
CDH	congenital diaphragmatic hernia
CEDKA	cerebral edema and diabetic ketoacidosis
CF	cystic fibrosis
CFTR	cystic fibrosis transmembrane conductance regulator
CHD	congenital heart disease
CHEOPS	Children's Hospital of Eastern Ontario pain scale

CI	confidence interval
CK	creatine kinase
CKD	chronic kidney disease
CLS	child life specialist
CMV	cytomegalovirus
COHb	carboxyhemoglobin
COPD	chronic obstructive pulmonary disease
CPAP	continuous positive airway pressure
CPP	cerebral perfusion pressure
CPSP	Canadian Paediatric Surveillance Program
CRH	corticotrophin-releasing hormone
CRP	C-reactive protein
CSF	cerebrospinal fluid
CTA	CT angiography
CTV	CT venogram

D

DAT	direct antiglobulin test
DDAVP	desmopressin
DFA	direct florescent antibody
DI	diabetes insipidus
DIC	disseminated intravascular coagulation
DIP	distal interphalangeal
DKA	diabetic ketoacidosis
DM	diabetes mellitus
DMSA	dimercaptosuccinic acid
DMT	*N,N*-dimethyltryptamine
DRUJ	disruption of the distal radioulnar joint
D-TGA	D-transposition of the great arteries
DVT	deep vein thrombosis
DWI	diffusion-weighted imaging

E

EBV	Epstein-Barr virus
ECG	electrocardiogram
ECMO	extracorporeal membrane oxygenation
ED	emergency department
EDTA	ethylenediamine tetraacetic acid
eFAST	extended focused assessment with sonography for trauma
EIA	enzyme immunoassay
EM	erythema multiforme
EMG	electromyography
ERIG	equine rabies immunoglobulin
ESI	Emergency Severity Index
ET	exfoliative toxin
ETN	erythema toxicum neonatorum

F

FAST	focused assessment with sonography for trauma
FEV_1	forced expiratory volume in 1 second
FFP	fresh frozen plasma
FiO_2	fraction of inspired oxygen
FOOSH	fall onto an outstretched hand
FSGS	focal segmental glomerulosclerosis
FSH	follicle-stimulating hormone

G

GAS	group A *Streptococcus* (group A beta-hemolytic streptococci)
GBL	gamma butyrolactone

GBS	group B *Streptococcus*
GBS	Guillain-Barré syndrome
GCS	Glasgow Coma Scale
GER	gastroesophageal reflux
GERD	gastroesophageal reflux disease
GGT	gamma-glutamyl transferase
GHB	gamma-hydroxybutyric acid
GP	glycoprotein
GUD	genital ulcer disease

H

H2RA	histamine-2 receptor antagonist
HbA	normal adult hemoglobin, hemoglobin A
HbA1c	hemoglobin A1c
HbF	hemoglobin F
HBIg	hepatitis B immunoglobulin
HbS	hemoglobin S
HBsAg	hepatitis B surface antigen
HbSS	homozygous hemoglobin S
hCG	human chorionic gonadotropin
HEPA	high-efficiency particulate air
Hib	*Hemophilus influenzae* type b
HIT	Heparin-induced thrombocytopenia
HLH	hemophagocytic lymphohistiocytosis
HPF	high-power field
HPV	human papillomavirus
HR	heart rate
HRIG	human rabies immunoglobulin
HSP	Henoch-Schönlein purpura
HSV	herpes simplex virus
HUS	hemolytic uremic syndrome

I

IBD	inflammatory bowel disease
IBS	irritable bowel syndrome
ICA	internal carotid artery
ICP	intracranial pressure
ICU	intensive care unit
ID	intradermal
IDDM	insulin-dependent diabetes mellitus
Ig	immunoglobulin
IgA	immunoglobulin A
IgE	immunoglobulin E
IGRA	interferon gamma release assay
IM	intramuscular
IN	intranasal
INH	isonicotinylhydrazide (isoniazid)
INR	international normalized ratio
IO	intraosseous
IOP	intraocular pressure
IP	interphalangeal
ITP	immune thrombocytopenia purpura
IV	intravenous
IVC	inferior vena cava
IVIG	intravenous immunoglobulin

J

J-tube	jejunostomy tube

L

LDH	lactate dehydrogenase
LES	lower esophageal sphincter
LET	lidocaine, epinephrine, tetracaine
LH	luteinizing hormone
LKE	leukocyte esterase
LMA	laryngeal mask airway

LMWH	low–molecular weight heparin
LP	lumbar puncture
LV	left ventricle, left ventricular
LVH	left ventricular hypertrophy

M

mAChR	muscarinic acetylcholine receptor
MAP	mean arterial pressure
MCA	middle cerebral artery
MCL	medial collateral ligament
MCP	metacarpophalangeal
MCV4	meningococcal conjugate ACYW-135 vaccine
MDAC	multiple dose activated charcoal
MDI	metered dose inhaler
MRA	MR angiograph
MRSA	methicillin-resistant *Staphylococcus aureus*
MRV	MR venography
MSK	musculoskeletal
MSSA	methicillin-sensitive *Staphylococcus aureus*
MT	metatarsal

N

NAAT	nucleic acid amplification technology; nucleic acid amplification testing
NAC	N-acetylcysteine
nAChR	nicotinic acetylcholine receptor
NADH	nicotinamide adenine dinucleotide
NADP+	alcohol dehydrogenase
NADPH	nicotinamide adenine dinucleotide phosphate
NAI	nonaccidental injury
NAPQI	N-acetyl-p-benzoquinone imine
NASPGHAN	The North American Society for Pediatric Gastroenterology, Hepatology and Nutrition
NAT	nonaccidental trauma
NE	norepinephrine
NEC	necrotizing enterocolitis
NF	necrotizing fasciitis
NG	nasogastric
NIF	negative inspiratory force
NJ	nasojejunal
NMDA	N-methyl-D-aspartate
NMJ	neuromuscular junction
NNRTI	nonnucleoside reverse transcriptase inhibitors
NPO	*nil per os* (nothing by mouth)
NPV	negative predictive value
NRS-11	numerical rating scale
NRTI	nucleoside reverse transcriptase inhibitor
NS	normal saline
NSAIDs	nonsteroidal anti-inflammatory drugs
NT-proBNP	N-terminal pro b-type natriuretic peptide

O

OCD	obsessive compulsive disorder
OCP	oral contraceptive pill
OG	orogastric
OM	otitis media
OR	operating room
ORIF	open reduction and internal fixation
ORT	oral rehydration therapy

P

PA	posteroanterior
PABA	para amino benzoic acid
$PaCO_2$	partial pressure of arterial carbon dioxide
PaedCTAS	Canadian Triage and Acuity Scale Paediatric Guidelines

PAF	platelet activating factor
PALS	pediatric advance life support
PaO$_2$	partial pressure of arterial oxygen
PAT	pediatric assessment triangle
PCA	posterior cerebral artery
PCI	percutaneous coronary intervention
pCO$_2$	partial pressure of carbon dioxide
PCOS	polycystic ovary syndrome
PCR	polymerase chain reaction
PCT	procalcitonin
PCV13	pneumococcal conjugate vaccine
PDA	patent ductus arteriosus
PE	pulmonary embolus
PECARN	Pediatric Emergency Care Applied Research Network
PEF	peak expiratory flow
PEG	polyethylene glycol
PEM	pediatric emergency medicine
PEP	postencounter prophylaxis, postexposure prophylaxis
PGE1	prostaglandin E1
PICC	peripherally inserted central catheter
PICU	pediatric intensive care unit
PID	pelvic inflammatory disease
PJP	*Pneumocystis jirovecii* pneumonia
PMNs	polymorphonuclear leukocytes
PO	*per os* (orally, by mouth)
PO$_2$	partial pressure of oxygen
POCUS	point-of-care ultrasound
PPD	purified protein derivative
PPI	proton pump inhibitor
PPV	positive pressure ventilation
PPV23	pneumococcal polysaccharide vaccine
PR	rectally, by rectum
PRAM	pediatric respiratory assessment measure
PRBC	packed red blood cells
PRN	*pro re nata* (whenever necessary)
PT	prothrombin time
PTH	parathyroid hormone
PTT	partial thromboplastin time
PTU	propylthiouracil
PUD	peptic ulcer disease

R

R+M	routine and microscopy
RAA	renin-angiotensin-aldosterone
RBCs	red blood cells
RCo	ristocetin cofactor
ROSC	return of spontaneous circulation
RR	relative risk
RRT	renal replacement therapy
RSI	rapid sequence intubation
RSV	respiratory syncytial virus
RT-PCR	reverse transcription polymerase chain reaction
RV	right ventricle, right ventricular

S

SA	sinoatrial
SABA	short-acting beta agonist
SBI	serious bacterial infection
SBP	systolic blood pressure
SC	subcutaneous
SCD	sickle cell disease
SCFE	slipped capital femoral epiphysis

SCIWORA	spinal cord injury without radiological abnormality
ScvO$_2$	central venous oxygen saturation
SGA	small for gestation age
SI	sacroiliac
SIADH	symptom of inappropriate antidiuretic hormone
SIRS	systemic inflammatory response syndrome
SJS	Stevens-Johnson Syndrome
SLE	systemic lupus erythematosus
SMA	superior mesenteric artery
SMV	superior mesenteric vein
SpO$_2$	peripheral oxygen saturation
SSSS	staphylococcal scalded skin syndrome
STI	sexually transmitted infection
STSS	*Streptococcus* toxic shock syndromes
SVC	superior vena cava
SVT	supraventricular tachycardia

T

T$_3$	3,5,3'-triiodothyronine
T$_4$	thyroxine
TB	tuberculosis
TBI	traumatic brain injury
TBSA	total body surface area
TCA	tricyclic antidepressant
TCD	transcranial Doppler
TEN	toxic epidermal necrolysis
TGA	transposition of the great arteries
THC	tetrahydrocannabinol
tHUS	typical hemolytic uremic syndrome
TIA	transient ischemic attack
TIBC	total serum iron binding capacity
TIg	tetanus immunoglobulin
TLS	tumor lysis syndrome
TMP-SMX	trimethoprim-sulfamethoxazole
TMT	tarsometatarsal
TNF	tumor necrosis factor
tPA	tissue plasminogen activator
TPN	total parenteral nutrition
TSB	total serum bilirubin
TSH	thyroid-stimulating hormone (thyrotropin)
TST	tuberculin skin test
TTP	thrombotic thrombocytopenia purpura

U

UCL	ulnar collateral ligament
UFH	unfractionated heparin
URTI	upper respiratory tract infection
US	ultrasound
UTI	urinary tract infection

V

VAS	visual analogue scale
VBG	venous blood gas
VEGF	vascular endothelial growth factor
VOC	vasoocclusive crisis
VP	ventriculoperitoneal
VSD	ventricular septal defect
VTE	venous thromboembolism
vWD	von Willebrand disease
vWf	von Willebrand factor

W

WBC	white blood cell
WBI	whole bowel irrigation
WPW	Wolff-Parkinson-White

SI Unit / Conventional Unit Conversion Table

To convert from SI units to conventional units, multiply the value in SI units by the conversion factor listed in the table below.

Analyte	Normal range (SI units)	SI units	Conventional units	Conversion factor
C-reactive protein	0.76 – 28.5	mmol/L	mg/L	0.105
Hemoglobin	140 – 175	g/L	g/dL	0.100
Platelet count	150 – 350	units $\times$ 10^9/L	units $\times$ 10^3/μL	1.000
White cell count	4.5 – 11	units $\times$ 10^9/L	units $\times$ 10^3/μL	1.000
Chemistry				
Alanine transaminase (ALT)	0.17 – 0.68	μkat/L	U/L	59.880
Albumin	35 – 50	g/L	g/dL	0.100
Alkaline phosphatase	0.67 – 2.51	μkat/L	U/L	59.880
Amylase	0.46 – 2.23	μkat/L	U/L	59.880
Aspartate transaminase (AST)	0.34 – 0.82	μkat/L	U/L	59.880
Bicarbonate	21 – 28	mmol/L	mEq/L	1.000
Bilirubin	5 – 21	μmol/L	mg/dL	0.058
Blood Urea Nitrogen (BUN)	2.9 – 8.2	mmol/L	mg/dL	2.801
Calcium (ionized)	1.15 – 1.27	mmol/L	mg/dL	4.167
Creatinine	53 – 106	μmol/L	mg/dL	0.011
Lactate dehydrogenase	1.7 – 3.4	μkat/L	U/L	59.880
Magnesium	0.65 – 1.05	mmol/L	mEq/L	2.000
Phosphorus	0.81 – 1.45	mmol/L	mg/dL	3.096
Protein	60 – 80	g/L	g/dL	0.100
Random glucose	4 – 6	mmol/L	mg/dL	18.018
Uric acid	240 – 480	μmol/L	mg/dL	0.017
Toxicology				
Acetaminophen	–	μmol/L	μg/mL	0.151
Ethanol	< 4.3	mmol/L	mg/dL	4.606
Ethylene glycol (toxic)	> 5	mmol/L	mg/dL	6.207
Iron	10.7 – 26.9	μmol/L	μg/dL	5.587
Lead	< 0.5 – 1	μmol/L	μg/dL	20.704
Mercury	< 25	mmol/L	μg/L	0.201
Methanol	< 6.2	mmol/L	μg/mL	32.051
Salicylate	–	mmol/L	mg/L	138.122

Contributors

Tracy Lynn Akitt, BA, CLSt Dipl., CCLS
Certified Child Life Specialist, Clinical Leader
McMaster Children's Hospital
Hamilton Health Sciences
Hamilton, ON

Waleed Alqurashi, MD, MSc, FAAP, FRCPC
Assistant Professor, University of Ottawa
Department of Pediatrics and Emergency Medicine
Children's Hospital of Eastern Ontario (CHEO)
Ottawa, Ontario

Ahmed Alterkait, MD, MPH, FRCPC, FAAP
Pediatric Emergency Physician
Pediatric Emergency Division
Royal University Hospital
Saskatoon, Saskatchewan

Carlos R. Alvarez-Allende, MD
Pediatric Surgeon
Department of Surgery
Puerto Rico Children's Hospital
Bayamón, Puerto Rico

Qamar Amin, MD, MSc, FRCPC
Emergency Physician
Assistant clinical professor (Adj)
Department of Family Medicine
McMaster University
Hamilton, Ontario
Staff Physician
Sunnybrook Health Sciences Centre
Toronto, Ontario

Nicole Anderson, BSc, MD
General Pediatric Resident
Department of Pediatrics
University of Alberta
Edmonton, Alberta

Haley F. M. Augustine, MD, MScOT, BScH
Resident
Division of Plastic Surgery
McMaster University
Hamilton, Ontario

Emily Austin, MD
Staff Physician
Department of Emergency Medicine
St. Michael's Hospital
Toronto, Ontario

Iwona Baran, MD, FRCPC
Program Director, Pediatric Emergency Medicine Program
Department of Pediatrics, Division of Emergency Medicine
University of Toronto
Toronto, Ontario

Jouseph Osama Barkho, MD, BSc
Resident, Division of Plastic Surgery
McMaster University
Hamilton, Ontario

Bandar Baw, MD
Emergency Physician and Clinical Pharmacologist and Toxicologist
Associate Professor
Department of Medicine, McMaster University
Hamilton, Ontario

Mary E. Brindle, MD, MPH
Associate Professor of Surgery
Department of Surgery
Cumming School of Medicine
University of Calgary
Calgary, Alberta

David Bulir, BHSc, MD, PhD
Medical Resident
Division of Dermatology
Department of Medicine
Michael G DeGroote School of Medicine
McMaster University
Hamilton, Ontario

Kevin Chan, MD, MPH,
Chair and Associate Professor
Discipline of Pediatrics
Memorial University
St. John's, Newfoundland and Labrador

Melissa Chan, MD
Assistant Professor, Pediatric Emergency Medicine
Department of Pediatrics
University of Alberta
Edmonton, Alberta

Matthew Choi, MD, MPH
Associate Professor
Division of Plastic Surgery
McMaster University
Hamilton, Ontario

Sheryl Christie, MA, CLSt Dipl., CCLS
Certified Child Life Specialist
McMaster Children's Hospital
Hamilton Health Sciences
Hamilton, Ontario

Carmen Coombs, MD, MPH
Assistant Professor of Pediatrics
Division of Pediatric Emergency Medicine
Division of Child Advocacy
Children's Hospital of Pittsburgh of the University of
Pittsburgh Medical Center
Pittsburgh, Pennsylvania USA

Camila de Lima, MD
Pediatric Resident
Discipline of Pediatrics
Memorial University of Newfoundland
St. John's, Newfoundland and Labrador

Joanne Delaney, MD
Pediatric Resident
Discipline of Pediatrics
Memorial University of Newfoundland
St. John's, Newfoundland and Labrador

Andrew Dixon, MD, FRCPC
Program Director-Pediatric Emergency Medicine Residency
Associate Professor
Division of Pediatric Emergency Medicine
Department of Pediatrics, University of Alberta
Edmonton, Alberta

Jonathan Duff, MD, MEd
Associate Professor
Department of Paediatrics
University of Alberta
Edmonton, Alberta

Marcia Edmonds, MD, MSc
Clinical Associate Professor
Division of Emergency Medicine, Department of Medicine
University of Western Ontario
London, Ontario

Mohamed Eltorki, MBchB, FRCPC (PEM)
Clinical Assistant Professor
Pediatric Emergency Medicine
McMaster Children's Hospital

Andrea Estey, MD, FRCPC (PEM)
Assistant Clinical Professor
Department of Pediatrics
University of Alberta
Edmonton, Alberta, Canada

E. Vicky Fera, MSc., MBBCh, FRCPC
Clinical Physician
Department of Pediatric Emergency Medicine
The Hospital for Sick Children
University of Toronto
Toronto, Ontario

Eric Flynn, MD
Resident
Department of Emergency Medicine
University of Manitoba
Winnipeg, Manitoba

Aaron Guinn, MD, FRCPC
Lecturer
Department of Emergency Medicine
University of Manitoba
Winnipeg, Manitoba

Louise Guolla
Pediatric Resident
Discipline of Pediatrics
Memorial University of Newfoundland
St. John's, Newfoundland and Labrador

Jan Hanot, MD
Pediatric Intensivist, Anesthesiologist
Department of Pediatrics
University of Maastricht
Maastricht, the Netherlands

Krista Helleman, MD
Associate Professor
Department of Pediatrics
Western University
London, Ontario

Erik Hildahl, MD, FRCPC
Lecturer
Department of Emergency Medicine
University of Manitoba
Winnipeg, Manitoba

Chih-Ho Hong, MD
Dermatologist
Clinical Assistant Professor
University of British Columbia
Vancouver, British Columbia

Jo-Anna Hudson, MD, PhD
Pediatric Resident
Discipline of Pediatrics
Memorial University of Newfoundland
St. John's, Newfoundland and Labrador

Katrina F. Hurley, MD, MHI, FRCPC
Assistant Professor
Department of Emergency Medicine
Dalhousie University
Halifax, Nova Scotia

Elana Jackson, MA, CLSt Dipl., CCLS
Certified Child Life Specialist
McMaster Children's Hospital
Hamilton Health Sciences
Hamilton, Ontario

April J. Kam, MD, MScPH, FRCPC
Associate Professor
Division of Pediatric Emergency Medicine
Department of Pediatrics
McMaster Children's Hospital
McMaster University
Hamilton, Ontario

Anna Kempinska, MD, FRCPC
Assistant Professor
Division of Pediatric Emergency Medicine
Hospital for Sick Children
University of Toronto
Toronto, Ontario

Sarah Khan, BSc, MD, MSc, FRCPC
Assistant Professor
Department of Pediatrics
McMaster University
Hamilton, Ontario

Vidushi Khatri, BESc, MD
Department of Paediatrics
McMaster University
Hamilton, Ontario

Ian Kitai, MB, BCh, FRCPC
Staff Physician, TB Specialist
Department of Infectious Diseases
The Hospital for Sick Children
Associate Professor
Department of Paediatrics
University of Toronto
Toronto, Ontario

Eric Koelink, BMBS, FRCPC, Dip. Sport Med
Assistant Clinical Professor
Department of Pediatric Emergency Medicine, McMaster
Children's Hospital McMaster University
Hamilton, Ontario

Jennifer Y. Lam, MD
Pediatric surgery fellow
Department of Surgery
Cumming School of Medicine
University of Calgary
Calgary, Alberta

Rodrick Lim, MD
Associate Professor
Department of Paediatrics and Medicine
Schulich School of Medicine & Dentistry
Western University
London, Ontario

Vincent Lim, MD, FRCPC
Lecturer
Department of Emergency Medicine
University of Manitoba
Winnipeg, Manitoba

Sasha Litwin, MB, BCh, BAO, FRCPC
Staff Physician
Division of Emergency Medicine
Department of Paediatrics
Hospital for Sick Children
Toronto, Ontario

Hanyang Liu, BSc, MD
Resident, Division of Plastic Surgery
McMaster University
Hamilton, Ontario

Eman Loubani, MD, FAAP, FRCPC
Pediatric Emergency Physician
Assistant Professor, Western University
London, Ontario

David Lussier, MD
Resident
Department of Emergency Medicine
University of Manitoba
Winnipeg, Manitoba

Tim Lynch, MD
Associate Professor
Department of Pediatrics
Division of Emergency Medicine
Western University
London, Ontario

Fahad Masud
Department of Pediatrics
McMaster University
Hamilton, Ontario

Ahmed Mater, MD, FRCP
Paediatric Emergency Medicine
Department of Paediatrics, Royal University Hospital
Assistant Professor
University of Saskatchewan

Karen McAssey, BA, MD, MEd, FRCPC
McMaster Children's Hospital
Hamilton, Ontario

Sarah McKillop, MD, MSc, FRCPC
Assistant Professor
Department of Pediatrics
University of Alberta
Edmonton, Alberta

Shruti Mehrotra, MD, FRCPC (PEM, Paeds)
Consultant, Paediatric Emergency Dept
CPD Director & Assistant Professor
Children's Hospital, LHSC
Schulich School of Medicine & Dentistry
Western University
London, Ontario

Shabnam Minoosepehr, MD, MA, FRCPC
Associate Professor, Department of Paediatrics
University of Calgary
Calgary, Alberta

Amita Misir, MD, FRCPC, FAAP
Assistant Professor & Attending Physician
Department of Pediatrics & Division of Emergency Medicine
London Health Sciences Centre (Children's Hospital)
Western University, Schulich School of Medicine
London, Ontario

Shawn Mondoux, MD, MSc, FRCPC
Assistant Professor
Department of Medicine, Division of Emergency Medicine
McMater University
Institute of Health Policy, Management and Evaluation
University of Toronto
Hamilton, Ontario

Channy Muhn, MD, FRCPC
Clinical Professor
Division of Dermatology
Department of Medicine
Michael G DeGroote School of Medicine
McMaster University
Hamilton, Ontario

Samantha Woodrow Mullett, MD
Pediatric Resident
Department of Pediatrics
Memorial University of Newfoundland
St. John's, Newfoundland and Labrador

Ahmed Ali Nahari, MD
King Fahad Central Hospital
Jazan, Saudi Arabia

Joe Nemeth, MD, FCFP EM
Associate Professor, McGill University / University of Toronto
Emergency Medicine/Trauma Team Leader, Montreal General Hospital / Montreal Children's Hospital / The Hospital for Sick Children / St-Michael's Hospital
Director, Trauma Fellowship for the Emergency Medicine Physician, McGill University
Montreal, Quebec / Toronto, Ontario

Wesley Palatnick, MD, FRCPC
Professor
Department of Emergency Medicine
University of Manitoba
Winnipeg, Manitoba

Karen Paling, BA, CLSt Dipl., CCLS
Certified Child Life Specialist
McMaster Children's Hospital
Hamilton Health Sciences
Hamilton, ON

Zoë Piggott, MD, FRCP-C EM
Lecturer
Department of Emergency Medicine
University of Manitoba
Winnipeg, MB

Naveen Poonai, MSc, MD, FRCPC
Associate Professor, Paediatrics & Internal Medicine, Schulich School of Medicine & Dentistry
Associate Scientist, Child Health Research Institute
Research Director, Division of Paediatric Emergency Medicine
London, Ontario

Sowmith Rangu, MD
Chief Pediatric Resident
Discipline of Pediatrics
Memorial University of Newfoundland
St. John's, Newfoundland and Labrador

Sarah Reid, MD, FRCPC
Pediatric Emergency Physician
Children's Hospital of Eastern Ontario
Assistant Professor
Departments of Pediatrics and Emergency Medicine
University of Ottawa
Ottawa, Ontario

Michael Rieder, MD Ph.D FRCPC FAAP FRPC (Edinburgh)
CIHR-GSK Chair in Paediatric Clinical Pharmacology
Department of Paediatrics
University of Western Ontario
London, Ontario

Marina I. Salvadori, MD, FRCPC
Professor
Department of Paediatrics
Schulich School of Medicine and Dentistry
Western University
Division Head
Paediatric Infectious Diseases
Children's Hospital, London Health Sciences Center
London, Ontario

Suzan Schneeweiss, MD, MEd, FRCPC
Associate Professor
Department of Paediatrics
University of Toronto
Toronto, Ontario

Archna Shah, MBChB, FRCPC (PEM)
Clinical Assistant Professor, Discipline of Pediatrics, Memorial University
Pediatric Emergency Medicine Physician
Janeway Children's Hospital and Rehabilitation Centre
St. John's, Newfoundland

Christopher Skappak, MD, PhD
Resident Physician
Division of Emergency Medicine
McMaster University
Hamilton, Ontario

K. A. Sutherland, MD, MSc
Attending Physician
Department of Emergency Medicine
Vancouver General Hospital
Vancouver, British Columbia

Rahim Valani, MD, M Med Ed, MBA
Associate Professor of Medicine and Pediatrics
McMaster University
Hamilton, Ontario

Kenneth Van Dewark, BMSc, MD, FRCPC, MEd
Emergency Physician and Clinical Instructor
Vancouver General Hospital
Department of Emergency Medicine
University of British Columbia
Vancouver, British Columbia

David Warren, MD, CCFP(EM), FRCPC, FAAP
Associate Professor of Paeditrics
Medical Director Child Protection, LHSC
Western University
London, Ontario

Kirstin Weerdenburg, MD, FRCPC
Director of Pediatric Emergency Ultrasound, Research and Quality Assurance; Assistant Professor
Division of Emergency Medicine, IWK Health Centre;
Dalhousie University
Halifax, Nova Scotia

Laura Weingarten, MD, FRCPC
Clinical Assistant Professor
Department of Pediatrics
McMaster University
Hamilton, Ontario

Shelly Weiss, MD, FRCPC
Professor
Department of Paediatrics
University of Toronto
Toronto, Ontario

Patrick Weldon, MDCM, FRCPC
Staff Physician, Division of Emergency Medicine
Children's Hospital of Eastern Ontario
Lecturer, Department of Pediatrics
University of Ottawa
Ottawa, Ontario

Judy Wismer, BSc, MD, FRCPC
Associate Clinical Professor Dermatology
Michael G DeGroote School of Medicine
McMaster University
Hamilton, Ontario

Natalie L. Yanchar, MD, MSc, FRCSC
Clinical Professor in Surgery
Section of Pediatric Surgery
University of Calgary
Calgary, Alberta

Helen Yaworski, MD, FRCPC
Lecturer
Department of Emergency Medicine
University of Manitoba
Winnipeg, Manitoba

Index